The Management of Labour

FOURTH EDITION

The Management of Labour

FOURTH EDITION

Sir Sabaratnam Arulkumaran
Professor Emeritus, St George's University of London
Formerly President, International Federation of Gynecology and Obstetrics (FIGO)
British Medical Association, and Royal College of Obstetricians & Gynaecologists, UK

Gita Arjun
Former Senior Obstetrician & Gynaecologist, E V Kalyani Medical Centre
Director, E V Kalyani Medical Foundation, Chennai

Uma Ram
Director and Lead Consultant, Seethapathy Clinic and Hospital, Chennai
All India Chair, AICC RCOG

Universities Press

MANAGEMENT OF LABOUR, FOURTH EDITION

UNIVERSITIES PRESS (INDIA) PRIVATE LIMITED

Registered Office
3-6-747/1/A & 3-6-754/1, Himayatnagar, Hyderabad 500 029, Telangana, India
info@universitiespress.com; www.universitiespress.com

Distributed by
Orient Blackswan Private Limited

Registered Office
3-6-752, Himayatnagar, Hyderabad 500 029, Telangana, India

Other Offices
Bengaluru, Chennai, Guwahati, Hyderabad, Kolkata, Mumbai, New Delhi, Noida, Patna

First published 1996: Reprinted 1997 (twice), 2001 (twice), 2003
Second edition 2005: Reprinted 2006, (twice), 2007, 2008 (twice)
First Universities Press Impression 2008
Third edition 2011: Reprinted 2011, 2012, 2014, 2015, 2016, 2019, 2020, 2022, 2023 (twice)
Fourth edition 2025

ISBN 978-93-93330-82-6

Cover and book design

Cover image source: FREEPIK.com

502129

Typeset in IowanOldSt BT 10/12.5 pt *by*
e-Leaf Technologies, Chennai

Printed in India at
SDR Printers, Tronica City, Ghaziabad

Published by
Universities Press (India) Private Limited
3-6-747/1/A & 3-6-754/1, Himayatnagar, Hyderabad 500 029, Telangana, India

Contents

Preface to the Fourth Edition vii

Preface to the First Edition viii

Contributors ix

Section I: The Process of Labour

1. The Physiology of Labour 1
   Sheila Balakrishnan
2. Mechanics, Mechanism, and Stages of Labour 8
   Lakshmi Seshadri

Section II: Intrapartum Management

3. Respectful Obstetric Care and the Role of a Birth Companion 19
   Sirisha Rao G, Evita Fernandez
4. Management of the First and Second Stages of Normal Labour 30
   Gita Arjun
5. Management of the Third Stage of Labour 49
   Basab Mukherjee, Poushali Sanyal
6. Monitoring Labour: Partograph to Labour Care Guide 58
   Anandhi Venkatesan, Uma Ram
7. Episiotomy: What Does the Evidence Say? 74
   A Tamilselvi
8. Fetal Surveillance in Labour 83
   Sabaratnam Arulkumaran
9. Labour Analgesia 98
   M Subrahmanyam, Sailaja K
10. Immediate Postpartum Monitoring and Care (Including Postpartum Collapse) 111
   Jiji Elizabeth Mathews, Richa Sasmita Tirkey

Section III: Intrapartum Management of Complicated Labour

11. Abnormalities in the Latent Phase and the Active First Stage of Labour 124
   Kalaivani Ramalingam
12. Abnormalities in the Second Stage of Labour 134
   Manjiri Khare, Gauri Karandikar
13. Abnormalities in the Third Stage of Labour: Postpartum Hemorrhage and Retained Placenta 143
   Sam Ononge, Andrew D Weeks
14. Induction and Augmentation of Labour 163
   Shobana Mahadevan, Amritha Karthik
15. Identification and Management of Fetal Distress 177
   Sabaratnam Arulkumaran
16. Meconium-Stained Amniotic Fluid 193
   N Hephzibah Kirubamani
17. Management of Labour in Multiple Pregnancy 205
   Nashwa Eltaweel, Helena Blakeway, Asma Khalil
18. Obstructed Labour and Uterine Rupture 213
   Kanika Chopra, Manju Puri
19. Antibiotic Prophylaxis in Labour and Delivery 223
   Gita Arjun
20. Role of Ultrasound in the Labour Room 229
   Mariya Kovalenko, Sana Usman, Arwa Hanidu, Christoph Lees

Section IV: Operative Obstetrics

21. Operative Vaginal Delivery 241
   Tulika Singh, Samera A Khalil
22. Cesarean Section: Procedure and Technique 256
   Gita Arjun
23. Reducing Cesarean Section Rates 274
   Gita Arjun
24. Peripartum Hysterectomy 283
   V P Paily, G Raji Raj

Section V: Obstetric Skills

25. Prevention and Management of Perineal Trauma Occurring in Childbirth 296
Stergios K Doumouchtsis, Maria Patricia Roman

26. Vaginal Birth After Cesarean Delivery 307
Pranathi Reddy

27. Breech Delivery 317
Lakshmi Seshadri

28. Shoulder Dystocia 326
B S Susheela Rani

Section VI: Management of Obstetric Complications

29. Antepartum Hemorrhage 338
Nishita Mehta, Amarnath Bhide

30. Preterm Labour and Preterm Prelabour Rupture of Membranes 352
Sareena Gilvaz, Deepthi D Nair

31. Late Term and Postterm Pregnancy 369
Nozer Sheriar

32. Late Intrauterine Fetal Death and Stillbirth 380
A G Radhika, Richa Aggarwal

33. Management of Labour with a Growth-Restricted Fetus 392
Tony Tan

34. Management of Labour with Fetal Macrosomia 402
Manisha Madhai Beck, Nitin Alexander Abraham

35. Malpositions and Malpresentations (Other Than Breech) 410
Jyothi Unni

36. Management of Labour in Women with Fibroids 419
Gita Arjun

Section VII: Management of Labour with Medical Disorders

37. The Hypertensive Woman in Labour 425
Nuzhat Aziz, Sailaja Devi Kallur

38. Management of Labour in a Woman with Diabetes 439
Lakshmi Shanmugasundaram, Uma Ram

39. Other Medical Disorders: Cardiac Disorders, Antiphospholipid Syndrome, Hepatic Disorders, and Epilepsy 449
Tarakeswari S

Section VIII: Management of Labour with Current Infection

40. SARS-CoV-2 465
Sophie Relph, Pat O'Brien

41. Chickenpox 480
Mandira Dasgupta, Bhaskar Pal

42. HIV 489
Pallavi Chandra Ravula, Hemamalini Vadlamani

Section IX: Neonatal Care

43. Routine Care of the Newborn 500
Swathi Padankatti

44. Neonatal Resuscitation 512
V Lakshmi

Section X: The Puerperium

45. The Normal Puerperium 522
Mathangi Thirunavakkarasu

46. Abnormalities in the Puerperium 530
Muralidhar V Pai

Index 542

Preface to the Fourth Edition

Obstetricians in the 21st century are faced with a variety of clinical and therapeutic options. An understanding of sound clinical principles and a grounding in evidence-informed guidelines will help them navigate issues that they face in the labour room on a daily basis.

The fourth edition of *Management of Labour* strives to provide clear and well-defined recommendations that are based on contemporary data and established clinical principles. The ideal book should not only make knowledge easy to acquire and exciting but should help clinicians apply it in daily practice to best benefit the women under their care and their babies. The previous editions of this book have become entrenched in the obstetric world, particularly in India, and have helped innumerable postgraduates and clinicians provide exemplary care to labouring women.

A good physician never stops learning. Keeping oneself abreast of current knowledge is a lifelong process that involves years of dedication to the perusal of textbooks and journals and a commitment to gain insight from clinical experience. The young postgraduate or the practicing clinician can feel overwhelmed by the vast amount of information that is currently available. Assimilation of information is easier when it is put together in a concise, simple, and comprehensible format.

The editors of this book are privileged to have worked with numerous contributors who are experts in the field of obstetrics and who furnished this edition with information that is up-to-date and firmly grounded in evidence. We are deeply indebted to them for the enormous effort that they have put in and the time they carved out of their busy schedules. To enable the clinician to follow guidelines that suit the population they deal with, this book presents global data along with data from the Indian subcontinent.

To enable ease of learning and recall, the chapters have been carefully edited for consistency and uniformity, and contain boxes, tables, algorithms and illustrations. We hope that this is the kind of book that a clinician will keep at hand for immediate reference, be it in the consulting room or in the labour suite.

We are grateful to the publishers and their excellent editorial team for having supported us unstintingly in bringing out this book. We cannot but be grateful to our long-suffering spouses who encouraged and sustained us through long hours and looming deadlines.

We have been privileged to work with women who entrusted their pregnancies to us and from whom we gained a wealth of knowledge, learned about courage in the face of adverse situations, and participated in the unadulterated joy of motherhood. To these magnificent women, we dedicate this edition of *Management of Labour*!

Sir Sabaratnam Arulkumaran
Gita Arjun
Uma Ram

Preface to the First Edition

Passage through the birth canal is the shortest but possibly the most hazardous journey made by an individual in his or her life. Hypoxia, trauma and infection are inherent risks. The risks are increased if they are associated with preterm and postterm birth, prelabour rupture of the membranes or antepartum hemorrhage and when labour is induced as a consequence of medical or obstetric disorders in pregnancy. The mother faces problems of anxiety, pain, infection and if labour is prolonged, the possibility of operative delivery, trauma, postpartum hemorrhage and long-term morbidity. At times, she runs the risk of losing her life because of complications during childbirth. The women and babies who face these risks every day deserve care to the best of our ability. The art of intrapartum care has evolved and is evidence based. The knowledge of scientific principles should be available to everyone who provides care to the pregnant mother, a healthy baby and emotional satisfaction to those involved, including members of the family. These can be achieved by acquiring knowledge, skill and through compassionate team care with attention to details of the needs of the mother, the fetus and the process of labour.

This multi-author volume tries to achieve the goal of providing the knowledge of intrapartum management to the caregiver. It also covers closely related topics which may be of importance just prior to or just after the process of labour. Where possible, the book is adequately illustrated. The references cited in each chapter should prove especially useful as they provide recent knowledge in key areas of the field. As editors we have used our vast experience in the subject to fine tune each chapter. We hope that this book will serve the needs of many obstetricians, midwives and trainees who offer valuable care to the pregnant mother in labour.

S Arulkumaran
S S Ratnam
K Bhasker Rao

Contributors

A G Radhika
Senior Consultant, Department of Obstetrics and Gynecology, UCMS and GTB Hospital, New Delhi

A Tamilselvi
Senior Consultant Urogynaecologist, Madras Medical Mission Hospital, Chennai

Amarnath Bhide
Consultant & Reader in Fetal Medicine & Obstetrics, Fetal Medicine Unit, Lanesborough Wing, St. George's Hospital, London, UK

Amritha Karthik
Consultant OBGYN, Seethapathy Clinic and Hospital, Chennai

Anandhi Venkatesan
Junior Consultant, Seethapathy Clinic and Hospital, Chennai

Andrew D Weeks
Consultant Obstetrician, Liverpool Women's Hospital, UK; Professor of Internal Maternal Health, Department of Women's and Children's Health, University of Liverpool, UK

Arwa Hanidu
Queen Charlotte's and Chelsea Hospital, Imperial Healthcare NHS Trust, London, UK

Asma Khalil
Fetal Medicine Unit, St George's Hospital, London, UK; Vascular Biology Research Centre, Molecular and Clinical Sciences Research Institute, St George's University of London, London, UK

B S Susheela Rani
Director, Manjushree Speciality Hospital, Bengaluru, India

Basab Mukherjee
Consultant Obstetrician and Gynecologist, Woodlands Multispecialty Hospital, Kolkata, India

Bhaskar Pal
Senior Consultant, Obstetrics and Gynecology, Apollo Multispeciality Hospital, Kolkata, India

Christoph Lees
Queen Charlotte's and Chelsea Hospital, Imperial Healthcare NHS Trust, London, UK; Institute of Reproductive and Developmental Biology, Department of Metabolism, Digestion and Reproduction, Imperial College London, London, UK; Department of Development and Regeneration, Belgium

Deepthi D Nair
Assistant Professor, Department of Obstetrics and Gynecology, Jubilee Mission Medical College and Research Institute, Thrissur, Kerala, India

Evita Fernandez
Chairperson, Fernandez Foundation, Hyderabad, Telangana, India

G Raji Raj
Senior Consultant, Obstetrics and Gynecology, Rajagiri Hospital, Aluva, Kerala, India

Gauri Karandikar
Director, Karandikar Hospital, Nashik, India

Gita Arjun
Former Senior Obstetrician and Gynaecologist, E V Kalyani Medical Centre; Director, E V Kalyani Medical Foundation, Chennai, India

Helena Blakeway
Imperial College London, UK

Hemamalini Vadlamani
Consultant Obstetric Physician, Fernandez Hospital, Hyderabad, India

Jiji Elizabeth Mathews
Professor and Head of the Department, Department of Obstetrics and Gynecology, Christian Medical College Hospital Vellore, Tamil Nadu, India

Jyothi Unni
Director, Department of Obstetrics and Gynecology, Jehangir Hospital, Pune, India

Kalaivani Ramalingam
Pursuing Masters in Medical Law and Ethics, Dundee, UK

Kanika Chopra
Associate Professor, Department of Obstetrics and Gynaecology, Lady Hardinge Medical College, New Delhi, India

Lakshmi Seshadri
Former Professor, Department of Obstetrics and Gynaecology, Christian Medical College Hospital, Vellore, Tamil Nadu, India

Lakshmi Shanmugasundaram
Consultant OBGYN, Frimley Park Hospital, Surrey

M Subrahmanyam
Head, Department of Anaesthesia, Rainbow Hospitals, Hyderabad, India

Mandira Dasgupta
Professor and Head, Department of Obstetrics and Gynecology, Deben Mahata Government Medical College, Purulia, West Bengal, India

Manisha Madhai Beck
Professor and Head, Fetal Medicine Unit, Department of Obstetrics and Gynecology, Christian Medical College, Vellore, India

Manjiri Khare
Consultant in Maternal–Fetal Medicine, Clinical Tutor, Department of Clinical education; Programme Director for sub-specialty training programme in maternal-fetal medicine, University Hospitals of Leicester, NHS Trust, UK; Honarary Senior lecturer, University of Leicester, UK

Manju Puri
Director Professor, Department of Obstetrics and Gynaecology, Lady Hardinge Medical College, New Delhi, India

Maria Patricia Roman
Department of Obstetrics and Gynaecology, Epsom and St. Helier University Hospitals NHS Trust, Epsom, UK, St. George's University of London, London, UK, Laboratory of Experimental Surgery and Surgical Research "N.S. Christeas", National and Kapodistrian University of Athens, Medical School, Athens, Greece, School of Medicine, American University of the Caribbean, Cupecoy, Sint Maarten, School of Medicine, Ross University, Miramar, FL, USA, 2nd Department of Obstetrics and Gynaecology, "Iuliu Hatieganu" University of Medicine and Pharmacy Cluj-Napoca, Romania

Mariya Kovalenko
Queen Charlotte's and Chelsea Hospital, NHS Trust, London, UK

Mathangi Thirunavakkarasu
Consultant, Seethapathy Clinic and Hospital, Chennai, India

Muralidhar V Pai
Dean, Sikkim Manipal Institute of Medical Sciences, Sikkim, India

N Hephzibah Kirubamani
Professor, Saveetha Medical College, Chennai, India

Nashwa Eltaweel
Division of Biomedical Science, Warwick Medical School, University of Warwick, University Hospital of Coventry and Warwickshire, England

Nishita Mehta
Senior Clinical Fellow in Fetal Medicine, Fetal Medicine Unit, Royal Free Hospital, UK

Nitin Alexander Abraham
Assistant Professor, Department of Obstetrics and Gynecology, Christian Medical College, Vellore, Tamil Nadu, India

Nozer Sheriar
Consultant Obstetrician and Gynecologist, Breach Candy, Mumbai and PD Hinduja and Holy Family Hospital, Mumbai; Technical Advisor, Southeast Asia Region, World Health Organisation; Board Member, Guttmacher Institute and Centre for Catalysing Change

Nuzhat Aziz
Consultant Obstetrician, Head of Obstetric Emergencies Department, Fernandez Hospital, Hyderabad, India

Pallavi Chandra Ravula
Consultant Obstetrician, Fernandez Hospital, Hyderabad, India

Pat O'Brien
Consultant in Obstetrics & Gynaecology, Institute for Women's Health, University College London Hospitals, London, UK; The Royal College of Obstetricians and Gynaecologists, London, UK

Poushali Sanyal
Consultant Obstetrician, Gynaecologist & Laparoscopic Surgeon, Woodlands Multispecialty Hospital, Bellevue Clinic and AMRI Mukundapur Hospital, Kolkata, India

Pranathi Reddy
Clinical Director, Obstetrics and Gynaecology at Rainbow Hospital for Women and Children, Hyderabad, India

Richa Aggarwal
Professional and academic positions Professor, Department of Obstetrics and Gynecology, UCMS and GTB Hospital, New Delhi, India

Richa Sasmita Tirkey
Assistant Professor, Department of Obstetrics and Gynecology, Christian Medical College and Hospital, Vellore, India

Sabaratnam Arulkumaran
Professor Emeritus, St George's University of London; formerly President, International Federation of Gynecology and Obstetrics (FIGO), British Medical Association, and Royal College of Obstetricians & Gynaecologists, UK

Sailaja Devi Kallur
Consultant obstetrician, Medical Director Unit 2, Fernandez Hospital, Hyderabad, India

Sailaja K
Head, Department of Anaesthesia, Care Hospital, HiTech City Branch, Hyderabad, India

Sam Ononge
Senior Lecturer, Department of Obstetrics & Gynaecology, Makerere University College of Health Sciences; Consultant Obstetrician and Gynaecologist, Kawempe National Referral and Teaching Hospital, Kampala, Uganda

Samera Khalil
MBBS, BSc (Hons), Medical student at the Hull York Medical School

Sana Usman
Queen Charlotte's and Chelsea Hospital, Imperial Healthcare NHS Trust, London, UK, Institute of Reproductive and Developmental Biology, Department of Metabolism, Digestion and Reproduction, Imperial College London, London, UK; City Hospital, Sandwell and West Birmingham NHS Trust, UK

Sareena Gilvaz
Prof and HOD, Department of Obstetrics and Gynecology, Jubilee Mission Medical College and Research Institute, Thrissur, Kerala, India

Sheila Balakrishnan
Former Professor and Head of the Department of Reproductive Medicine, Govt. Medical College, Trivandrum, India

Shobana Mahadevan
Consultant OBGYN, Seethapathy Clinic and Hospital, Chennai, India

Sirisha Rao G
Consultant Obstetrician and Gynaecologist, Fernandez Hospital, Hyderabad, India

Sophie Relph
Subspecialist Trainee, Maternal and Fetal Medicine, Institute For Women's Health, University College London Hospitals, London, UK

Stergios K Doumouchtsis
Consultant obstetrician, gynecologist, and subspecialist; Urogynaecologist, Department of Obstetrics and Gynaecology, Epsom and St Helier University Hospitals NHS Trust; Honorary Senior Lecturer, St George's University of London, UK

Swathi Padankatti
Senior Consultant and Head, Department of Pediatrics and Neonatology, Sundaram Medical Foundation, Dr Rangarajan Memorial Hospital, Chennai, India

Tarakeswari S
Lead Senior Consultant, Obstetric Medicine, National NBE Webinar coordinator in speciality of High-Risk Pregnancy and Perinatology

Tony Tan
Consultant Obstetrician and Gynaecologist, Tony Tan Women and Fetal Clinic, Mount Alvernia Hospital, Singapore; Medical Director, Alvernia Obstetric Screening Centre, Mount Alvernia Hospital, Singapore; Chairman, Maternal Fetal Medicine Section, College of Obstetricians and Gynaecologists, Faculty of Academy of Medicine

Tulika Singh
Consultant obstetrician with special interest in fetal medicine at Mid Yorks NHS Trust

Uma Ram
Director and Lead Consultant, Seethapathy Clinic and Hospital, Chennai, India; All India Chair, AICC RCOG

V Lakshmi
Senior Consultant and HOD, Dr Mehta's Multispeciality Hospitals and Samraksha Neonatal Care, Chennai, India

V P Paily
Senior Consultant and HOD, Obstetrics and Gynecology, Rajagiri Hospital, Aluva, Kerala, India

CHAPTER 1

The Physiology of Labour

SHEILA BALAKRISHNAN

INTRODUCTION

Labour is characterised by painful uterine contractions leading to progressive effacement and dilatation of the cervix, resulting in fetal descent and expulsion of the fetus, placenta, and membranes. Understanding the physiology and pharmacokinetics of labour helps in managing labour more efficiently and assists in stimulating or inhibiting labour with pharmacological agents.

The physiological processes regulating the initiation and maintenance of labour are still not well-defined, unlike parturition in animals—most notably, sheep. Labour in humans is not preceded by dramatic changes in the maternal concentrations of estradiol and progesterone such as those seen in sheep. Fetal cortisol, which plays a major role in labour in sheep, is unlikely to play a major role in human labour.

Theories to Explain Labour Initiation

There are three theories to explain the initiation of labour:

- A functional decrease in the factors that were maintaining uterine quiescence
- The synthesis of factors that induce labour
- The triggering of a signal by the mature fetus to initiate labour

It is possible that the three processes together play a major role in the initiation of labour and the parturition cascade.

PHASES OF LABOUR

Labour consists of four phases (Table 1.1). These phases reflect the change from the maintenance of myometrial relaxation and cervical structural integrity to cervical softening and ripening, progressive uterine contractions, cervical effacement and dilatation, delivery of the fetus and placenta, and recovery to the non-pregnant state. This chapter deals mainly with the first two phases.

Phase 1 or Quiescence

This phase constitutes 95% of the entire pregnancy and is characterised by quiescence of the uterine smooth muscle with maintenance of cervical structural integrity. This lack of contractility continues till the end of pregnancy. However, some low-intensity myometrial contractions are

Table 1.1 Phases of labour and mediators

Phase	Characteristics	Mediators
Quiescent phase	• Acontractility of the uterine smooth muscle • Maintenance of cervical structural integrity	• Progesterone • Prostacyclin • Relaxin
Activation phase	Transition from quiescence to active labour	Relative increase in the estrogen–progesterone ratio
Stimulation phase	Includes active labour	• Prostaglandins • Oxytocin • Relaxin
Involution phase	Uterus and cervix return to their normal state and integrity	• Oxytocin • Local factors

felt during the third trimester which do not cause cervical dilatation. These are called **Braxton–Hicks contractions.**

The vascularity of the myometrium increases throughout pregnancy and provides nutrient and gas exchange for the fetus as well as for energy expenditure to meet the requirements of labour.

Mechanisms involved in uterine contractions

Uterine contractions are brought about by the following mechanisms:

- **Interaction between actin and myosin:** This is catalysed by the enzyme myosin light chain kinase.
- **Intracellular calcium**: Myosin light chain kinase is activated by calcium, which results in the lowering of intracellular calcium-promoted uterine quiescence.
- **Contraction-associated proteins (CAPs)**: Low levels of CAPs (oxytocin receptor, prostaglandin F receptor, and connexin-43) reduce the occurrence of uterine contractions.
- **Caspase 3**: This is an anticontractile molecule which inhibits the action of CAPs.
- **G protein-coupled receptors**: These receptors combine with hormones such as luteinising hormone (LH) and cortisol-releasing hormone (CRH) and maintain uterine relaxation.

The mechanisms involved in uterine quiescence are regulated by **progesterone, relaxin, corticotropin-releasing hormone, prostacyclin, and hCG**.

> **Key Point**
>
> Progesterone causes uterine quiescence.
> **Clinical significance**—It is used to prevent preterm labour.

Cervical softening in phase 1

The cervix sustains cervical competence which has to act against gravity. It also maintains the epithelial barrier which helps protect the uterus and its contents from infection. In the non-pregnant state, the cervix is closed and firm. Towards the end of pregnancy, the cervix becomes soft and distensible. The cervix has a high ratio of fibroblasts to smooth muscle cells, and the extracellular matrix (ECM) contributes significantly to the overall cervical tissue.

Cervical softening is an active process and balances cervical competence against structural changes in the ECM to increase compliance. The ECM is made up of collagens, matricellular proteins, glycosaminoglycans, proteoglycans, and elastic fibres. Specifically, collagen processing is altered such that mature cross-linked collagen fibrils are replaced with loosely-linked fibrils. Thus, the collagen becomes less stiff and more compliant [1].

> **Key Point**
>
> Cervical softening is an active process in which cervical competence is balanced against structural changes in the ECM to increase compliance.

Phase 2 or Activation

This phase involves the transition from quiescence to active labour and is brought about by a relative increase in the **estrogen–progesterone ratio**, which gradually occurs in the last weeks of pregnancy.

At this time, the myometrium becomes more responsive to signalling and as the level of progesterone decreases, the uterine contractility increases. Along with this, cervical tissue compliance and distensibility increase.

This phase commences in the last few weeks of pregnancy. There is no clear-cut progesterone withdrawal in humans. However, there is a **functional progesterone withdrawal** as the myometrium and cervix become refractory to the inhibitory action of progesterone.

Myometrial changes in phase 2

In phase 2, there is a shift in the expression of proteins favouring uterine quiescence to the expression of CAPs [2], which increase uterine sensitivity to stimulatory agents.

The **lower uterine segment** develops from the isthmus. It becomes differentiated from the upper segment, and each segment performs different roles near term and in labour. There is differential expression of prostaglandin receptors and CAPs in the upper and lower segments [3].

Oxytocin receptors also increase in the myometrium. Oxytocin increases the amplitude and duration of myometrial contractions. Contractility is caused by the following:

- Enhanced actin–myosin interaction
- Heightened excitability of the myometrial cells and promotion of intracellular cross-talk
- Increased intracellular calcium

Agents that induce contractions act on the myometrial cells to augment calcium levels. For example, prostaglandin F2-alpha (PGF2-alpha) and oxytocin bind to their receptors to release calcium from the sarcoplasmic reticulum.

Cervical ripening in phase 2

The cervix plays a dual role—remaining firm and closed in pregnancy and softening, effacing, and dilating in labour. In phase 2, there are changes in the connective tissue that lead to cervical ripening. This transition from softening to ripening begins weeks or days prior to labour.

The cervix in the non-pregnant state is mainly composed of collagen bundles tightly packed and embedded in ground substance consisting of glycosaminoglycans (GAGs). The GAGs form complexes with proteins called proteoglycans.

> **Key Point**
>
> The firmness of the cervix in the non-pregnant state is chiefly due to the collagen fibrils, which are tightly packed together as bundles. The main glycosaminoglycans in the cervix are dermatan sulfate and chondroitin sulfate, which are hydrophobic (repel water) and cause the cervix to remain firm.

As pregnancy advances, the proportion of collagen decreases. By late pregnancy, the cervix becomes soft and compliant. This is further exaggerated in labour when the cervix becomes elastic and plastic. All these changes are due to changes at the molecular level. As pregnancy advances, the composition of the GAGs gets altered, resulting in the accumulation of water in between the collagen fibrils. This destabilises the collagen fibrils and reduces their mechanical strength, contributing to cervical ripening [4,5].

> **Key Point**
>
> Cervical ripening occurs due to the replacement of dermatan and chondroitin sulphates with hyaluronic acid. Hyaluronic acid contributes to the accumulation of water within the cervix, which destabilises the collagen fibrils and contributes to cervical ripening.

Collagen remodelling by enzymes

Collagenase and leukocyte esterase are enzymes that decrease the concentration of collagen in phase 2 [6]. In addition, they also cause the remodelling of collagen.

Prostaglandins and cervical ripening

Cervical ripening is induced by prostaglandins, which have a direct effect on the production of procollagenase, which is a precursor of collagenase. This is why intracervical prostaglandins produce cervical changes without inducing uterine contractions.

> **Key Point**
>
> PGE2 causes cervical softening.
> **Clinical significance**—It is used for cervical ripening.

Phase 3 or Stimulation

This phase includes active labour and is mediated by **prostaglandins**, **oxytocin,** and **relaxin**. There are progressive uterine contractions with associated cervical effacement and dilatation culminating in the expulsion of the fetus. This complex process involving the mother, fetus, and the placenta is known as the **parturition cascade.**

Role of the fetus

The fetus produces dehydroepiandrosterone sulphate (DHEAS) and 16 (OH) DHEAS, which in turn, are converted to estradiol and estriol by the placenta. Fetal cortisol stimulates the production of prostaglandins and oxytocin, potent uterine stimulants, by the placenta.

Role of the placenta

The placenta produces key hormones and substances that regulate uterine contractions and play a pivotal role in the initiation of labour. The placenta cannot convert progesterone to estrogen, but it can produce estrogens from DHEAS and 16 (OH) DHEAS. The following are key placental hormones:

- Estrogen
- Progesterone
- Placental corticotropin-releasing hormone
- Contraction-associated proteins (CAPs)
- Prostaglandins
- Oxytocin

Regular and strong uterine contractions in labour occur due to myometrial electrical coupling via **gap junctions**. Cellular signals controlling myometrial contraction and relaxation are effectively transferred between cells through gap junctions [2]. The expression of CAPs in the myometrium increases towards the onset of labour.

> **Key Point**
>
> Cellular signals controlling uterine contraction and relaxation are transferred between cells through gap junctions. These gap junctions enable the myometrium to act as a syncytium.

Progesterone inhibits gap junctions and promotes quiescence by inhibiting the contraction-associated protein expression. Towards the end of pregnancy, there is an integration of different regulatory pathways, and this leads to the release of the inhibition of connexin-43 and oxytocin receptor levels. This promotes uterine contractions [7,8]. Nearing labour, progesterone activity decreases and estrogen activity increases. This, in turn, increases the gap junctions between myocytes and synchronises contractions [9].

The levels of progesterone do not drop dramatically at term as was thought earlier. There is only a functional progesterone withdrawal. This has been discussed earlier in this chapter.

> **Key Point**
>
> Estrogen and prostaglandins induce the formation of gap junctions, while progesterone inhibits it. Braxton–Hicks contractions in the late third trimester may represent patches of uterine activity due to inadequate gap junction connectivity.

Role of the mother

The maternal pituitary and decidua actively participate in the process of labour. Oxytocin, the most important uterine stimulant responsible for maintaining uterine contractions, is produced by the maternal pituitary [10]. Estrogens stimulate and progesterone inhibits the development of oxytocin receptors in the myometrium [11].

In addition to the myometrium, oxytocin and oxytocin receptors are found in the amnion, chorion, and decidua, where they stimulate prostaglandin synthesis. Studies in vitro have shown that oxytocin treatment of **human amnion cells** stimulates prostaglandin E2 (PGE2) synthesis, whereas the treatment of **human decidua cells** with oxytocin causes increased PGF2-alpha synthesis. Oxytocin increases prostaglandin production, activating cytoplasmic phospholipase A_2 which causes the release of arachidonic acid [12].

The effect of oxytocin on the uterus is marked in late pregnancy and during labour [13]. The benefits of oxytocin antagonists like atosiban in preterm labour strengthen the evidence that oxytocin may have an important role to play in initiating labour.

It is not clear whether prostaglandins influence oxytocin receptors. However, in clinical practice, it is found that the amplitude and frequency of uterine contractions are higher when oxytocin is administered after prostaglandins as compared to cases in which oxytocin is administered alone. Hence, it is postulated that prostaglandins may have a stimulatory effect on the synthesis of oxytocin receptors.

Key Point

The sensitivity of the myometrium to circulating oxytocin increases with advancing gestation and peaks at parturition. Oxytocin promotes the synthesis and release of PGF2-alpha from the uterine decidua, which results in myometrial contractility. It is postulated that prostaglandins may have a stimulatory effect on the synthesis of oxytocin receptors.

Role of prostaglandins

The decidua synthesises prostaglandins—'the final common pathway' in the onset of human labour. In spontaneous labour, both prostaglandins and their metabolites increase in circulation [14]. Prostaglandins are lipid molecules with different hormone-like actions.

Prostaglandin synthesis

In humans, the majority of prostaglandins are produced in the amnion and decidua. The sensitivity of the myometrium to prostaglandins increases at term due to an increase in the number of myometrial receptors. Both PGE2 and PGF2-alpha can increase the sensitivity of the myometrium to circulating oxytocin by increasing the production of oxytocin receptors. The amnion is an important source of amniotic fluid prostaglandins. These have a critical role in activating the cascade of events that leads to the rupture of membranes.

Prostaglandins are produced from plasma membrane-derived arachidonic acid by the action of phospholipases (Fig. 1.1). The enzymes type 1 and 2 prostaglandin H synthase convert arachidonic acid to the intermediary prostaglandin H2. By means of prostaglandin isomerases, PGH2 is converted into active prostaglandins. These include prostaglandin F2-alpha, which has a predominant effect on the uterine myometrium, and prostaglandins E2 and I2 (PGE2, PGI2), which chiefly affect the cervix. Prostaglandins increase both the resting tone of the uterine myometrium as well as the amplitude and duration of myometrial contractions.

Greer et al. [15] have shown that following the administration of PGE2 for cervical ripening and labour induction, there is an associated increase in PGF2-alpha as well, which coincides with the onset of uterine contractions.

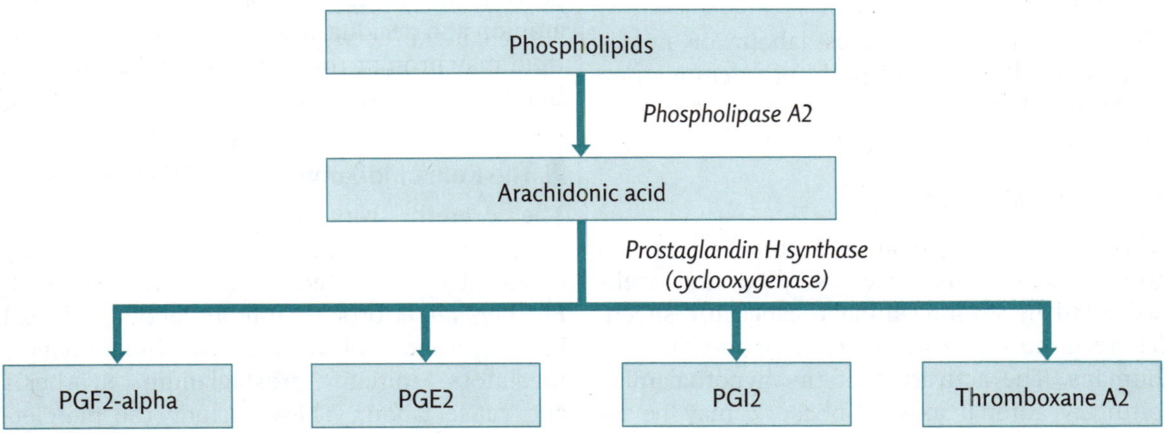

Fig. 1.1 Prostaglandin synthesis
PGE2, prostaglandin E2; *PGF2-alpha*, prostaglandin F2-alpha; *PGI2*, prostaglandin I2

The synthesis of PGF2-alpha is **suppressed in pregnancy to maintain quiescence**. This persists throughout pregnancy, and the suppression has to be withdrawn as a requisite for labour to ensue.

> **Key Point**
>
> Prostaglandins are capable of inducing myometrial contractions at all gestational ages.
> **Clinical significance**—Prostaglandins are widely used for the termination of pregnancy at any gestational age.

Phase 4 or Involution

The recovery of the uterus throughout the puerperium is referred to as phase 4.

INITIATION OF LABOUR

The events that disable the mechanisms maintaining uterine quiescence and recruit factors promoting uterine activity are listed below [16].

Progesterone Withdrawal

There is no clear-cut progesterone withdrawal in humans. However, there is a functional progesterone withdrawal. The myometrium and cervix become refractory to the inhibitory action of progesterone.

Oxytocin

Whether oxytocin initiates labour or not is not established as studies do not demonstrate an increase in the oxytocin level at the onset of labour.

Fetal Endocrine Signals

The existence of fetal endocrine signals to initiate labour has been studied and well-validated in several animals, especially sheep. There is no clear-cut evidence of the same in humans. The activation of the hypothalamic–pituitary–adrenal axis in phase 2 may be an important component of the initiation of labour in humans.

Towards the end of pregnancy, the levels of CRH-binding protein decline, leading to high levels of bioavailable CRH. Placental CRH may enhance the production of fetal cortisol, which in turn, has a positive feedback effect on the placenta to produce more CRH. The placenta and fetus influence the timing of the onset of labour by an endocrine cascade.

There is evidence to show that placental sulphatase deficiency and fetal anencephaly may be associated with prolonged pregnancy. In anencephaly, abnormal function of the fetal brain–pituitary–adrenal axis results in a deficiency of 19-carbon steroids.

Uterine Stretching

Fetal growth and uterine stretching are important contributors to uterine activation in phase 2. Uterine stretching increases the expression of connexin-43 and oxytocin receptors. The fact that multiple gestation and pregnancies complicated by hydramnios have a higher risk of preterm labour is corroborative of the role of uterine stretching.

Fetal Lung Surfactant

A surfactant protein produced by the fetal lung is required for lung maturation. It has been postulated that a surfactant produced by the amnion and decidua and present in the amniotic fluid may prompt the signalling of pathways in human myometrial cells [17].

The Role of Inflammatory Mediators

The preterm rupture of membranes with occult or obvious infection (chorioamnionitis) is usually associated with preterm labour. Further, all efforts to inhibit labour will fail in the presence of an infection. Inflammatory mediators initiate prostaglandin synthesis and cause labour. These include the platelet-activating factor, interleukins (especially IL-6), and tumour necrosis factor (TNF) [18].

Relationship Between Oxytocin and Prostaglandins

As labour sets in, there is an increase in the local estrogen–progesterone ratio, or at least, a functional withdrawal of progesterone as previously described. This leads to the synthesis of oxytocin by the decidua and increased oxytocin receptor expression in the myometrium. This will then stimulate the synthesis and release of prostaglandins from the fetal membranes and decidua, which in turn, will further increase oxytocin release. Thus, a positive feedback loop is set into motion. Both oxytocin and prostaglandins have a synergistic role in the initiation and maintenance of labour.

CONCLUSION

The maintenance of pregnancy and the onset of labour are both controlled by opposing factors which strike a delicate balance. The initiation and maintenance of labour are governed by complex mechanisms which are still not very clear in humans. Cervical ripening and an increase in myometrial contractility are the basic processes governing labour, which in turn, are controlled by different mechanisms.

REFERENCES

1. Yoshida K, Jiang H, Kim M, et al. Quantitative evaluation of collagen crosslinks and corresponding tensile mechanical properties in mouse cervical tissue during normal pregnancy. *PLoS One*. 2014. 9(11):e112391.
2. Solan JL, Lampe PD. Spatio-temporal regulation of connexin 43 phosphorylation and gap junction dynamics. *Biochem Biophys Acta Biomembr*. 2018. 1860(1):83.
3. Astle S, Thornton S, Slater DM. Identification and localisation of prostaglandin E2 receptors in upper and lower segment human myometrium during pregnancy. *Mol Hum Reprod*. 2005. 11(4):279.
4. Uldgberg N, G Ekman, A Malmstrom, K Olsson, U Umsten. Ripening of the human uterine cervix related to changes in collagenolytic activity. *Am J Obstet Gynecol*. 1983. 47 (6): 662-6.
5. Akgul Y, Word RA, Ensign LM, Yamaguchi Y, Lydon J, Hanes J, Mahendroo M. Hyaluronan in cervical epithelia protects against infection-mediated preterm birth. *J Clin Invest*. 2014. 124(12):5481-9.
6. Koay TS, CK Too, FC Greenwood, Bryant-Greenwood GD. Relaxin stimulates collagenase and plasminogen activator secretion by dispersed human amnion and chorion cells in vitro. *J Clin Endocrinol Metabol*. 1983. 56 (6):1332-4.
7. Mendelson CR, Gao L, Montalbano AP. Multifactorial regulation of myometrial contractility during pregnancy and parturition. *Front Endocrinol* (Lausanne). 2019. 10:714.
8. Peavey MC, Wu SP, Li R, et al. Progesterone receptor isoform B regulates the Oxtr-Plcl2-Trpc3 pathway to suppress uterine contractility. *Proc Natl Acad Sci* USA. 2021. 118(11): e2011643118.
9. Smith R, Imtiaz M, Banney D, Paul JW, Young RC. Why the heart is like an orchestra and the uterus is like a soccer crowd. *Am J Obstet Gynecol*. 2015. 213(2):181–5.
10. Thornton S, JM Davison, PM Bayllis. Plasma oxytocin during the third stage of labour: Comparison of natural and active management. *BMJ*. 1988. 297:167-69.
11. Alexandrova M and MA Soloff. Oxytocin receptors and parturition I: Control of oxytocin receptor concentration in rat myometrium at term. *Endocrinology*. 1980. 106:730-35.
12. Bennett PR, Slater D, Sullivan M, Elder MG, Moore GE. Changes in amniotic arachidonic acid metabolism associated with increased cyclo-oxygenase gene expression. *Br J Obstet Gynaecol*. 1993. 100(11):1037–42.
13. Kao CY. Electrical properties of uterine smooth muscle. *Biology of the Uterus*. RM Wynn and W Jollie (Eds). 2nd ed. New York: Plenum Medical. 1977. 423-96.
14. Brennecke SP, BM Castle, LM Demers, AC Turnbull. Maternal plasma prostaglandin E_2 metabolite levels during human pregnancy and parturition. *Br J Obstet Gynaecol*. 1985. 92 (4):345-9.
15. Greer IA, M McLaren, AA Calder. Plasma prostaglandin E_2 and prostaglandin F_2a metabolite levels following the vaginal administration of PGE_2 for the induction of labour. *Acta Obstet et Gynecol Scand*. 1990. 69:621-66.
16. Norwitz ER, Robinson JN, Challis JR. The control of labor. *N Engl J Med*.1999. 341:660.
17. Toyoshima K, Narahara H, Furukawa M, et al. Platelet-activating factor. Role in fetal lung development and relationship to normal and premature labor. *Clin Perinatol*. 1995. 22(2):263.
18. Szekeres-Bartho J, P Varga, AS Pasca. Immunologic factors contributing to the initiation of labor-lymphocyte reactivity in term and threatened preterm delivery. *Am J Obstet Gynecol*. 1986. 155 (1):108-12.

CHAPTER 2

Mechanics, Mechanism, and Stages of Labour

LAKSHMI SESHADRI

INTRODUCTION

Normal labour and unaided vaginal delivery, though considered to be the most common mode of childbirth worldwide, constitute a complex process involving the fetus, the maternal pelvis, maternal forces, and endocrine factors.

DEFINITION OF NORMAL LABOUR

The World Health Organization (WHO) defines normal birth as spontaneous in onset, low-risk at the start of labour and remaining so throughout labour and delivery. The infant is born spontaneously in the vertex position between 37 and 42 completed weeks of pregnancy. After birth, the mother and infant are in good health [1]. In other words, normal labour is a complex process in which the fetus and the placenta are expelled through the vagina at term, aided by uterine contractions, cervical effacement and dilatation, and maternal expulsive efforts.

MECHANICS OF LABOUR

In normal labour, the fetal presentation is vertex. However, the largest diameter of the fetal vertex does not occupy the largest diameter of the maternal pelvis. The diameters of the maternal pelvis vary at different levels. At the pelvic brim, the largest diameter is the transverse diameter but at the outlet, it is the anteroposterior diameter. Hence, the fetus has to move down the birth canal and rotate to negotiate the various pelvic diameters. This is achieved by the complex interaction between the **maternal forces** (powers), the **maternal pelvis** (passage), and the **fetus** (passenger).

> **Key Point**
>
> The mechanics of labour are complex and involve key factors such as uterine contractions, the diameters and configuration of the maternal pelvis, and fetal size, presentation, position, and attitude. The progress of labour can be affected by an abnormality in any one or more of these key factors.

Maternal Forces (Powers)

Uterine activity is the most important maternal force and is generated by the myometrium. The frequency, duration, and intensity of maternal force are the three characteristics that determine the progress of labour. Uterine contractions increase in frequency and intensity as labour progresses.

Frequency and duration

Uterine contractions occur once in 5–10 minutes and last for 20–30 seconds in the latent phase of labour. As labour progresses, the frequency of contractions increases gradually to once in 2–3 minutes, with each contraction lasting for 30–60 seconds in the active phase. In the second stage of labour, contractions occur once every 1–2 minutes and last for 60–90 seconds. Three to five contractions in 10 minutes are considered 'adequate' for the normal progress of labour.

Intensity

Palpation of the uterus is used to clinically assess the intensity of contractions (see **Chapter 4**,

Management of the first and second stages of normal labour). External tocodynamometry can give a qualitative estimate of uterine contractions but cannot measure the exact intensity. Though the intensity of contractions can be measured using an intrauterine pressure catheter (IUPC)—the pressure being expressed in Montevideo units (MVU)—the measurement of intrauterine pressure is not used in routine clinical practice. An intensity of 200–250 MVU is considered adequate in active labour [2].

Formation of the upper and lower uterine segments

Upper and lower segments of the uterus are formed as labour progresses. The isthmus, which is a small, insignificant segment of the uterus in the non-pregnant state, becomes the lower segment in late pregnancy and labour (Fig. 2.1). The active upper segment becomes thicker, and the passive lower segment becomes thinner and stretches to receive the fetus, which is then pushed down through the vagina and delivered.

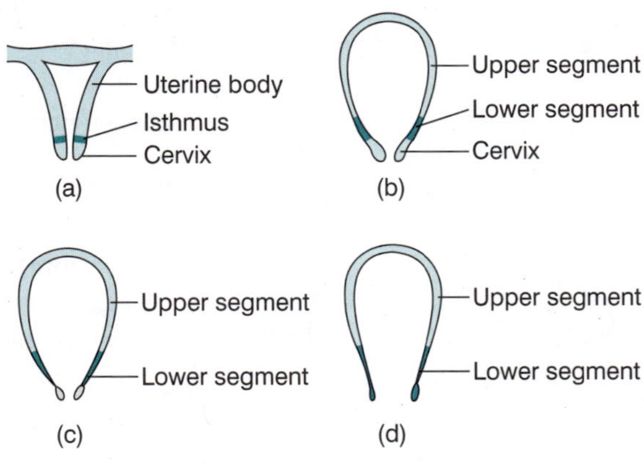

Fig. 2.1 Formation of the lower segment of the uterus: (a) The isthmus is a small segment in the non-pregnant uterus, (b) it stretches to become the lower segment in pregnancy, (c) this becomes thinner and stretches further, and (d) the fully effaced cervix is incorporated into the lower segment

Hydrostatic pressure exerted by the amniotic fluid aids in cervical dilatation. Maternal voluntary expulsive forces help in the second stage of labour.

Changes in the cervix

Cervical changes occur as a result of uterine contractions. The two fundamental changes are cervical **effacement** and **dilatation.** Effacement is the shortening of the cervix from about 3 cm to a paper-thin rim. This is accompanied by the dilatation of the cervix. In a nullipara, the dilatation may begin only after the cervix is fully effaced. On the other hand, in a multipara, the two proceed simultaneously. Only after the cervix is fully dilated (10 cm) can the fetal head pass through it.

Maternal Pelvis (Passage)

The fetus has to pass through the maternal pelvis which consists of four bones—the ilium, ischium, pubis, and sacrum. The bony pelvis is divided into the **false** and **true** pelvis. The line of demarcation between the two is referred to as the **pelvic inlet** or **pelvic brim**. The true pelvis is shaped like a truncated cylinder and is divided into three planes—the **pelvic inlet, midpelvis,** and **the pelvic outlet** (Fig. 2.2). The important diameters in the pelvis at these planes are listed in Table 2.1.

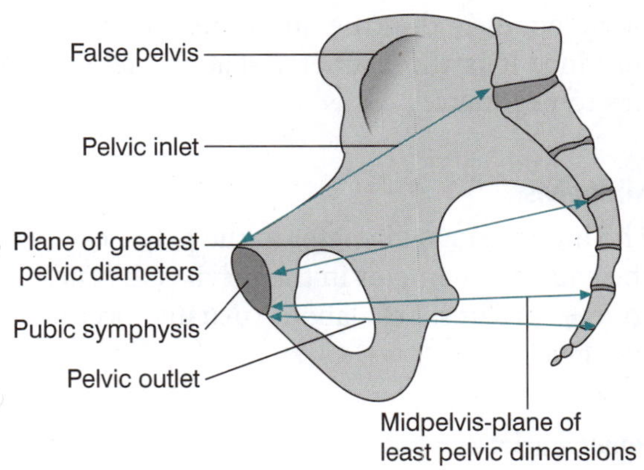

Fig. 2.2 Pelvic cavity, lateral view: The plane of the least dimensions is at the level of ischial spines and the fourth and fifth sacral vertebrae. The interischial spinous diameter (transverse diameter) is the smallest diameter that the fetal head has to pass through (10 cm).

Table 2.1 The diameters of the pelvis

Plane of the pelvis	Diameter	Measurement (cm)
Pelvic inlet	Anteroposterior • Diagonal conjugate • Obstetric conjugate Transverse Oblique	 12 10.5 13.5 12.5
Midpelvis	Anteroposterior Transverse	12 10
Pelvic outlet	Anteroposterior Transverse	12 10.5

Pelvic inlet

At the inlet, the transverse diameter is the largest diameter, and the anteroposterior diameter is the smallest (Fig. 2.3a). Hence, the head enters the pelvis with its engaging diameter in the transverse diameter of the pelvis.

There are three anteroposterior diameters at the pelvic inlet (Fig. 2.3b). Of these, the **obstetric conjugate** (the linear distance between the sacral promontory and the internal edge of the pubic bone) is the true anteroposterior diameter since it is the diameter that the fetal head has to negotiate.

Midpelvis

The interspinous diameter in the pelvic cavity is the smallest diameter in the pelvis. Obstruction to the progress of labour usually occurs at this level.

Pelvic outlet

The anteroposterior diameter is the largest at the outlet (Fig. 2.4). Therefore, the head has to rotate to bring its engaging diameter to lie in the anteroposterior diameter at the outlet for delivery to occur.

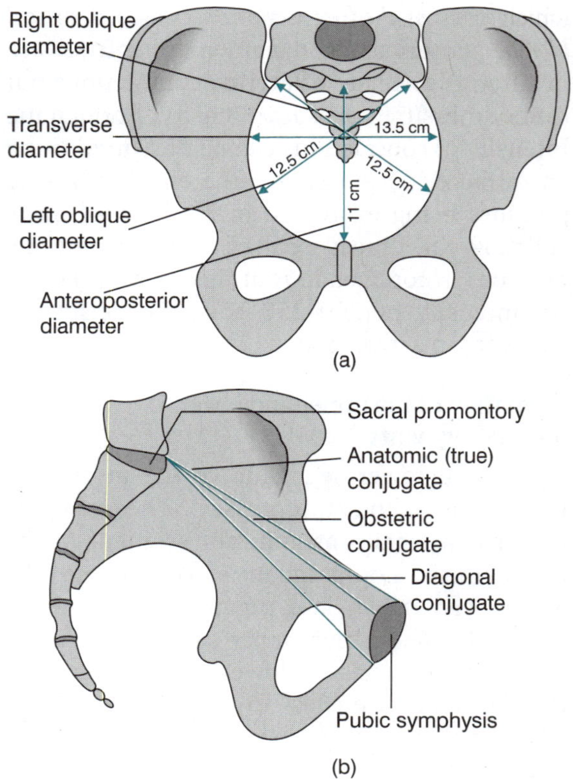

Fig. 2.3 (a) The diameters of the pelvic inlet and (b) the three anteroposterior diameters of the pelvic inlet

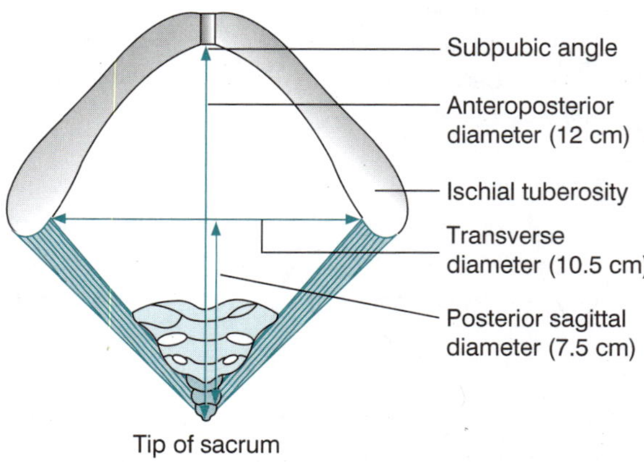

Fig. 2.4 The diameters of the pelvic outlet

Predicting the risk of cephalopelvic disproportion

The **critical limit values** for the various diameters of the pelvis are the cut-off diameters below which the risk of cephalopelvic disproportion (CPD) increases, depending on the fetal size [3]. These values can be obtained by computed tomography (CT) or magnetic resonance imaging (MRI) [4]. However, in current practice, these methods of measurement are not used routinely due to the lack of evidence of benefit. Clinical pelvimetry by vaginal examination is the method currently recommended for predicting or confirming CPD, though it is becoming a lost art [5].

Key Point

Though the diameters of the pelvis can be measured accurately using CT and MRI, these methods are not recommended in routine obstetric practice. Clinical pelvimetry by vaginal examination is the method currently recommended for predicting or confirming CPD.

Classification of the female pelvis

Based on the shape of the pelvis, Caldwell and Moloy classified the female pelvis into four parent types—**gynecoid, android, platypelloid, and anthropoid**. (Fig. 2.5) [6]. The most salient features of these types and their effects on labour are presented in Table 2.2.

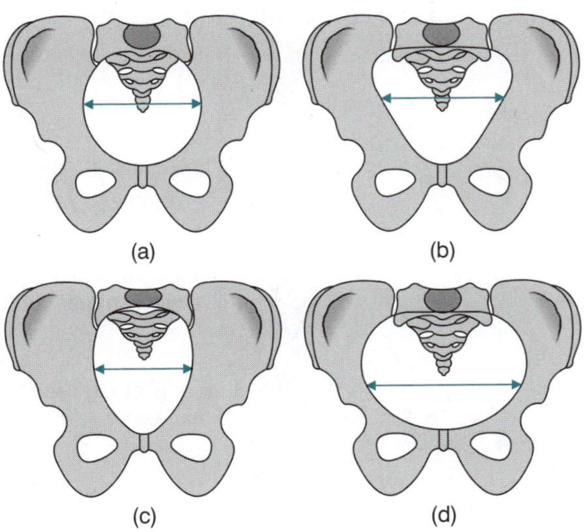

Fig. 2.5 The four parent types of pelvises—(a) gynecoid, (b) android, (c) anthropoid, and (d) platypelloid

Table 2.2 Salient features of pelvic types and their effects on labour

Pelvic type	Salient features	Effects on labour
Gynecoid	Classic female pelvis	Normal labour
Android	• Male type • Narrow forepelvis • Convergent side walls	• High risk of CPD • Deep transverse arrest
Anthropoid	• Exaggerated oval inlet • Narrow transverse diameter	Delivery as occipitoposterior
Platypelloid	Narrow anteroposterior diameter	• Asynclitism • Face presentation

Fetus (Passenger)

The fetus, for obvious reasons, plays a major role in labour. The fetal variables that must be taken into consideration are the following:

- Lie
- Presentation
- Attitude
- Position
- Size
- Descent
- **Fetal lie** refers to the position of the long axis of the fetus in relation to the long axis of the mother. It may be longitudinal, oblique, or transverse (Fig. 2.6). The fetal lie must be longitudinal, and presentation must be vertex for normal labour to ensue.
- **Fetal presentation** refers to the fetal part that directly overlies the pelvic inlet and is determined by the lie of the fetus and the presenting part.

  Longitudinal lie with the head in the lower pole is referred to as a **cephalic presentation**. Cephalic presentation may be vertex, face, or brow, depending on the attitude of the fetal head. When the buttock is the presenting part, it is known as **breech presentation**. Transverse lie results in **shoulder presentation.**
- **Attitude** of the fetal head refers to the degree of flexion or extension of the fetus. When the

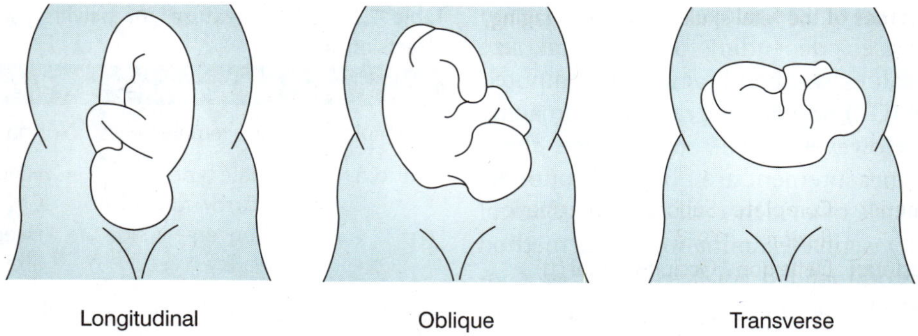

Fig. 2.6 Types of fetal lie

head is completely flexed, the presentation is **vertex**. In the occipitoposterior position, the head is deflexed. A partially extended head results in a **brow presentation** and when the head is completely extended, it results in a **face presentation** (Fig. 2.7).

- The **engaging diameter** of the fetal skull would depend on the position and attitude (Fig. 2.8). An occipitoanterior position with the vertex in complete flexion is the most favourable (Fig. 2.7a). The engaging diameter is increased when the head is in deflexion (Fig. 2.7b). Hence, there are increased chances of prolonged labour, operative vaginal delivery, and cesarean section [7]. The attitudes of the fetal skull and their engaging diameters are presented in Table 2.3.
- **Fetal size** is a crucial factor in labour. The risk of cephalopelvic disproportion increases when the fetal weight increases.
- **Descent of the presenting part** occurs with uterine contractions during labour. It is expressed in terms of the 'fifths' of the fetal head palpable above the pubic symphysis.

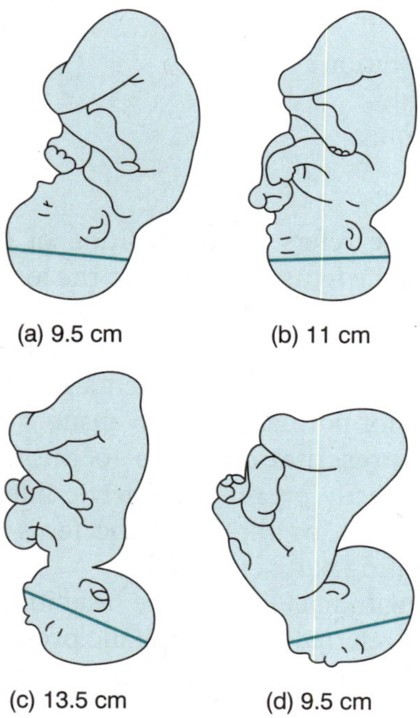

Fig. 2.7 Attitudes of the fetal head and presentations—(a) complete flexion – vertex, (b) deflexion – occipitoposterior, (c) partial extension – brow, and (d) complete extension – face

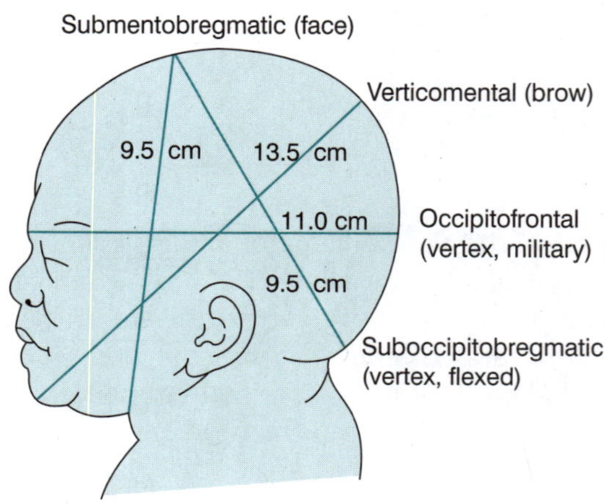

Fig. 2.8 The diameters of the fetal head

Table 2.3 Attitudes of the fetal skull and their engaging diameters

Presentation	Attitude	Engaging diameter (cm)
Vertex • Occipitoanterior • Occipitoposterior	 Complete flexion Deflexion	 Suboccipitobregmatic (9.5) Occipitofrontal (11)
Face	Complete extension	Submentobregmatic (9.5)
Brow	Partial extension	Verticomental (13.5)

MECHANISM OF NORMAL LABOUR

Normal labour is not a simple process of the fetus passing straight through the pelvis—the maternal pelvis is irregular in shape, and the diameters of the fetal skull vary with the attitude and position. Due to this asymmetry, the fetal skull has to negotiate the pelvis through a series of **cardinal movements**.

The bony reference point in vertex presentation is the occiput. The occiput may occupy the anterior, posterior, or lateral position in the pelvis on the left or right side, giving rise to one of six possible positions: left or right occipitoanterior (LOA or ROA), left or right occipitoposterior (LOP or ROP), or left or right occipitotransverse (LOT or ROT) as shown in Fig. 2.9.

Engagement

Cardinal movements in labour begin with the engagement of the vertex. This refers to the passage of the widest diameter of the presenting part through the pelvic inlet (Fig. 2.10a and b). The widest diameter in vertex presentation is the **biparietal diameter**. Since the occiput is at the same level as the parietal eminences in a well-flexed head, when the head engages, the occiput also enters the pelvic cavity and only the sinciput is palpable abdominally. When the head is engaged, the leading bony part of

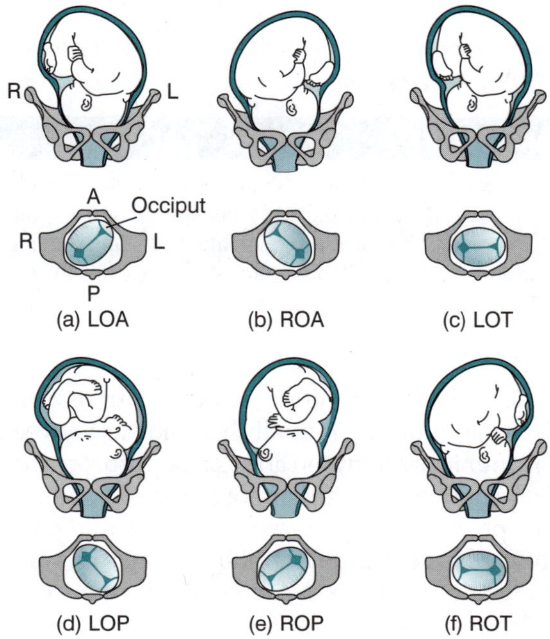

Fig. 2.9 Fetal positions in vertex presentation

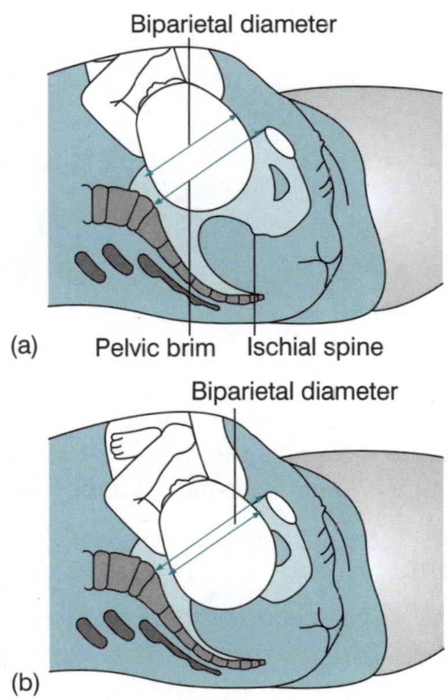

Fig. 2.10 Engagement of the fetal vertex : (a) The biparietal diameter is above the pelvic brim and (b) when it has crossed the pelvic inlet, the leading bony part is at the level of the ischial spines

the vertex is at the level of the ischial spines [8]. Engagement may occur by 38 weeks in primigravid women.

Key Point

In vertex presentation, when the head is engaged, the occiput is not palpable on second pelvic grip and only the sinciput is palpable. On vaginal examination, the leading part of the vertex is at the level of the ischial spines.

Asynclitism

When the fetal position is occipitotransverse, the sagittal suture normally lies midway between the pubic symphysis and sacral promontory. To negotiate the anteroposterior diameter of the pelvic inlet, the vertex may tilt laterally (towards the symphysis pubis or sacrum), and the sagittal suture may be more anterior or posterior, as shown in Fig. 2.11. This is known as **asynclitism.** This can occur in normal labour but can occasionally lead to dystocia.

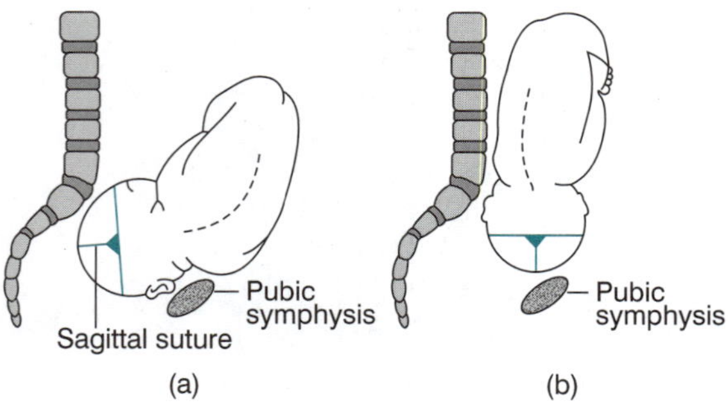

Fig. 2.11 Asynclitism: (a) In anterior asynclitism, the sagittal suture is towards the sacral hollow and (b) the sagittal suture is towards the pubic symphysis

Descent

Descent of the presenting part occurs as labour progresses, aided by uterine contractions. Descent is assessed by abdominal palpation and expressed in terms of 'fifths' of the fetal head palpable above the pubic symphysis. This is referred to as **Crichton's manoeuvre** and is described in **Chapter 4**, *Management of the first and second stages of normal labour.* When the head is engaged and only the sinciput is felt, it is 1/5th palpable. When the head descends further and no part of the head is felt abdominally (0/5), further assessment of descent is done by vaginal examination.

Flexion

Flexion of the fetal head occurs as the head descends (Fig. 2.12a). Mild degrees of deflexion are corrected, and the head flexes until the chin touches the chest wall. Flexion is brought about by the resistance offered by soft tissues such as the pelvic floor and the cervix and by the bony pelvis.

Internal Rotation

The head enters the pelvic inlet in the transverse or oblique diameter and must rotate to the anteroposterior diameter in order to be born. This is known as **internal rotation**. The occiput rotates anteriorly towards the pubic symphysis to bring the suboccipitobregmatic diameter in line with the anteroposterior diameter of the midpelvis and the widest part of the fetal head to the widest part of the pelvis (Fig. 2.12b). This rotation is brought about by the curve of the levator ani muscle, impetus of the ischial spines, and the shape of the bony pelvis.

Extension

At the pelvic outlet, the birth canal curves anteriorly. The fetal occiput hitches under the pubic symphysis, the head extends, and the bregma, nose, mouth, and chin are born in that order (Fig. 2.12c).

Restitution

The fetal head rotates back so that the occiput is lateral once again.

External Rotation

External rotation of the fetal head is the outward manifestation of the internal rotation

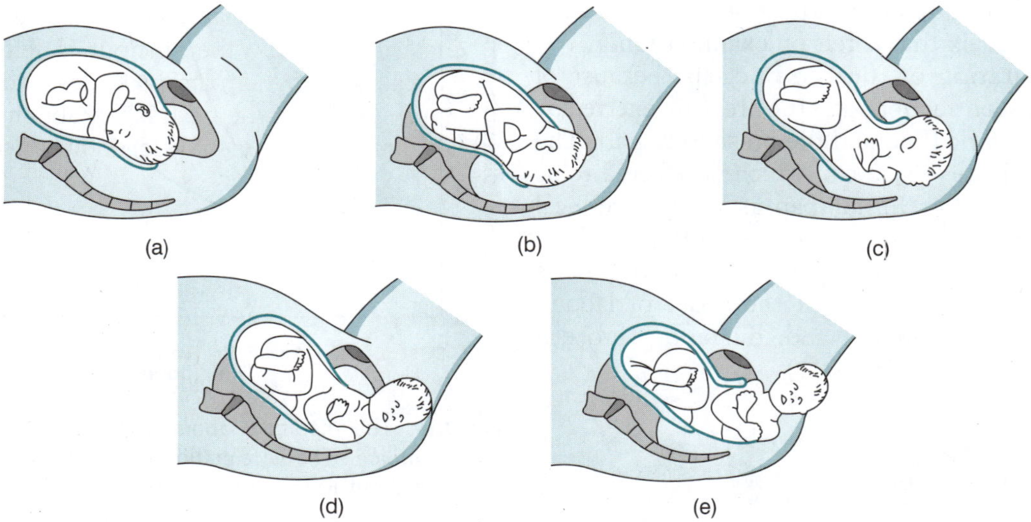

Fig. 2.12 Mechanism of normal labour: (a) Flexion, (b) internal rotation, (c) extension, (d) external rotation, and (e) delivery of the shoulders

of the fetal shoulder, which now rotates to engage in the opposite oblique diameter of the pelvis. Restitution and external rotation occur as a continuous movement (Fig. 2.12d). One of the shoulders, now referred to as the anterior shoulder, hitches under the pubic symphysis and the posterior shoulder is born first, followed by the anterior shoulder (Fig. 2.12e). The delivery of the rest of the fetus follows.

STAGES OF LABOUR

In preparation for the onset of labour, under the influence of various hormones, changes occur in the genital tract a few weeks before labour. This is referred to as **prelabour** or **the preparatory stage of labour**. The uterus falls forward and the cervix becomes soft and 'ripe'.

Labour is divided into three stages:

- **First stage**: This is the stage of cervical dilatation which begins with the onset of uterine contractions and the beginning of cervical changes and ends with the full dilatation of the cervix.
- **Second stage**: This is the stage of expulsion of the fetus and begins with full cervical dilatation and ends with the delivery of the baby.
- **Third stage**: This is the stage of expulsion of the placenta and extends from the delivery of the fetus to the delivery of the placenta, followed by the contraction and retraction of the uterus.

First Stage of Labour

Regular, painful uterine contractions mark the onset of labour. It may be difficult to establish the exact time of the onset of labour because it is based on the woman's perception of the onset of painful contractions. In this stage, the uterus becomes elongated, and the horizontal diameter decreases as the vertical length increases. This results in fetal axis pressure, thrusting the lower pole of the fetus downward.

Changes in the cervix are an essential part of the first stage of labour and are mandatory for the progress of labour and delivery. **Cervical effacement** or 'taking up' of the cervix refers to the shortening and thinning of the cervix. The cervix is pulled and incorporated into the lower uterine segment. The cervix is about 4 cm in length at the onset of labour but is not palpable when it is fully effaced. **Effacement** is expressed as the percentage of cervical length that is taken up or in terms of the actual length of the cervix that is felt on examination.

Dilatation of the cervix occurs because of uterine contractions and the pressure exerted by the amniotic fluid and the presenting part. The cervix dilates to 10 cm, which is referred to as **full dilatation**. In nulliparous women, cervical effacement usually takes place first, followed by dilatation. In multiparas, the internal os is usually partially open at the onset of labour. Cervical effacement and dilatation proceed simultaneously (Fig. 2.13).

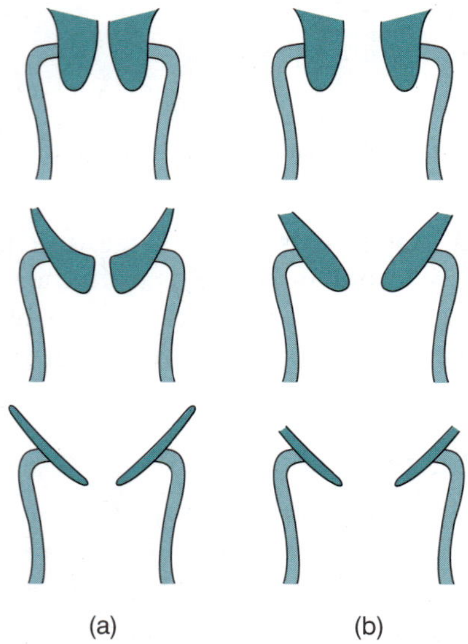

Fig. 2.13 Cervical effacement—(a) in a nulliparous woman and (b) in a multipara

The mucus plug that occludes the cervix is expelled as the cervix effaces and dilates. This mucosanguinous discharge seen in the first stage of labour is known as **'show'**.

Phases of the first stage of labour

Friedman, in 1954, established the criteria for normal labour progression [9,10]. The labour curve he proposed has long been accepted as the standard for the assessment of labour progression. This labour curve was later modified by Zhang (Fig. 2.14) based on contemporary data

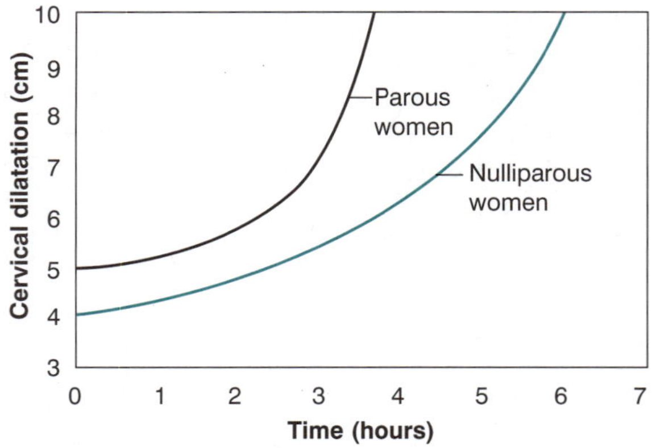

Fig. 2.14 The modified labour curve in a nullipara and multipara—The acceleration of cervical dilatation starts at about 6 cm for multiparous women; there is no clear point where cervical dilatation accelerates for nulliparous women and there is no deceleration phase

from the Consortium on Safe Labour [11]. This has been adopted by the World Health Organization and other professional bodies. Based on the labour curve, the first stage of labour is divided into the **latent** and **active** phases.

The latent phase

The WHO defines the latent phase of the first stage of labour as the period of time characterised by painful uterine contractions and variable changes in the cervix, including some degree of effacement and slow progression of dilatation up to 5 cm for first and subsequent labours [12]. No standard has been established for the duration of this stage; it may extend up to 20 hours in primigravid women.

Key Points

- The active phase of labour begins at 5 cm dilatation according to the WHO's current definition.
- Labour progression is more rapid after 6 cm dilatation in multiparous women.

The active phase

The WHO defines the active phase of the first stage of labour as the period of time characterised by regular painful uterine contractions, a substantial degree of cervical effacement, and more rapid cervical dilatation from 5 cm to full dilatation for first and subsequent labours [13]. The median duration of the active phase is 4 hours in first labours and 3 hours in subsequent labours but can extend up to 12 hours in first labours and 10 hours in subsequent labours.

The rate of cervical dilatation increases after 5 cm and accelerates progressively [14]. The labour curves are different for nulliparous and multiparous women. The sharp increase in the rate of dilatation which occurs from 6 cm in multiparous women does not occur in nulliparas [12]. The mean duration of the active phase is also longer in nulliparous women.

During the active phase of labour, the lower uterine segment develops further, the presenting part descends, and the bag of membranes is formed. Towards the end of the first stage, the bag of membranes may rupture.

Second Stage of Labour

Once the cervix is fully dilated, the presenting part is pushed into the vagina, and delivery occurs. The uterine contractions are stronger and occur more frequently. This is accompanied by bearing down efforts by the mother. The median duration of the second stage is 20 minutes in multiparas and 50 minutes in nulliparas but can extend to 2 hours in a multipara and 3 hours in a nullipara.

Phases of the second stage of labour

The second stage of labour is divided into two phases. Normally, it is difficult to differentiate between the two.

- **Phase 1—passive phase or phase of descent:** Rapid descent of the presenting part occurs during this phase, which extends from the full dilatation of the cervix to the onset of active pushing.
- **Phase II—active phase or phase of expulsion:** The presenting part reaches the pelvic floor and the bearing down pains begin. If this phase is prolonged, fetal hypoxia and damage to the pelvic floor muscles and fascia can occur. Close monitoring of the fetal heart rate and maternal condition is mandatory during this phase of the second stage.

Prolongation of the second stage is associated with increased risk of postpartum hemorrhage, infection, cesarean section, and difficult instrumental delivery [14].

Key Point

'Pushing pains' mark the beginning of the active phase of the second stage. Prolongation of this phase is associated with maternal and fetal morbidity.

Third Stage of Labour

Contraction of the uterus causes placental separation. This can begin at the centre of the placenta or at the edges, and progress to the separation of the entire placenta. With further contractions of the uterus, the placenta is expelled. The bleeding from the torn ends of the blood vessels is arrested by the contraction and retraction of the uterus. The criss-cross fibres of the middle layer of the uterine myometrium compress the blood vessels. Clots that are formed in the vessels further occlude the vessels to control the bleeding.

The median duration of the third stage of labour is 6–8 minutes. When it exceeds 30 minutes, the risk of complications such as postpartum hemorrhage and the need for manual removal of the placenta increase [15,16].

CONCLUSION

Knowledge of the mechanics and mechanisms of labour is crucial in the management of delivery. Awareness and familiarity with this core information allow the clinician to assess and evaluate the prolongation or arrest of labour. Even in this era of imaging technology, abdominal and digital vaginal examination of the labouring woman is the gold standard and enables the clinician to bring about better outcomes for the woman and her child.

REFERENCES

1. World Health Organization. Maternal and Newborn Health/Safe Motherhood Unit. Care in normal birth: A practical guide. WHO Press. Geneva. 1996.
2. Caldeyro-Barcia R, Sica-Blanco Y, Poseiro J, et al. A quantitative study of the action of synthetic oxytocin on the pregnant human uterus. *J Phramacol Exp Ther*. 1957. 121:18-31.
3. Joyce D, Giwa-Osagie F, Stevenson G. Role of pelvimetry in active management of labour. *Br Med J*. 1975. 4:505.
4. Morris C, Heggie J, Acton C. Computed tomography in pelvimetry: Accuracy and radiation dose compared with conventional pelvimetry. *Australas Radiol*.1993. 37:186.
5. Maharaj D. Assessing cephalopelvic disproportion: Back to basics. *Obstet Gynecol Surv*. 2010. 65(6):387.
6. Caldwell W, Moloy H. Anatomical variations in the female pelvis and their effect in labor, with a suggested classification. *Am J Obstet Gynecol*. 1933. 26:479.
7. Cheng Y, Shaffer B, Caughey A. Associated factors and outcomes of persistent occiput posterior position: A retrospective cohort study from1976 to 2001. *J Matern fetal Neonatal Med*. 2006. 19 (9):563.
8. Caldwell W, Moloy H, D'Esopo D. A roentgenologic study of the mechanism of engagement of the fetal head. *Am J Obstet Gynecol*. 1934. 28:824-841.
9. Friedman E. Primigravid Labor. *Obstet Gynecol*. 1955. 6:567.
10. Friedman E. Labor in multiparas: A graphicostatistical analysis. *Obstet Gynecol*. 1956. 8:691.
11. Zhang J, Landy HJ, Branch DW, Burkman R, Haberman S, Gregory KD, et al. Contemporary patterns of spontaneous labor with normal neonatal outcomes. Consortium on Safe Labor. *Obstet Gynecol*. 2010. 116:1281–7.
12. WHO recommendations: Intrapartum care for a positive childbirth experience. World Health Organization. WHO Press. Geneva. 2018.
13. Zhang J, Troendle J, Yancey M. Reassessing the labor curve in nulliparous women. *Am J Obstet Gynecol*. 2002. 187:824.
14. American College of Obstetricians and Gynecologists (College). Society for Maternal-Fetal Medicine. Caughey A, Cahill A, et al. Safe prevention of the primary caesarean delivery. *Am J Obstet Gynecol*. 2014. 210930:179-193.
15. Combs C, Laros R Jr. Prolonged third stage of labor: Morbidity and risk factors. *Obstet Gynecol*. 1991. 77:863.
16. Magann E, Lannaeu G. Third stage of labor. *Obstet Gynecol Clin North Am*. 2005. 32(2):323.

CHAPTER 3

Respectful Obstetric Care and the Role of a Birth Companion

SIRISHA RAO G, EVITA FERNANDEZ

RESPECTFUL OBSTETRIC CARE

INTRODUCTION

Pregnancy and childbirth are natural physiological events that are significant and life-changing for women. The journey to motherhood should be joyous and life-affirming. It is unfortunate that an experience as powerful and life-transforming as childbirth is dominated by a climate of fear—fear of pain, fear for the well-being of the mother and her baby, the fear of being mistreated, and the fear of death [1,2].

Key Point

Childbirth is a significant event in the life of a woman with lasting emotional consequences.

The increasing number of women delivering in health facilities has not resulted in a concomitant improvement in maternal and neonatal outcomes because of the poor quality of care secondary to incompetent care providers, inadequate infrastructure, and an acute lack of evidence-based practices [3]. Women may receive care that is **too little, too late**, or **too much, too soon**. Many others may receive no care, particularly adolescents, unmarried pregnant women, immigrants, refugees, women belonging to ethnic or religious minorities, women living in poverty, informal urban settlements, or fragile states, and those facing humanitarian crises [4]. Care that is too much and too soon escalates health costs in facility births and amounts to disrespectful care [5].

Key Point

Women who have little or no access to care include adolescents, unmarried pregnant women, immigrants, refugees, women belonging to ethnic or religious minorities, women living in poverty, informal urban settlements, or fragile states, and those facing humanitarian crises.

Disrespect and abuse of women in childbirth are widespread. Mistreatment during labour can lead to reduced use of maternity care provided for women and is one of the underlying causes of the slow reduction in the global maternal mortality ratio [6]. Disrespect is a belittling experience and indicates apathy and a lack of quality and accountability in the health system.

LaQshya, a Labour Room Quality Improvement Initiative introduced by the National Health Mission, Ministry of Health and Family Welfare, Government of India [7], has advocated for respectful and humane treatment during labour.

COMPONENTS OF DISRESPECT AND ABUSE

To understand what respectful obstetric care comprises, it is essential to recognise the various components of disrespect and abuse. This can range from verbal insults to physical assault and from neglect to non-consensual interventions. The 2014 bulletin issued by the World

Health Organization (WHO) defined disrespect and abuse in childbirth as "interactions or facility conditions that local consensus deems to be humiliating or undignified, and those interactions or conditions that are experienced as or intended to be humiliating or undignified" [8]. The Respectful Maternity Care Charter: Universal Rights for Women and Newborns by the White Ribbon Alliance (Table 3.1) clarifies the ambit of women's rights and addresses the issue of disrespect and abuse [9]. This charter recognises the power of human rights and focuses on the promotion of values rather than purely clinical outcomes.

Key Point

Safe motherhood refers not only to the prevention of morbidity and mortality but also to respect for women's basic human rights.

Women's Perceptions and Maternal Satisfaction

Childbirth Connection's Listening to Mothers initiative aims to understand the viewpoint of pregnant women and use this knowledge to improve maternity care [10]. A total of 2400 pregnant women participated in Survey III, which was carried out in 2013. The results indicated that 59% of these women were not given a choice with regard to episiotomy; 8–23% experienced pressure to opt for one of many interventions; and 20% of black and Hispanic women reported racial discrimination.

The results of the Dignity Survey, 2013, which included the experiences of 1100 women and midwives with UK Maternity Care [11], were as follows:

- Only 68% of women were given a choice regarding the place of birth.
- 31% did not feel in control of their birth experience.
- 15% were unhappy with the availability of pain relief and 10% were unhappy with the choice of pain relief.
- 23% were unhappy about not being given a choice of position during labour.
- 20% said healthcare professionals did not always introduce themselves.
- 18% felt that their health professionals did not listen to them.

Table 3.1 The universal rights of women and newborns [9]

Category of disrespect and abuse	Corresponding right
Physical abuse	Freedom from harm and ill-treatment
Non-consensual care	Right to information, informed consent and refusal, and respect for choices and preferences, including the right to the companionship of choice during maternity care, and refusal of medical procedures
Non-confidential care	Privacy and confidentiality
Non-dignified care (including verbal abuse)	Dignity, respect
Discrimination based on specific attributes	Equality, freedom from discrimination, equitable care
Abandonment or denial of care	Right to timely healthcare and to the highest attainable level of health
Detention in facilities	Liberty, autonomy, self-determination, and freedom from arbitrary detention
Separation of the newborn from the mother	Right of the child to be with parents or guardians
Denial of birth registration or nationality	Right of the child to identity and nationality from birth
Prevention from accessing nutrition, clean water or a healthy environment	Right to adequate nutrition and clean water

- 12% did not consider that they had consented to medical procedures.
- 24% of women who had an instrumental birth said they had not consented to the procedures performed.

Respect for basic human rights and courteous treatment are important determinants of maternal satisfaction and may be perceived as more important than the technical competence of providers. Women's birth experiences are most profoundly shaped by the attitudes of their caregivers and the sense of control they feel during childbirth [12,13]. The influences of pain, pain relief, and intrapartum medical interventions on satisfaction are not as powerful as the influences of the attitudes and behaviours of the caregivers [12]. Women in low- and middle-income countries may prefer to give birth at home with a traditional birth attendant due to the fear of abuse at health facilities [14].

With 'guidance compliance' taking priority, i.e., uncompromising conformity to guidelines, there is a reluctance to support women's choices, leading to dehumanisation and disrespectful care. **Evidence provided by clinical research can inform but can never replace individual clinical expertise or patients' values** [15]. Therefore, care must be individualised, and this should form the basis for informed choice.

> **Key Point**
>
> The lack of satisfaction among labouring women stems largely from the attitudes and behaviours of the caregivers [12]. Women in low- and middle-income countries may avoid health facilities and prefer to give birth at home with a traditional birth attendant due to fear of abuse [14].

Implementing Respectful Maternal Care

Data from a systematic review of five studies suggest that multi-component respectful maternity care policies could increase women's experiences of good quality and respectful care. These policies help reduce the incidence of disrespectful or abusive behaviours including physical abuse by staff [16].

Caring for the Carers

Caring for the carers includes ensuring that staff are duly respected and promptly paid, able to do their job well, have access to supplies, clean water, and well-maintained equipment, have the potential for updating their skills and for personal development, and have the provision of mentorship and dispute resolution [17].

KEY COMPONENTS OF RESPECTFUL OBSTETRIC CARE

Respectful maternity care is a basic human right, ensuring every woman who births will have a positive birth experience. It does not matter if she has a vaginal birth or a cesarean delivery. What matters is that every woman, regardless of her education or socio-economic status, feels respected and listened to and is given the freedom to make choices and/or be involved in decision-making regarding her birthing experience. **Kindness and compassion matter to all, and honesty is an integral component of true compassion.**

> **Key Point**
>
> Dignity and respectful care are key components of maternal satisfaction.

Themes of Respectful Maternity Care

In a review of data from 67 qualitative studies on care during pregnancy and childbirth in 32 countries, 12 themes of respectful maternity care were derived [17]:

1. Freedom from harm and mistreatment
2. Maintaining privacy and confidentiality
3. Preserving women's dignity
4. Prospective provision of information and seeking informed consent
5. Ensuring continuous access to family and community support
6. Enhancing the quality of the physical environment and resources
7. Providing equitable maternity care
8. Engaging with effective communication
9. Respecting women's choices, which strengthens their ability to give birth

10. Availability of competent and motivated human resources
11. Provision of efficient and effective care
12. Continuity of care

The authors of the review concluded that the perceptions of women were consistent globally. The authors proposed the following strategies to promote respectful care:

- **At the individual level:** Essential human rights
- **At the health facility level**: Skilled healthcare providers to ensure continuity of care and adequate infrastructure
- **At the health system level:** Formulation of respectful care indicators and policies to ensure compliance

Box 3.1 outlines the general principles that should guide interactions with women in labour [18,19].

Box 3.1 General principles for caregiver–parturient interaction [18,19]

- All women in labour should be treated with respect.
- The woman should be in control of and involved in what is happening to her.
- Caregivers should courteously introduce themselves and always wear identity badges.
- The general principles of good communication should be used.
- When performing an initial assessment of a woman in labour, her preferences and emotional and psychological needs should be considered.
- A care plan should be agreed upon, including guidance about whom the woman should contact in the facility and when.
- The birth plan should be discussed or reinforced if one is already in place.
- Pain management strategies should be explored.
- The woman's informed consent, privacy, dignity, and comfort must be ensured before all procedures and observations, focusing on her rather than technology and documentation.
- Clinical wisdom and experience must be balanced with protocols, guidelines, and manuals.
- The woman should be involved in any handover of care to another professional.
- Adequate staffing should be ensured to sustain continuity of care.

Key Point

Women in high-income settings expressed a desire to be involved in decision-making more than those in low- and middle-income settings [17]. Women in LMICs should be encouraged and empowered to participate in decision-making.

STEPS TO PROMOTE AND SUSTAIN RESPECTFUL MATERNITY CARE

Overcoming Tokophobia: The Fear of Pregnancy and Childbirth

Fear begets fear and contributes to the release of stress hormones. Just as catecholamines shut down labour when an animal seeking to deliver in a quiet, secluded spot feels threatened, the progress of labour is slowed or arrested when a labouring woman does not feel safe or protected [20]. Conversely, labour is facilitated when the production of oxytocin is upregulated by the presence of kind and caring attendants and pleasant sensory stimulation of the skin [1].

Undeniably, fear has emerged as the driving principle in maternity care practice. The fear that healthcare providers feel is directly and indirectly transferred to the women they serve, contributing to **defensive practice**. The challenges plaguing maternity services are immense because helping women birth their babies involves anxiety and stress for healthcare workers. There is global pressure on maternity care workers due to a rising birth rate in many countries and increased medical and social complexities of the women using maternity services [1]. With the increasing demands on maternity services, it is imperative to help women overcome fear by creating a **trust-based relationship** in which childbirth is not dreaded [1].

Key Point

Labour is facilitated when the production of oxytocin is upregulated by the presence of kind and caring attendants. The progress of labour is slowed down or arrested when a labouring woman does not feel safe and protected.

Antenatal Education

Information is power and the key to resisting over-medicalisation [1]. Women and couples attending childbirth preparation classes are empowered with knowledge and confidence and are well-motivated to enjoy a birth without interventions.

Childbirth classes differ in their focus and philosophy, but all types provide valuable lessons for labour, delivery, and postpartum issues. Extending support to fathers through education and engaging them in interactions will enable them to empower their partners during pregnancy and childbirth and be better parents in the future [1].

Information on diet and exercise

A healthy diet and exercise ensure physical fitness. Women are encouraged to exercise as this can build stamina, alleviate aches and pains, and relieve stress. In addition to other advantages such as a reduction in gestational diabetes mellitus and preeclampsia, women who exercise during pregnancy have decreased cesarean and operative vaginal deliveries and a shorter postpartum recovery time [21].

Planning a safe and comfortable birth

Childbirth education can help women develop plans so that their labour and birth can unfold optimally and in the safest way possible. Analgesia options can be explored early in the prenatal period. The woman's expectations can be gauged, and her belief in her own innate ability to give birth can be strengthened. A **birth plan** is a practice of making decisions about labour, birth, and postpartum procedures before labour begins, and is a means for pregnant women and their partners to express their choices.

Avoiding Unnecessary Interventions in Spontaneous Births

Birthing is a natural process, and the vast majority of labours have the potential to be uncomplicated. While hospitals provide life-saving interventions, over-medicalisation causes women to lose control of their births. Modern obstetric care subjects mothers to institutional routines which may instil anxiety and adversely affect the progress of labour. Research has demonstrated an increase in prophylactic and unnecessary interventions without a concomitant reduction in perinatal mortality [22].

In the quest for reducing mortality and morbidity and the ensuing interventions, **quality of care must not take a backseat; rather, it should be at the forefront.** Used appropriately, interventions can be life-saving procedures. However, unnecessary interventions cause more harm than good [23].

> **Key Point**
>
> Increasing interventions in spontaneous labour has not demonstrated a resultant decrease in perinatal mortality [22]. Unnecessary interventions cause more harm than good [23].

Providing Midwifery Care

Obstetric care is especially crucial for women with high-risk pregnancies and may be life-saving in a number of situations. However, with its risk-oriented approach and reliance on technology, obstetric practice is associated with an increasing number of interventions that may only sometimes be beneficial. On the contrary, midwifery highlights the normalcy of pregnancy, labour, and childbirth and focuses on the importance of providing relationship-based respectful care; this is the need of the hour, especially for the vast majority of women whose pregnancies and labours are uncomplicated. The term **'midwife', translated as 'being with the woman', describes a professional companion; this concept of companionship is unique to midwifery.**

Women who receive midwifery care (and develop a trust-based relationship) are more positive about their birth experience and less dissatisfied with interventions because of better support and communication than women who receive other models of care [24]. Midwifery-led care has been reported to be a low-cost option for high-quality care with the best outcomes and lowest rates of interventions [25,26]. Women who receive care from a midwife have a slightly higher probability of spontaneous vaginal birth. They also have comparable adverse maternal and fetal outcomes as women who receive other models of care [26].

Key Point

Midwifery-led care is a low-cost option for high-quality care with the best outcomes and the lowest rates of interventions [25]. Ideally, all pregnant women should be offered midwifery care and support during labour and childbirth.

ENDEAVOURS BY THE WHO, NATIONAL GOVERNMENTS, AND NGOS

The WHO released a statement on respectful maternity care in 2014—"Every woman has the right to the highest attainable standard of health, which includes the right to dignified, respectful healthcare throughout pregnancy and childbirth" [27]. The organisation proposed an action plan to prevent and eliminate disrespect and abuse during facility-based childbirth (Box 3.2).

With the Government of India prioritising respectful maternity care, the **Hamara Swasthya, Hamari Awaaz** campaign was launched by the White Ribbon Alliance India in 2016 [28]. This soon became a global effort—the What Women Want campaign—with more than a million women from 114 countries voicing their opinions. **All women, irrespective of education, socio-economic status, caste, or creed, had one common demand—to be treated with dignity and without discrimination when in labour.**

The Ministry of Health and Family Welfare, Government of India, in December 2018, launched the **LaQshya programme for public healthcare facilities**, a quality improvement initiative for the labour room and maternity operation theatre [7]. The main objectives of this programme are as follows:

- Reducing maternal and newborn morbidity and mortality
- Improving quality of care during delivery and the immediate postpartum period
- Enhancing the satisfaction of beneficiaries, promoting positive birthing experiences, and providing **respectful maternity care (RMC)** to all pregnant women attending public health facilities

Box 3.2 The WHO's action plan to eliminate disrespect during childbirth [27]

- Generating greater support from governments and development partners for research and action on disrespect and abuse
- Initiating, supporting, and sustaining programmes designed to improve the quality of maternal health care, with a strong focus on respectful care as an essential component of quality care
- Emphasising the rights of women to dignified and respectful healthcare throughout pregnancy and childbirth
- Generating data related to respectful and disrespectful care practices, systems of accountability, and meaningful professional support
- Involving all stakeholders including women in efforts to improve the quality of care and eliminating disrespectful and abusive practices

The International Childbirth Initiative

Launched in 2018 by professional associations (including the International Confederation of Midwives, International Federation of Gynecology and Obstetrics, White Ribbon Alliance for Safe Motherhood, International Childbirth Education Association, and others), the International Childbirth Initiative [29] provided 12 steps (Table 3.2) for implementing respectful care during childbirth to the mother–baby–family triad [30].

Table 3.2 The 12 Steps to Safe and Respectful Mother–Baby–Family Maternity Care (adapted from The International Childbirth Initiative [29])

Steps	Performance indicators
1. **Provide respect, dignity, and informed choice** (Provision of information; effective communication in a culturally sensitive manner; involving the woman in decision-making; right to informed consent)	• Feedback mechanisms for addressing complaints (e.g., through a complaint box) • Grievance mechanism • The charter on 'Respectful Maternity Care: The universal rights of women and newborns' is displayed at facilities • Local observers • Questionnaires and interviews for recipients of care (pregnant women)
2. **Provide free or affordable care with cost transparency** (Access to non-discriminatory and free or affordable care; counselling about anticipated financial costs; bribes forbidden)	• Care should not be refused, and women and newborns should not be detained after care due to the inability to pay • Surveys and interviews • Informational posters displaying relevant costs
3. **Routinely provide Mother–Baby–Family maternity care**	• Knowledge about this model assessed through questionnaires and interviews with care providers • Questionnaires and interviews to confirm that these methods are being practised
4. **Offer continuous support**	• Posters stating that birth companions are welcome • Local observers • Questionnaires and interviews for recipients of care
5. **Provide pain relief measures** (See **Chapter 9**, *Labour analgesia*)	• Protocols about comfort measures and pain relief measures • Assessment of the knowledge of these protocols through questionnaires and interviews with care providers • Local observers • Questionnaires and interviews for recipients of care
6. **Provide evidence-based practice** (See **Chapter 4**, *Management of the first and second stages of normal labour*)	• Posters displaying mobility in labour, and birthing positions • Tools for facilitating birthing positions • Privacy walls and curtains • Evidence of staff training • Questionnaires and interviews for recipients of care
7. **Avoid harmful practices**	• Facility rates of procedures within accepted international ranges • Questionnaires and interviews for recipients of care
8. **Enhance wellness and prevent illness**	• Posters on prenatal and postnatal education • Care providers to be up-to-date • Women's questionnaires and interviews
9. **Provide emergency care and transport**	• Written policies and guidelines for transport • Proof of ongoing education and training for all emergency procedures • Observers • Women's questionnaires and interviews

(Continued . . .)

Table 3.2 **Continued**

Steps	Performance indicators
10. Have a supportive human resource policy (Staff safety, security, and positive work environment)	• Staff surveys and interviews
11. Provide a care continuum	• Written policies for collaboration and care transfer • Surveys, interviews
12. Promote breastfeeding and skin-to-skin contact	• Posters displaying breastfeeding and skin-to-skin contact • Sufficient space and beds large enough for mother and baby for rooming-in • Local observers • Women's questionnaires and interviews

THE ROLE OF A BIRTH COMPANION

INTRODUCTION

Birth companions are persons who provide continuous one-on-one support to women experiencing labour and childbirth. Historically, women have been attended to and supported by other women during labour and birth. However, a birth companion could be her partner, a friend, a family member, a doula, a midwife, or any person the labouring woman feels comfortable having with her (Fig. 3.1). A birth companion can assist in the following ways [30]:

- By providing information and facilitating communication between the mother and the caregiver
- By advocating for the woman and articulating her wishes
- By assessing labour progress, advising on coping techniques, and comforting the woman with massages
- By providing emotional support and reassurance

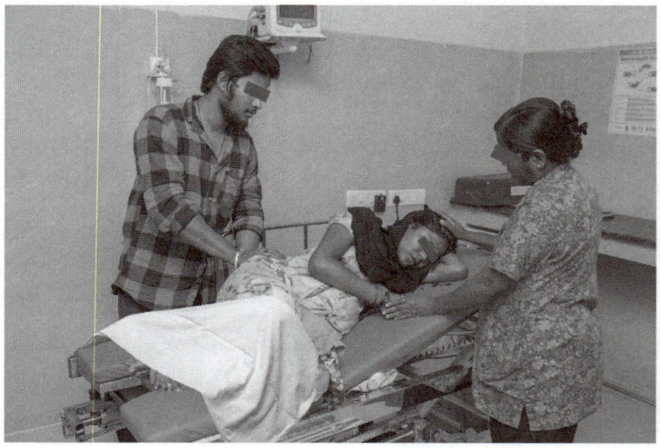

Fig. 3.1 Birth companionship provided by the partner and the midwife (*Image courtesy:* Dr Sirisha Rao, Fernandez Hospital, Hyderabad)

PRIVACY AND SUPPORT IN LABOUR

Privacy does not mean being alone; rather, it implies not being unduly disturbed and feeling protected and safe as labour progresses. The birth companion provides this support.

Privacy also includes maintaining and protecting the woman's modesty. Even in the most low-resource areas, a curtain or screen should be provided to protect the woman's privacy. The upper half of the woman's body should be clothed and the lower half should be covered with a sheet. Even in the poorest setting, a woman can be covered with an old *sari*. Non-medical staff members (especially males) should not be allowed to wander in and out of the labour room.

The Right to a Birth Companion

No woman should be denied the right to a birth companion. This is her fundamental human right and she should be encouraged to have support from the birth companion(s) of her choice [18]. The WHO promotes labour companionship as a core element of care for improving maternal and infant health, and the WHO Safe Childbirth Checklist encourages a companion to be present at birth [31].

In February 2016, the Ministry of Health and Family Welfare, Government of India, issued an order to allow birth companions during childbirth in public health facilities, stating that 'the presence of a female relative during labour is a low-cost intervention that has proved to be beneficial to women in labour' [32].

A large cross-sectional study in 18 tertiary public sector healthcare facilities in India provides information about the status of birth companionship in the country [33]. As part of the study, care providers were interviewed to understand the challenges they faced with the provision of respectful care. The results revealed that **less than 50% of women were accompanied by a birth companion.** The reasons cited for this were hospital policy, restrictions of space, overloaded health facilities, and privacy concerns for other women in the labour ward.

Evidence Regarding Birth Companionship

A systematic review of the Cochrane Database [34], which included 27 trials from 17 countries and involved more than 15,000 women in a wide range of settings and circumstances, found that **women who received continuous support during labour were more likely to have the following:**

- Spontaneous vaginal births
- Shorter labours
- Decreased cesarean and instrumental vaginal births
- Decreased use of analgesia
- Lower incidence of low 5-minute Apgar scores
- Lesser likelihood of negative birth experiences

The review summarised the gathered evidence as follows:

- Women wanted their birth companion to be compassionate and trustworthy.
- Birth companionship helped women to have a positive birth experience.
- Doulas often met with women during the antenatal period, which helped them develop a rapport.

Factors that negatively impact the implementation of birth companionship

These factors include the failure to recognise the benefits of birth companionship, care provider resistance to integrating lay companions, space constraints, and the perceived increase in the risk of infection. The reviewers concluded that further research is needed in training lay birth companions during the antenatal period and designing labour rooms in low-resource settings that would permit a birth companion without encroaching on the privacy of other birthing women [30].

THE WAY FORWARD

- Respectful maternity care indicators need to be developed.
- Respectful maternity care should be made a part of the curriculum for OBGYN residents, midwives, and all those involved in maternity care.

CONCLUSION

Women want a positive childbirth experience that fulfils or exceeds their personal and sociocultural beliefs and expectations [35]. This includes giving birth to a healthy baby in a clinically and psychologically safe environment with respectful maternity care, and continuity of practical and emotional support from a birth companion and kind, technically competent clinical staff.

REFERENCES

1. Byrom S, Downe S (Eds). *The Roar Behind the Silence.* Pinter and Martin. 2015. London.
2. Lothian JA. Safe, healthy birth: What every pregnant woman needs to know. *J Perinat Educ.* 2009. 18(3): 48-54.
3. Austin A, Langer A, Salam RA, Lassi ZS, Das JK, Bhutta ZA. Approaches to improve the quality of maternal and newborn health care: An overview of the evidence. *Reprod Health.* 2014. 11 (suppl 2): S1.
4. Maternal Health. An Executive Summary for The Lancet's Series. September 2016. Available at https://www.thelancet.com/pb/assets/raw/Lancet/stories/series/maternal-health-2016/mathealth2016-exec-summ.pdf. Accessed 24 April 2023.
5. Miller S, Abalos E, Chamillard M, Ciapponi A, Colaci D, Comande D, et al. Beyond too little, too late and too much, too soon: A pathway towards evidence-based, respectful maternity care worldwide. The Lancet Maternal Health Series. *Lancet.* 2016. 388 (10056): 2176-2192.
6. Freedman LP, Kruk ME. Disrespect and abuse of women in childbirth: Challenging the global quality and accountability agendas. *Lancet.* 2014. 384(9948): e42-4.
7. National Health Mission. Labour Room and Quality Improvement Initiative. Available at https://nhm.gov.in/index1.php?lang=1&level=3&sublinkid=1307&lid=690. Accessed 24 April 2023.
8. Freedman LP, Ramsey K, Abuya T, Bellows B, Ndwiga C, Warren CE, et al. Defining disrespect and abuse of women in childbirth: A research, policy and rights agenda. Bulletin of the WHO. 2014. 92: 915-917.
9. The White Ribbon Alliance. Respectful maternity care: The universal rights of women and newborns. Available at https://whiteribbonalliance.org/wp-content/uploads/2022/05/WRA_RMC_Charter_FINAL.pdf. Accessed 24 April 2023.
10. Report of the Third National U.S. Survey of Women's Childbearing Experiences. Available at https://www.birthbythenumbers.org/united-states-2/listening-to-mothers-surveys/ Accessed 24 April 2023.
11. Dignity in Childbirth. Available at https://www.birthrights.org.uk/campaigns-research/dignity-in-childbirth/#:~:text=Only%2068%25%20of%20women%20and,the%20choice%20of%20pain%20relief. Accessed 24 April 2023.
12. Hodnett ED. Pain and women's satisfaction with the experience of childbirth: A systematic review. *Am J Obstet Gynecol.* 2002. 186: S160-72.
13. Dzomeku MV. Maternal satisfaction with care during labour: A case study of the Mampong-Ashanti district hospital maternity unit in Ghana. *Int J Nursing Midwifery.* 2011. 3(3): 30-34.
14. Bohren MA, Hunter EC, Munthe-Kaas HM, Souza JP, Vogel JP, Gulmezoglu AM. Facilitators and barriers to facility-based delivery in low- and middle-income countries: A qualitative evidence synthesis. *Reprod Health.* 2014. 11(1): 71.
15. Sackett DL, Rosenberg WC, Gray JAM. Evidence-based medicine: What it is and what it isn't. *BMJ.* 1996. 312(7023): 71-2.
16. Downe S, Lawrie TA, Finlayson K, Oladapo OT. Effectiveness of respectful care policies for women using routine intrapartum services: A systematic review. *Reprod Health.* 2018. 15: 23.
17. Shakibazadeh E, Namadian M, Bohren MA, et al. Respectful care during childbirth in health facilities globally: A qualitative evidence synthesis. *BJOG.* 2018. 125(8): 932-942.
18. National Institute for Health and Care Excellence. Intrapartum care for healthy women and babies. Guideline CG. 2014. 190.
19. WHO recommendation on respectful maternity care during labour and childbirth. 2018. WHO, Geneva.
20. Lothian JA. Do not disturb: The importance of privacy in labour. *J Perinat Educ.* 2004. 13 (3):4-6.
21. The American College of Obstetricians and Gynecologists. Physical activity and exercise during pregnancy and the postpartum period. Committee Opinion No. 650. 2015.
22. Dahlen HG, Tracy S, Tracy M, Bisits A, Brown C, Thornton C. Rates of obstetric intervention and associated perinatal mortality and morbidity among low-risk women giving birth in private and public hospitals in NSW (2000-2008): A linked data population-based cohort study. *BMJ Open.* 2014. 4 (5): e004551.
23. Jansen L, Gibson M, Bowles BC, Leach J. First do no harm: Interventions during childbirth. *J Perinat Educ.* 2013. Spring; 22(2): 83-92.
24. McCourt C. Technologies of birth and models of midwifery care. Revista da Escola de Enfermagem da USP. 2014. 48(spe), 168-177.
25. Renfrew MJ, McFadden A, Bastos MH, Campbell J, Channon AA, Cheung NF, et al. Midwifery and quality care: Findings from a new evidence-informed framework for maternal and newborn care. *Lancet.* 2014. 384: 1129-45.
26. Sandall J, Soltani H, Gates S, Shennan A, Devane D. Midwife-led continuity models versus other models of care for childbearing women. *Cochrane Database of Systematic Reviews.* 2016. Issue 4. Art. No.: CD004667.
27. WHO. The prevention and elimination of disrespect and abuse during facility-based childbirth. World Health Organization. Geneva. 2014. WHO/RHR/14.23.
28. White Ribbon Alliance. Government of India embeds respectful maternity care in its priorities. Available at

https://whiteribbonalliance.org/stories/government-of-india-embeds-respectful-maternity-care-in-its-priorities/ Accessed 24 April 2023.

29. Lalonde A, Herschderfer K, Pascali-Bonaro D, Hanson C, Fuchtner C, Visser GHA. The International Childbirth Initiative: 12 steps to safe and respectful MotherBaby-Family maternity care. *Int J Gynaecol Obstet.* 2019. 146(1):65-73.
30. Bohren MA, Berger BO, Munthe-Kaas H, Tuncalp O. Perceptions and experiences of labour companionship: a qualitative evidence synthesis. *Cochrane Database of Systematic Reviews.* 2019. Issue 3. Art. No.: CD012449.
31. WHO. Safe Childbirth Checklist. Available at http://apps.who.int/iris/bitstream/10665/199179/1/WHO_HIS_SDS_2015.26_eng.pdf?ua=1. Accessed 24 April 2023.
32. Government of India. Ministry of Health and Family Welfare. Health Ministry allows birth companions during delivery in public health facilities. Available at https://pib.gov.in/newsite/PrintRelease.aspx?relid=136801. Accessed 24 April 2023.
33. Singh S, Goel R, Gogoi A, Caleb-Varkey L, Manoranjini M, Ravi T, Rawat D. Presence of birth companion—a deterrent to disrespectful behaviours towards women during delivery: An exploratory mixed-method study in 18 public hospitals of India. *Health Policy and Planning.* 2021. 36(10): 1552-1561.
34. Bohren MA, Hofmeyr GJ, Sakala C, Fukuzawa RK, Cuthbert A. Continuous support for women during childbirth (review). *Cochrane Database Syst Rev.* 2017. Issue 7. Art. No.: CD003766.
35. WHO recommendations on intrapartum care for a positive childbirth experience. Available at https://apps.who.int/iris/bitstream/handle/10665/260178/9789241550215-eng.pdf Accessed 27 April 2020.

CHAPTER 4

Management of the First and Second Stages of Normal Labour

GITA ARJUN

INTRODUCTION

Labour is defined as regular, painful contractions that progressively increase in frequency and duration, resulting in the effacement and dilatation of the cervix.

Normal birth is defined as the spontaneous birth of an infant in the vertex position between 37 and 42 weeks of pregnancy after the spontaneous onset of labour in a low-risk pregnancy that remains low-risk throughout labour and delivery. After birth, the mother and infant are in good condition [1].

Adherence to protocols and processes in the labour room will ensure a good outcome for the mother and child in the majority of labouring women.

This chapter deals with specific evidence-based recommendations for the management of labour and delivery in a woman who is full-term (≥37 weeks) and has a singleton pregnancy with the fetus in vertex presentation.

RESPECTFUL MATERNITY CARE

Every woman in labour expects and deserves respectful maternity care. The maintenance of the woman's dignity, modesty, and privacy is paramount. She and her birth companion should be addressed with courtesy. Communication should be clear and empathetic throughout the process of labour and delivery (see **Chapter 3**, *Respectful obstetric care and the role of a birth companion*).

> **Key Point**
>
> It is important for the labouring woman to receive respectful, empathetic treatment and obstetric care right from the initial presentation to the facility.

DEFINITIONS

First Stage of Labour

The first stage of labour begins with the onset of regular contractions and ends with full cervical dilatation. This stage of labour has two phases—the **latent phase** and the **active phase.**

For more than 50 years, the progress of labour was measured based on data derived by Friedman in the 1950s. The **Friedman curve** has long been accepted as the standard for the assessment of labour progression. However, recent studies have questioned the Friedman curve. Data from the Consortium on Safe Labor [2] have provided newer definitions of the latent and active phases of labour. The World Health Organization and other professional bodies have adopted these recommendations [3,4].

Latent phase

The latent phase is a period of time characterised by painful uterine contractions that may or may not be regular. There are variable changes in the cervix, including some degree of effacement and slow progression of dilatation up to 5 cm for first and subsequent labours.

Active phase

The active first stage is a period of time characterised by regular painful uterine contractions, a substantial degree of cervical effacement, and more rapid cervical dilatation from 5 cm [3] to full dilatation for first and subsequent labours.

The active phase is also the maximal slope in the rate of change of cervical dilatation over time and often does not start until at least 6 cm in multiparous women [2,4]. There is no clear point at which cervical dilatation accelerates for nulliparous women (Fig. 4.1).

Key Point

The median duration of the **active first stage** is 5.3 hours in nulliparas and 3.8 hours in multiparas [2]. The WHO [3] defines the duration of the active phase as 4 hours in first labours and 3 hours in second and subsequent labours, when the reference starting point is 5 cm cervical dilatation. However, both the labouring woman and the obstetrician should be aware that the duration of the active first stage may vary, but usually does not extend beyond 12 hours in first labours, and beyond 10 hours in subsequent labours.

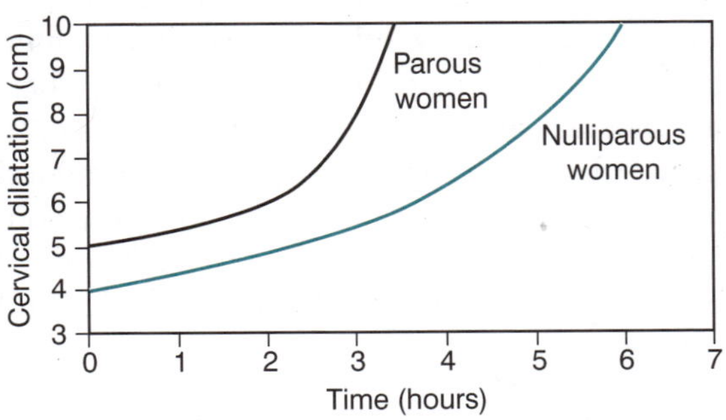

Fig. 4.1 Contemporary patterns of spontaneous labour [2]: The acceleration of cervical dilatation starts at about 6 cm for multiparous women; there is no clear point where cervical dilatation accelerates for nulliparous women and there is no deceleration phase

Second Stage of Labour

The second stage of labour begins with full cervical dilatation and ends with the delivery of the baby.

Third Stage of Labour

The third stage of labour extends from the delivery of the baby to the expulsion of the placenta.

For the sake of uniformity, the above definitions will be adopted throughout the chapter.

TIMING OF ADMISSION TO THE HOSPITAL

When a **healthy, low-risk** pregnant woman presents to the hospital in spontaneous labour, an initial assessment is made to determine whether she is in labour or not.

Diagnosis of Labour

It may not always be easy to differentiate false labour from true labour. The differences between the two are listed in Table 4.1.

If it is not clear that the woman is in labour, she should be encouraged to walk around or relax, and her cervix should be reassessed after 2–4 hours, depending on the regularity and intensity of uterine contractions. If there is no progress in effacement or dilatation, the woman may be discharged if the following criteria are met:

- Intact membranes
- Cervical dilatation <3 cm
- No cervical change or contractions at the end of two hours' observation
- Normal fetal heart rate (FHR) tracing

If the woman lives far from the facility or has no reliable means of transportation back to the facility, she may be observed for a longer period of time.

If she is in labour (as indicated by regular, painful contractions and cervical dilatation >3 cm), the woman should be admitted to the hospital and supported appropriately. Though the active first stage of labour is defined as

Table 4.1 **Differences between false labour and true labour**

	False labour	True labour
Timing of contractions	• Often irregular with irregular intervals • May be continuous and without a break	• Occur at regular intervals • Increase in frequency
Strength of contractions	• Variable intensity	• Increase in intensity over time
Change with ambulation	• Contractions may stop when the woman walks or rests • May even stop with a change of position	• Contractions continue despite ambulation
Location of pain	• Usually felt only in the front, especially the lower abdomen	• Usually starts in the back and moves to the front • Moves from the top of the uterus downwards
Cervical changes	• Effacement and dilatation will not be progressive	• Progressive effacement and dilatation of cervix
Response to sedation	• Contractions stop • Pain is relieved	• Contractions continue

beginning at 5 cm of cervical dilatation, there is no reason to delay admission till that dilatation is reached.

If the woman lives close to the hospital and wants to wait at home for active labour to start, she should be allowed to do so [5].

ADMISSION TO THE LABOUR ROOM/WARD

It is reasonable to delay admission to the labour room till the woman is in the **active stage of labour**. She can be observed in the room or ward until a vaginal examination confirms cervical dilatation of 5 cm.

WHO SHOULD DELIVER A WOMAN WITH A LOW-RISK PREGNANCY?

Intrapartum care for a low-risk pregnant woman can be provided by an obstetrician or a trained, qualified midwife. In India, this depends on whether the woman is delivering in a public or private facility, in an urban or rural setting. Nurses, midwives, and trained birth attendants provide healthcare in the most vulnerable, isolated, and hard-to-reach communities in India. The Government of India [6] has formulated a policy decision to roll out midwifery services in the country to be able to reach more women requiring care in labour and delivery.

A systematic review of the Cochrane Database [7] showed that the psychological support provided by midwives led to women being more likely to be satisfied with their care. There was also a significant reduction in interventions such as episiotomy, instrumental birth, and the use of pain relief. In addition, there was a reduction in preterm birth below 37 weeks, fetal loss before and after 24 weeks, and neonatal death.

REVIEW OF ANTENATAL RECORDS AND OBTAINING RELEVANT HISTORY

Review of Antenatal Records

It is important to review a pregnant woman's antenatal records for the following:

- Antenatal risk factors
- Complications in a previous pregnancy, labour, or delivery

Key Points

- The woman's antenatal records must be available in the labour room.
- Her blood group and Rh type must be clearly noted.
- Any medical/obstetric complications must be reviewed.
- Any allergies must be documented.

Obtaining Relevant History

A detailed history should include the following:

- Time of onset of contractions
- Frequency and duration of contractions
- Presence of show
- Bleeding (in larger quantities than show)
- Leakage of amniotic fluid (either as a gush or as a slow trickle)
- The presence or absence of fetal movements

INITIAL EXAMINATION ON ADMISSION

The initial examination includes the recording and documentation of vital signs including maternal pulse, blood pressure, and temperature.

An **abdominal examination** should be performed to evaluate the fetal lie, presentation, and position. The timing and intensity of uterine contractions should be noted. Fetal well-being should be confirmed by the presence of a normal fetal heart rate.

A **vaginal digital examination** is important to assess cervical effacement and dilatation. The presence or absence of membranes should be documented.

Abdominal Examination

An initial examination of the abdomen will help determine the following:

- Fetal lie and presentation
- Estimated fetal weight

Fetal lie and presentation

The lie of the fetus refers to the position of the long axis of the fetus in relation to the mother.

In the **longitudinal lie**, the long axis of the fetus is parallel to that of the mother. When the long axis of the fetus is perpendicular to the mother's long axis, it is called a **transverse lie.** In the **oblique lie,** the long axis of the fetus lies at an oblique angle to the mother's long axis.

The presentation of the fetus is determined by the fetal lie and the presenting part. A longitudinal lie with the head in the lower pole is called a **vertex** or **cephalic** presentation. A longitudinal lie with the buttocks in the lower pole is called a **breech** presentation. Other presentations such as **shoulder** presentation (common in transverse lie), **face** presentation and **brow** presentation are better diagnosed on vaginal examination.

Estimation of fetal weight

The accuracy of fetal weight estimation is of key importance in the planning and management of labour and the mode of delivery. Macrosomia may result in morbidity in both the mother and the neonate. Even an average-sized fetus may cause cephalopelvic disproportion in a small-built mother.

Clinical vs. sonographic estimate of birth weight

With experience, clinicians can estimate fetal weight by physical examination using Leopold's manoeuvres. In a randomised controlled study, Hendrix et al. [8] concluded that in women in labour at term, clinical estimates had significantly higher accuracy than ones derived sonographically. Similarly, Preyer et al. [9], in a prospective blinded observational study, did not observe significantly better accuracy of ultrasound as compared to Leopold's manoeuvres in women who are of normal weight. Sonographic estimation was, however, more accurate in women with a high BMI.

If a late third-trimester sonographic estimation of fetal weight is available, it should be correlated with clinical assessment. Selective sonographic screening for macrosomia may be useful in the following circumstances [10]:

- Maternal diabetes (particularly in poorly controlled diabetes)

- Previous macrosomic newborn (with a history of complicated labour and delivery)
- Previous shoulder dystocia

It is important to keep in mind that a sonographic estimated fetal weight >4000 g (or the 90th centile) has only 22% sensitivity and 90% specificity for subsequent shoulder dystocia [11]. For further details, see **Chapter 34**, *Management of labour with a macrosomic fetus*.

Vaginal Examination

The initial vaginal examination helps determine the following:

- Cervical effacement and dilatation
- Presence or absence of membranes
- Presence or absence of meconium
- Clinical assessment of pelvic capacity

> **Key Points**
>
> **Gentle and respectful vaginal examination**
> - The woman should be informed about the procedure and her consent should be obtained.
> - She should gently be prepared for the possible discomfort she will face during the procedure.
> - The woman should be kept covered with a sheet during the examination and attention should be paid to maintaining her modesty.
> - The digital examination should be performed gently and with adequate lubrication.
>
> (See **Chapter 3**, *Respectful obstetric care and the role of a birth companion.*)

The digital examination must be performed with aseptic precautions. The well-lubricated index and middle fingers of the gloved hand are used.

> **Key Point**
>
> A vaginal examination should be deferred in the presence of excessive bleeding (until placenta previa is ruled out).

Cervical effacement

Effacement is expressed either as a percentage of the length of the cervix that is taken up (e.g., 50% or 80%) or in terms of the actual length of the cervix below the presenting part (e.g., 3 cm or 2 cm).

Cervical dilatation

The assessment of cervical dilatation is an essential part of monitoring the progress of labour. With increasing uterine contractions and the pressure exerted by the amniotic fluid and the presenting part, the cervix dilates to 10 cm by the end of the first stage of labour.

Presence or absence of membranes

The woman may or may not be aware of the amniotic membranes rupturing. If she has ruptured membranes prior to admission, she may give a history of one of the following:

- Gush of fluid
- Continuous trickle
- Intermittent discharge

On examination, amniotic fluid may be seen leaking out of the vagina. Digital examination may reveal absent membranes.

> **Key Points**
>
> - A digital examination should not be performed when membranes have ruptured in the absence of labour pains (prelabour rupture of membranes or PROM).
> - It is important to note the time of rupture of membranes (ROM). Once the membranes have ruptured, it is best to deliver the baby within 12–24 hours [12,13].

Clinical assessment of pelvic capacity

A mismatch between the size of the fetal head and that of the maternal pelvis leads to **cephalopelvic disproportion (CPD)**, resulting in a 'failure to progress' in labour for mechanical reasons. Though clinical pelvimetry still has a place in obstetrics for predicting or confirming CPD, it has become a lost art [14].

> **Key Point**
>
> On initial digital examination, the **ischial spines** should be assessed. If they are flat, the chances of deep transverse arrest are low. The presence

of prominent ischial spines should alert the obstetrician to the possibility of a deep transverse arrest due to mid-pelvic contraction.

PREPARATION FOR DELIVERY

Enema

There is no evidence to support the routine administration of an enema prior to delivery [15]. However, if the woman is constipated and requests an enema, she might be given one for the sake of comfort during labour.

Key Point

If a woman complains of an urge to pass motion, a vaginal examination should be performed to ensure that the urge is not due to the fetal head lying low in the vagina and exerting rectal pressure.

Shaving of Pubic Hair and the Perineum

There is no evidence to support routinely shaving the pubic hair or the perineum [16]. The perineum alone may be shaved in the area below the fourchette if an episiotomy is being considered or deemed to be necessary or if a tear is being sutured. This is only to make it easier to place sutures and prevent discomfort to the mother from hair being caught in sutures.

MANAGEMENT OF THE FIRST STAGE OF LABOUR

SUPPORTIVE MEASURES

The first stage of labour can last for a few hours. It is important to support the woman through this stage and keep her comfortable and hydrated. Pain relief is an important supportive measure. A birth companion is essential for the woman's well-being, and all labour rooms should support the inclusion of one (see **Chapter 3**).

Bladder Emptying

The woman should be encouraged to empty her bladder at least every two hours or as often as she wants during labour. Catheterisation is usually not indicated.

Oral Intake

The Practice Guidelines for Obstetric Anesthesia [17] and the ACOG [18] recommend the following:

Liquids

Pregnant women who are considered low-risk (no antenatal or intrapartum complications) may be allowed to have sips of water/non-particulate fruit juices during labour.

If oral fluids are being restricted because of an increased risk of cesarean birth, then maintenance intravenous fluids—5% dextrose in 0.45% saline, normal saline, or lactated Ringer's solution—can be administered. Though it has been suggested that IV fluids in labour can reduce the length of labour, this was not borne out in a study that compared high-dose intravenous fluids, with or without dextrose, in nulliparous women who presented in active labour [19].

Solids

It is best for women in active labour to avoid solid foods [18].

Antibiotics

Prophylactic antibiotics

Vaginal delivery is **not** an indication for routine antibiotic prophylaxis (see **Chapter 19**, *Antibiotic prophylaxis in labour and delivery*).

Endocarditis prophylaxis is not recommended for women with cardiac lesions since the rate of bacteremia is low with vaginal delivery.

Therapeutic antibiotics

Antibiotics are indicated when chorioamnionitis is suspected due to the presence of the following signs and symptoms:

- Maternal temperature of ≥38°C
- Foul-smelling vaginal discharge
- Ruptured membranes >18 hours
- Maternal tachycardia >100/minute

- Fetal tachycardia >160/minute
- Uterine tenderness

After taking a high vaginal smear for culture and sensitivity, the woman should be started on any of the following [20]:

- Ampicillin 2 g intravenously every six hours PLUS gentamicin 5 mg/Kg once daily OR
- Cefoxitin 2 g IV every 8 hours OR
- Ampicillin–sulbactam 3 g IV every six hours OR
- Piperacillin–tazobactam 3.375 g IV every 6 hours or 4.5 g every 8 hours

The antibiotic regimen is continued until the woman is afebrile for 48 hours.

MATERNAL ACTIVITY

The woman should be allowed to walk, sit, or lie down according to her preference. Walking during the first stage neither improves nor worsens active labour but certainly is not harmful to the woman or the fetus [21].

PAIN RELIEF

Analgesia should be offered to all women in labour. Most women are aware that labour is painful and are frightened and anxious even before labour begins. However, they believe and hope that they will be given pain relief. In the majority of cases, there is a mismatch between women's expectations and their actual experience [22].

The options available for pain relief in labour should be discussed with the woman/couple during the antenatal period (see **Chapter 9**, *Labour analgesia*).

MONITORING FETAL RESPONSE TO LABOUR

Monitoring fetal heart rate and well-being is absolutely essential throughout labour (see **Chapter 8**, *Fetal surveillance in labour*).

MONITORING THE FREQUENCY AND INTENSITY OF UTERINE CONTRACTIONS

Monitoring of uterine contractions is a very important aspect of monitoring the progress of labour. The easiest method of monitoring contractions is to palpate the uterine fundus by placing the palm of the hand flat on the abdomen and timing the contractions.

Timing and Frequency

A contraction is timed from the onset of the hardening of the uterus to when the uterine muscle relaxes.

The frequency of contractions is documented as the number of contractions per 10 minutes. In the late active phase, there are usually 3–4 contractions over 10 minutes, each lasting 45–60 seconds. If a cardiotocograph (CTG) is available, uterine contractions are recorded using external tocodynamometry.

Intensity

A contraction is considered **mild** or **weak** if it lasts <20 seconds and if the fundus can be indented by the examining fingers. A **moderate** contraction lasts for 20–40 seconds, and the fundus feels firm at the height of the contraction. A contraction is considered **strong** if it lasts >40 seconds and the uterine fundus cannot be indented by the examining fingers throughout the contraction.

MONITORING THE PROGRESS OF LABOUR

Progress in the first stage of labour is assessed by both abdominal and vaginal examinations.

Abdominal Examination

Along with assessing uterine contractions, abdominal examination is useful for gauging the descent of the fetal head.

Descent and engagement of the fetal head

The degree of descent and engagement of the head is assessed by feeling how many 'fifths' of the head are palpable above the brim of the pelvis. Five fingers of the examining hand are placed on the abdomen with the ulnar or radial border of the hand in line with the pubic symphysis **(Crichton's manoeuvre)**. The number of fingers required to cover the part of the head above the symphysis is equal to the number of fifths of head palpable (Fig. 4.2).

Five-fifths of the head palpable means that the whole head is above the inlet of the pelvis. When a small part of the head is below the brim of the pelvis and can be lifted out of the pelvis with a deep pelvic grip, it is said to be **four-fifths palpable**. At **three-fifths,** the head cannot be lifted out of the pelvis. On performing a deep pelvic grip, the fingers will move outwards from the neck of the fetus, then inwards before reaching the pelvic brim. **Two-fifths** of the head palpable means that most of the head is below the pelvic brim; at this degree, on performing a deep pelvic grip, the fingers only splay outwards from the fetal neck to the pelvic brim. When the head is **one-fifth** palpable, only the sinciput is felt. This denotes that the occiput has entered the pelvic brim and that the lowermost bony point of the head is at the level of the ischial spines, indicating the **engagement of the head.**

Vaginal Examination

On vaginal examination, the following should be noted:

- Effacement and dilatation of the cervix
- Station of the presenting part
- Degree of flexion
- Caput formation
- Moulding
- Status of membranes

Frequency and timing of intrapartum vaginal examination

This depends on how labour is progressing. Generally, vaginal examination is performed at the following intervals:

- At two- to four-hour intervals in the first stage (more frequently if labour seems to be progressing fast)
- When the woman feels the urge to push (to determine whether the cervix is fully dilated)
- At 15- to 30-minute intervals in the second stage
- Prior to administering analgesia/anesthesia
- In the presence of FHR abnormalities (to evaluate for complications such as cord prolapse and uterine rupture)

Cervical effacement and dilatation

Vaginal digital examination is performed to document effacement and dilatation as labour progresses. Dilatation of the cervix to 10 cm (full dilatation) marks the end of the first stage of labour.

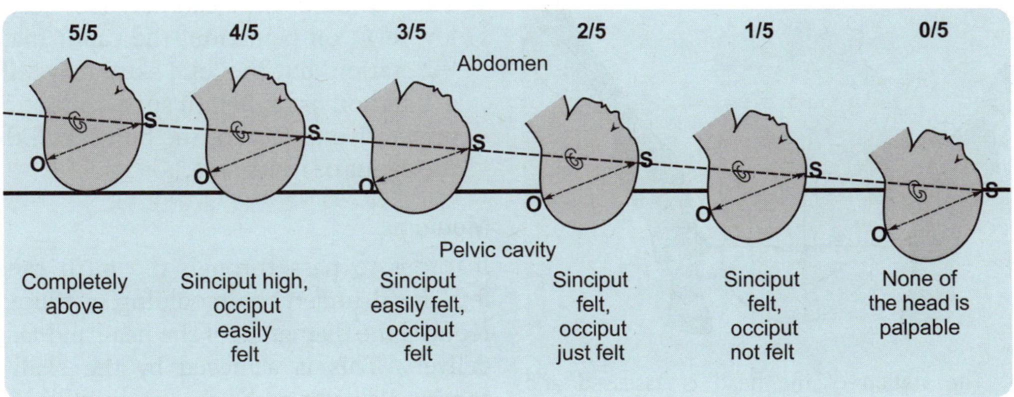

Fig. 4.2 Diagrammatic representation of the descent of the presenting part in 'fifths': Five fingers of the examining hand are placed on the abdomen to cover the part of the fetal head that is above the pubic symphysis: the descent of the fetal head is expressed in fifths depending on the number of fingers that can cover the head abdominally

Fetal descent and station

Fetal descent is recorded by assessing the fetal station, which is the relationship of the fetal head to the ischial spines. It is measured in centimetres above (-) or below (+) the ischial spines (Fig. 4.3).

Since the distance between the leading edge of the skull and the BPD is shorter than the distance between the spines and the pelvic brim, it can be assumed that the largest diameter of the head (BPD) has passed through the pelvic brim when the lowest part of the baby's skull has reached the ischial spines. The head is now considered to be **engaged**.

Fetal position

Fetal position (Fig. 4.4) is the relationship of the occiput to the quadrants of the pelvis, for example, left occipitoanterior (LOA) or right occipitoanterior (ROA). To assess the fetal position, the sagittal suture is palpated first. The examiner's fingers follow the sagittal suture to the **Y-shaped posterior fontanelle** to identify the **occiput,** and then in the opposite direction to identify the **diamond-shaped anterior fontanelle**. Knowing the position of the fetal occiput is extremely important for the management of labour.

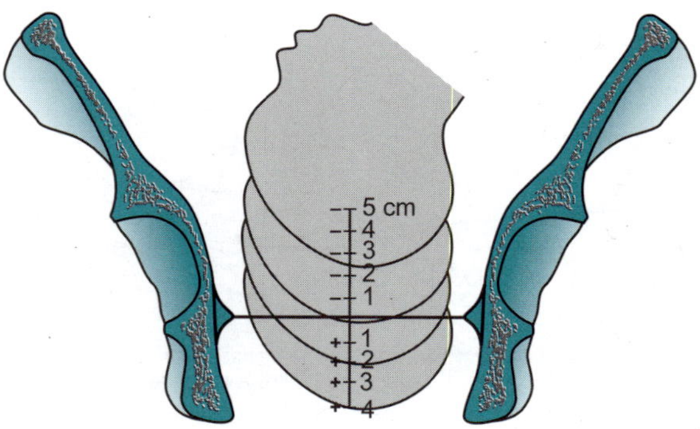

Fig. 4.3 The station of the head is assessed and documented based on its relationship to the ischial spines (in this image, the lowest part of the baby's skull has reached the ischial spines and the head is considered to be engaged)

Apart from assessing fetal position, it is possible to establish whether the fetal head is **flexed** or **deflexed**—information that is important for determining presentation and managing delivery. **Flexion** is determined by the portion of the sagittal suture and the fontanelle that is felt on vaginal examination. When the head is well-flexed (**vertex presentation**), the posterior fontanelle is easily felt and the anterior fontanelle is not felt or is felt with difficulty (Fig. 4.5a). If the anterior and posterior fontanelles are felt with equal ease at either end of the sagittal suture or if the anterior fontanelle is felt more easily, then the head is said to be **deflexed** (**brow** or **face presentation**) (Fig. 4.5b).

Caput succedaneum

As labour progresses, a small edematous portion develops on the most dependent portion of the head, especially the part pressed against the cervix. This is called the caput succedaneum. It usually disappears spontaneously within 24–48 hours of delivery.

In prolonged labour, the caput can become significantly large. A large caput may cause the following problems:

- It may be difficult to feel the sutures, making it hard to determine the fetal position.
- The station of the head may feel deceptively low, e.g., on palpation, the caput may be at +2 station, but the fetal skull may still be at +1 station or higher. In such a situation, it is imperative to feel for the bony skull through the caput or to its side.

Moulding

In order to pass through the birth canal, the fetal head undergoes moulding, a process that reduces the diameters of the head and facilitates delivery. This is achieved by the skull bones coming closer to each other or even overlapping. Some degree of moulding is physiological and occurs often when the head negotiates the mid-pelvis. In obstructed labour, the moulding can

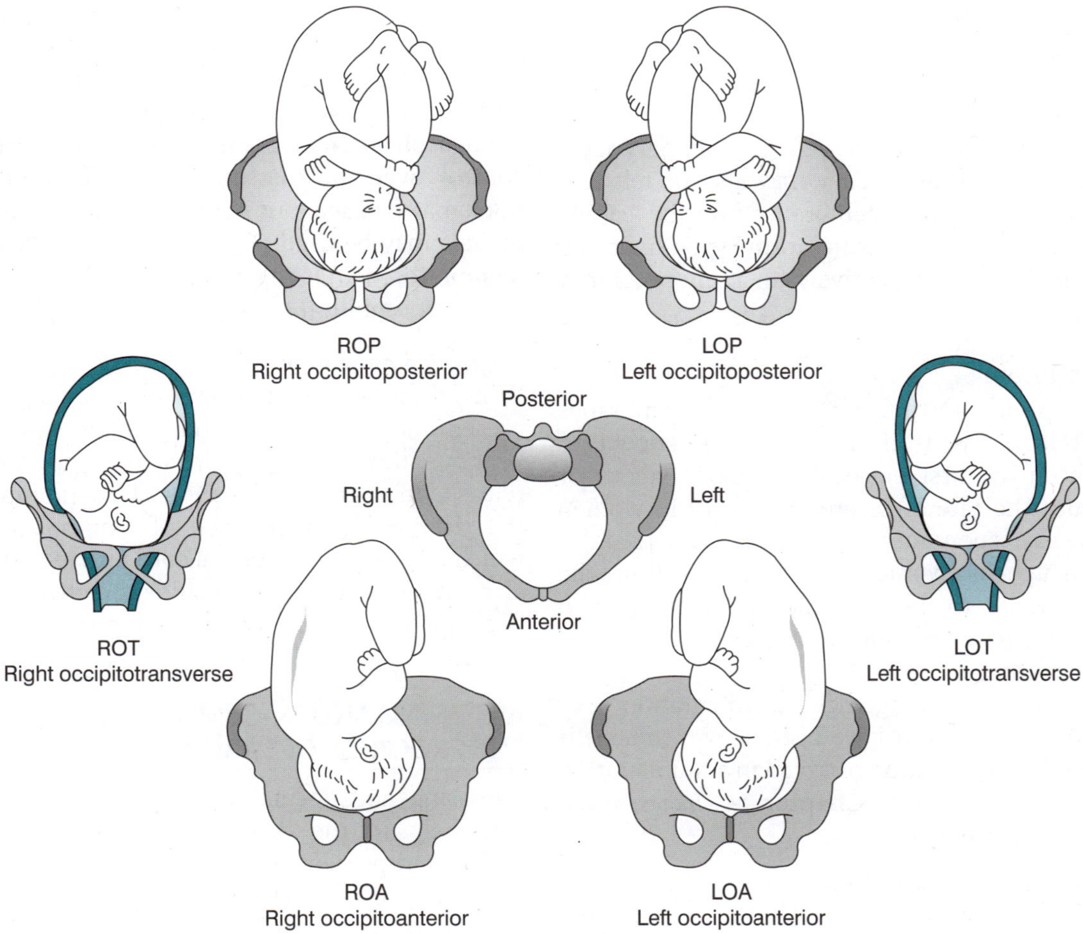

Fig. 4.4 Determining fetal position—on vaginal examination, the fetal position is determined by the relationship of the occiput to the quadrants of the pelvis; for example, in occipitotransverse positions, the occiput is pointing directly to the left or right side of the pelvis

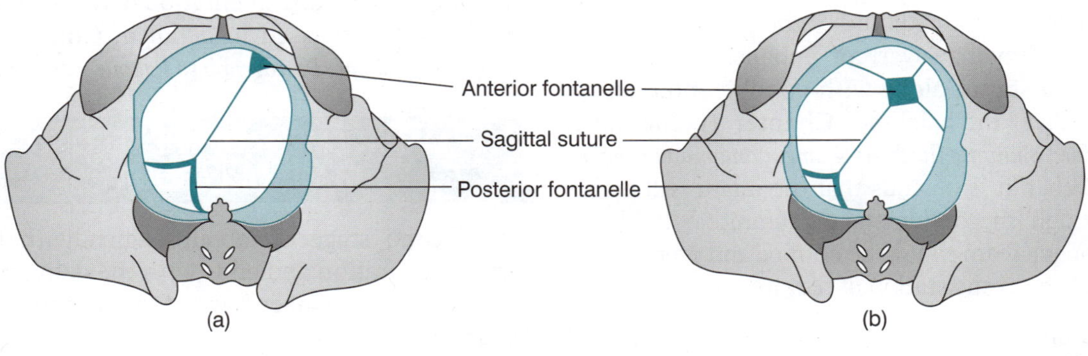

Fig. 4.5 Determining the extent of flexion of the fetal head on vaginal examination—(a) when the head is well-flexed, the Y-shaped posterior fontanelle is easily felt, and the diamond-shaped anterior fontanelle is felt with difficulty and (b) when the head is deflexed, both the anterior and posterior fontanelles are felt with equal ease

be severe, and the overlapping bones cannot be moved apart by digital pressure.

Status of the membranes

The membranes can be felt as a slippery layer over the fetal head. They may also be felt as a soft or tense bag of membranes over the leading part. The membranes can rupture spontaneously during labour; alternatively, an amniotomy may be performed.

Amniotomy

Amniotomy (artificial rupture of membranes [AROM]) by itself has not been shown to shorten the first or second stage of labour or reduce the rate of cesarean delivery in women who have spontaneous onset of labour [23].

In high-risk women, an amniotomy allows the obstetrician to check for meconium that, when present, may warrant enhanced monitoring of fetal status.

Women undergoing augmentation or induction of labour have been shown to benefit from the combination of oxytocin administration and amniotomy (see **Chapter 14**, *Induction and augmentation of labour*).

Presence or absence of meconium

When the amniotic fluid is clear, it is a reassuring sign. When the amniotic fluid is mildly meconium-stained and the fetal heart rate is normal, labour can be observed without any intervention. The presence of solid elements in meconium-stained fluid or the presence of thick meconium may warrant enhanced monitoring of fetal status, along with possible intervention to deliver the baby (see **Chapter 16**, *Meconium-stained amniotic fluid: Assessment and management*).

When it is obvious that the infant will deliver through meconium-stained amniotic fluid, the neonatal team should be notified and preparations made for resuscitation, if required [24].

Technique

An amniotomy should be performed under strict aseptic precautions. It is best done after 3–4 cm cervical dilatation and with an engaged presenting part. The author suggests using the left hand for vaginal examination and the right hand to perform the amniotomy (for right-handed physicians) because this allows better control over the instrument. An amniotomy hook may be used, but if it is not available, Allis forceps may be used. The fetal heart rate must be monitored after the amniotomy to recognise an occult umbilical cord prolapse.

Controlled amniotomy

When there is polyhydramnios or an unengaged presenting part, the examining fingers must be kept over the amniotomy site so that the fluid is released in a controlled manner. This minimises the risk of a sudden gush of amniotic fluid which may lead to umbilical cord prolapse. This also allows the operator to guide the unengaged head so that it drops gently into the pelvis as the fluid is released.

ASSESSING AND DOCUMENTING THE PROGRESS OF LABOUR

Assessing and documenting events in labour may help in the diagnosis of dysfunctional labour and prevent obstructed labour. Cervical dilatation, descent of the presenting part, uterine contractions, maternal vital signs, oxytocin augmentation, and fetal parameters such as fetal heart rate, the presence of meconium, and moulding of the head are recorded on a **partograph**. The documentation of the progress of labour is discussed in detail in **Chapter 6,** *Monitoring labour: Partograph to Labour Care Guide*.

MANAGEMENT OF THE SECOND STAGE OF LABOUR

The second stage of labour begins with full cervical dilatation and ends with the delivery of the infant. The management of the second stage of labour includes the following:

- Identifying the onset of the second stage
- Helping the woman with expulsive efforts

- Preparation for delivery
- Conduct of delivery

IDENTIFYING THE ONSET OF THE SECOND STAGE

The second stage begins when the cervix is fully dilated. The fetal head descends and presses against the rectum. At this point, the woman gets an uncontrollable urge to bear down. She will flex her knees and start pushing down during contractions. Very often, the woman will say she 'wants to pass motion' because of rectal pressure from the baby's head.

Key Point

Occasionally, the fetal head will be so low in the birth canal that the woman will start bearing down even before the cervix is fully dilated. When the vaginal examination reveals a cervical dilatation <10 cm, it is best to turn the woman on her side. She should be instructed to take short, panting breaths during contractions so that she does not bear down. Pushing against a partially dilated cervix can lead to cervical edema and a delay in delivery.

HELPING THE WOMAN WITH EXPULSIVE EFFORTS

In the second stage, uterine contractions increase in frequency and intensity. At this stage, the woman has to supplement the involuntary urge to push with a voluntary effort to deliver the baby. Expulsive forces are dependent on the contraction of the diaphragm and abdominal wall muscles.

The woman's expulsive efforts must be continually supported so that she can have a quick and safe delivery. A birth companion is invaluable in the second stage of labour, especially when the woman needs to push.

Pushing During the Second Stage of Labour

If the vaginal examination reveals a fully dilated cervix, the woman may be encouraged to begin pushing. Sometimes, at full dilatation, the head will not yet have descended and so, the woman may not have the urge to push. In such cases, we can wait for the descent of the head before the woman is encouraged to push.

Key Point

Persistent anterior lip of the cervix

Occasionally, the last centimetre of the cervix will not dilate and will be caught anteriorly between the fetal head and the symphysis pubis. If the woman continues to push against such a cervix, it can become edematous and friable. To prevent this, the cervical lip is gently pushed backwards during a contraction until it slips over the fetal head and behind the symphysis pubis. The examining fingers are used to hold the cervix above the head until the fetal head descends beyond the cervix with maternal pushing.

Position for pushing

Women spontaneously assume positions that they are most comfortable with during the course of labour. They can be encouraged to adopt any position as long as it allows appropriate maternal and fetal monitoring and treatment [18]. Two systematic reviews of the Cochrane Database compared various positions in which women pushed during the second stage of labour without epidural analgesia [25] and with epidural analgesia [26]. The reviews compared upright positions (sitting, squatting, kneeling) versus lying positions (lateral, semi-recumbent, lithotomy, Trendelenburg) and found that no position was clearly superior.

The lithotomy position or semi-recumbent (head and torso at an angle of >30–45°) is usually recommended for pushing or giving birth. These positions are also convenient when fetal manipulation is required or when operative delivery is needed.

Key Point

Though upright positions may marginally decrease the duration of the second stage, they are associated with increased blood loss of >500 mL and possibly, an increased rate of second-degree tears [25].

Technique for pushing

Women should be advised to pull back their knees, tuck in their chin, take a deep breath, bear down with a closed glottis at the start of a contraction (Valsalva technique), and push for 8–10 seconds, with an average of 2–3 pushes per contraction. The birth companion can help with timing the duration of the push and can support the mother's head, neck, and shoulders as she bears down. The duration of the second stage of labour is shorter with Valsalva pushing [27].

However, a systematic review of the Cochrane Database compared spontaneous to Valsalva pushing in the second stage of labour and found no clear differences in the duration of the second stage, spontaneous vaginal delivery, episiotomy, perineal lacerations, or duration of pushing [28].

Key Point

With the data not conclusive on the superiority of either the Valsalva technique or spontaneous pushing with an open glottis, the mother may be encouraged to use whichever technique she prefers.

Pushing with epidural analgesia

Women who have received epidural analgesia may not get the urge to push after reaching full dilatation. In this situation, data support pushing when full dilatation is confirmed by digital examination [29], as opposed to earlier data suggesting delayed pushing (starting 60–90 minutes after full dilatation). In a systematic review and meta-analysis, Di Mascio et al. [30] observed that delayed pushing was associated with a higher incidence of chorioamnionitis and low umbilical cord pH.

Perineal massage while the woman is pushing

Perineal massage is performed by moving two fingers of the lubricated gloved hand from side to side over the fourchette with mild, downward pressure. This has been shown to reduce severe perineal trauma and the need for episiotomy when compared to the 'hands-off' approach [31].

Gentle stretching and massaging of the introitus during the second stage of labour marginally reduces the incidence of third- and fourth-degree tears [32] (see **Chapter 25**, *Prevention and management of perineal trauma occurring in childbirth*).

Manual Rotation of Fetal Head in the Second Stage of Labour

The frequency of the occiput posterior (OP) position in labour is approximately 20% and, of this, 5% persistently remain posterior until the end of labour. Persistent occiput posterior (POP) is associated with increased rates of maternal and newborn morbidity.

Persistent posterior and transverse positions are associated with the arrest of labour and as a consequence, higher rates of cesarean section and instrumental deliveries.

Manual rotation can convert 90% of OP or transverse arrest situations to occiput anterior (OA) [33]. Manual rotation after the onset of the second stage of labour is more likely to be successful if it is performed before arrest occurs. Manual rotation is more successful in multiparous women.

After manual rotation, delivery can occur spontaneously or with the use of forceps or a ventouse (see **Chapter 21**, *Operative vaginal delivery*).

Technique of digital or manual rotation

The bladder should be emptied before proceeding with manual rotation. It is best to drop the lower end of the labour bed and place the woman at the edge of the bed in a dorsal lithotomy position with the hips flexed and legs supported in stirrups. This allows the obstetrician to have better access to the fetal head [34].

Digital rotation

The author prefers digital rotation as it is easy to perform and less uncomfortable for the woman than other methods. The vertex must be carefully palpated to identify the posterior fontanelle and the parietal bones. The exact position of the occiput is easy to identify if this is done.

The index and middle fingers are used to locate and apply counterclockwise pressure on the posterior edge of the upper parietal bone at the lambdoid suture, and the head is gently rotated till the occiput reaches the anterior position (Fig. 4.6). The rotation is performed during a contraction and with the woman pushing down so that the digital rotation assists the physiological rotation of the head. Quite often, as soon as the rotation is achieved, the vertex will descend rapidly, and delivery will occur.

The rotation may also be performed to achieve an occiput anterior position for forceps or ventouse application.

Manual rotation

For manual rotation from the left occiput posterior (LOP) position, the operator's right hand is placed in the vagina, palm up. Four fingers are placed against the left side of the fetal head. The thumb is placed on the right side of the opposite parietal bone (Fig. 4.7). The fetal head is slightly pushed up, flexed, and rotated counterclockwise to the left occiput anterior (LOA) position or OA position by pronation of the right hand [34]. The left hand is used if the fetal head is in the right OP position and the direction of rotation is exactly reversed.

Persistent occipitoposterior position may often be associated with significant moulding and caput formation. The vertex may appear to be low in the pelvis even though the biparietal diameter is above the spines (unengaged). Manual/digital rotation followed by a difficult instrumental delivery in this situation is dangerous; a cesarean is the better option.

Fetal Heart Rate Monitoring in the Second Stage

The frequency of fetal heart rate monitoring should increase in the second stage of labour. Intermittent auscultation is recommended every 5 minutes during the second stage of labour and after each contraction when the woman is pushing [35]. If a woman is on continuous CTG monitoring, the FHR tracings should be reviewed every 15 minutes in the second stage in low-risk pregnancies, and every 5 minutes in higher-risk pregnancies [36] (see **Chapter 8**, *Fetal surveillance in labour*).

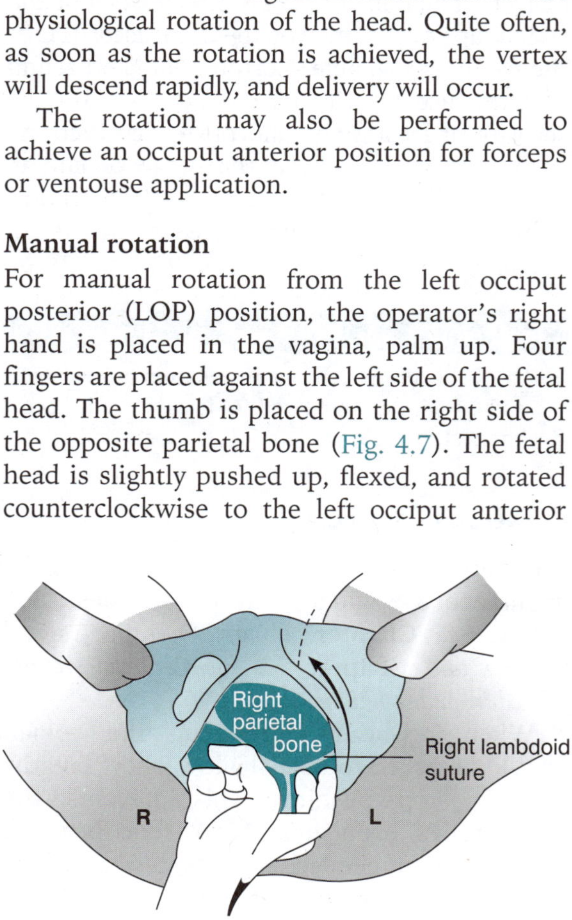

Fig. 4.6 Digital rotation of the left occiput posterior to left occiput anterior: The index and middle fingers are used to locate and apply counterclockwise pressure on the posterior margin of the right parietal bone at the right lambdoid suture

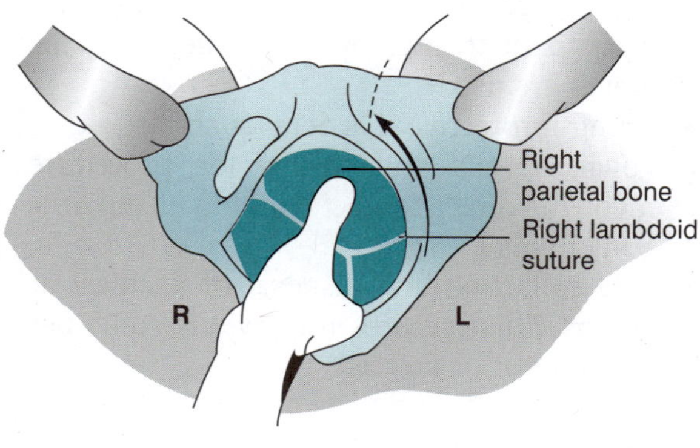

Fig. 4.7 Manual rotation of the left occiput posterior to left occiput anterior: With the palm of the right hand facing up, four fingers are placed along the left side of the fetal head with the thumb on the right side; while gently disengaging the fetal head, the operator rotates the occiput counterclockwise into the anterior segment of the pelvis

EPISIOTOMY

The routine use of episiotomy is not recommended (see **Chapter 7**, *Episiotomy: What does the evidence say?*).

PREPARING FOR VAGINAL DELIVERY

Aseptic Precautions

The obstetrician should wear a waterproof apron underneath a sterile cloth gown or a disposable waterproof gown. Sterile gloves are mandatory. A cap and mask are not mandatory but do protect the obstetrician from being splashed with bodily fluids and are a part of universal precautions.

The perineum should be cleaned with cotton pads soaked in water. Subsequently, a povidone–iodine or chlorhexidine solution can be used to clean the perineal area.

Universal Precautions

All staff in the labour room must be aware of the universal precautions to prevent infection or the spread of HIV, hepatitis B, and other blood-borne infections. Universal precautions include the following:

- Hand hygiene before and after contact with every patient, regardless of whether or not gloves are used
- Using protective barriers such as gloves, gowns/aprons and masks for procedures involving direct contact with blood and other body fluids
- Safe collection and disposal of needles and sharps (this requires impervious containers that cannot be pierced)
- Following the correct procedures for the care of a needlestick injury (the area should be washed with soap and water, the needle disposed safely, and immediate post-exposure prophylaxis given)
- Covering all cuts and abrasions with waterproof dressings
- Cleaning up spills of blood and other body fluids with 1 part bleach in 10 parts of water
- Segregation of waste and proper disposal of contaminated waste

Maternal Position for Delivery

If the woman is on a labour table, dropping the end flap will provide access to the perineum and fetus, especially if fetal manipulation is required. If the fetal heart rate has stayed normal and no fetal manipulation is required, the woman may deliver in the lateral position or partial sitting position. Obstetricians need training to be able to deliver women in alternative birthing positions.

Stirrups may or may not be used, according to the facilities available. Corton et al. [37] found that the use of stirrups did not increase the severity of lacerations and obstetric outcomes such as a prolonged second stage of labour, forceps delivery, and cesarean birth. Similarly, infant outcomes were unaffected by the use of stirrups.

Key Point

The use of stirrups has not been shown to have any disadvantages as compared to delivering on a bed without stirrups [37].

CONDUCT OF DELIVERY

The important techniques involved in a spontaneous vaginal delivery are described below. See **Chapter 21** for *Operative vaginal delivery* and **Chapter 22** for *Cesarean section: Procedure and technique*.

When the head is crowning, the woman should be asked to take shallow, short breaths and to stop pushing. This prevents the uncontrolled expulsion of the fetal head. It is also recommended that expulsive efforts are applied between contractions rather than during a contraction.

Manual Perineal Protection (MPP) and the Modified Ritgen Manoeuvre

Perineal support and the modified Ritgen manoeuvre (fingers placed between the maternal anus and coccyx to actively lift the fetal chin anteriorly) have been traditionally used to reduce the occurrence of significant perineal trauma during childbirth. Perineal support has been found to be protective against obstetric anal sphincter injuries [38,39,40,41]. However, a meta-analysis [42] found no clear reduction in obstetric anal sphincter injuries. Another meta-analysis [43] was unable to show a clear benefit of Ritgen manoeuvre in preventing severe perineal trauma.

In the modified Ritgen manoeuvre, one hand is used to maintain the head in a flexed position and control the speed of crowning, and the other hand is used to gently ease the perineum away from the fetal face. Some obstetricians support the perineum with a surgical pad (Fig. 4.8). Once the fetal head delivers, external rotation (restitution) occurs spontaneously. It is important that perineal support be maintained until the shoulders are delivered to avoid perineal injury.

Delivery of the Shoulders

Once the head is delivered, a hand is placed on either side of the head, and gentle downward traction is applied toward the woman's sacrum as she pushes. The anterior shoulder will slip under the symphysis pubis and will be delivered (Fig. 4.9a).

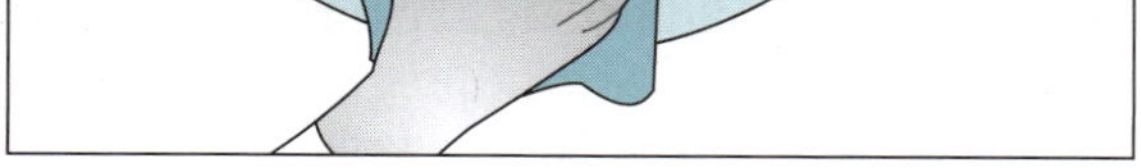

Fig. 4.8 As the head is delivered, one hand controls the head and gently flexes it so that there is no sudden expulsion; the other hand supports the perineum and gently slips the perineum away from the fetal face

The posterior shoulder is then delivered by upward traction (Fig. 4.9b). Care should be taken to perform these manoeuvres without undue stretching of the woman's perineum and the fetal neck to avoid perineal injury and/or traction injuries to the brachial plexus. The delivery is then completed spontaneously as the rest of the fetal body is delivered.

Nuchal Cord (Cord Around the Neck)

The presence of the cord around the neck at birth is common—1 of 4 babies is born with this. Most often, there is a single loop of cord around the neck but 2, 3, and 4 loops may also be seen wrapped around the neck. As the head is delivered, the loose loop of the cord is slipped over the head by the obstetrician and the baby is delivered.

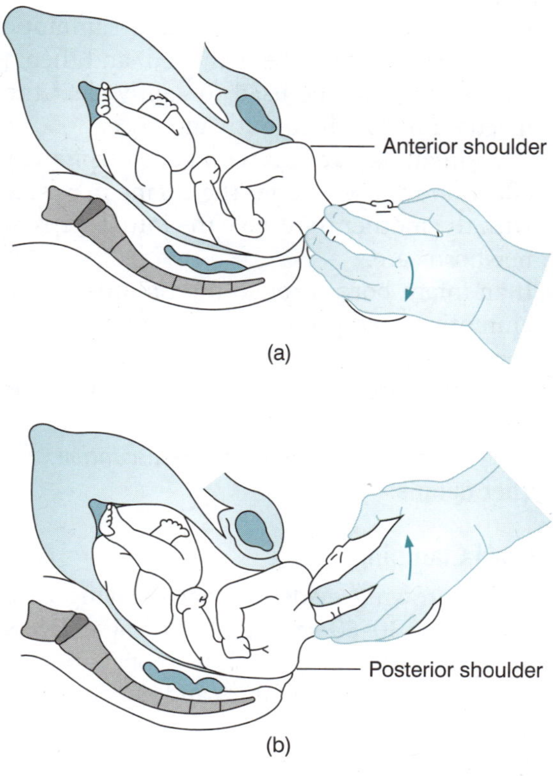

Fig. 4.9 Delivery of (a) the anterior shoulder and (b) the posterior shoulder

Occasionally, the cord may be tightly wrapped around the neck. In such a situation, the cord is doubly clamped and transected between the clamps. This allows the delivery of the fetal head.

IMMEDIATE CARE OF THE NEWBORN

Oropharyngeal Suctioning

For a baby born after 35 weeks, the mouth and nose can be wiped at birth with a towel [44]. This is an alternative (and equally effective method) to oronasopharyngeal suctioning, which may be required only if the baby has excessive secretions.

For a baby born through meconium-stained fluid, it was traditionally recommended that the mouth and nose be suctioned as soon as the head is delivered and before the delivery of the shoulders. However, recent guidelines [24] state the following:

- In cases of meconium-stained amniotic fluid, the infant can be delivered, and then a bulb syringe can be used to gently clear the meconium from its mouth and nose.
- If the infant is vigorous with good respiratory effort and muscle tone, the infant may stay with the mother to receive the initial steps of newborn care.
- If an infant born through meconium-stained amniotic fluid presents with poor muscle tone and inadequate breathing efforts, the initial steps of resuscitation should be completed under a radiant warmer.

See **Chapter 44,** *Neonatal resuscitation,* for further details.

Cord Clamping

There is growing evidence that delaying cord clamping for 30–60 seconds following delivery increases early hemoglobin concentration and iron stores in infants and is therefore recommended [45,5].

However, delayed cord clamping also causes a 40% increase in the risk of neonatal jaundice requiring phototherapy. Therefore, delayed cord clamping should be considered only as long as access to phototherapy is available [46]. Phototherapy increases the cost of hospitalisation, which is a consideration in low-resource countries.

In preterm babies, delayed clamping can cause cardiac overload but could reduce the risk of death before discharge in preterm babies [47]. Current recommendations are to delay umbilical cord clamping in vigorous term and preterm infants for at least 30–60 seconds after birth [45].

Cleaning and Bathing

The baby should be dried with a towel and laid on the mother's chest. A bath can be given after 6 hours and may be delayed up to 24 hours.

See **Chapter 43,** *Routine care of the newborn,* for further management of the newborn.

MANAGEMENT OF THE THIRD STAGE OF LABOUR

The placenta is delivered by active management of the third stage of labour. Active management consists of the following measures:

- Prophylactic administration of a uterotonic agent before the delivery of the placenta
  - Oxytocin 10 units IM or in an IV infusion
  - Methylergometrin (Methergine) 0.25 mg IV or IM
- Controlled traction of the umbilical cord after cord clamping and transection
- Uterine massage

See **Chapter 5**, *Management of the third stage of labour,* for a detailed description.

CONCLUSION

The process of childbirth is a natural part of life for women who choose to be pregnant. However, it carries possible risks for the pregnant woman and the newborn. Hence, it is important for every individual providing care for the labouring woman to know the steps involved in a labour that progresses normally. Every effort should be made to ensure a good outcome for the mother and child.

REFERENCES

1. WHO. Maternal and Newborn Health/Safe Motherhood Unit. Care in normal birth: A practical guide. World Health Organization. WHO Press. Geneva. 1996.
2. Zhang J, Landy HJ, Branch DW, Burkman R, Haberman S, Gregory KD, et al. Contemporary patterns of spontaneous labor with normal neonatal outcomes. Consortium on Safe Labor. *Obstet Gynecol*. 2010. 116:1281–7.
3. WHO recommendations: Intrapartum care for a positive childbirth experience. World Health Organization. WHO Press. Geneva. 2018.
4. American College of Obstetricians and Gynecologists (ACOG). Safe prevention of the primary cesarean delivery. Obstetric Care Consensus No. 1. *Obstet Gynecol*. 2014 (reaffirmed 2017). 123:693–711.
5. WHO recommendation on labour ward admission policy. World Health Organization. WHO Press. Geneva. 2018a.
6. Guidelines on midwifery services in India. Ministry of Health and Family Welfare, Government of India. 2018. https://nhm.gov.in/New_Updates_2018/NHM_Components/RMNCHA/MH/Guidelines/Guidelines_on_Midwifery_Services_in_India.pdf.
7. Sandall J, Soltani H, Gates S, et al. Midwife-led continuity models versus other models of care for childbearing women. *Cochrane Database Syst Rev*. 2016. Issue 4. Art. No.: CD004667.
8. Hendrix NW, Grady CS, Chauhan SP. Clinical vs. sonographic estimate of birth weight in term parturients. A randomized clinical trial. *J Reprod Med*. 2000. 45(4):317-22. PMID: 10804488.
9. Preyer O, Husslein H, Concin N, et al. Fetal weight estimation at term—ultrasound versus clinical examination with Leopold's manoeuvres: A prospective blinded observational study. *BMC Pregnancy Childbirth*. 2019. 11;19(1):122.
10. Abramowicz, Abramowicz JS, Ahn TJ. Fetal macrosomia. Levine D (Ed). *UpToDate*. Waltham, MA. 2022.
11. Moraitis AA, Shreeve N, Sovio U et al. Universal third-trimester ultrasonic screening using fetal macrosomia in the prediction of adverse perinatal outcome: A systematic review and meta-analysis of diagnostic test accuracy. *PLoS Med*. 2020. 17:e1003190.
12. Seaward PG, Hannah ME, Myhr TL, et al. International Multicentre Term Prelabor Rupture of Membranes Study: Evaluation of predictors of clinical chorioamnionitis and postpartum fever in patients with prelabor rupture of membranes at term. *Am J Obstet Gynecol*. 1997. 177:1024.
13. Bellussi F, Livi A, Diglio J, et al. Timing of induction for term prelabor rupture of membranes and intravenous antibiotics. *Am J Obstet Gynecol*. 2021. 3:100245.
14. Maharaj D. Assessing cephalopelvic disproportion: Back to the basics. *Obstet Gynecol Surv*. 2010. 65:387.
15. Reveiz L, Gaitán HG, Cuervo LG. Enemas during labour. *Cochrane Database Syst Rev*. 2013. Issue 7. Art. No.: CD000330.
16. Basevi V, Lavender T. Routine perineal shaving on admission in labour. *Cochrane Database Syst Rev*. 2014. Issue 11. Art. No.: CD001236.
17. Practice Guidelines for Obstetric Anesthesia: An Updated Report by the American Society of Anesthesiologists Task Force on Obstetric Anesthesia and the Society for Obstetric Anesthesia and Perinatology. *Anesthesiology*. 2016. 124(2):270-300.
18. ACOG Committee on Obstetric Practice. Committee Opinion No. 766. Approaches to limit intervention during labor and birth. 2019. *Obstet Gynecol*.
19. Fong A, Serra AE, Caballero D, et al. A randomized, double-blinded, controlled trial of the effects of fluid rate and/or presence of dextrose in intravenous fluids on the labor course of nulliparas. *Am J Obstet Gynecol*. 2017. 217:208.e1.
20. Tita ATN. Prenatal care: Intra-amniotic infection (clinical chorioamnionitis). Berghella V (Ed). *UpToDate*. Waltham, MA. 2022.
21. Bloom SL, McIntire DD, Kelly MA, et al. Lack of effect of walking on labor and delivery. *N Engl J Med*. 1998. 339:76.
22. Lally JE, Murtagh MJ, Macphail S, et al. More in hope than expectation: A systematic review of women's expectations and experience of pain relief in labour. *BMC Med*. 2008. 6, 7.
23. Smyth RM, Markham C, Dowswell T. Amniotomy for shortening spontaneous labour. *Cochrane Database Syst Rev*. 2013. Issue 6. Art. No.: CD006167.
24. ACOG Committee on Obstetric Practice. Committee Opinion No. 689: Delivery of a newborn with meconium-stained amniotic fluid. *Obstet Gynecol*. 2017. 129:e33.
25. Gupta JK, Sood A, Hofmeyr GJ, Vogel JP. Position in the second stage of labour for women without epidural anaesthesia. *Cochrane Database Syst Rev*. 2017. Issue 5. Art. No.: CD002006.
26. Walker KF, Kibuka M, Thornton JG, Jones NW. Maternal position in the second stage of labour for women with epidural anaesthesia. *Cochrane Database Syst Rev*. 2018. Issue 11. Art. No. CD008070.
27. Prins M, Boxem J, Lucas C, Hutton E. Effect of spontaneous pushing versus Valsalva pushing in the second stage of labour on mother and fetus: A systematic review of randomised trials. *BJOG*. 2011. 118:662.

28. Lemos A, Amorim MMR, Dornelas de Andrade A, et al. Pushing/bearing down methods for the second stage of labour. *Cochrane Database Syst Rev.* 2017. Issue 3. Art. No.: CD009124.
29. Cahill AG, Srinivas SK, Tita ATN, Caughey AB, Richter HE, Gregory WT, et al. Effect of immediate vs. delayed pushing on rates of spontaneous vaginal delivery among nulliparous women receiving neuraxial analgesia: A randomized clinical trial. *JAMA.* 2018. 320:1444–54.
30. Di Mascio D, Saccone G, Bellussi F, Al-Kouatly HB, Brunelli R, Benedetti Panici P, Liberati M, D'Antonio F, Berghella V. Delayed versus immediate pushing in the second stage of labor in women with neuraxial analgesia: A systematic review and meta-analysis of randomized controlled trials. *Am J Obstet Gynecol.* 2020. 223(2):189-203.
31. Funai EF, Norwitz ER. Labor and delivery: Management of the normal second stage. Prabhu M (Ed). *UpToDate.* Waltham, MA. 2022.
32. Aquino CI, Guida M, Saccone G et al. Perineal massage during labor: A systematic review and meta-analysis of randomized controlled trials. *J Matern Fetal Neonatal Med.* 2020. 33:1051.
33. Le Ray C, Serres P, Schmitz T, et al. Manual rotation in occiput posterior or transverse positions: Risk factors and consequences on the cesarean delivery rate. *Obstet Gynecol.* 2007. 110:873.
34. Barth WH Jr. Clinical Expert Series. Persistent Occiput Posterior. *Obstet Gynecol.* 2015. 125:695–709.
35. Lewis D, Downe S. FIGO Intrapartum Fetal Monitoring Expert Consensus Panel. FIGO consensus guidelines on intrapartum fetal monitoring: Intermittent auscultation. *Int J Gynecol Obstet.* 2015. 131(1):9–12.
36. American College of Obstetricians and Gynecologists. ACOG Practice Bulletin No. 106. Intrapartum fetal heart rate monitoring: Nomenclature, interpretation, and general management principles. *Obstet Gynecol.* 2009 (reaffirmed 2021). 114:192.
37. Corton MM, Lankford JC, Ames R, McIntire DD, Alexander JM, Leveno KJ. A randomized trial of birthing with and without stirrups. *Am J Obstet Gynecol.* 2012. 207(2):133. e1–133.e1335.
38. Hals E, Øian P, Pirhonen T, Gissler M, et al. A multicenter interventional program to reduce the incidence of anal sphincter tears. *Obstet Gynecol.* 2010. 116:901-908.
39. Laine K, Skjeldestad FE, Sandvik L, et al. Incidence of obstetric anal sphincter injuries after training to protect the perineum: Cohort study. *BMJ Open.* 2012. 2(5), e001649.
40. Fretheim A, Odgaard-Jensen J, Røttingen JA, et al. The impact of an intervention programme employing a hands-on technique to reduce the incidence of anal sphincter tears: Interrupted time-series reanalysis. *BMJ Open.* 2013. 3(10): e003355.
41. Jansova M, Kalis V, Rusavy Z, et al. Fetal head size and effect of manual perineal protection. *PLoS One.* 2017. 12:e0189842.
42. Bulchandani S, Watts E, Sucharitha A, et al. Manual perineal support at the time of childbirth: A systematic review and meta-analysis. *BJOG.* 2015. 122:1157.
43. Aquino CI, Saccone G, Troisi J, et al. Is Ritgen's maneuver associated with decreased perineal lacerations and pain at delivery? *J Matern Fetal Neonatal Med.* 2020. 33:3185.
44. Kelleher J, Bhat R, Salas AA, et al. Oronasopharyngeal suction versus wiping of the mouth and nose at birth: A randomised equivalency trial. *Lancet.* 2013. 382:326.
45. ACOG Committee on Obstetric Practice. Committee Opinion No. 684: Delayed umbilical cord clamping after birth. *Obstet Gynecol.* 2017a. 129:e5.
46. McDonald SJ, Middleton P, Dowswell T, Morris PS. Effect of timing of umbilical cord clamping of term infants on maternal and neonatal outcomes. *Cochrane Database Syst Rev.* 2013. Issue 9. Art. No.: CD004074.
47. Rabe H, Gyte GML, Díaz-Rossello JL, Duley L. Effect of timing of umbilical cord clamping and other strategies to influence placental transfusion at preterm birth on maternal and infant outcomes. *Cochrane Database Syst Rev.* 2019. Issue 9. Art. No.: CD003248.

CHAPTER 5

Management of the Third Stage of Labour

BASAB MUKHERJEE, POUSHALI SANYAL

INTRODUCTION

The third stage of labour is the shortest among the four stages. However, it has immense clinical significance as complications in this stage, particularly postpartum hemorrhage, can lead to significant morbidity and mortality.

DEFINITION

The third stage of labour begins with the complete delivery of the newborn and ends with the complete delivery of the placenta with the membranes [1].

> **Key Point**
>
> The third stage of labour is considered **prolonged** if the placenta and membranes are not delivered within 30 minutes with active management and within 60 minutes with physiological management [2].

PHYSIOLOGICAL PROCESSES IN THE THIRD STAGE OF LABOUR

- Separation of the placenta
- Descent of the placenta
- Expulsion or birth of the placenta

Separation of the Placenta

At the onset of labour, the placenta is usually attached to the upper uterine segment. The placenta is approximately 20 cm in diameter. During the first stage, there is almost no reduction in the area of attachment of the placenta. During the second stage, as the strength and frequency of uterine contractions increase along with successive retractions of the uterine musculature, there is a slight but sustained reduction in the area of placental attachment.

Immediately after the baby is born, the uterus becomes discoid in shape. Due to the retraction of the uterine muscles, the upper segment is disproportionately thickened (Fig. 5.1a), whereas the lower segment is flabby and folded into itself several times. The surface area of placental

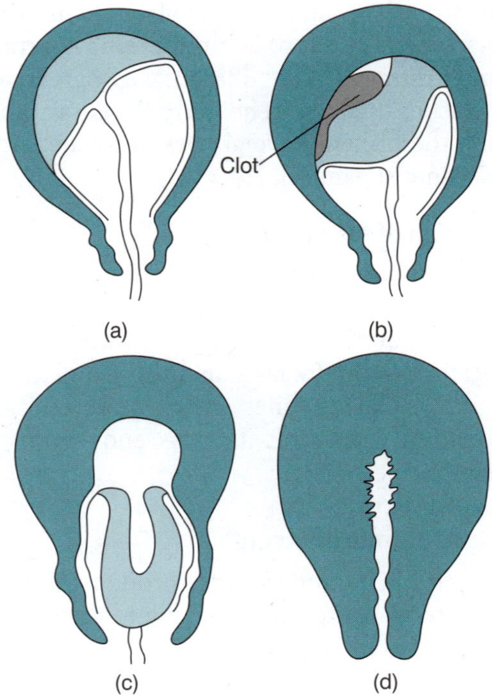

Fig. 5.1 The phases of the third stage of labour: (a) Contraction and retraction of the uterus, (b) formation of a retroplacental clot, (c) placental separation and descent, and (d) the appearance of the uterus after placental expulsion

attachment is reduced by more than half. The placenta, an inelastic structure, buckles up on itself due to the reduction in its attachment area. This produces a shearing force that acts between the placenta and its site of uterine attachment, resulting in placental separation. The plane of separation is through the spongy layer of the decidua basalis [3].

There are two mechanisms of placental separation:

- **Matthew Duncan** or **marginal separation**: Marginal separation is the more common of the two mechanisms. The placenta separates at its margin, and as uterine contractions increase, it continues to separate until it detaches completely from the uterus.
- **Schultze** or **central separation:** Placental separation starts from the centre of its attachment site. Uterine sinuses over this area open up and blood collects behind the placenta (Fig. 5.1b). As the uterus contracts and retracts, the placenta progressively detaches from it. The retroplacental blood and the placental weight result in the entire placenta separating [3].

Separation of the membranes

The membranes attached to the lower uterine segment separate along with the placenta when the lower uterine segment is stretched. This separation is chiefly facilitated by the placental weight. The membranes detach more easily as the placenta separates and descends from the upper uterine segment.

Descent of the Placenta

The placenta now descends through the birth canal after separation, partly due to gravity and partly due to its own weight (Fig. 5.1c).

Placental Expulsion or Delivery

After the placenta has completely separated, it is pushed down into the lax lower uterine segment due to forceful uterine contraction and retraction. Then, it is expelled out of the birth canal by maternal bearing down efforts or by manual methods (Fig. 5.1d). Placental expulsion is usually followed by a gush of approximately 200 mL of blood.

> **Key Point**
>
> Placental separation usually takes place within 5 minutes of the end of the second stage. 90% of placentae are expelled within 15 minutes of birth [4].

CLINICAL FEATURES OF PLACENTAL SEPARATION

After the delivery of the baby, before placental separation, the uterus becomes discoid in shape and is firm to feel. The height of the fundus comes down to or slightly below the level of the umbilicus. There may be a small amount of vaginal bleeding, but there is no lengthening of the cord noted, till the placenta actually separates. The signs of placental separation are recognised by abdominal and vaginal examination.

Per Abdomen

- The uterus becomes firm, globular, and ballottable.
- The height of the uterine fundus is slightly raised.
- There is suprapubic bulging.

Per Vaginum

- There is a gush of vaginal bleeding.
- There is lengthening of the umbilical cord.

MECHANISM OF HEMOSTASIS OF THE PLACENTAL BED

After the placenta has separated, the uterine sinuses, through which blood from ovarian and uterine vessels circulates, are torn open. The uterus attempts to occlude these vessels and prevent blood loss by completely retracting. As a result, the arterioles passing through the interlacing muscle layers of the myometrium are forcibly clamped. This mechanism of hemostasis is called the **living ligature**. Additionally, as pregnancy is a hypercoagulable state, there is a natural thrombosis of the torn vessels, which stops the bleeding. Moreover, as the walls of the uterus are opposed to each other following expulsion, this also helps to stop blood loss.

MANAGEMENT OF THE THIRD STAGE OF LABOUR

The third stage of labour can be managed by two distinct approaches:

- Active management
- Physiological or expectant management

Active Management

Active management of the third stage of labour (AMTSL) [5] is a bundle of interventions that are instituted after the birth of the baby to minimise the risk of postpartum hemorrhage (PPH) and the need for blood transfusion.

The main component of AMTSL is the use of **uterotonics** to ensure effective uterine contractions, help in early separation and expulsion of the placenta, and result in a well-contracted uterus [2]. It is a key step in preventing PPH, the most common cause of maternal death worldwide, especially in low-resource countries.

In line with WHO recommendations, the three main **components** of AMTSL are as follows:

- **Uterotonics** are used to prevent PPH. The recommended uterotonic for the prevention of PPH is oxytocin (10 IU IV/IM) given within one minute of the birth of the baby [5].
- **Delayed clamping of the umbilical cord** is recommended. A waiting time of 60 seconds to a maximum of 180 seconds postdelivery or after the cessation of umbilical cord pulsation is the recommended approach (see the section on *Delayed cord clamping* below).
- **Controlled cord traction (CCT)** is the recommended method of placental delivery for vaginal births in the presence of a skilled birth attendant. This applies to cesarean delivery as well. If a skilled birth attendant is not present, CCT is generally not recommended [6,7]. While CCT does not significantly reduce bleeding compared to spontaneous placental separation, it does reduce the duration of the third stage.

Postpartum assessment of uterine tone by abdominal examination for early identification of uterine atony is universally recommended.

Uterine massage

It is not clear whether uterine massage is effective in further reducing PPH [8]. In under-resourced areas where uterotonics may not always be available, uterine massage is a simple and inexpensive intervention, performed by repetitive massaging or squeezing movements after the delivery of the placenta.

Though sustained uterine massage is no longer a recommended intervention for the prevention of PPH in women who have already been administered oxytocin [9], a recent meta-analysis [10] did not find good-quality studies to either support or refute uterine massage. As a simple intervention, it may be a life-saving one in under-resourced areas. If the uterus becomes flabby, gentle massaging makes the uterus firm and expels retained blood clots from the uterus.

> **Key Points**
>
> - The use of uterotonics is the most important component of AMTSL followed by delayed cord clamping.
> - Controlled cord traction is recommended in the presence of a skilled birth attendant.
> - Sustained uterine massage is no longer recommended, though it may be useful when uterotonics are not available.
> - It is important to examine the placenta for completeness of expulsion.

Uterotonics

Oxytocin is the WHO-recommended uterotonic for AMTSL for all births. It is administered as a dose of 10 IU IM or in an IV infusion. The uterotonics that are available for use are listed in Table 5.1.

A network meta-analysis that compared different agents for the prevention of PPH has shown that oxytocin, in combination with methylergometrine or misoprostol is very effective [11].

Key Points

- Oxytocin is the uterotonic of choice for AMTSL. Along with ergometrine or misoprostol, it is effective in preventing PPH.
- Carbetocin is as effective as oxytocin, but its cost restricts its routine use. Heat stability is its biggest advantage, but it must be borne in mind that not all brands available in India are heat-stable.

The WHO Champion trial [12] compared carbetocin with oxytocin and found that carbetocin was not inferior to oxytocin for the prevention of PPH.

Delayed cord clamping (DCC)

The ideal time for clamping the cord is the subject of ongoing research, but the WHO recommends delaying cord clamping for 1–3 minutes in all stable term and preterm babies while initiating routine newborn care. Current research has also suggested that where adequate thermoregulation and initial resuscitation can be safely undertaken with an intact cord, it may even be possible to delay clamping whilst performing these interventions [13].

Delayed cord clamping is usually advised after at least 30–60 seconds [14] for term births

Table 5.1 Uterotonics recommended for AMTSL

Uterotonic	Oxytocin	Misoprostol	Methylergometrine	Carbetocin
Properties	Nonapeptide with a half-life of 30 minutes	PGE1 analogue	Semisynthetic ergot alkaloid derived from lysergic acid	Newer long-acting analogue of oxytocin with uterotonic and antihemorrhagic properties
Advantages	• Rapidly metabolised • Quick onset of action (30 seconds on IV administration) • Action can be controlled	• Cheap • Stable at room temperature • Long shelf life • Easy to store	• Produces a sustained, tetanic uterine contraction stronger than oxytocin • Has a longer duration of action than oxytocin (2–3 hours)	• Heat-stable (can be kept at room temperature) • Does not require cold chain • Single dose, long-acting • Half-life 4–10 times longer than oxytocin • Duration of action is 2 hours
Limitations	• Causes nausea and water intoxication at high doses • Requires cold storage at 2–8°C as it is heat-labile	• Incidence of uterine tachysystole and diarrhea noted • Contraindicated with previous cesarean scar	• Higher incidence of retained placenta • Contraindicated in women with heart failure, severe hypertension	• Expensive • Not readily available in public healthcare facilities • Causes headache, dizziness, pruritus, nausea, vomiting
Dosage	10 IU IM or 10–40 IU in IV infusion after birth of baby	600 mcg rectally after delivery of baby	0.2 mg IM/slow IV within 1 minute of the birth of the baby	100 mcg as a single dose slow IV injection over 1 minute or IM injection to be given as soon as possible after the birth of the baby

and at least 30 seconds for babies delivered at <34 weeks. Canadian guidelines recommend cord clamping after 60–120 seconds for preterm babies [15].

According to FIGO, delayed cord clamping that is carried out in the first minute in preterm infants that are born before 34 weeks of pregnancy can improve neonatal hematologic indices. It may also reduce neonatal mortality without increasing any other types of neonatal morbidity [16].

Delaying cord clamping for at least 1 minute after birth allows time for a passive physiological transfer of warm, oxygenated, fetal blood from the placenta to the baby at the time of birth (the process of 'placental transfusion') [15,17,18]. Delayed clamping of the cord by three minutes or until cessation of cord pulsation has been shown to reduce the incidence of anemia in the newborn baby [14]. This benefit is of particular importance in LMICs [19].

In full-term babies, delayed cord clamping improves both short- and long-term outcomes and shows a favourable score in fine motor and social skills. However, there is insufficient evidence to determine how much delay in clamping the umbilical cord benefits the baby the most. Until further trials and publications come up, a delay in cord clamping of 30 to 120 seconds seems to be justified for full-term babies.

In terms of maternal outcomes, if delayed umbilical cord clamping is practised, there is no increase in the risk of postpartum hemorrhage or blood transfusion [14,16]. Moreover, postpartum maternal hemoglobin levels are also not affected by delayed cord clamping as compared to immediate umbilical cord clamping [14].

Twin pregnancy

Many of the trials that evaluated the effects of delayed umbilical cord clamping did not include multifetal pregnancies. Therefore, there is little information regarding the safety and efficacy of delayed cord clamping in this group.

- ***Dichorionic twins***: A delay in umbilical cord clamping for at least 30–60 seconds after birth is recommended in vigorous term and preterm infants [14].
- ***Monochorionic twins***: DCC should **not** be practised for monochorionic twins because acute and large inter-twin blood transfusion with unpredictable direction of transfusion may occur during labour and birth [20].

Controlled cord traction (CCT)

Techniques of controlled cord traction

Modified Brandt–Andrews method

The manoeuvre is described below (Fig. 5.2):

- The umbilical cord is clamped close to the perineum (once the cord pulsation stops), and the cord is held with one hand.
- The other hand is placed above the mother's pubic bone, and the uterus is stabilised by applying counterpressure on the abdomen.
- With every strong uterine contraction, a gentle downward and backward pull is applied on the cord to deliver the placenta. The abdominal hand is used to apply counterpressure on the uterine fundus.

In between two consecutive contractions, the cord is gently held. No pull is applied till the uterus becomes well-contracted again.

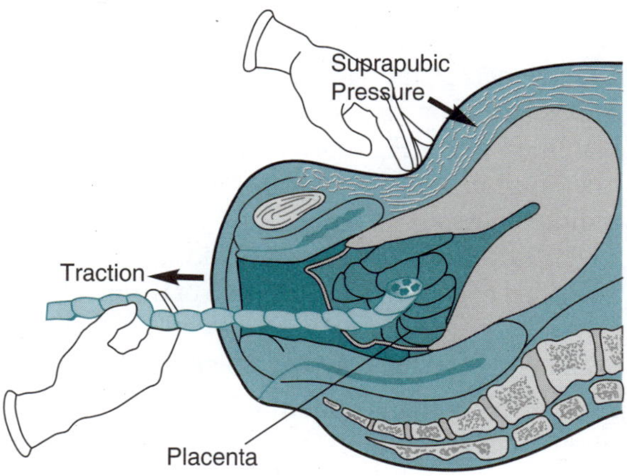

Fig. 5.2 Controlled cord traction and delivery of the placenta using the modified Brandt–Andrews manoeuvre

Crede's manoeuvre

In this technique, the cord is held in a fixed position without applying any pressure on it while the hand on the abdomen applies cephalad pressure on the fundus. In case of an accidental tear of the umbilical cord, it is important to stay calm. The gloved right hand should be introduced vaginally into the uterine cavity to gently check for the plane of separation, grasp the placenta and draw it out. Meanwhile, the left hand should keep a firm guarding pressure over the uterine fundus to prevent uterine inversion.

Delivery of the membranes

The membranes are slowly stripped off from the uterine bed, facilitated by the rotating movement of the placenta as the operator grasps the placenta and brings it out by rotating both hands.

Examination of the placenta to ensure complete removal

After the placenta is delivered, it is placed on a tray, and both its surfaces are examined to see if any placental lobes or cotyledons have been left behind. The maternal surface is examined first to note any missing cotyledons and placental anomalies (Fig. 5.3). The maternal surface appears shaggy as it is covered with the spongy layer of the decidua basalis. If there is any gap between the cotyledons, it implies a missing cotyledon, thereby necessitating uterine exploration. The fetal surface or the shiny placental surface is examined next (Fig. 5.4). The fetal membranes (the amnion and the chorion) are examined for completeness.

The cut surface of the umbilical cord is also examined to confirm the presence of three vessels.

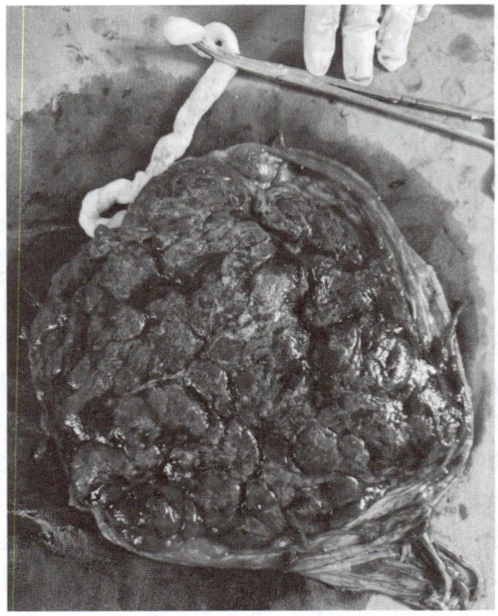

Fig. 5.3 The maternal surface of the placenta with all cotyledons present, confirming that there are no retained placental bits

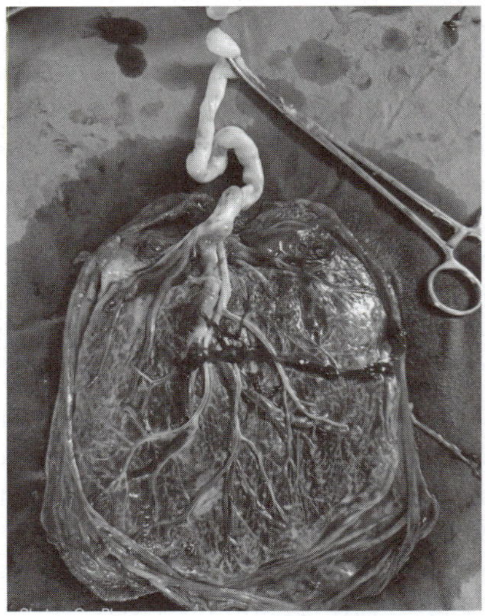

Fig. 5.4 Examination of the shiny fetal surface of the placenta to inspect for completeness of delivery of the fetal membranes

Examining for cuts, tears, and bleeding

The complete management of the third stage of labour includes the examination of the vagina and perineum for tears or lacerations.

The labia are gently separated, and the lower vagina and perineum are inspected for lacerations that might need to be repaired for the prevention of further blood loss. The paraurethral region is carefully inspected for tears which sometimes occur after a vaginal delivery and cause third-stage hemorrhage. It is good practice to perform a rectal exam to identify anal sphincter injury.

With each delivery, and especially after instrumental deliveries, it is important to visualise the cervix. To do this, the cervix is ideally held with two sponge-holding forceps, and the entire cervix, including the angles, is checked for tears (further details can be found in **Chapter 6**, *Prevention and management of perineal trauma occurring in childbirth*, and the section on *Genital tract injuries and hematomas* in **Chapter 46**, *Abnormalities in the puerperium*).

As after any surgical procedure, it is essential to check that no cotton swabs or sponges are left in the vagina postdelivery.

Advantages of AMTSL

The advantages of AMTSL are most significant in women at high risk of PPH [2].

- In a randomised controlled prospective trial, the mean postpartum hemoglobin concentration was significantly higher in the active management group. Falls of hemoglobin levels of >3 g/dL were also less common in this group [21].
- It helps reduce the incidence of PPH and the necessity of interventions to manage PPH [2].
- It reduces the need for blood transfusion [2].
- The duration of the third stage of labour did not significantly decrease with ATMSL in a meta-analysis [2], though Yildirim and colleagues [21] found it significantly reduced in the active management group.

Key Point

AMTSL reduces the risk of PPH of >1000 mL and >500 mL besides reducing the need for blood transfusion and additional uterotonics.

Limitations of AMTSL

- AMTSL is used with caution in women with rheumatic heart diseases for fear of cardiac overload.
- Severe preeclampsia and eclampsia are relative contraindications to the use of AMTSL.
- There is a 2% chance of retained placenta, which might require manual removal of the placenta.

Role of AMTSL in twins

AMTSL, if used correctly, is extremely beneficial in preventing PPH in twins. It should be initiated only after the second twin has been delivered [7].

Uterotonics must be administered only after the second twin is born. The dose of oxytocin remains the same (10 IU IM/IV). Inadvertent administration of uterotonics after the birth of the first twin places the second baby in grave danger of asphyxia as a result of the spasmodic contraction of the uterus. Hence, it is important to rule out twin pregnancies in all emergency unbooked deliveries.

Physiological or Expectant Management of the Third Stage of Labour

The chief principle of expectant management is a 'hands off' approach, where signs of placental separation are awaited, and the placenta is expelled spontaneously or with the help of gravity, maternal efforts, or sometimes with contractions induced by nipple stimulation. Physiological management—also known as conservative management—is popular in some northern European countries and in midwife-led units and home births in the UK.

Physiological management is characterised by the following:

- No routine use of uterotonic drugs
- No clamping of the cord until the cord pulsation has ceased
- Complete delivery of the placenta with the aid of maternal effort

There can be variations within expectant management. After the delivery of the placenta, it is examined in a way similar to that in AMTSL to ensure that there are no retained cotyledons in the uterus.

It is important to remember that with physiological management, the frequency of retained placenta is higher—only 80% of placentae being expelled within 30 minutes, whereas with AMTSL, 98% of placentae are delivered. If there is hemorrhage or failure to deliver the placenta within one hour of expectant management, or an increased risk of PPH, one should implement active management of the third stage. Expectant management of the third stage is not appropriate for women who have risk factors for PPH.

Umbilical cord milking

Umbilical cord milking or stripping can be considered a method of increasing placental blood transfusion to the newborn rapidly, usually in less than 15–20 seconds. It is shown to be beneficial in circumstances where the 30–60-second delay in clamping the cord might be a little too long—for instance, when the infant needs immediate resuscitation or when the mother is hemodynamically unstable. However, milking of the cord has not yet been studied in detail.

Though the requirements for inotropic support and transfusions are reduced by cord milking, there is no overall reduction in morbidity and mortality of the preterm neonate. In neonates born before 28 weeks, cord milking is **not** recommended because of its increased association with intraventricular hemorrhage [22].

The Resuscitation Council UK recommends umbilical cord clamping after at least 60 seconds, but if this is not possible, suggests that cord milking may be an option in babies born after 28 weeks' gestation [23].

Placental cord drainage

Placental cord drainage involves releasing the cord clamp on the maternal side of the umbilical cord so that the blood from the placental side is allowed to drain, thereby decreasing the size of the placenta. No clinical benefit has been identified with this technique, and there is no reduction in PPH or retained placenta [24].

COMPLICATIONS OF THE THIRD STAGE OF LABOUR

- Delayed delivery of the placenta or retained placenta
- Postpartum hemorrhage
- Uterine inversion

Retained placenta and postpartum hemorrhage are dealt with in detail in **Chapter 13**, *Abnormalities in the third stage of labour: Postpartum hemorrhage and retained placenta.* Uterine inversion is discussed in **Chapter 46**, *Abnormalities in the puerperium*.

CONCLUSION

The delivery of the placenta and prevention of PPH are the most important aspects of the management of the third stage of labour. It is very important to simultaneously ensure skin-to-skin contact between the baby and the mother, and early initiation of breastfeeding.

REFERENCES

1. National Institute for Health and Care Excellence. *Intrapartum Care for Healthy Women and Babies, Guideline CG190.* London: National Institute for Health and Care Excellence. 2014. Updated in 2022.
2. Begley CM, Gyte GML, Devane D, et al. Active versus expectant management for women in the third stage of labour. *Cochrane Database Syst Rev.* 2019. Issue 2. Art. No.: CD00741.
3. Konar H, Dutta DC. *D C Dutta's Textbook of Obstetrics Including Perinatology & Contraception.* 10th Edition. 2023. Jaypee Brothers Medical Publishers, New Delhi.
4. Jangsten E, Mattsson LA, Lyckestam I, et al. A comparison of active management and expectant management of the third stage of labour: A Swedish randomised controlled trial. *BJOG.* 2011. 118(3):362–9.
5. WHO recommendations for the prevention and treatment of postpartum haemorrhage. World Health Organization. Geneva. 2012.
6. Deneux–Tharaux C, Sentilhes L, Maillard F, et al. Effect of routine controlled cord traction as part of the active management of the third stage of labour on postpartum haemorrhage: Multicentre randomised controlled trial (TRACOR). *BMJ (Clinical Research Ed.).* 2013. 346: f1541.
7. Gulmezoglu AM, Lumbiganon P, Landoulsi S, et al. Active management of the third stage of labour with and without controlled cord traction: A randomised, controlled, non–

inferiority trial. [Erratum appears in *Lancet*. 2012 May 5;379(9827):1704]. *Lancet*. 2012. 379(9827):1721–7.
8. Hofmeyr GJ, Abdel-Aleem H, Abdel-Aleem MA. Uterine massage for preventing postpartum haemorrhage. *Cochrane Database Syst Rev*. 2013. Issue 7. Art no.: CD006431.
9. Escobar MF, Nassar AH, Theron G, et al. FIGO recommendations on the management of postpartum hemorrhage 2022. *Int J Gynecol Obstet*. 2022. 157 (Suppl. 1): 3–50.
10. Saccone G, Caissutti C, Ciardulli A, et al. Uterine massage as part of active management of the third stage of labour for preventing postpartum haemorrhage during vaginal delivery: A systematic review and meta-analysis of randomised trials. *BJOG*. 2018. 125:778.
11. Gallos ID, Williams HM, Price MJ, et al. Uterotonic agents for preventing postpartum haemorrhage: A network meta-analysis. *Cochrane Database Syst Rev*. 2018. Issue 4. Art. no.: CD011689.
12. Widmer M, Piaggio G, Nguyen TMH, Osoti A, Owa OO, Misra S, et al. Heat-stable carbetocin versus oxytocin to prevent hemorrhage after vaginal birth. *N Engl J Med*. 2018. 379(8):743–752.
13. Delayed umbilical cord clamping for improved maternal and infant health and nutrition outcomes. World Health Organization [Internet]. 2018. Available from: https://www.who.int/nutrition/publications/guidelines/cord_clamping/en/
14. American College of Obstetricians and Gynaecologists. *Delayed Umbilical Cord Clamping after Birth*. Committee Opinion Paper No. 814. Vol 136. No. 6. 2020.
15. Macdonald Sarah D, et al. SOGC Practice Guideline No 424: Umbilical cord management in preterm and term infants. *J Obstet Gynaecol Can* 2022;44(3): 313–322.
16. Bianchi A, Jacobsson B, Mol BW. FIGO good practice recommendations on delayed umbilical cord clamping. *Int J Gynecol Obstet*. 2021. 155:34–36.
17. Tarnow-Mordi W, Morris J, Kirby A, et al. Delayed versus immediate cord clamping in preterm infants. *N Engl J Med*. 2017. 377: 2445–2455.
18. Rabe H, Gyte GM, Díaz-Rossello JL, Duley L. Effect of the timing of umbilical cord clamping and other strategies to influence placental transfusion at preterm birth on maternal and infant outcomes. *Cochrane Database Syst Rev*. 2019. Issue 9. Art. no.: CD003248.
19. Fogarty M, Osborn DA, Askie L, et al. Delayed vs early umbilical cord clamping for preterm infants: A systematic review and meta-analysis. *Am J Obstet Gynecol*. 2018. 218:18.
20. Chasen ST. Twin pregnancy: Labor and delivery. Simpson LL (Ed). *UpToDate*. 2022. Waltham, MA.
21. Yildirim D, Ozyurek SE, Ekiz A, et al. Comparison of active vs. expectant management of the third stage of labor in women with low risk of postpartum hemorrhage: A randomized controlled trial. *Ginekologia Polska*. 2016. 87(5):399–404.
22. Basile S, Pinelli S, Micelli E, et al. Milking of the Umbilical Cord in Term and Late Preterm Infants. *Biomed Res Int*. 2019. 9185059.
23. Resuscitation Council UK. Newborn resuscitation and support of transition of infants at birth Guidelines [Internet]. Resuscitation Council UK. 2021. Available from: https://www.resus.org.uk/library/2021-resuscitation-guidelines/newborn-resuscitation-and-support-transition-infants-birth.
24. Soltani H, Poulose TA, Hutchon DR. Placental cord drainage after vaginal delivery as part of the management of the third stage of labour. *Cochrane Database Syst Rev*. 2011. Issue 9. Art. no.: CD004665.

CHAPTER 6

Monitoring Labour

Partograph to Labour Care Guide

ANANDHI VENKATESAN, UMA RAM

INTRODUCTION

Labour and childbirth are natural biological processes with relatively few complications in most healthy women. However, for some women, the process is more difficult, and medical assistance may be necessary to ensure safe delivery.

Globally, labour complications account for more than a third of all maternal deaths, half of all stillbirths, and a quarter of all neonatal deaths [1,2]. These severe outcomes are usually seen when women deliver alone or with the assistance of semi-skilled birth attendants. In India, women giving birth at home without access to skilled care are a significant cause for concern [3].

Some adverse outcomes are the result of inadequate monitoring and delays in interventions and can be prevented by interventions undertaken in a timely manner [4]. Hence, it is necessary to have a tool to track the progress of labour, monitor the mother and child, and identify women in need of assistance during labour.

The **partograph** (or **partogram**) is a visual record of the progress of labour. Such monitoring helps to ensure the safety of both mother and baby. However, a systematic review of the Cochrane Database [5] found no conclusive evidence to support the effectiveness of the partograph in standard labour management.

This chapter provides an overview of the evolution of the traditional partograph and an understanding of how it evolved into a **Labour Care Guide**. Additionally, this chapter provides guidance on how to use the WHO Labour Care Guide effectively in managing labour.

EVOLUTION OF THE PARTOGRAPH

Friedman Labour Curve

In 1954, Friedman published the first labour progression curve, which influenced obstetric practice for over five decades [6]. Until the mid-1950s, the progress of labour was primarily evaluated by its duration. According to Friedman, normal cervical dilatation during the active phase was 1.2 cm/hour for nulliparous women and 1.5 cm/hour for multiparous women. **If cervical dilatation was slower than 1 cm/hour, labour was considered to be protracted** or **prolonged**.

Nevertheless, this approach was ineffective in identifying when interventions were necessary or optimal. Based on Friedman's original work, Philpott and Castle developed the partograph nearly two decades later [7,8].

The 1 cm of dilatation per hour 'rule' for what was considered 'normal labour' led to O'Driscoll and colleagues proposing the **'active management of labour'** (AML) protocol during the 1970s. AML was a set of interventions suggested for women whose labour did not advance at the rate considered normal [9,10].

The linear 1 cm per hour cervical dilatation rate has been found to be unrealistic in many populations [11]. Its general application may lead to unnecessary interventions during labour. Recent studies have questioned the Friedman curve, and contemporary data has produced a smoother curve, with the acceleration of cervical dilatation in the active stage, starting at 5–6 cm [12] (see **Chapter 4**, *Management of the first and second stages of normal labour*).

Key Point

Friedman's labour progression curve, which was the first to be published, was based on observations noted from 500 women, 73% of whom were moderately or deeply sedated. The rate of dilatation of 1 cm per hour has since been questioned, and the Friedman curve is now considered flawed.

WHO Partographs

Composite partograph

Following the WHO Safe Motherhood initiative, the WHO Composite Partograph (Fig. 6.1) was introduced in 1994, which included a latent phase of eight hours and an active phase that began at 3 cm. The graph depicted the duration of labour in hours (X axis) and cervical dilatation in centimetres (Y axis). Additionally, maternal and fetal parameters were recorded, including the level of the presenting part (in fifths of the fetal head palpable above the pelvic brim) rather than the station, the fetal heart rate, the frequency, duration, and strength of uterine contractions, and the colour of the amniotic fluid. Moreover, maternal temperature, blood pressure, pulse rate, and drugs administered to her were also recorded.

The graph included an **alert line** with a slope of 1 cm/hour and an **action line** 4 hours to the right and parallel to the alert line. The action line indicated whether progress was satisfactory or not. The line of acceptable progress was conventionally based on the slowest 10th percentile of cervical dilatation observed in women who progressed without intervention and delivered normally. However, there was a grace period before interventions were deemed necessary—based on a parallel line placed 1–4 hours to the right of the action line. This helped identify abnormal labour, based on which, women could be referred to tertiary care centres at the appropriate time [7,8].

Drawbacks

There were difficulties in demonstrating the transition from the latent to active phase in this partograph. Prolonged latent phases resulted in increased interventions in the form of cesarean sections.

Modified partograph

A modified WHO partograph (Fig. 6.2) was introduced by WHO in 2000 to overcome the difficulty of identifying the latent phase. In this graph, latent phase representation was omitted, and the active phase started at 4 cm. When the action line is crossed, the labour is assessed, and augmentation with oxytocin is started, if indicated.

It is to be noted that the **alert line** and **action line** are recorded when the woman is in the active phase of labour. The WHO partograph does not differentiate between nulliparous and multiparous women.

Colour-coded partograph

The WHO simplified partograph, with colour-coded zones, was introduced for ease of use and interpretation. The area to the left of the alert line is coloured green, representing normal progress, while the area to the right of the action line is coloured red, indicating significantly slow progress. The area between the alert and action line is coloured amber, indicating a need for vigilance.

The colour-coded partograph is more user-friendly than the composite partograph and is easier to use for documentation in busy labour wards in resource-poor areas.

RATIONALE FOR CHANGING THE PARTOGRAPH

In overcrowded labour wards in low- or middle-income countries (LMICs), intrapartum monitoring with the partograph is a time-consuming task that is often not performed or is performed incorrectly [13]. Skilled birth attendants have also

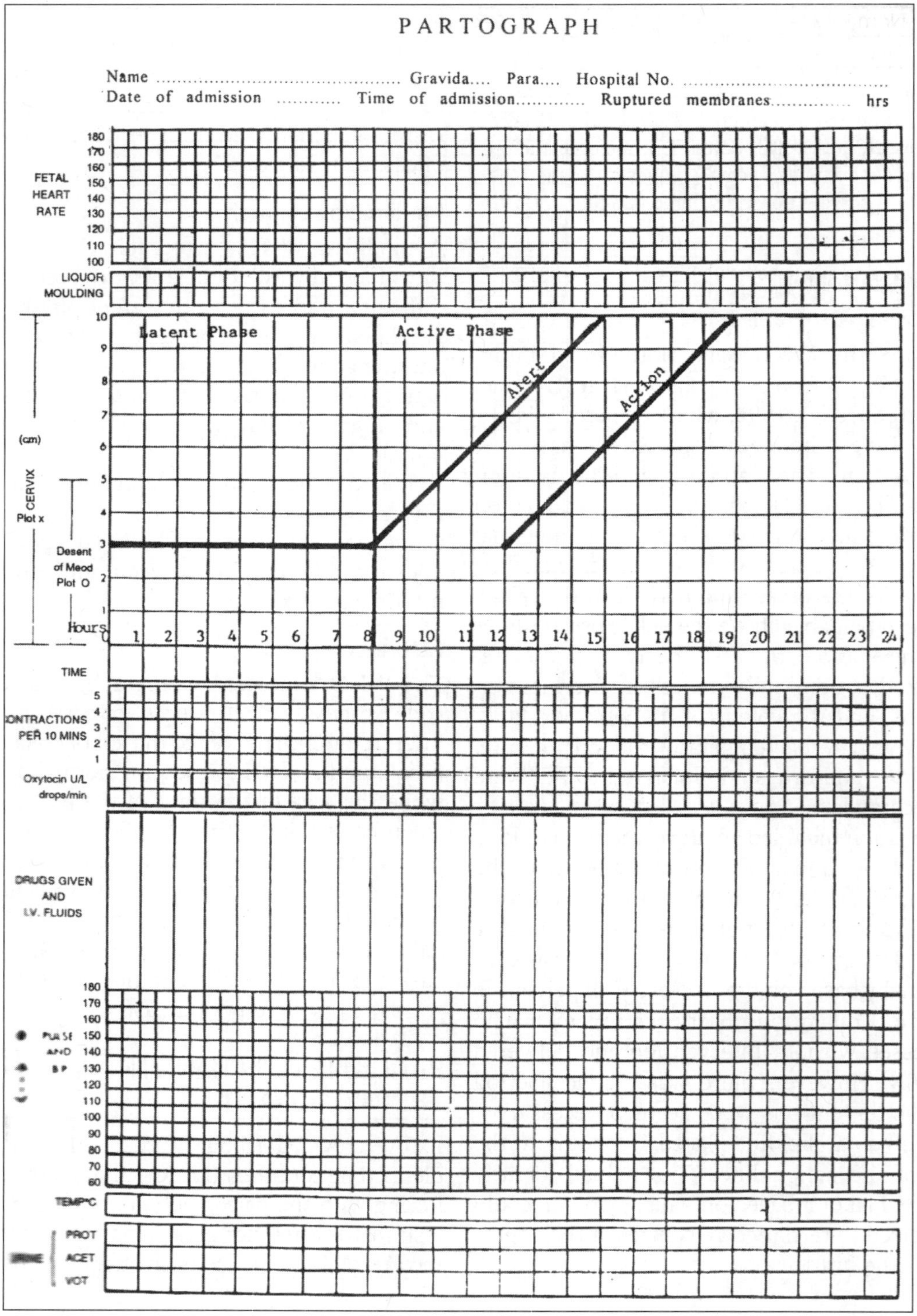

Fig. 6.1 The World Health Organization's composite partograph

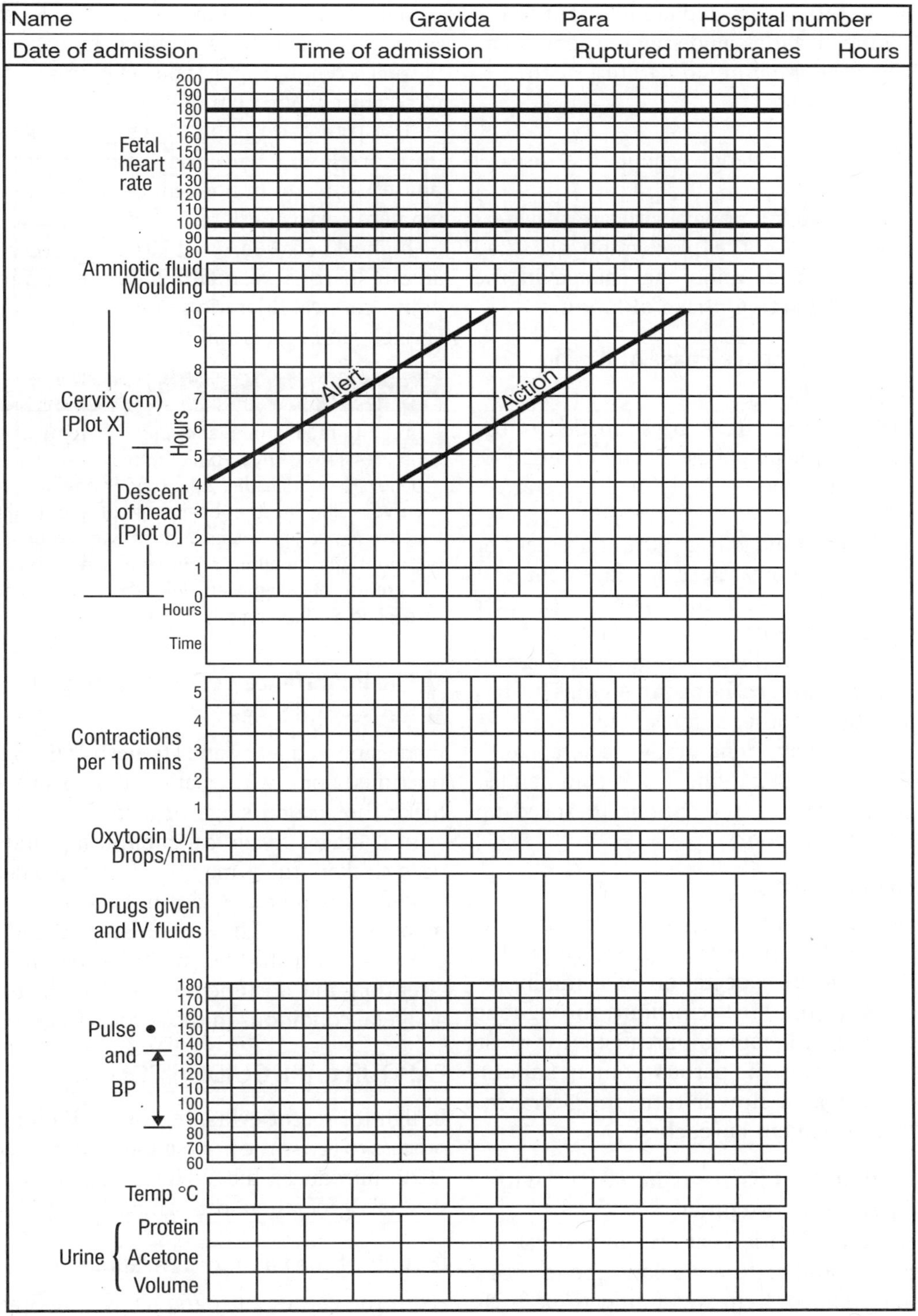

Fig. 6.2 The World Health Organization's modified partograph

not 'bought into' its use and are reluctant to use it [14]. Some obstacles hindering the appropriate use of the partograph in LMICs are [15,16]:

- Time constraints
- Staff shortages
- Insufficient knowledge about the use of partographs
- Negative attitude among healthcare providers

The evolution of the partograph also had to take into consideration the change in the definition of the **active phase of labour**.

Redefining the Active Phase of the First Stage of Labour

Significant changes have been made to the definition of the active phase of labour. In 2000, Rouse and colleagues [17] defined the start of the active phase at:

- 4 cm dilatation and at least 90% effacement **or**
- 5 cm dilatation regardless of effacement

In 2010, Zhang and colleagues [12], after studying contemporary patterns of labour, defined the start of the active phase at **6 cm of cervical dilatation, rather than 4 cm.** This has been validated by other studies [18].

Since labour may not naturally accelerate until 5 cm of cervical dilatation, it is recommended not to use medical interventions to speed up labour before this point.

Duration of the first stage

A recent systematic review of seven observational studies that included 99,971 births [19] concluded that an expectation of a minimum cervical dilatation of 1 cm/hour throughout the first stage of labour is unrealistic for most healthy nulliparous and parous women. **Labour will progress at a slower rate until cervical dilatation of 5–6 cm is reached.**

Cervical dilatation patterns in women with normal perinatal outcomes

When cervical dilatation patterns in nulliparous women were studied, the median time to progress from 2 cm to 3 cm was found to be 5.28 hours. This reduces to 2 hours to dilate from 3 to 4 cm and 1.42 hours from 4 to 5 cm [20]. Some women may take much longer; even in parous women, it may take as long as 14 hours to advance from 3 cm to 4 cm.

The transition point at which labour speeds up (correlating with the onset of the 'active phase') is 5 cm. In both nulliparous and parous women, cervical dilatation rates were found to be highest between 7 and 10 cm and were higher among parous women. Before the transition point, cervical dilatation patterns appear highly variable and individual.

> **Key Point**
>
> In both nulliparous and parous women, labour progression is hyperbolic rather than linear (as believed for decades following Friedman's labour curve)—slow at the beginning of the traditional active phase and faster in the advanced first stage. Labour abnormalities requiring intervention should therefore be diagnosed only after the woman has reached a dilatation of 5–6 cm [18,21,22].

The Importance of Documenting the Second Stage

Increasing frequency and strength of uterine contractions along with maternal expulsive efforts make the second stage of labour a particularly critical stage. If clinical monitoring and alertness slacken, there may be poor outcomes. The modified partograph does not include or document progress in the second stage of labour. In contrast, the Labour Care Guide requires close attention and documentation of both maternal and fetal conditions in the second stage.

LABOUR CARE GUIDE (LCG)

In light of recent evidence, the WHO initiated a process to revise the partograph, and in December 2020, introduced the WHO Labour Care Guide, the 'next generation' partograph (Fig. 6.3).

Aims of the Labour Care Guide

As in the earlier partographs, the LCG aims to monitor and document the well-being of the woman, the fetus, and the progress of labour. The most important difference is that the documentation on the LCG starts when the woman has reached a cervical dilatation of 5 cm (active phase of the first stage of labour).

For whom should the LCG be used?

The LCG can be used for all healthy pregnant women who are in labour. High-risk women may need extra monitoring and care. When women arrive in the labour unit, they should undergo an initial assessment to see if labour has truly started and to determine the stage of labour.

When should documentation start on the LCG?

Documentation should be started on the LCG when the woman enters the active phase of the first stage of labour (≥5 cm cervical dilatation), regardless of her parity and membrane status. Although the LCG should not be started during the latent phase, the woman should be monitored and receive labour support and care during this stage. Fetal well-being too should be monitored and documented in the latent phase.

Where should the LCG be used?

It can be used at all levels of care in health-care facilities.

LCG vs. WHO's Modified Partograph

The chief differences between the modified WHO partograph and the LCG are listed in Table 6.1.

Table 6.1 Differences between WHO's modified partograph and the Labour Care Guide [24]

Modified WHO partograph	WHO Labour Care Guide
The active phase begins at a cervical dilatation of 4 cm	The active phase starts from 5 cm of cervical dilatation
The 'alert' and 'action' lines are fixed at 1 cm/hour	Every centimetre of cervical dilatation has a time limit based on evidence
There is no provision for the monitoring of the second stage	There is a separate section for the second stage, and monitoring is increased
A lack of documentation of supportive care	Labour companionship, oral fluid intake, pain relief, and posture are clearly recorded
Keeps track of uterine contraction strength, duration, and frequency	• Measures the duration and frequency of uterine contractions • Strength of uterine contractions is no longer recorded as it is hard to quantify and standardise clinically
Except for cervical dilatation alerts and action lines, there is no clear requirement to respond to deviations from expected observations	Ensures that any deviation from expected observations of any labour parameter is highlighted, and the provider records the corresponding response

LCG USE AND DOCUMENTATION

Sections of the LCG

The LCG has seven sections (Fig. 6.3). Section 1 is completed at confirmation of the active phase of labour. Sections 2–7 of the LCG are completed as labour progresses. All observations are documented on a **horizontal time axis** and a **vertical reference values axis** to look for any deviation from the normal. In addition, the column provided for the **second stage allows the user** to continue recording observations from the first stage, except for cervical dilatation assessments, which end with the first stage.

For every observation, an alert parameter has been defined. If any observation reflects an alert parameter, a shared decision-making process is necessary, i.e., a decision is made after discussing the current situation with the woman in labour and her birth companion.

Key Point

The focus of the LCG is on action-oriented labour and shared decision-making with the labouring woman.

Assessment and Implementation

A health provider should use a consistent approach to ensure that the LCG is applied

WHO LABOUR CARE GUIDE

Section 1

Name	Parity	Labour onset	Active labour diagnosis [Date]
Ruptured membranes [Date	Time]		Risk factors

Alert Column

Section			Time	:	:	:	:	:	:	:	:	:	:	:	:	:	:	:
			Hours	1	2	3	4	5	6	7	8	9	10	11	12	1	2	3
			ALERT	← ACTIVE FIRST STAGE →												← SECOND STAGE →		
Section 2	SUPPORTIVE CARE	Companion	N															
		Pain relief	N															
		Oral fluid	N															
		Posture	SP															
Section 3	BABY	Baseline FHR	<110, ≥160															
		FHR deceleration	L															
		Amniotic fluid	M+++, B															
		Fetal position	P, T															
		Caput	+++															
		Moulding	+++															
Section 4	WOMAN	Pulse	<60, ≥120															
		Systolic BP	<80, ≥140															
		Diastolic BP	≥90															
		Temperature °C	<35.0, ≥37.5															
		Urine	P+++, A++															
Section 5	LABOUR PROGRESS	Contractions per 10 min	≤2, >5															
		Duration of contractions	<20, >60															
		Cervix [Plot X] 10																
		9	≥2h													In active first stage, plot 'X' to record cervical dilatation. Alert triggered when lag time for current cervical dilatation is exceeded with no progress. In second stage, insert 'P' to indicate when pushing begins.		
		8	≥2.5h															
		7	≥3h															
		6	≥5h															
		5	≥6h															
		Descent [Plot 0] 5																
		4																
		3																
		2																
		1																
		0																
Section 6	MEDICATION	Oxytocin (U/L, drops/min)	<60, ≥120															
		Medicine	<80, ≥140															
		IV fluids	≥90															
Section 7	SHARED DECISION-MAKING	ASSESSMENT																
		PLAN																
		INITIALS																

INSTRUCTIONS: CIRCLE ANY OBSERVATION MEETING THE CRITERIA IN THE 'ALERT' COLUMN; ALERT THE SENIOR MIDWIFE OR DOCTOR AND RECORD THE ASSESSMENT AND ACTION TAKEN. IF LABOUR EXTENDS BEYOND 12H, PLEASE CONTINUE ON A NEW LABOUR CARE GUIDE.

Abbreviations: Y – Yes, N – No, D – Declined, U – Unknown, SP – Supine, MO – Mobile, E – Early, L – Late, V – Variable, I – Intact, C – Clear, M – Meconium, B – Blood, A – Anterior, P – Posterior, T – Transverse, P+ – Protein, A+ – Acetone

Fig. 6.3 WHO Labour Care Guide (from WHO Labour Care Guide User's Manual [23])

systematically. This is done by using the following plan:

- ***Assess:*** Check the woman's and baby's well-being and labour progress
- ***Record:*** Keep track of labour observations
- ***Check reference threshold:*** Compare labour observations with alert values
- ***Plan:*** Inform the woman, come to a shared decision on what interventions are necessary, and document accordingly

This approach should be used at every assessment. Observations that meet the alert values should be circled to ensure that they are not overlooked. However, reference thresholds are intended as early warning signals and do not replace expert clinical judgement. Moreover, each woman's preferences and expectations should be respected while making decisions. Decisions should be based on an overall assessment of the woman and her baby and not on individual parameters.

Time axis

On the time axis, the first row, labelled **'Time'**, indicates the actual time of each observation, while the second row, **'Hours'**, indicates how many hours have elapsed since the start of the active phase of labour (Fig. 6.4). Each column represents one clock hour in the 'Time' row. The column represents the actual time in hours and minutes.

If labour extends past 12 hours, a second LCG should be commenced. Time should be recorded using a 12-hour (am and pm) or 24-hour format (00.00 to 24.00), depending on local norms and preferences.

> **Key Point**
>
> While using the framework of the LCG, good clinical judgement and the woman's preferences should be taken into account when managing individual labour.

Section 1: Identifying information and labour characteristics at admission

This section documents the woman's name and the characteristics of labour that are important for labour management, including parity, mode of labour onset, time of diagnosis of active labour, date and time of rupture of membranes, and any risk factors associated with labour. As soon as the diagnosis of active labour is confirmed, this section should be completed.

Section 2: Supportive care

This section documents the presence of a birth companion, non-pharmacological and pharmacological pain relief measures, oral fluids, and the position of the mother. These supportive measures should be offered and evaluated continuously during labour. However, for documentation, observations should be recorded every hour. The steps required to complete Section 2 are illustrated in Fig. 6.5 and 6.6).

> **Key Point**
>
> Women and their companions should be clearly informed about any procedure performed, the results of the physical examination, and the next course of action to enable shared decision-making (see **Chapter 3**, *Respectful obstetric care and the role of a birth companion*).

↓ (at 14:00)

Time	07:00	08:00	09:00	10:00	11:00	12:00	13:00	14:00	:	:	:	:		14:05	15:05	:
Hours	1	2	3	4	5	6	7	8	9	10	11	12		1	2	3
	First stage of labour													Second stage of labour		

Fig. 6.4 Time axis indicating actual time and hours in labour—at 14:00 hours or 2.00 pm (arrow), the woman has reached full dilatation and has completed the first stage of labour

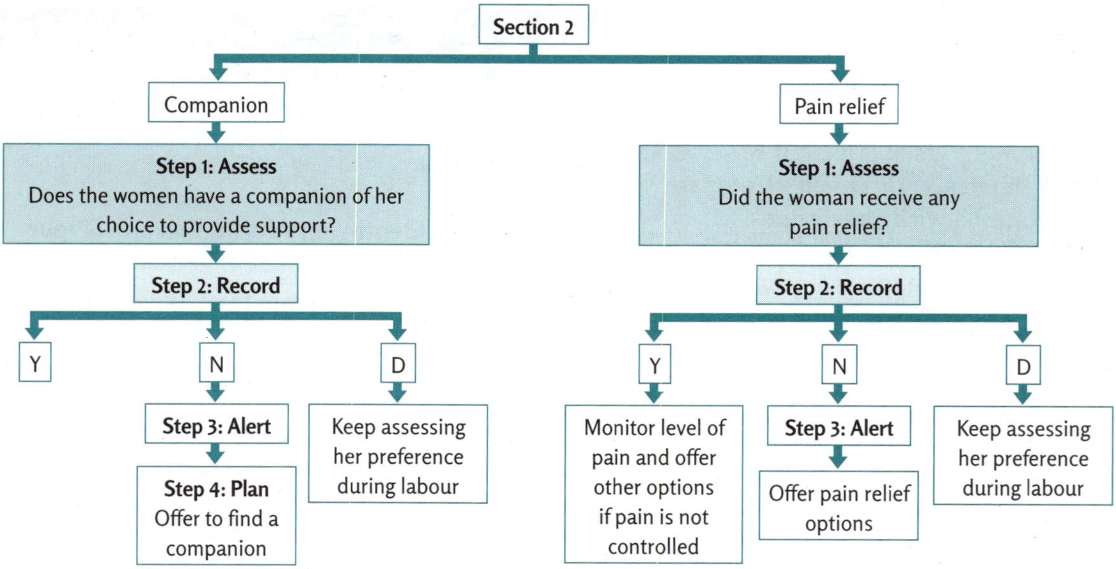

Fig. 6.5 Section 2—Recording the presence of a birth companion and the method of pain relief *Y*, yes; *N*, no; *D*, declines

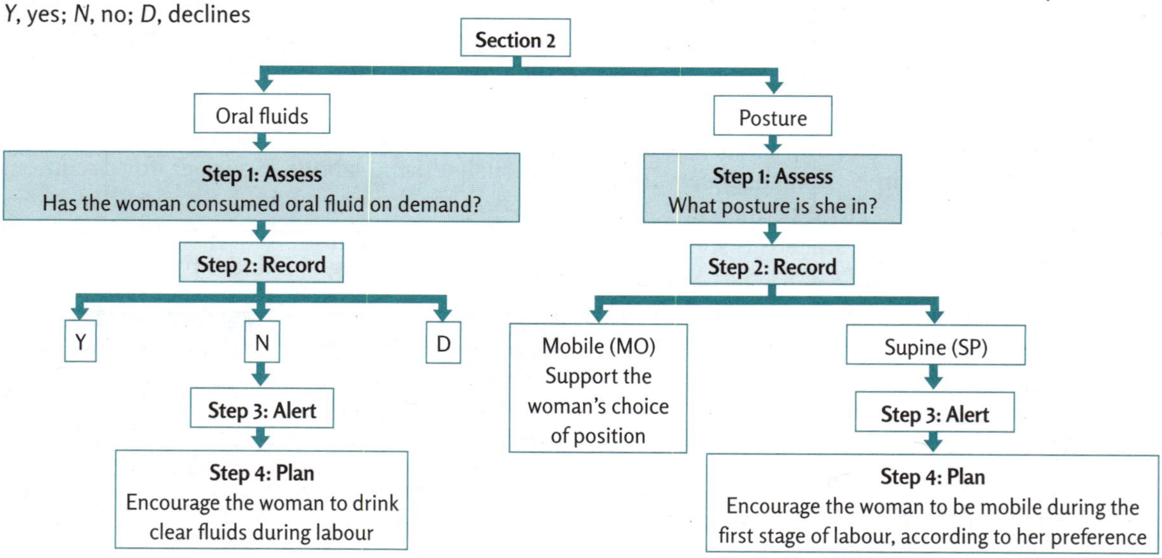

Fig. 6.6 Section 2—Recording the administration of oral fluids and mobility during the first stage of labour *Y*, yes; *N*, no; *D*, declines

Section 3: Fetal assessment

Fetal assessment is conducted every 30 minutes. Fetal heart rate monitoring is performed every 15–30 minutes, and the baseline heart rate and type of deceleration (if present) are noted (see **Chapter 8,** *Fetal surveillance in labour*). An alert is raised if FHR is <110 bpm or >160 bpm or for prolonged decelerations.

The colour of the liquor, fetal position, the presence or absence of caput and moulding are noted and compared with alert parameters. The WHO Labour Care Guide user care manual has standardised the nomenclature to be used by healthcare workers [23]. The abbreviations for recording non-numerical findings for Section 3 are presented in Tables 6.2 and 6.3.

Fig. 6.7 demonstrates how to record Sections 2 and 3 using these abbreviations.

Table 6.2 Abbreviations for non-numerical observations for Section 3 of the LCG [23] – I

Observations	Abbreviations used
FHR decelerations	N=No
	E=Early
	L=Late
	V=Variable
Fetal position	A=Any occiput-anterior position
	P=Any occiput-posterior position
	T=Any occiput-transverse position

Table 6.3 Abbreviations for non-numerical observations for Section 3 of the LCG [23] – II

Observations	Abbreviations used
Amniotic fluid	I=Intact membranes
	C=Membranes ruptured; clear fluid
	M=Meconium-stained fluid (Record as +, ++. +++ to represent non-significant, medium, and thick meconium, respectively)
	B=Bloodstained fluid
Caput	0 (None)
	+
	++
	+++ (Marked)
Moulding	0 (None)
	+ (Sutures apposed)
	++ (Sutures overlapping but reducible)
	+++ (Sutures overlapping and non-reducible)

WHO LABOUR CARE GUIDE

Name: **Parity** 1 **Labour onset** INDUCED **Active labour diagnosis Date:** 13/09/2023

Ruptured membranes {Date 13/09/2023 **Time** 09:00**}** **Risk factors** GESTATIONAL DIABETES MELLITUS

ACTIVE FIRST STAGE

		Time	07:00	08:00	09:00	10:00	11:00	12:00	13:00	14:00	:	:	:	:
		Hours	1	2	3	4	5	6	7	8	9	10	11	12
		ALERT												
SUPPORTIVE CARE	Companion	N	(N)	(N)	Y	Y	Y	Y	Y	Y				
	Pain relief	N	(N)	(N)	Y	Y	Y	Y	Y	Y				
	Oral fluid	N	Y	Y	Y	Y	Y	Y	Y	Y				
	Posture	SP	MO	(SP)	(SP)	MO	MO	(SP)	(SP)	(SP)				
BABY	Baseline FHR	<110, ≥160	138, 140	136, 142	136, 144	134, 150	152, 148	140, 138	136, 130	142, 144				
	FHR deceleration	L	N, N	V, N	N, N	V, N	N, N	N, N	N, N	N, N				
	Amniotic fluid	M+++, B	I		C				C	C				
	Fetal position	P, T	(P)		(P)				(T)	(T)				
	Caput	+++	O		O				O	O				
	Moulding	+++	O		O				O	O				

SECOND STAGE

	14:05		15:05		:	
Hours	1		2		3	
Companion	Y		Y			
Pain relief	Y		Y			
Oral fluid	Y		Y			
Posture	(SP)		(SP)			
Baseline FHR	136, 132	144, 142	138, 140	136, 134		
FHR deceleration	N, N	E, E	E, E	E, E		
Amniotic fluid				C		
Fetal position				A		
Caput				O		
Moulding				O		

Fig. 6.7 Completed Sections 2 and 3, which document information regarding the supportive care provided to the woman and fetal well-being (*Data courtesy*: Seethapathy Clinic and Hospital, Chennai)

Section 4: Care of the woman

The woman's well-being is documented with monitoring of pulse, blood pressure, temperature, and urine output, which are recorded every four hours. They are compared with alert parameters.

The alert thresholds are presented in Table 6.4. If an alert threshold is reached, an intervention should be initiated to correct the underlying cause. A senior obstetrician should be informed. An example of how to record Section 4 is shown in Fig. 6.8.

Table 6.4 Alert parameters for completing Section 4 of the LCG (adapted from the WHO LCG manual [23])

Monitored parameter	Alert thresholds
Pulse	<60 bpm, ≥120 bpm
Systolic BP	<80 mmHg, ≥140 mmHg
Diastolic BP	≥90 mmHg
Temperature	<35.0°C, ≥37.5°C
Urine	Presence of 2+ proteinuria or 2+ ketonuria

BP, blood pressure; *bpm*, beats per minute

WHO LABOUR CARE GUIDE

Name: **Parity 1** **Labour onset** INDUCED **Active labour diagnosis** **Date:** 13/09/2023

Ruptured membranes {Date 13/09/2023 **Time** 09:00**}** **Risk factors** GESTATIONAL DIABETES MELLITUS

ACTIVE FIRST STAGE

		Time	07:00	08:00	09:00	10:00	11:00	12:00	13:00	14:00	:	:	:	:
		Hours	1	2	3	4	5	6	7	8	9	10	11	12
		ALERT												
SUPPORTIVE CARE	Companion	N	(N)	(N)	Y	Y	Y	Y	Y	Y				
	Pain relief	N	(N)	(N)	Y	Y	Y	Y	Y	Y				
	Oral fluid	N	Y	Y	Y	Y	Y	Y	Y	Y				
	Posture	SP	MO	(SP)	(SP)	MO	MO	(SP)	(SP)	(SP)				
BABY	Baseline FHR	<110, ≥160	138, 140	136, 142	136, 144	134, 150	152, 148	140, 138	136, 130	142, 144				
	FHR deceleration	L	N, N	V, N	N, N	V, N	N, N	N, N	N, N	N, N				
	Amniotic fluid	M+++, B	I		C				C	C				
	Fetal position	P, T	(P)		(P)				(T)	(T)				
	Caput	+++	O		O				O	O				
	Moulding	+++	O		O				O	O				
WOMAN	Pulse	<60, ≥120	84				94							
	Systolic BP	<80, ≥140	116				126							
	Diastolic BP	≥90	86				88							
	Temperature °C	<35.0, ≥37.5	36.5				36.9							
	Urine	P++, A++	–/–				–/–							

SECOND STAGE

		14:05	15:05	:
	Hours	1	2	3
SUPPORTIVE CARE	Companion	Y	Y	
	Pain relief	Y	Y	
	Oral fluid	Y	Y	
	Posture	(SP)	(SP)	
BABY	Baseline FHR	136, 132; 144, 142	138, 140; 136, 134	
	FHR deceleration	N, N; E, E	E, E; E, E	
	Amniotic fluid		C	
	Fetal position		A	
	Caput		O	
	Moulding		O	
WOMAN	Pulse			
	Systolic BP			
	Diastolic BP			
	Temperature °C			
	Urine			

Fig. 6.8 Completed Section 4, which documents information regarding maternal well-being (*Data courtesy:* Seethapathy Clinic and Hospital, Chennai)

Section 5: Labour progress

This section records the progress of labour and is extremely useful in identifying abnormal progression. Labour progress is monitored by documenting the frequency and duration of contractions, cervical dilatation, and the descent of the baby's head (see **Chapter 4**). Any abnormal finding or alert parameter is verified for the next 10 minutes. A persistent alert parameter warrants action.

Findings are marked as **X** in the cells corresponding to **time** and **cervical dilatation** during the active first stage of labour. During the second stage, **P** is used to indicate the beginning of **pushing**. As a general rule, a vaginal examination should be performed every four hours unless otherwise indicated. Descent is measured abdominally and marked as **O** in the cells corresponding to the **time** and **level of descent**.

Fetal station is described as 5/5, 4/5, 3/5, 2/5, 1/5, and 0/5 by abdominal palpation. Assessment of fetal station should be performed before the vaginal examination and repeated every four hours. If the duration of the active phase exceeds 12 hours, another LCG can be added. Table 6.5 lists the alert values for the progress of labour in Section 5.

An example of how to record Section 5 is shown in Fig. 6.9.

Table 6.5 Alert values for the progress of labour, which are entered in Section 5 of the LCG [23]

Monitored parameter	Alert thresholds
Contractions per ten minutes	<2, >5
Duration of contraction	<20 seconds, >60 seconds
Cervical dilatation—first stage	5 cm = ≥6 h (cervical dilatation remains at 5 cm for 6 or more hours)
	6 cm = ≥5 h (cervical dilatation remains at 6 cm for 5 or more hours)
	7 cm = ≥3 h (cervical dilatation remains at 7 cm for 3 or more hours)
	8 cm = ≥2.5 h (cervical dilatation remains at 8 cm for 2.5 or more hours)
	9 cm = ≥2 h (cervical dilatation remains at 9 cm for 2 or more hours)
Duration of second stage	≥3 h in nulliparous women
	≥2 h in multiparous women

Note: There are no thresholds described for the descent of the fetal head.

LABOUR PROGRESS

Contractions per 10 min		≥2, >5	5 ¦ 4	4 ¦ 2	2 ¦ 3	4 ¦ 4	4 ¦ 4	4 ¦ 4	4 ¦ 5	4 ¦ 4				
Duration of contractions		≥20, >60	45 ¦ 20	15 ¦ 10	15 ¦ 15	40 ¦ 45	25 ¦ 30	40 ¦ 50	45 ¦ 50	45 ¦ 50				
Cervix B [Plot X]	10									X				
	9	≥2h												
	8	≥2.5h							X					
	7	≥3h												
	6	≥5h												
	5	≥6h	X		X									
Descent [Plot O]	5													
	4		O											
	3				O									
	2													
	1								O					
	0									O				

Contractions per 10 min	4 ¦ 4	5 ¦ 4	4 ¦ 4	4 ¦ 4		
Duration of contractions	45 ¦ 40	45 ¦ 50	45 ¦ 40	50 ¦ 50		
Pushing	P ¦ P	P ¦ P	P ¦ P	P ¦ P		
Descent 5						
Descent 4						
Descent 3						
Descent 2						
Descent 1						
Descent 0	O					

In active first stage, plot X to record cervical dilatation. Alert triggered when lag time for current cervical dilatation is exceeded with no progress. In second stage, insert P to indicate when pushing begins.

Fig. 6.9 Completed Section 5, which documents information regarding the progress of labour (*Data courtesy*: Seethapathy Clinic and Hospital, Chennai)

For further details regarding the management of abnormal progression of labour, see **Chapter 11**, *Abnormalities in the latent phase and the first stage of labour,* and **Chapter 12**, *Abnormalities in the second stage of labour*.

Section 6: Medication

This section records the administration of IV fluids and the medications the woman receives in labour, especially oxytocin. 'Y' denotes 'yes' and 'N' denotes 'no' on the LCG. The amount of oxytocin administered is recorded in units per litre (U/L) and/or drops per minute (drops/min). The name, dosage, and route of administration of any further medication that is being administered to the woman during the active first or second stage of labour is documented.

Section 7: Shared decision-making

This section aims to facilitate continuous communication with the woman and her birth companion using simple terms. Communication should be in a language that the woman understands. Clear explanations of procedures, their intended purpose, and the findings of the examinations should be provided to the woman, and the subsequent course of action made clear to enable shared decision-making. It is important to take the woman's preference into consideration and allow her to make an informed decision.

The overall assessment and any additional findings important for labour monitoring are recorded. The plan following the assessment is recorded and may include the following:

- Continuation of routine monitoring
- Augmentation of labour with oxytocin infusion
- Any procedures such as artificial rupture of membranes
- Assisted birth with vacuum or forceps
- The need for CTG monitoring or review of CTG in a specified time period
- Cesarean section

Fig. 6.10 shows a completed Labour Care Guide chart.

Evaluating the LCG

To evaluate the usability, acceptability, and feasibility of the WHO LCG, a multicountry evaluation was conducted among maternity care practitioners in clinical settings [25].

Providers' experience

The majority of practitioners who evaluated the LCG found the following:

- It improved their ability to meet women's unique labour needs.
- It improved the targeting of interventions and reduced unnecessary interventions.
- It facilitated critical thinking and clinical handovers.
- Although some found it challenging initially, they reported that, with usage, they became comfortable with the new tool.
- The numerical representation was found to be more precise and accurate but also more time-consuming than the modified WHO partograph.
- The lack of alerts and action lines made it harder to understand how to respond to the information on the LCG; a greater understanding of the LCG was said to be required for its effective use.
- There was not enough space to make notes.
- The LCG helped practitioners provide supportive, patient-centred care, thus strengthening their relationships with women during birth.

Satisfaction scores

On completing questionnaires about their experiences with the LCG, practitioners agreed or strongly agreed that they were able to use it (96%) and complete it correctly (94.2%). In their final assessment, 75.7% of practitioners agreed they were satisfied with the LCG design overall. Usability scores ranged from 22.5 to 95, with a median score of 67.5 [25].

WHO LABOUR CARE GUIDE

Name: **Parity** 1 **Labour onset** INDUCED **Active labour diagnosis Date:** 13/09/2023

Ruptured membranes {Date 13/09/2023 **Time** 09:00**}** **Risk factors** GESTATIONAL DIABETES MELLITUS

ACTIVE FIRST STAGE

		ALERT	07:00	08:00	09:00	10:00	11:00	12:00	13:00	14:00	:	:	:	:
	Hours		1	2	3	4	5	6	7	8	9	10	11	12
SUPPORTIVE CARE	Companion	N	(N)	(N)	Y	Y	Y	Y	Y	Y				
	Pain relief	N	(N)	(N)	Y	Y	Y	Y	Y	Y				
	Oral fluid	N	Y	Y	Y	Y	Y	Y	Y	Y				
	Posture	SP	MO	(SP)	(SP)	MO	MO	(SP)	(SP)	(SP)				
BABY	Baseline FHR	<110, ≥160	138, 140	136, 142	136, 144	134, 150	152, 148	140, 138	136, 130	142, 144				
	FHR deceleration	L	N, N	V, N	N, N	V, N	N, N	N, N	N, N	N, N				
	Amniotic fluid	M+++, B	I		C				C	C				
	Fetal position	P, T	(P)		(P)				**T**	**T**				
	Caput	+++	O		O				O	O				
	Moulding	+++	O		O				O	O				
WOMAN	Pulse	<60, ≥120	84				94							
	Systolic BP	<80, ≥140	116				126							
	Diastolic BP	≥90	86				88							
	Temperature °C	<35.0, ≥37.5	36.5				36.9							
	Urine	P++, A++	–/–				–/–							
LABOUR PROGRESS	Contractions per 10 min	≥2, >5	5, 4	4, 2	2, 3	4, 4	4, 4	4, 4	4, 5	4, 4				
	Duration of contractions	≥20, >60	45, 20	15, 10	15, 15	40, 45	25, 30	40, 50	45, 50	45, 50				
	Cervix [Plot X] 10									X				
	9	≥2h												
	8	≥2.5h							X					
	7	≥3h												
	6	≥5h												
	5	≥6h	X		X									
	Descent [Plot O] 5													
	4		O											
	3				O									
	2													
	1								O					
	0									O				
MEDICATION	Oxytocin (U/l, drops/min)		N	N	8	16	16	16	16	16				
	Medicine		N	N	N	N	N	N	N	N				
	IV fluids		N	N	N	N	N	N	N	N				
SHARED DECISION-MAKING	ASSESSMENT		PAIN RELIEF REQUIRED	PAIN RELIEF REQUIRED	CONTRACTIONS NOT ADEQUATE	NORMAL PROGRESS	NORMAL PROGRESS	NORMAL PROGRESS	NORMAL PROGRESS	NORMAL PROGRESS				
	PLAN		CONTINUOUS FETAL HEARTRATE MONITORING	EPIDURAL OFFERED	ARTIFICIAL RUPTURE OF MEMBRANES & SYNTOCINON AUGMENTATION		CONTINUOUS FETAL HEART RATE MONITORING		CONTINUOUS FETAL HEART RATE MONITORING					
	INITIALS		LA	LA	SR	SR	SR	SR	SR	SR				

SECOND STAGE

	14:05	15:05	:
Hours	1	2	3
Companion	Y	Y	BIRTH
Pain relief	Y	Y	
Oral fluid	Y	Y	
Posture	(SP)	(SP)	
Baseline FHR	136, 132 / 144, 142	138, 140 / 136, 134	
FHR deceleration	N, N / E, E	E, E / E, E	
Amniotic fluid		C	
Fetal position		A	
Caput		O	
Moulding		O	
Pulse			
Systolic BP			
Diastolic BP			
Temperature °C			
Urine			
Contractions per 10 min	4, 4 / 5, 4	4, 4 / 4, 4	
Duration of contractions	45, 40 / 45, 50	45, 40 / 50, 50	
Pushing	P, P / P, P	P, P / P, P	
Descent 0	O		
Oxytocin (U/l, drops/min)	16	16	
Medicine	N	N	
IV fluids	N	N	
ASSESSMENT	NORMAL PROGRESS	NORMAL PROGRESS	
PLAN	ENCOURAGE PUSHING	FETAL HEARTRATE MONITORING ENCOURAGE PUSHING	
INITIALS	SR	SR	

In active first stage, plot X to record cervical dilatation. Alert triggered when lag time for current cervical dilatation is exceeded with no progress. In second stage, insert P to indicate when pushing begins.

Fig. 6.10 A completed LCG, which has documented the progress of labour, including interventions and outcomes (*Data courtesy:* Seethapathy Clinic and Hospital, Chennai)

Unanswered questions

The LCG makes provisions for documentation only after the onset of active labour, which is at 5 cm. There are no provisions for the monitoring of women until they reach this point in labour. In many busy units, this may result in a large number of women with regular contractions who may be admitted to the labour unit with inadequate monitoring. More importantly, there is no guidance on how to identify a protracted latent phase, how to manage the same, and how and where to provide care for women who request pain relief or have fetal heart rate abnormalities at this early phase of labour.

Strategies of LCG Implementation in Labour Wards

To ensure the successful implementation and effective management of the LCG, both residents and staff nurses should be trained in its usage. The results of the implementation of the guide should be audited using indicators such as satisfaction rates, completion rates, neonatal outcomes, and cesarean rates. Feedback should also be gathered from staff, women who have undergone labour, and their families to ensure that the guide is meeting its objectives.

CONCLUSION

Over the last 50 years, significant changes have been made in how evidence-based, respectful intrapartum care can be provided for the labouring woman. As a tool to monitor labour progress, the partograph has undergone many changes since its introduction in the 1970s. The WHO Labour Care Guide is the culmination of research, knowledge synthesis, consultation, field testing, and refinement in our understanding of the normal progress of labour.

REFERENCES

1. Say L, Chou D, Gemmill A, Tunçalp Ö, Moller AB, Daniels J, Gülmezoglu AM, Temmerman M, Alkema L. Global causes of maternal death: A WHO systematic analysis. *Lancet Glob Health*. 2014. 2(6):e323–33.
2. Lawn JE, Blencowe H, Waiswa P, Amouzou A, Mathers C, Hogan D, et al. Lancet's Ending Preventable Stillbirths Series study group. Lancet Stillbirth Epidemiology investigator group. Stillbirths: Rates, risk factors, and acceleration towards 2030. *Lancet*. 2016. 387(10018): 587–603.
3. Ou CY, Yasmin M, Ussatayeva G, Lee MS, Dalal K. Maternal delivery at home: Issues in India. *Adv Ther*. 2021. 38(1):386–398.
4. World Health Organization. Trends in maternal mortality 2000 to 2017: Estimates by WHO, UNICEF, UNFPA, World Bank Group and the United Nations Population Division: Executive summary. 2019. WHO, Geneva. Available at https://iris.who.int/handle/10665/327596.
5. Lavender T, Cuthbert A, Smyth RM. Effect of partograph use on outcomes for women in spontaneous labour at term and their babies. *Cochrane Database Syst Rev*. 2018. Issue 8. Art. No.:CD005461.
6. Friedman E. The graphic analysis of labor. *Am J Obstet Gynecol*. 1954. 68(6):1568–75.
7. Philpott RH, Castle WM. Cervicographs in the management of labour in primigravidae. I. The alert line for detecting abnormal labour. *J Obstet Gynaecol Br Commonw*. 1972. 79(7):592–8.
8. Philpott RH, Castle WM. Cervicographs in the management of labour in primigravidae. II. The action line and treatment of abnormal labour. *J Obstet Gynaecol Br Commonw*. 1972. 79(7):599–602.
9. O'Driscoll K, Stronge JM, Minogue M. Active management of labour. *Br Med J*. 1973. 3(5872):135-7.
10. O'Driscoll K, Meagher D, Boylan P. *Active management of labor, the Dublin experience*. 3rd ed. 1993. Aylesbury. England: Mosby.
11. Orji E. Evaluating progress of labor in nulliparas and multiparas using the modified WHO partograph. *Int J Gynaecol Obstet*. 2008. 102(3):249–52.
12. Zhang J, Landy HJ, Branch DW, et al. Contemporary patterns of spontaneous labor with normal neonatal outcomes. *Obstet Gynecol*. 2010. 116:1281.
13. Yisma E, Dessalegn B, Astatkie A, Fesseha N. Completion of the modified World Health Organization (WHO) partograph during labour in public health institutions of Addis Ababa, Ethiopia. *Reprod Health*. 2013. 10:23.
14. Gans-Lartey F, O'Brien BA, Gyekye FO, Schopflocher D. The relationship between the use of the partograph and birth outcomes at Korle-Bu teaching hospital. *Midwifery*. 2013. 29(5):461–7.
15. Qureshi ZP, Sekadde-Kigondu C, Mutiso SM. Rapid assessment of partograph utilisation in selected maternity units in Kenya. *East Afr Med J*. 2010. 87(6):235–41.
16. Opiah MM, Ofi AB, Essien EJ, Monjok E. Knowledge and utilization of the partograph among midwives in the

Niger Delta Region of Nigeria. *Afr J Reprod Health*. 2012. 16(1):125–32.

17. Rouse DJ, Owen J, Hauth JC. Criteria for failed labor induction: Prospective evaluation of a standardized protocol. *Obstet Gynecol*. 2000. 96(5 Pt 1):671–7.
18. Caughey AB. Is Zhang the new Friedman: How should we evaluate the first stage of labor? *Semin Perinatol*. 2020. 44(2):151215.
19. Oladapo OT, Diaz V, Bonet M, Abalos E, Thwin SS, Souza H, et al. Cervical dilatation patterns of 'low-risk' women with spontaneous labour and normal perinatal outcomes: A systematic review. *BJOG*. 2018. 125(8): 944–954.
20. Oladapo OT, Souza JP, Fawole B, Mugerwa K, Perdoná G, Alves D, et al. Progression of the first stage of spontaneous labour: A prospective cohort study in two sub-Saharan African countries. *PLoS Med*. 2018. 15(1):e1002492.
21. Caughey AB, Cahill AG, Guise JM, Rouse DJ. American College of Obstetricians and Gynecologists, Society for Maternal-Fetal Medicine. Safe prevention of the primary cesarean delivery. *Am J Obstet Gynecol*. 2014. 210:179–93.
22. Abalos E, Oladapo OT, Chamillard M, Díaz V, Pasquale J, Bonet M, Souza JP, Gülmezoglu AM. Duration of spontaneous labour in 'low-risk' women with 'normal' perinatal outcomes: A systematic review. *Eur J Obstet Gynecol Reprod Biol*. 2018. 223:123–132.
23. WHO Labour Care Guide: User's manual. 2020. WHO, Geneva.
24. Hofmeyr GJ, Bernitz S, Bonet M, et al. WHO next-generation partograph: Revolutionary steps towards individualised labour care. *BJOG*. 2021. 128: 1658–1662.
25. Vogel JP, Comrie-Thomson L, Pingray V, et al. Usability, acceptability, and feasibility of the World Health Organization Labour Care Guide: A mixed-methods, multicountry evaluation. *Birth*. 2021. 48(1):66-75.

CHAPTER 7

Episiotomy: What Does the Evidence Say?

A TAMILSELVI

INTRODUCTION

Episiotomy is defined as a surgical incision to enlarge the vaginal opening for obstetrical purposes during the birth process. A common intrapartum intervention performed around the world, it involves surgical incision of the skin, subcutaneous tissue, vaginal mucosa, and perineal muscles.

Episiotomy as a means to facilitate difficult childbirth was first proposed by Ould in 1742 [1]. Once vaginal birth became a hospital-based event, episiotomy became the norm in most vaginal deliveries based on the belief that it reduced maternal and fetal morbidity before any evidence could substantiate its use in routine practice.

The true value of routine episiotomy at vaginal birth has been questioned in the past few decades, and the associated complications and outcome measures have been evaluated. Since the 1990s, several trials have assessed the short- and long-term outcomes of episiotomy in different populations and varying settings. In the last two decades, guidelines have been developed by various professional bodies with the aim of standardising the practice of episiotomy.

In this chapter, evidence regarding the current use of episiotomy, the recommended technique, the suturing principles, and the outcomes are dealt with.

PREVALENCE

The prevalence of episiotomy varies in different parts of the world; an accurate estimation of global episiotomy rates is difficult due to disparities in data collection in different countries. The prevalence of episiotomy in 11 low- and middle-income countries (LMICs), in the context of the overuse of an obstetric intervention, varied from 17.4–91.8% [2]. Within a country as well, there may be wide variations in the episiotomy rate depending on the delivery unit and its size and location and the experience of the caregiver. In India, a study calculating the prevalence rates of episiotomy across 18 tertiary care obstetric units found the rate to be 63.4%. Nulliparous women were found to be 8.8 times more likely to undergo episiotomy than multiparous women [3].

> **Key Point**
>
> In 1996, the World Health Organization (WHO) recommended an episiotomy rate of **10%** for vaginal deliveries [4]. In 2018, the new guidelines stated that routine/liberal use of episiotomy is 'not recommended', instead of categorically recommending the selective/restricted use of episiotomy. It acknowledged that though there is no evidence currently to establish the need for episiotomy in routine vaginal birth, an 'acceptable' rate of episiotomy is difficult to determine [5].

RESTRICTED USE OF EPISIOTOMY

Systematic reviews [6,7] comparing the routine and restricted use of episiotomy identified that women in the restrictive episiotomy group were more likely to have the following:

- An intact perineum with no posterior perineal lacerations
- A lower incidence of third- and fourth-degree lacerations

- Anterior labial lacerations, though these had less need for suturing
- 30% less risk of severe perineal/vaginal trauma when there was no instrumental delivery

There was similar or little effect on Apgar scores and no difference in perineal infection [7]. The severity of pain was similar in both groups at 10 days postdelivery and at three months.

Women with episiotomy were more likely to report pain with intercourse three months after delivery. There is no evidence to suggest that sexual function is improved by episiotomy or that those who have had an episiotomy are slower to resume intercourse.

Key Point

Episiotomy confers no short- or long-term benefit with regard to urinary continence, fecal continence, and pelvic floor defects. It was found to confer no benefit within three months of delivery. One study that evaluated these parameters at three years found no significant difference between the routine and restricted groups [8]. There is no data for periods longer than 3 years.

Indications for Episiotomy

An episiotomy is indicated when the caregiver believes that enlarging the birth outlet will facilitate the delivery of the fetus and benefit the woman or her baby. The clinical decision should take into consideration the potential adverse outcomes associated with the procedure.

Though there is not enough evidence to justify routine episiotomy, clinical judgement may dictate the need for an episiotomy in the situations listed below [9]:

- To expedite delivery in the presence of a non-reassuring fetal status in the second stage of labour
- To reduce the duration of the second stage in cases of maternal heart disease or severe anemia
- To gain more space for manoeuvres such as those needed for shoulder dystocia, breech delivery, and assisted vaginal delivery

Key Point

The routine use of episiotomy in vaginal deliveries should be discouraged, as no reduction in maternal or fetal morbidity has been identified with routine use. Selective or restrictive episiotomy should be practised in all labour rooms, with regular auditing of the indications for episiotomy.

TYPES OF EPISIOTOMIES

There are two main types of episiotomies in practice—**midline** and **mediolateral** episiotomy. In midline episiotomy, two fingers are placed between the presenting part and the perineum, and a vertical incision is made in the midline of the perineum, from the posterior fourchette towards the anus, up to the external anal sphincter, but not including it (Fig. 7.1). In the mediolateral type, the perineal incision starts at the midline of the posterior fourchette and continues downward and laterally, with the scissors directed towards the ipsilateral ischial tuberosity (Fig. 7.2). It can be performed either on the right or left side, depending on the preference of the birth attendant, with no advantage of one side over the other.

Mediolateral vs. Midline Episiotomy

Mediolateral episiotomy is most commonly used globally whereas midline episiotomy is more commonly practised in the United States.

- ***Mediolateral episiotomy:*** In a mediolateral episiotomy, the bulbospongiosus muscle, bulb of the vestibule, and superficial transverse perineal muscles are incised. The American College of Obstetricians and Gynecologists recommends that if an episiotomy is needed, a mediolateral episiotomy should be preferred over the midline episiotomy as the latter is associated with an increased risk of anal sphincter injury [9].
- ***Midline episiotomy:*** In a midline episiotomy, the connective tissues of the perineal body and overlying skin are incised up to the superior margin of the external anal sphincter

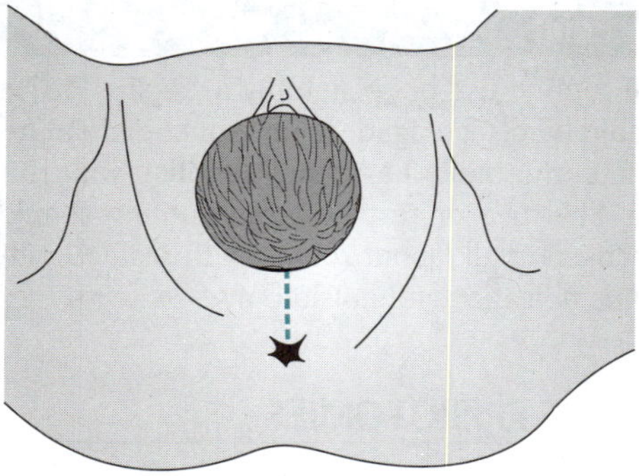

Fig. 7.1 Midline episiotomy

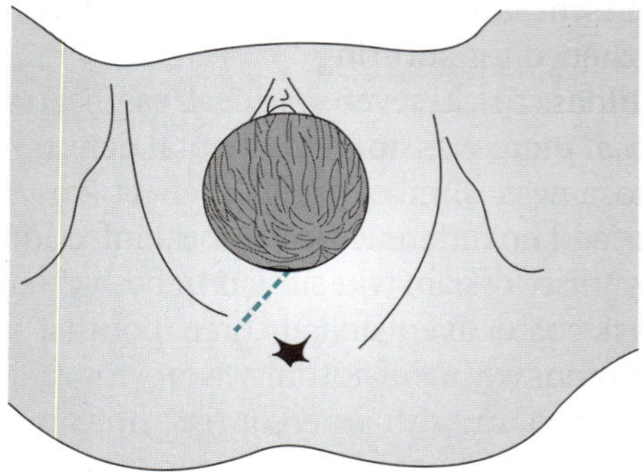

Fig. 7.2 Mediolateral episiotomy (right)

(EAS). Though the suggested advantages of median episiotomy are easy repair, better healing, lesser scarring, and better cosmetic appearance, the extension of this type of episiotomy is more likely to cause **obstetric anal sphincter injury (OASI)** [10,11,12]. OASI is an important factor in the subsequent development of anal incontinence, a devastating sequel of vaginal delivery.

There is no difference between mediolateral and midline episiotomy in outcomes such as blood loss, vaginal hematoma, and infection.

Key Point

When indicated, a mediolateral episiotomy is recommended instead of a midline one [9]. It can be performed either on the right or the left side depending on the preference of the obstetrician/midwife, though repair of an incision on the woman's left side is mechanically easier for a right-handed operator.

EPISIOTOMY TECHNIQUE

When an episiotomy is indicated, the technique adopted should adhere to certain parameters—the timing of the incision, adequate anesthesia, the appropriate type, and correct incision angle and length. A Mayo's scissor or a straight scissor is used to make the incision in a single cut. The incision should extend approximately 4 cm into the perineum.

Timing of Episiotomy

The episiotomy should be timed along with the crowning of the head in cephalic presentation, i.e., when 3–4 cm diameter of the fetal head is visible at contraction and does not recede.

Anesthesia

It is vital to administer an anesthetic before making any incision—this applies to the episiotomy incision as well. In some women, an already-sited epidural serves the purpose well. In the absence of this, either a pudendal block or local anesthetic infiltration to the perineum should be considered. Even if the woman has received epidural analgesia, supplementing it with local anesthetic infiltration is helpful in providing additional pain relief.

- ***Pudendal block:*** In this method. either 1% lidocaine or 0.5% bupivacaine, with or without adrenaline 1:200,000, is used for anesthesia. Two fingers are inserted between the fetal head and the lateral vaginal wall. The ischial spine with the adjacent sacrospinous ligament is identified by palpation. The pudendal needle with the guard is then inserted between the vagina and the fingers, directed towards the ischial spine. After setting the needle guard at 1–1.5 cm from the tip, the pudendal needle is inserted into the sacrospinous ligament within 1 cm of the ischial spine. 5–10 mL of local anesthetic is then injected (after aspiration to rule out venipuncture).

- ***Local perineal infiltration:*** 5–10 mL of 1–2% lidocaine is commonly used. Two fingers are placed between the fetal head and vagina in the direction of the intended mediolateral episiotomy. The needle is then inserted at the posterior fourchette, between the perineal skin and vaginal mucosa (not through the perineal skin) and directed laterally. Lidocaine is injected, but only after aspiration confirms no entry into a blood vessel (Fig. 7.3). The anesthetic is best administered at the height of a uterine contraction so that the woman does not feel the needle.

Angle of Episiotomy

In mediolateral episiotomy, the incision begins in the midline of the posterior fourchette and extends laterally towards the ipsilateral ischial tuberosity. The mediolateral episiotomy should begin within 3 mm of the midline in the posterior fourchette and is directed laterally at an angle of 60 degrees from the midline towards the ischial tuberosity.

Mediolateral episiotomy has not been shown to eliminate sphincter injury completely, with

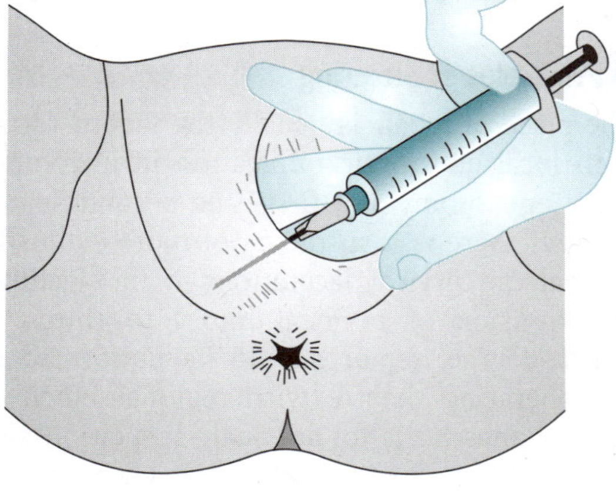

Fig. 7.3 Local anesthetic infiltration

the quoted OASI rate varying from 1.1–7.7% [6]. When the mediolateral episiotomy is performed inappropriately, it is shown to be an independent risk factor for OASI, chiefly from the angle of the episiotomy [13].

It is important to remember that the incision angle of an episiotomy and the suture angle (measured after repair) are significantly different due to the edema and deformation of perineal tissues at crowning. Studies have shown that a mediolateral episiotomy with an incision angle of 60 degrees at the time of crowning results in a suture angle of 45 degrees after repair. This is associated with a low incidence of anal sphincter injuries, anal incontinence, and perineal pain [14].

To accurately achieve the 60 degree incision angle at mediolateral episiotomy, several techniques have been evaluated, one of which is the **episcissor**, which is used in the United Kingdom (Fig. 7.4). These are adapted surgical scissors with 5 cm long blades and a guide limb mounted at the pivotal point of the blade so that the angle between the blade and the guide limb is constantly 60 degrees. With the guide limb aligned in the vertical axis and directed towards the anus at crowning, the perineal incision is made at or around 60 degrees (Fig. 7.5).

Apart from the angle of mediolateral episiotomy, other factors such as the length and depth of episiotomy also influence the risk of OASI.

> **Key Point**
>
> The incision angle of a mediolateral episiotomy should be at or around 60 degrees at the time of crowning and the length should be at least 4 cm to reduce the risk of OASI.

REPAIR OF EPISIOTOMY

Basic surgical principles and optimal technique should be observed during episiotomy repair to reduce both short- and long-term maternal morbidity. Adequate lighting and analgesia are essential. It is important that the operator

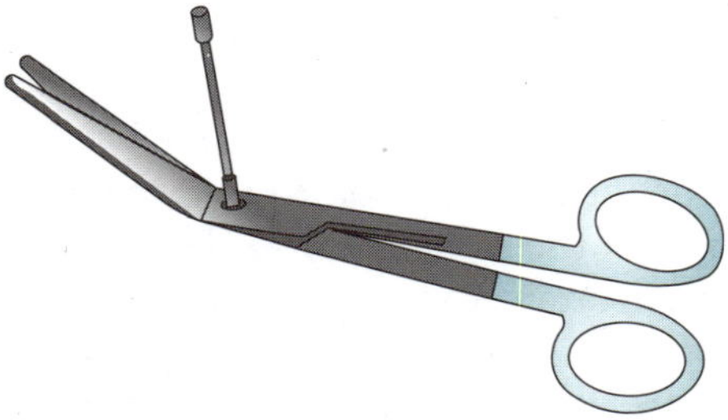

Fig. 7.4 Episcissor

is trained or, if in training, is supervised when performing an episiotomy repair.

Examination

Examination is the first step in assessing the extent of episiotomy and any other vaginal, cervical, peri-urethral, or perineal lacerations. It is a combination of visual inspection, vaginal and rectal examination, and digital rectal examination intended to assess anal sphincter integrity and rule out button-hole tears in the rectum. A systematic examination, with a focus on rectal examination has been shown to improve the detection rate of third- and fourth-degree perineal tears which are collectively referred to as obstetric anal sphincter injuries (OASI) [15].

A visual inspection of the periurethral area, the lateral vaginal walls for paravaginal tears, and the posterior vagina and perineum for extension of the episiotomy and any other perineal lacerations is followed by palpation of the external anal sphincter (EAS).

At the end of the examination, the extent of perineal injury should be classified as per the WHO classification devised by Sultan in 1999 [16] and adopted by the WHO, RCOG, and the International Consultation on Incontinence.

Under this classification, perineal injury is classified into four degrees, with third-degree injury involving the anal sphincter complex and fourth-degree injury involving the rectum along with the sphincter complex (see **Chapter 25**, *Prevention and management of perineal trauma occurring in childbirth*, for further details).

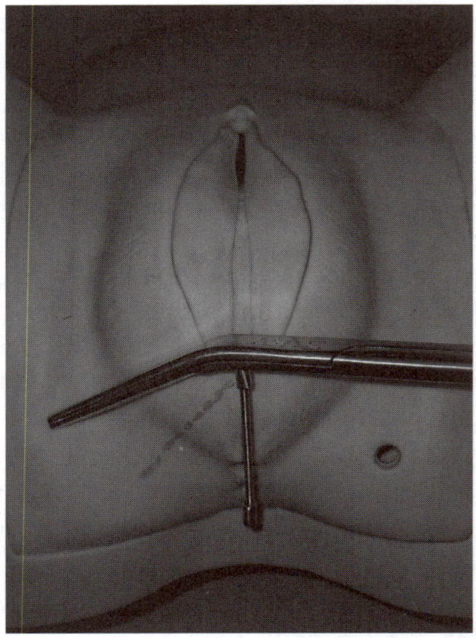

Fig. 7.5 Angle of incision with episcissor: The guide limb is aligned in the vertical axis, directed towards the anus, ensuring an incision angle of 60 degrees. Post delivery, the episiotomy will be at a 45-degree angle (dotted red line). (Image courtesy: Dr A Tamilselvi, Institute of Reproductive Health, Madras Medical Mission, Chennai)

On examination, if there is any uncertainty about the severity of a third-degree perineal tear, it is recommended that the laceration be classified under a higher grade rather than a lower one.

Episiotomy with no extension is similar to a second-degree perineal tear.

Principles of Suturing

The place of repair is usually the labour room, with local anesthetic infiltration in uncomplicated episiotomy and first- and second-degree tears. If there is a suspicion of more extensive vaginal or cervical lacerations with bleeding, or extension of perineal injury to third- or fourth-degree, repair should be performed in the operating theatre with regional block or general anesthesia for adequate relaxation (see **Chapter 25** for further details). In each of these settings, appropriate instruments should be available for the type of repair planned.

Suture material

The choice of the appropriate suture material for episiotomy repair has been evaluated extensively in randomised controlled trials (RCT) and meta-analyses, comparing catgut, polyglycolic acid, and polyglycolic acid rapid sutures [17,18,19,20].

Catgut, a natural absorbable suture material which was used widely in the past, maintains its 60% tensile strength for 7–10 days and is absorbed in 90 days. **Polyglycolic acid** (Polyglactin 910), a synthetic absorbable suture material, loses its original tensile strength in 4–5 weeks and is completely absorbed in 56–70 days. **Polyglycolic acid rapid suture** (Polyglactin 910 rapid) has rapid absorption, with a loss of original tensile strength in 10–14 days and complete absorption in 42 days.

In a systematic review of the Cochrane Database comparing catgut with standard synthetic sutures in episiotomy repair, the outcomes measured were perineal pain, the need for analgesia, and wound healing [21]. Compared to catgut, standard synthetic sutures were associated with less pain up to three days after delivery and less analgesia requirement up to ten days postpartum. Wound dehiscence was more common with catgut sutures, and the need for suture removal was greater with standard absorbable synthetic sutures (Polyglactin 910) as compared to rapid absorbable synthetic sutures (Polyglactin 910 rapid).

> **Key Point**
>
> The existing evidence suggests polyglycolic acid rapid sutures offer many short-term advantages in terms of pain and wound healing.

Technique

- Episiotomy suturing begins with the identification of the apex in the vaginal mucosa, with the first suture **being placed 1 cm beyond the apex to include any retracted vessel.** This is referred to as the **anchoring stitch.**
- The vaginal mucosa is then approximated in a continuous non-locking fashion up to the hymenal ring. The anatomical landmarks, such as the hymenal ring and the vermilion border (where the vaginal mucosa and the skin meet), should be identified and reapproximated accurately.
- The needle is then directed downward at the fourchette, and using the same suture material, the perineal muscles are re-approximated with a continuous non-locking technique (Fig. 7.6a). The first suture is placed through the superficial bulbocavernosus muscle on each side in a 'V' configuration, commonly referred to as the **'crown stitch'**.
- Finally, the perineal skin is approximated, starting from the lower edge of the skin incision, the sutures being placed in the subcutaneous layer on either side, directed towards the vagina up to the hymenal ring (**Fig. 7.6b**). The repair is completed with a knot just proximal to the hymenal ring.

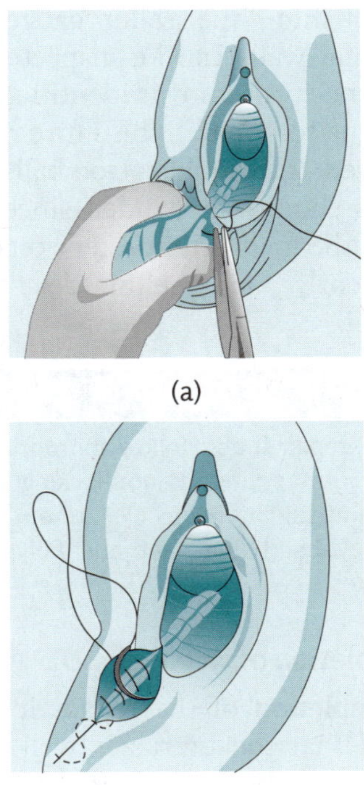

(a)

(b)

Fig. 7.6 (a) The vaginal mucosa suturing is completed and the perineal muscles are being sutured and (b) approximation of skin with subcutaneous sutures

- In this technique, both knots are placed within the vaginal mucosa with no knot over the perineal skin. The tissues in each layer are approximated without undue tension at repair. The tension is transferred through the whole length of a single suture.
- The subcutaneous placement of skin sutures avoids nerve endings. Evidence indicates that with the continuous non-locking technique, there is less pain, decreased analgesia use, and lesser need for suture removal; moreover, the repair is cost-effective with lesser suture material used [22,23].
- On analysing the continuous and interrupted techniques with dyspareunia as an outcome, statistically, no significant difference was noted between the two [24].
- To keep the field of suturing clear of blood, a sterile roller gauze or large tampon may be used. This is gently inserted into the vagina after the cervix has been inspected. While pushing the roller gauze upwards, the vaginal walls can be inspected, and the apex of the episiotomy is identified. Once the suturing is completed, the entire roller gauze is removed. Individual cotton balls and small tampons should be avoided since they may result in the inadvertent retention of one and consequently, foul-smelling discharge a few days later.

Key Point

Episiotomy repair should follow appropriate surgical principles with continuous non-locking suturing of all layers and subcutaneous closure of the perineal skin, using absorbable synthetic Polyglactin 910 rapid sutures.

At Completion of Repair

At the completion of the repair, it should be ascertained that the uterus is well contracted and no abnormal bleeding is present. Any roller gauze or tampon placed in the vagina should be removed. Inspection of the periurethral areas, vaginal and digital rectal examination should be repeated, along with counting of all swabs and instruments used in the repair.

Documentation of the delivery details, along with a clear description of the repair is important. This should include the indication for the episiotomy, type of episiotomy performed, and extension of injuries (pictorial representation if possible), degree of injury as per WHO classification, place of repair, analgesia used, the technique used, with suture material for each layer, and pre- and post-procedure examination findings.

Key Point

Post-repair documentation is an important clinical risk management exercise. Postnatal care of repair and subsequent follow-up is essential.

Antibiotic Prophylaxis

Prophylactic antibiotics have not been shown to reduce the risk of wound infection in women with uncomplicated vaginal delivery with episiotomy. In the absence of risk factors, prophylactic antibiotics are not recommended for the prevention of wound infection in women with first- and second-degree perineal tears and episiotomy even in low-resource areas [27,28]. See **Chapter 19**, *Antibiotic prophylaxis in labour and delivery*, for further details.

Use of Postpartum Analgesics

NSAIDs are the first choice for perineal pain relief. A systematic review of the Cochrane Database showed that NSAIDs provided 50% more relief than paracetamol [25]. Ibuprofen 400 mg orally every 6–8 hours as needed provides significant relief in the first postpartum week.

Apart from these analgesics, other agents that have been studied for pain relief include topical lidocaine gel and cold compress using ice packs. There is limited evidence to support the application of cool packs to the perineum for pain relief, but some women do find this method useful when they apply the packs at regular intervals [26]. The duration of analgesic use should be as per the woman's requirement with frequent examination of the perineum in case of extended analgesic use.

Postnatal Perineal Care

Before discharge from the facility, women (with or without episiotomy) should be educated on how to keep the perineal area clean. They should be advised on the following:

- Washing the perineum with water for cleaning; it is important to stress the need to avoid routine use of any antiseptic solutions
- Changing sanitary pads at regular intervals
- Bathing or showering daily and maintaining proper hand hygiene to reduce the risk of infection
- Avoiding constipation by consuming a fibre-rich diet and adequate fluids
- Recognising warning signs to identify wound infection, wound breakdown, or hematoma

At the postnatal visit, pelvic floor exercises, resumption of sexual activity, and contraception are discussed.

CONCLUSION

In the context of vaginal delivery, episiotomy is an intervention that appears to have been overused. With selective and appropriate use of episiotomy, maternal morbidity is expected to reduce worldwide. Understanding the proper technique of performing an episiotomy, identifying anal sphincter injuries, and teaching the correct surgical principles of repair in both episiotomy and OASI are important aspects of obstetric training.

REFERENCES

1. Ould F. *Treatise of midwifery*. 1742. Nelson and Connor. Dublin, Ireland.
2. Miller S, Abalos E, Chamillard M, Ciapponi A, Colaci D, Comandé D, et al. Beyond too little, too late and too much, too soon: A pathway towards evidence-based, respectful maternity care worldwide. *Lancet*. 2016. 388:2176-2192.
3. Singh S, Thakur T, Chandhiok N, Dhillon BS. Pattern of episiotomy use and its immediate complications among vaginal deliveries in 18 tertiary care hospitals in India. *Indian J Med Res*. 2016. 143(4):474-80.
4. World Health Organization Division of Family Health Maternal Health and Safe Motherhood. Care in normal birth: A practical guide. Report of a technical working group. 1996. WHO, Geneva.
5. World Health Organization. Intrapartum care for a positive childbirth experience. 2017. WHO, Geneva. https://www.who.int/reproductivehealth/publications/intrapartum-care-guidelines/en/.
6. Hartmann K, Viswanathan M, Palmieri R, Gartlehner G, Thorp J, Lohr KN. Outcomes of routine episiotomy: a systematic review. *JAMA*. 2005. 4;293(17):2141-8.
7. Jiang H, Qian X, Carroli G, Garner P. Selective versus routine use of episiotomy for vaginal birth. *Cochrane Database Syst Rev*. 2017. Issue 2. Art. No.: CD000081.
8. Fritel X, Schaal JP, Fauconnier A, Bertrand V, Levet C, Pigné A. Pelvic floor disorders 4 years after first delivery: A comparative study of restrictive versus systematic episiotomy. *BJOG*. 2008. 115(2):247-52.
9. Prevention and management of obstetric lacerations at vaginal delivery. ACOG Practice Bulletin No. 198. American College of Obstetricians and Gynecologists. *Obstet Gynecol*. 2018. 132:e87–102.
10. Coats PM, Chan KK, Wilkins M, Beard RJ. A comparison between midline and mediolateral episiotomies. Obstetrical & Gynecological Survey. 1981. 36(2):p 80-81.
11. Sooklim R, Thinkhamrop J, Lumbiganon P, Prasertcharoensuk W, Pattamadilok J, Seekorn K, et al. The outcomes of midline versus medio-lateral episiotomy. *Reprod Health*. 2007. 4:10.
12. Pergialiotis V, Vlachos D, Protopapas A, Pappa K, Vlachos G. Risk factors for severe perineal lacerations during childbirth. *Int J Gynaecol Obstet*. 2014. 125:6–14.
13. Andrews V, Sultan AH, Thakar R, Jones PW. Risk factors for obstetric anal sphincter injury: A prospective study. *Birth*. 2006. 33: 117– 22.
14. Kalis V, Ladsmanova J, Bednarova B, Karbanova J, Laine K, Rokyta Z. Evaluation of the incision angle of mediolateral episiotomy at 60 degrees. *Int J Gynecol Obstet*. 2011. 112:220–4.
15. Andrews V, Sultan AH, Thakar R, Jones PW. Occult anal sphincter injuries—myth or reality? *BJOG*. 2006. 113: 195-200.
16. Sultan A H. Obstetrical perineal injury and anal incontinence. *Clin Risk*. 1999. 5: 193-196.
17. Joseph K, Shantha B, Prakash S. Comparative study of episiotomy repair: Absorbable synthetic versus chromic catgut suture material. *Journal of Obstetrics and Gynecology of India*. 2008. 1;58(6):495-9.
18. Bharathi A, Reddy DD, Kote GS. A prospective randomized comparative study of vicryl rapide versus

chromic catgut for episiotomy repair. *Journal of clinical and diagnostic research (JCDR)*. 2013. 7(2):326.

19. McElhinney BR, Glenn DR, Dornan G, Harper MA. Episiotomy repair: Vicryl versus vicryl rapide. *The Ulster Medical Journal*. 2000. 69(1):27.
20. Viswanathan M, Hartmann K, Palmieri R, Lux L, Swinson T, Lohr KN, et al. The use of episiotomy in obstetrical care: A systematic review—summary. AHRQ_Evidence Report Summaries. 2005.
21. Kettle C, Dowswell T, Ismail KMK. Absorbable suture materials for primary repair of episiotomy and second-degree tears. *Cochrane Database of Systematic Reviews*. 2010, Issue 6. Art. no.: CD000006.
22. Kettle C, Dowswell T, Ismail KM. Continuous and interrupted suturing techniques for repair of episiotomy or second-degree tears. *Cochrane Database Syst Rev*. 2012. Issue 11. Art. no. :CD000947.
23. Sanson C, Papin S, Pierre F, Gachon B. Perineal suture practices. Are they up to date with the evidence-based medicine data: A local experience into a university maternity? *J Gynecol Obstet Hum Reprod*. 2020. 49(5):101634.
24. Schnittka E M, Lanpher N W, Patel P. Postpartum dyspareunia following continuous versus interrupted perineal repair: A systematic review and meta-analysis. *Cureus*. 2022. 14(9): e29070.
25. Wuytack F, Smith V, Cleary BJ. Oral non-steroidal anti-inflammatory drugs (single dose) for perineal pain in the early postpartum period. *Cochrane Database Syst Rev*. 2016. Issue 7. Art. no.:CD011352
26. East CE, Dorward ED, Whale RE, Liu J. Local cooling for relieving pain from perineal trauma sustained during childbirth. *Cochrane Database Syst Rev*. 2020. Issue 10. Art. no.:CD006304.
27. Mohamed N, Hanafy M, Mahmoud N. Effect of post episiotomy antibiotics on maternal infectious morbidity (clinical trial). *Journal of Recent Advances in Medicine*. 2022. 3(1): 31-37.
28. Garala NJ, Nambiar SS. Prophylactic antibiotics in patients with episiotomy following normal vaginal delivery: A randomised clinical trial. *International Journal of Reproduction, Contraception, Obstetrics and Gynecology*. 2019. 8(10):3846-52.

CHAPTER 8

Fetal Surveillance in Labour

SABARATNAM ARULKUMARAN

INTRODUCTION

Labour involves contractions of the uterus (**power**) leading to the dilatation of the cervical canal and the descent of the head, resulting in the delivery of the fetus (**passenger**) through the pelvis (**passage**).

The fetus receives its oxygen and nutrition through the umbilical cord (from the placenta) which floats in the amniotic fluid. The placenta receives oxygen and nutrition from and excretes its waste products into the maternal retroplacental pool of blood. Uterine contractions of labour intermittently cut off the blood perfusion via the umbilical cord vessels or reduce blood flow into the retroplacental area, thus reducing the exchange of gases and essential nutrition to the fetus.

In labour, uterine contractions and fetal heart rate (FHR) are monitored to detect fetal compromise. Where facilities are available, pregnancies known to be at high risk are offered continuous observation of the FHR and uterine contractions by cardiotocography (CTG). This is done electronically and is termed **electronic fetal monitoring (EFM)**.

This chapter deals with intrapartum fetal surveillance (IPFS), which is performed chiefly to detect possible hypoxia/asphyxia.

PATHOPHYSIOLOGY OF FETAL COMPROMISE

During the process of labour and delivery, the fetus may be subjected to the insults of **hypoxia, infection,** and **trauma**. Although most labours are not associated with complications, they may arise at any time and may cause compromise to the mother or fetus. Most complications may be anticipated and managed adequately.

Hypoxemia, Hypoxia, and Asphyxia

Cardiotocography is sensitive in picking up any stress to the fetus such as cord compression (**variable decelerations**), head compression (**early decelerations**), or a reduced retroplacental pool of blood (**late decelerations**). With decelerations, initially, there is **hypoxemia**—a lack of oxygen in the blood. When the fetus develops **hypoxia**, i.e., a lack of oxygen in the tissues with the decelerations—there is a rise in the baseline fetal heart rate due to a catecholamine surge. When hypoxia continues and results in **asphyxia**, i.e., hypoxia and metabolic acidosis in the tissues, there is a marked reduction in the baseline variability due to its effect on the autonomic nervous system.

Key Points

- **Hypoxemia:** Lack of oxygen in the blood
- **Hypoxia:** Lack of oxygen in the tissues
- **Asphyxia:** Hypoxia and metabolic acidosis in the tissues

The decision for delivery depends on the degree of concern based on the following:

- FHR pattern
- Physiological reserve of the fetus
- Parity
- Current cervical dilatation
- The rate of progress of labour

In the presence of suspected fetal compromise, the baby is delivered by cesarean section in the first stage of labour and by forceps or vacuum-assisted delivery in the second stage of labour. Instrumental vaginal delivery (IVD) may occasionally be associated with complications. Complications are usually minor, but rarely, they can result in severe morbidity or mortality. Attention and care in labour are directed towards anticipating, avoiding, and managing these problems. Despite meticulous care, however, fetal morbidity does occur.

METHODS OF INTRAPARTUM FETAL SURVEILLANCE (IPFS)

The methods available for evaluating and assessing fetal response to labour include the following:

- **Fetal heart rate monitoring**
  - Intermittent auscultation (IA)
    - Pinard fetoscope
    - Handheld Doppler device
  - Cardiotocography (CTG)/electronic fetal monitoring (EFM)
    - Intermittent (when required)
    - Continuous
- **Fetal scalp blood sampling**
  - Scalp pH
  - Fetal lactate concentration
- **Fetal electrocardiography**

INTERMITTENT AUSCULTATION (IA)

Globally, IA is the common mode of IPFS. It is the accepted modality for monitoring a low-risk pregnancy in labour even in high-income countries (HICs) and is quite often the only method available for fetal heart rate monitoring in many medical facilities in low- and middle-income countries (LMICs) [1].

IA is accomplished with either a Pinard stethoscope or a handheld Doppler ultrasound device. It is undertaken immediately after a contraction and is carried out for one minute, then every 15 minutes. The fetal heart rate is recorded as a single figure on the partograph, along with accelerations or decelerations, if heard.

FIGO Guidelines on IA

A strict protocol for intermittent auscultation has been recommended by the FIGO consensus guidelines on intrapartum fetal monitoring [2]. These guidelines must be followed to ensure that the maximum benefit is obtained from fetal heart rate monitoring (Table 8.1).

Low nurse-to-patient ratios may make this difficult to practice in busy labour and delivery suites, but this protocol should be adhered to as closely as possible to avoid missing fetal hypoxia.

Table 8.1 Recommended protocol for intermittent auscultation based on FIGO consensus guidelines on intrapartum fetal monitoring [2]

Intermittent auscultation	Recommendation
Intervals between auscultation	• 1st stage of labour—every 15–30 minutes • 2nd stage of labour—every 5 minutes • During pushing—after each contraction
Duration	• Each auscultation should last for at least 1 minute • If an abnormality is noted, auscultate over at least 3 contractions
Timing	• Auscultate during a uterine contraction and continue for at least 30 seconds after the contraction
Documentation	• Record the baseline FHR (e.g., 130 beats per minute) and the presence or absence of accelerations or decelerations

Intelligent Structured Intermittent Auscultation (ISIA)

ISIA has been introduced recently to implement evidence-based fetal heart monitoring for low-risk women [3,4]. Studies over the years have shown that CTG offers no benefit to low-risk women and may, in fact, even cause harm [5,6].

The concept of ISIA uses the following principles:

- **On initial assessment in labour,** a correct baseline rate is identified—excluding accelerations and decelerations—by listening when there are no fetal movements or contractions.
- **Fetal health** is assessed by listening to accelerations at the time of fetal movements.
- **Fetal compromise** is identified by listening immediately after a contraction to pick up late or prolonged variable decelerations where the FHR recovers to the baseline rate later than the end of a contraction.
- **Any rise in the baseline rate** is identified on sequential recording of baseline FHR.
- **CTG recording** is initiated if any rise in baseline FHR and/or decelerations are auscultated and persist over the next two or three contractions.

Decelerations and accelerations are detected by counting the FHR in 10 second epochs/periods [3,4]. If FHR decelerations are heard, continuous observation of the FHR is advised over the next two contractions. If repeated decelerations and/or a rise in the baseline rate are observed, then EFM is preferable with a re-evaluation of the risk factors. If the CTG trace is normal after 20 minutes, monitoring can revert to IA unless a high-risk factor was identified when continuous EFM was initiated [3].

Maternal pulse

The maternal pulse is palpated at the time of FHR auscultation to make sure it is distinct from the FHR. Maternal pulse is counted for one minute hourly and is recorded on the partograph. Whenever there are any concerns about the FHR (low or high) the maternal pulse should be palpated/monitored simultaneously to differentiate between the maternal and fetal heart rates.

Interval between auscultations

During the second stage of labour, intermittent auscultation of the FHR is performed every 5 minutes, immediately after a contraction, and the FHR is counted for 1 minute. If intermittent auscultation indicates possible FHR abnormalities during the second stage, CTG should be commenced but can revert to intermittent auscultation if the trace is normal after 20 minutes [3].

Calculating the fetal heart rate accurately

Listening for less than one minute and then multiplying by a factor to calculate the heart rate for 60 seconds may produce erroneous readings if the counting for 10 or 15 seconds was not accurate since the error is multiplied six or four times respectively (Fig. 8.1). **Counting in 10- or 15-second epochs/periods for a total of 60 seconds provides more accurate FHR and facilitates the identification of accelerations and decelerations.**

Doppler Device With Graphic Display

More recently, handheld Doppler devices equipped with a display for the FHR have become available (Fig. 8.2). These devices detect the FHR and display it digitally in numbers and present the FHR pattern as a graphical trace. The traces obtained can be annotated and stored in a microchip within the machine; this data can be retrieved for review or to be transferred to a central unit.

The Doppler device with graphic display has an advantage over a digital display Doppler as the observer can determine the baseline heart rate more accurately and visualise features like variability, accelerations, and decelerations. The carer should have the skills to assess baseline FHR and the presence of decelerations if the technology is not available. Whether the graphic display feature improves neonatal outcomes remains to be proven.

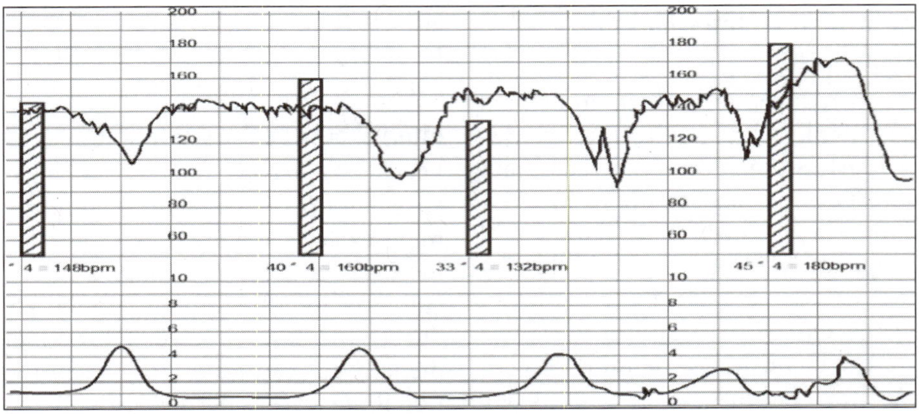

Fig. 8.1 A CTG tracing shows that counting for 15 seconds and multiplying by four provides erroneous fetal heart rate as represented by the shaded bars (*Image courtesy*: Prof. Sabaratnam Arulkumaran)

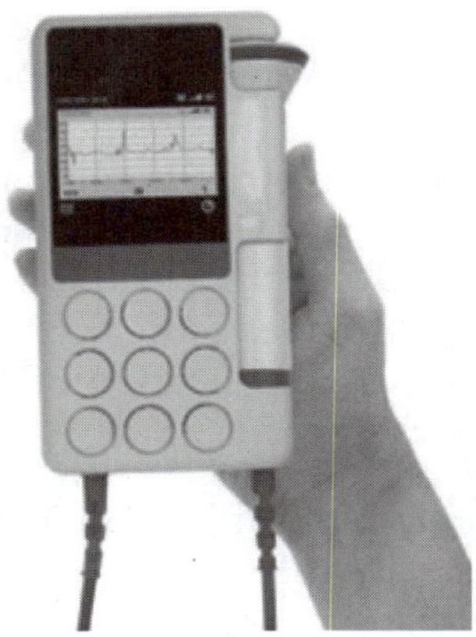

Fig. 8.2 Handheld Doppler with graphic display and memory to store FHR traces (*Image courtesy*: Prof. Sabaratnam Arulkumaran)

CARDIOTOCOGRAPHY (CTG)/ ELECTRONIC FETAL MONITORING (EFM)

Evidence is lacking to develop an ideal intrapartum fetal surveillance (IPFS) scheme to improve perinatal outcomes in high-risk pregnancies. Practice guided by expert consensus and obstetric culture recommends **admission CTG** and **continuous CTG** in high-risk women. The available epidemiological evidence points to poor outcomes with antepartum and intrapartum high-risk factors, and hence, these pregnancies need to be monitored by EFM (Table 8.2) [7,8].

A mismatch exists between international guidelines and what is locally achievable in

Table 8.2 Indications for the use of continuous electronic fetal monitoring

Maternal risk factors	Fetal risk factors	Intrapartum risk factors
• Previous cesarean delivery • Hypertension • Postterm pregnancy • Prolonged rupture of membranes (>24 hours) • Induced labour • Diabetes • Antepartum hemorrhage (placental abruption) • Medical disorders such as systemic lupus erythematosus	• Fetal growth restriction • Prematurity • Oligohydramnios • Abnormal Doppler artery velocimetry • Multiple pregnancy • Intrauterine infection	• Oxytocin augmentation • Vaginal bleeding in labour • Maternal pyrexia • Fresh meconium-stained liquor • Abnormalities on IA • Maternal request

IA, intermittent auscultation

low-resource settings, especially where EFM is not available. This being the case, intermittent auscultation should be undertaken for high-risk as well low-risk women.

Interpretation of CTG

The time of onset and rate of progression of hypoxia can be predicted by analysing the different CTG patterns. It is also possible to predict the type of neurological injury based on the patterns of CTG that give rise to hypoxia. The discussion of this topic in **Chapter 15**, *Identification and management of fetal distress* explains these issues.

In this chapter, we deal with the individual characteristics that constitute the CTG and how the analysis of all these features provides meaningful clinical information. There are four essential features in the interpretation of the FHR trace recorded by electronic fetal monitors [9,10,11]:

- Baseline fetal heart rate
- Accelerations
- Decelerations
- Baseline variability

Baseline FHR

The **baseline FHR** of a term fetus is 110–160 beats/minute (bpm) and can be read from the CTG recording by drawing a line across the trace over 10 minutes, excluding accelerations and decelerations. Each fetus will exhibit a unique baseline rate. It is important to know the following definitions of baseline FHR:

- Normal baseline FHR 110–160 bpm
- Moderate bradycardia 100–109 bpm
- Moderate tachycardia 161–180 bpm
- Abnormal bradycardia <100 bpm
- Abnormal tachycardia >180 bpm

Key Point

Hypoxic fetuses may have a normal baseline FHR of 110–160 bpm, but the absence of accelerations and a baseline variability of <5 bpm for >40 minutes should raise suspicion.

Accelerations

An acceleration is an abrupt rise in the FHR from the baseline for >15 beats for a duration of >15 seconds and is associated with a fetus that is **not** acidotic [10]. Accelerations are usually associated with fetal movements. The presence of two such accelerations in a 15-minute period of a CTG trace is referred to as a 'reactive trace'.

A **reactive CTG** (Fig. 8.3) indicates a non-hypoxic fetus and confirms the integrity of the somatic or voluntary nervous system, i.e., centres that control fetal movement. Accelerations and normal baseline variability are the hallmarks of a healthy fetus.

A confluence of accelerations may cause difficulties in CTG interpretation but can be identified by observing prolonged episodes of fetal movements. With time, an accelerative trace is likely to settle to a quiet epoch and show cyclicity (see the section below *on Cyclicity of the FHR due to normal behavioural states from the late preterm*).

Key Point

Accelerations and normal baseline variability are hallmarks of fetal health and reassure that the fetus is not hypoxic.

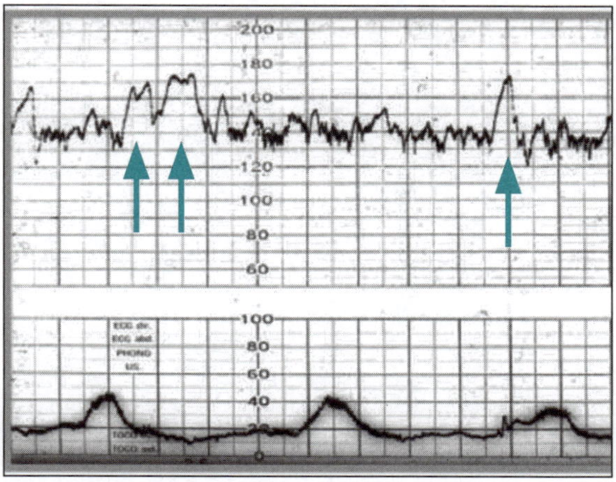

Fig. 8.3 A reactive trace with accelerations (arrows) and normal baseline variability (*Image courtesy*: Prof. Sabaratnam Arulkumaran)

Decelerations

Decelerations are temporary but distinct decreases of the baseline fetal heart rate for >15 bpm and lasting for >15 seconds. The absence of significant decelerations (≥15 bpm for ≥15 secs) with contractions indicates that there is no stress to the fetus. The shapes of the decelerations vary as well as their relationship to contractions. Decelerations indicate transient stress to the fetus. Based on the shape and timing of decelerations to the contractions, one can identify the cause of the stress [6].

> **Key Point**
>
> During labour, if decelerations are absent, asphyxia is unlikely.

Early decelerations

Early decelerations are 'mirror images' of contractions, i.e., the onset and offset of the decelerations mirror the onset and offset of the contractions and they are usually <40 bpm in depth. They are reflective of **head compression** and hence, are seen in the late first and second stages of labour (Fig. 8.4).

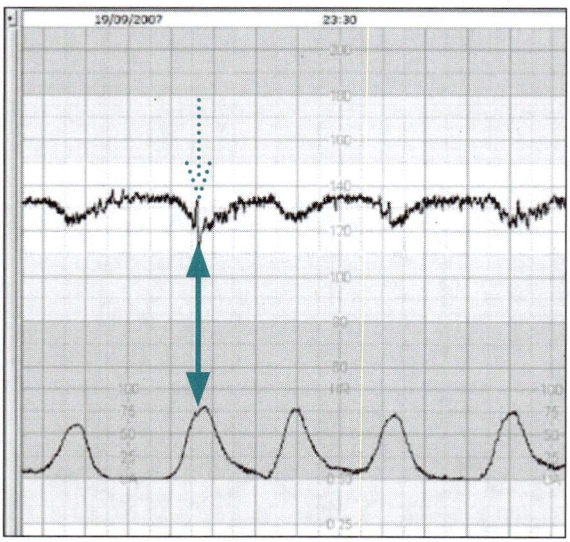

Fig. 8.4 Early decelerations (dotted arrow) which mirror the uterine contraction (bold arrow) (*Image courtesy*: Prof. Sabaratnam Arulkumaran)

Variable decelerations

Variable decelerations exhibit a precipitous fall and quick recovery of FHR. They vary in shape and size and can be periodic, i.e., associated with contractions, or they can be episodic, i.e., not associated with uterine contractions. They occur due to **cord compression** and are alleviated, at times, by a change in maternal position or amnioinfusion. There is a slight increase in the FHR just before and just after the deceleration due to baroreceptor-mediated cardiac activity associated with umbilical vein and arterial compression, which is described as '**shouldering**' (Fig. 8.5). Variable decelerations are seen in cases with reduced amniotic fluid.

Late decelerations

Late decelerations start after contractions have commenced. There is a lag of >20 seconds between the onset of the contraction to the onset of the deceleration i.e., the acme of the contraction to the nadir of the deceleration. They occur due to reduced retroplacental perfusion, which affects fetal oxygenation (Fig. 8.6).

Prolonged deceleration

A prolonged deceleration is an abrupt decrease in FHR to <80 bpm [12,13]. It is termed **suspicious** if it lasts <3 minutes and **pathological** if it lasts >3 minutes. Prolonged decelerations of <80 bpm for >3 minutes may be due to a reversible or non-reversible cause. Urgent intervention is mandated for **abruption, cord prolapse,** and **scar rupture**.

> **Key Point**
>
> Abruption, cord prolapse, and scar rupture can give rise to acute hypoxia and should be suspected clinically in the presence of prolonged decelerations.

Sinusoidal pattern

A sinusoidal pattern resembles a sine wave with regular oscillations of the baseline and no variability. This smooth, undulating pattern, **lasting for at least 10 minutes**, may have physiological causes which are transient—e.g., thumb sucking.

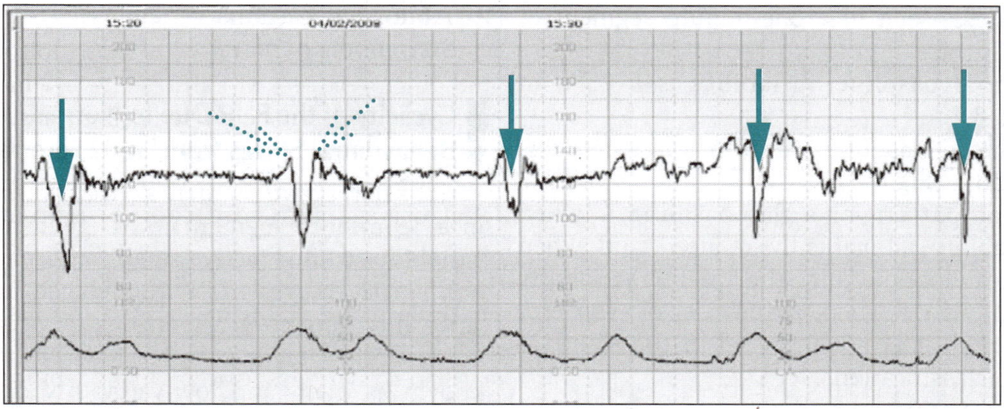

Fig. 8.5 Variable decelerations (bold arrows) with shouldering (dotted arrows) (*Image courtesy*: Prof. Sabaratnam Arulkumaran)

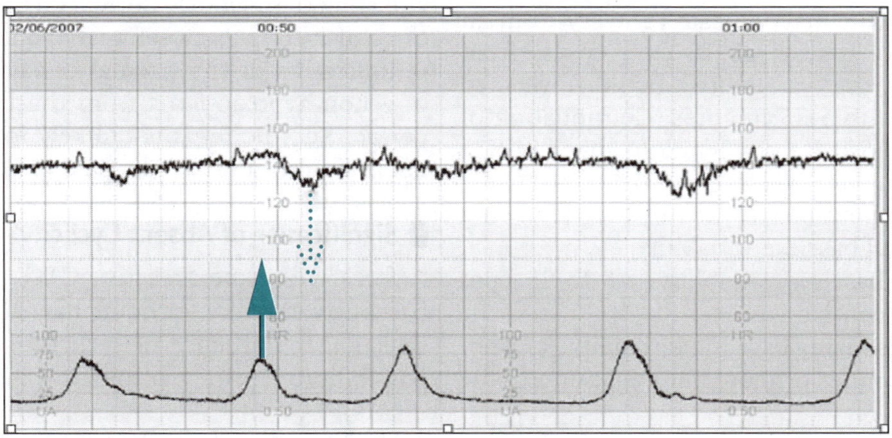

Fig. 8.6 Late decelerations—there is a lag of >20 seconds between the acme of the contraction (bold arrow) to the nadir of the deceleration (dotted arrow) (*Image courtesy*: Prof. Sabaratnam Arulkumaran)

If prolonged, such a pattern could have a pathological cause—**fetal anemia associated with Rh iso-immunisation** or **fetomaternal transfusion**. Inquiry of recent fetal movements, evaluation of the clinical situation, physical or acoustic stimulation, ultrasound for ascites, measurement of blood flow velocity in the middle cerebral artery by Doppler, blood group antibodies, and the Kleihauer–Betke test may be useful to identify fetal anemia and decide on therapy or delivery based on the period of gestation [5].

> **Key Point**
>
> A transient sinusoidal pattern may be physiological. However, a prolonged sinusoidal pattern is usually associated with significant fetal anemia.

Baseline variability

Baseline variability is the 'wiggliness' of the baseline. The ascending limb is due to the sympathetic activity and the descending limb is due to the parasympathetic activity of the baby's autonomic nervous system. Baseline variability is assessed by measuring the bandwidth of the 'wiggliness' seen in a one-minute segment of the FHR trace.

- **Normal baseline variability** is 5–25 bpm (Fig. 8.7c).
- **Reduced baseline variability** is when it is <5 bpm (Fig. 8.7b).
- **Silent pattern** or a **flat baseline** is when variability is markedly reduced and when one cannot determine the baseline variability (Fig. 8.7a). This pattern is of concern, although it is not included in the standard CTG classifications.
- **Saltatory pattern** is rare and is said to be present when the variability is >25 bpm (Fig. 8.7d). It occurs due to an overdrive of the sympathetic and parasympathetic activity. This may indicate recovery from an episode of acute hypoxia. On recovery from hypoxia, the variability should revert to normal within 25 minutes. Continuation of this pattern with decelerations may indicate continuing hypoxia.

It is important to know the following definitions of baseline variability:

- **Normal** baseline variability: >5 to 25 bpm between contractions
- **Non-reassuring** baseline variability: <5 bpm for 40 minutes or more but <90 minutes
- **Abnormal** baseline variability: <5 bpm for 90 minutes or more

Cyclicity of the FHR Due to Normal Behavioural States from Late Preterm

Periods of reactive segments (two accelerations in a 15-minute segment) with good baseline variability (called 'active sleep') alternate with non-reactive segments with reduced baseline variability and no accelerations or occasional accelerations (called 'quiet sleep') and are known as high- and low-variability cycles or '**cycling**' (Fig. 8.8). Periods of reduced variability can be normal in a healthy fetus during fetal sleep. A review of the CTG in such a situation will show a previously normal CTG and periods of 'fetal cycling' between rest and activity. This is indicative of the normal behavioural state of a non-hypoxic fetus from the late preterm period, i.e., the fetus is unlikely to have had a neurological injury in the past [6].

Significance of Absent Cyclicity

A fetus with a non-reactive CTG and reduced baseline variability for hours may be hypoxic or infected; the absence of cyclicity suggests the possibility of prior neurological injury. In the

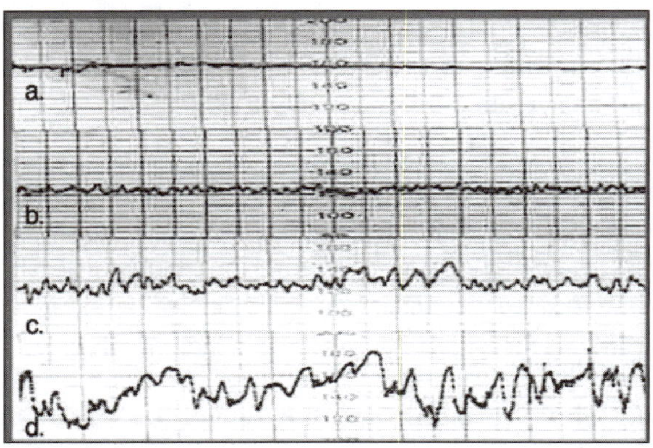

Fig. 8.7 The different patterns of baseline variability: (a) Silent pattern or flat baseline, (b) reduced baseline variability (<5 bpm), (c) normal baseline variability (5–25 bpm), and (d) saltatory variability (>25 bpm) (*Image courtesy*: Prof. Sabaratnam Arulkumaran)

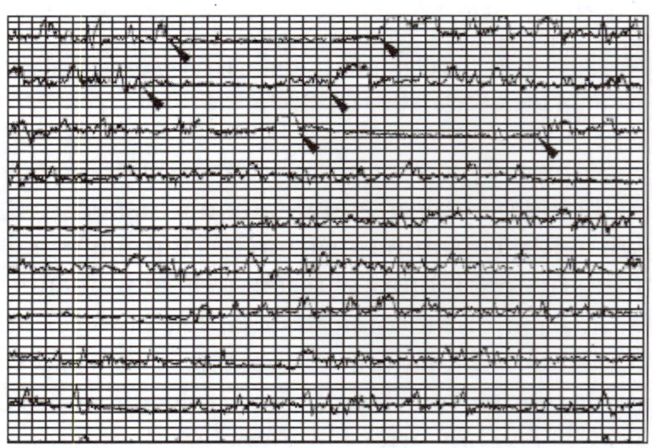

Fig. 8.8 A CTG trace showing repeated episodes of quiet (segments with reduced baseline variability and no accelerations) and active (segments with accelerations and good baseline variability) epochs/periods representing a cycling pattern

absence of baseline variability, repeated shallow late decelerations constitute an ominous tracing (Fig. 8.9).

> **Key Point**
>
> In the presence of baseline variability of <5 bpm, even shallow decelerations (<15 bpm) are ominous in a non-reactive trace.

Uterine Contractions

The recording of uterine contractions is important for assessing the progress of labour. The recording of contractions is essential to detect **hyperstimulation** when the uterus is stimulated with oxytocin or prostaglandins. The presence of >5 contractions in 10 minutes in two successive 10-minute periods or averaged over a 30-minute period is called **tachysystole.**

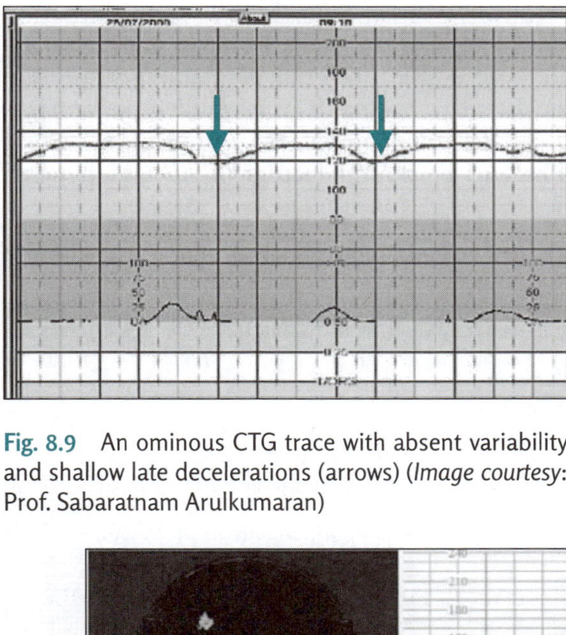

Fig. 8.9 An ominous CTG trace with absent variability and shallow late decelerations (arrows) (*Image courtesy*: Prof. Sabaratnam Arulkumaran)

Recording of uterine contractions is also important because decelerations of the FHR trace are defined in relation to them. Contractions can be assessed by the following methods:

- Palpation
- External tocodynamometer
- Intrauterine pressure catheter

The **frequency** of uterine contractions and the approximation of their **duration** are acceptable when recorded by palpation or an external tocodynamometer. The **amplitude** of contractions is reliable when measured by intrauterine catheters, but they are invasive and do not have any clinical advantage over external measurements.

Current external tocodynamometers have infrared sensors that can record the contractions and the maternal pulse at the same time (Fig. 8.10a and b).

CLINICAL CLASSIFICATION OF CTG BASED ON THE FOUR FEATURES

Based on the description of each of the four components of the FHR and the recorded contractions, the traces are classified as **normal,**

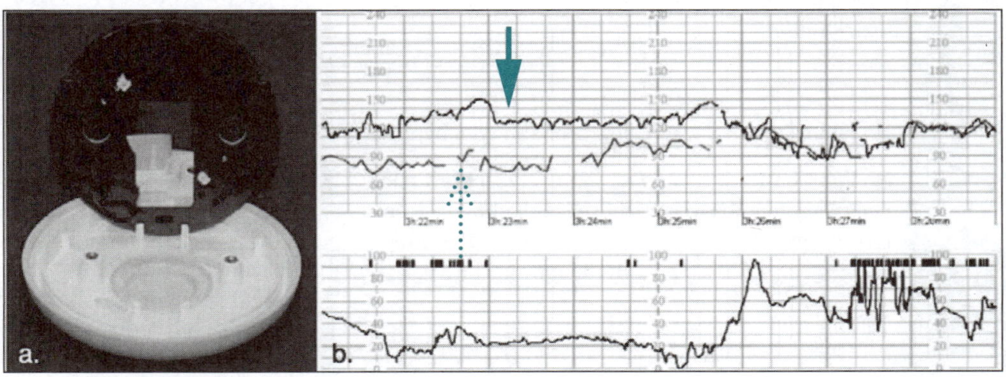

Fig. 8.10 (a) A smart pulse tocodynamometer that records uterine contractions and maternal pulse and (b) CTG trace using the smart pulse tocodynamometer showing maternal pulse (**dotted** arrow), fetal heart rate (bold arrow) in the upper panel and uterine contractions in the lower panel (*Image courtesy*: Prof. Sabaratnam Arulkumaran)

suspicious, or **pathological**. There are several classifications including ones put forth by the American College of Obstetricians and Gynecologists (ACOG) [5], the Royal Australian and New Zealand College of Obstetricians and Gynaecologists (RANZOG) [15], the National Institute of Clinical Excellence in the UK [9], and the International Federation of Gynaecology and Obstetrics (FIGO) [16]. The author of this chapter encourages the use of the FIGO classification (Table 8.3) because of its universal acceptance, even in countries that have their own system of classification [16].

The progress of labour, as signified by increasing frequency, duration, and strength of contractions and the impact of cumulative contractions on the umbilical arterial and retroplacental blood flow, leads to progressive changes in the features of the CTG. These changes need to be examined every 30 minutes in conjunction with the clinical situation, especially for any newly developing risk factors (e.g., the use of oxytocin and the appearance of bleeding or meconium).

> **Key Point**
>
> Hypoxia can be worsened by oxytocin, epidural analgesia, and difficult operative deliveries.

Normal CTG

All four parameters should fall within the reassuring category. Normal baseline variability of 5–25 bpm suggests good integrity of the autonomic nervous system. Accelerations that occur with fetal movements indicate an intact somatic nervous system. The risk of fetal hypoxia or acidosis with a normal CTG is unlikely. False negatives (poor outcome despite a normal CTG) are likely to be due to factors other than hypoxia

Table 8.3 Intrapartum cardiotocography—FIGO classification criteria, interpretation, and recommended management [16]

	Normal[a]	Suspicious	Pathological
Baseline	110–160 bpm	Lacking at least one characteristic of normality but with no pathological features	<100 bpm
Variability	5–25 bpm		• Reduced variability • Increased variability • Sinusoidal pattern
Decelerations	No repetitive[b] decelerations		• Repetitive[b] late or prolonged decelerations for >30 min (or >20 min if reduced variability) • Deceleration >5 min
Interpretation	No hypoxia	Low probability of hypoxia	High probability of hypoxia
Clinical management	No intervention necessary to improve fetal oxygenation state	Action to correct reversible causes if identified, close monitoring or adjunctive methods	• Prompt correction of reversible causes and adjunctive methods; if these are not possible, expedite delivery • In acute situations, (abruption, scar rupture, cord prolapse)—immediate delivery

a. The presence of accelerations reassures that the fetus is not hypoxic/acidotic. The absence of accelerations during labour is of uncertain significance.

b. Decelerations are considered repetitive if they are associated with >50% of uterine contractions.

such as intrauterine infection and fetal congenital or metabolic abnormalities.

Suspicious or Pathological CTG

FHR features in isolation, with the exception of late decelerations, are not reliable in predicting poor neonatal outcomes, i.e., CTG is highly sensitive for flagging possible fetal hypoxia/acidemia but its specificity is low. False positive rates are high even in the presence of multiple abnormalities. Nelson et al. found a false positive rate as high as 99.8% even in the presence of late decelerations or reduced variability [17].

Key Point

CTG is highly sensitive for flagging possible fetal hypoxia/acidemia but its specificity is low. False positive rates are high even in the presence of multiple abnormalities on the trace [17].

Features in isolation unlikely to be associated with significant acidosis

- Moderate bradycardia (100–109 bpm)
- Moderate uncomplicated tachycardia (161–180 bpm) in the presence of accelerations
- Absence of accelerations
- Variable decelerations without complicating features of rebound tachycardia
- Variable decelerations followed by late deceleration or late recovery

Features that may be associated with acidosis

The risk of acidosis is higher with an increasing number of non-reassuring features and with the severity or duration of the abnormality.

- Fetal tachycardia of >180 bpm or a rising baseline even within the normal range associated with reduced variability may be an ominous sign of fetal hypoxia where the fetus tries to increase oxygen delivery to vital organs by increasing cardiac output. Subsequent cardiac decompensation may eventually occur with a fall in the baseline.
- Reduced baseline variability <5 bpm for longer than 90 min with complicated or atypical variable or late decelerations are likely to be associated with acidosis [18].

Management of suspicious or pathological CTG

The appearance of a suspicious or pathological trace does not always demand urgent delivery. The underlying cause of the pathological FHR pattern should be identified. Simple measures such as the following may help to restore a normal CTG:

- Changing maternal position
- Treating hypotension or pyrexia
- Reducing or stopping oxytocin
- Tocolysis if there is hyperstimulation

Differentiating normal from abnormal CTG

Identifying **normal** (reactive, cycling trace) and **severely abnormal** pre-terminal traces (e.g., prolonged deceleration <80 bpm for >3 minutes or FHR trace with no variability and shallow late decelerations) is easy. If all four features are abnormal, pathology and the likelihood of acidosis is more common.

Difficulties arise in deciding to take corrective action in the presence of suspicious or pathological traces **with only one or two non-reassuring features**.

Key Point

When all four features on a CTG trace are abnormal (abnormal baseline, poor or absent variability, absence of accelerations, and presence of significant decelerations), fetal pathology and the likelihood of acidosis is more likely.

Decision to intervene

The decision to intervene is made by incorporating the clinical risk factors, the CTG pattern, current cervical dilatation, and the rate of progress of labour and parity. These are important considerations to avoid over-intervention without fetal compromise. Education, training, clinical experience, and the use of adjunctive methods to evaluate fetal health are helpful in this process [19].

Key Point

Hypoxia and acidosis may develop faster with an abnormal trace in women with scanty, thick meconium, fetal growth restriction, or intrauterine infection with pyrexia, and those who are pre- or postterm.

The assessment of the pathological trace and the timing of interventions to avoid catastrophic injury are discussed in greater detail in **Chapter 15**, *Identification and management of fetal distress*.

Common Pitfalls in CTG Interpretation

Recording maternal FHR

'Accelerations' occurring with uterine contractions should raise suspicion. These are very likely to be maternal in origin. This often occurs in the late first stage or second stage of labour as the head descends and the probe gets placed near the maternal iliac vessels. When there is doubt, ultrasound will help locate the fetal heart and can also rule out fetal demise. In this situation, a fetal scalp electrode may be a better option for accurate recording of the FHR.

STANDARDS FOR EFM AND RECORD-KEEPING

To obtain the maximal benefit of using EFM and for avoiding medicolegal situations, various recommendations have been put forward by professional and national organisations. The recommendations from NICE and the RCOG are given in Table 8.4 [9].

Table 8.4 **Recommended standards for EFM and record-keeping** [9]

Standards	Recommendation
Document woman's details	• Name • Hospital number • Date and time of recording
Document date and time	• Correctly set the date and time on the EFM machine
Standardise settings	• Paper speed 1 cm/min • Sensitivity displays 20 bpm/cm • FHR range displays 50 to 210 bpm
Check and document at the start	• Maternal pulse rate (ensure distinct from fetal) • Maternal temperature
Systematic assessment of the CTG	Hourly
When asked to give an opinion on a CTG	• Note findings on both CTG trace and medical records • Document time, date, and signature of the physician
Documentation at birth	• Mode of delivery • Date and time of birth • Signature of healthcare professional
Risk management	• Store CTGs for 25 years • Make adequate provision for: – Safe storage (since graphs fade, photocopies should be taken) – Easy retrieval – Where possible, store electronically

ADMISSION CTG

Admission CTG with and without fetal acoustic stimulation was introduced with the purpose of identifying fetuses that were already hypoxic on admission or likely to develop hypoxia in the subsequent few hours [20,21]. It consists of a short (usually 20 minutes) recording of the FHR and uterine activity which is performed on the woman's admission to the labour ward.

It is based on the following principles:

- If the CTG is **reactive** with no decelerations, then the fetus is unlikely to develop hypoxia for at least the next 4 hours.
- If the CTG is **suspicious** or **pathological**, EFM should be continued and management should follow the steps described above

in the section on *Management of suspicious or pathological tracing*.

- If it shows a **grossly pathological** CTG, intervention should be undertaken to salvage the baby.

The concept of the admission test was introduced based on the results of prospective descriptive studies, but subsequent randomised controlled studies (RCTs) not only failed to show any benefits to neonatal outcome but also showed an increase in interventions in the form of continuous EFM, augmentation of labour, epidural analgesia, and operative delivery. In one RCT, the membranes were ruptured early (mean cervical dilatation <2 cm) and the women were randomised only if there was clear amniotic fluid [22].

Despite the absence of sufficient evidence based on RCTs [23,24], the practice of admission CTG continues as a routine in Scandinavian countries, whilst being selectively used in many units in the UK, at times when there is a lack of staff to perform intermittent auscultation every 15 minutes.

However, the principle of inquiring about fetal movements (FM) and listening for accelerations with FM and deceleration with contractions on admission has become embedded in practice in most units.

ADJUNCTIVE TESTS FOR THE EVALUATION OF FETAL CONDITION

Fetal Scalp Blood Sampling (FBS)

Fetal scalp blood sampling to measure pH or lactate is practised in many European countries but is becoming less favoured due to its invasive nature and the need for intermittent assessment [25,26]. NICE has taken an equipoise on the use of FBS and recommends digital fetal scalp stimulation.

Fetal Scalp Stimulation Test

In the presence of a non-reassuring FHR pattern, the scalp stimulation test is a reassuring technique for determining fetal reserves and ruling out fetal hypoxia and acidemia. It is based on prospective descriptive studies [27].

During a vaginal examination, the examiner strokes the fetal scalp with a finger, using firm pressure. This should elicit a fetal heart rate acceleration of ≥15 bpm above the baseline and lasting for ≥15 seconds.

Even without a CTG, the acceleration can be heard on a Doppler handheld device. When there are no spontaneous FHR accelerations, this test is easily performed and is immediately reassuring, especially in a low-resource setting.

Fetal Acoustic Stimulation Test (FAST)

The use of a fetal acoustic stimulation test has been reported to predict an acidotic pH. An artificial electronic larynx is used near the region of the fetal head to startle and wake up the fetus. If accelerations are noted in the CTG following the test, a pH of <7.2 with metabolic acidosis is unlikely [28].

ST Waveform Analysis

ST waveform analysis has become a useful adjunct to EFM [29,30]. However, it needs membrane rupture, the use of a fetal scalp electrode, and a maternal skin reference electrode for its application. To achieve good results, the operator should be able to manually interpret the CTG changes and correlate them with computer-detected and analysed ST changes. A systematic review of the Cochrane Database indicates a reduction in FBS and operative vaginal delivery but no difference in cesarean sections, metabolic acidosis, or neonatal encephalopathy [31].

CONCLUSION

Overdiagnosis of fetal hypoxia and acidosis fuelled by the fear of litigation results in rising cesarean rates. A failure to recognise the hypoxic fetus based on the CTG and clinical picture or delayed intervention results in intrapartum stillbirths, early neonatal deaths, and catastrophic injury to the newborn with lifelong neurological handicaps. Inadequate education and training, failure to consider the clinical picture, non-recognition of the severity of the pathological CTG, poor communication, and delay in intervention have been shown as factors that contribute to poor outcomes in the 'Each baby counts' report by the RCOG [32]. Computer-assisted technology, although promising, has not shown any improvement in perinatal outcomes [33].

REFERENCES

1. World Health Organization. 2018. WHO recommendation on intermittent fetal heart rate auscultation during labour. 2018. WHO, Geneva.
2. Lewis D and Downe S. FIGO consensus guidelines on intrapartum fetal monitoring: Intermittent auscultation. *International Journal of Gynecology & Obstetrics*. 2015. 131: 9-12.
3. Maude RM, Skinner JP, Foureur MJ. Intelligent Structured Intermittent Auscultation (ISIA): Evaluation of a decision-making framework for fetal heart monitoring of low-risk women. *BMC Pregnancy Childbirth* [Internet]. 2014. 14(1):184. Available from: https://doi.org/10.1186/1471-2393-14-184.
4. Intelligent Intermittent Auscultation in labour—e-learning for health care 2023. https://www.e-lfh.org.uk/programmes/intelligent-intermittent-auscultation-in-labour/.
5. ACOG Practice Bulletin No. 106: Intrapartum fetal heart rate monitoring: Nomenclature, interpretation, and general management principles. *Obstet Gynecol* [Internet]. 2009. 114(1):192–202. Available on insights.ovid.com.
6. Gibb D, Arulkumaran S. *Electronic fetal monitoring: Terminology and interpretation*—The basics. Chapter 4. Fetal monitoring in practice. Oxford: Elsevier Ltd. 2023. p.25-46.
7. Badawi N, Kurinczuk JJ, Keogh JM, et al. Antepartum risk factors for newborn encephalopathy: The Western Australia case-control study. *BMJ*. 1998. 317: 1549e53.
8. Badawi N, Kurinczuk JJ, Keogh JM, et al. Intrapartum risk factors for newborn encephalopathy: The Western Australian case-control study. *BMJ*. 1998; 317: 1554e8.
9. NICE guideline 229. 2022. https://www.nice.org.uk/guidance/ng229/chapter/Recommendations.
10. Beard RW, Filshie GM, Knight CA, Roberts GM. The significance of the changes in the continuous fetal heart rate in the first stage of labour. *The J of Obstetrics & Gynaecology of British Commonwealth*. 1971. 78:865 – 881.
11. Kubli FW, Hon EH, Khazin AF, Takemura H. Observations on heart rate and pH in the human fetus during labor. *Am J Obstet Gynecol* [Internet]. 1969. 104(8):1190–206.
12. Ingemarsson I, Arulkumaran S, Ratnam SS. Single injection of terbutaline in term labor: Effect on fetal pH in cases with prolonged bradycardia. *Am J Obstet Gynecol* [Internet]. 1985.153(8):859–65.
13. Leung TY, Chung PW, Rogers MS, Sahota DS, Lao TT-H, Chung TKH. Urgent cesarean delivery for fetal bradycardia. *Obstet Gynecol* [Internet]. 2009. 114(5).
14. Gibb D, Arulkumaran S. Chapter 12. Cardiotocographic interpretation—Additional clinical scenarios. Oxford: Elsevier Ltd. 2023. p.130-140.
15. The Royal Australian and New Zealand College of Obstetricians and Gynaecologists. Intrapartum Fetal Surveillance: Clinical guideline [Internet]. 2019. Available on https://ranzcog.edu.au/RANZCOG_SITE/media/RANZCOG-MEDIA/Women%27s%20Health/Statement%20and%20guidelines/Clinical-Obstetrics/IFS-Guideline-4thEdition-2019.pdf?ext=.pdf.
16. Ayres–de–Campos D, Spong CY, Chandraharan E. FIGO consensus guidelines on intrapartum fetal monitoring: Cardiotocography. *International Journal of Gynecology & Obstetrics*. 2015. 131: 13-24.
17. Nelson KB, Dambrosia JM, Ting TY, Grether JK. Uncertain value of electronic fetal heart rate monitoring in predicting cerebral palsy. *N Engl J Med*. 1996. 334: 613e8.
18. Williams KP, Galerneau F. Intrapartum fetal heart rate patterns in the prediction of neonatal acidemia. *Am J Obstet Gynecol* [Internet]. 2003. 188(3):820–3.
19. Chandraharan E, Arulkumaran S. Prevention of birth asphyxia: Responding appropriately to cardiotocograph (CTG) traces. *Best Pract Res Clin Obstet Gynaecol*. 2007. 4: 609e24.
20. Ingemarsson I, Arulkumaran S, Ingemarsson E, Tamby Raja RL, Ratnam SS. Admission test. A screening test for fetal distress in labour. *Obstet Gynecol*. 1986. 68:800-806.
21. Ingemarsson I, Arulkumaran S, Paul RH, Ingemarsson E, Tamby Raja RL, Ratnam SS. Fetal acoustic stimulation in early labour in patients screened with the admission test. *Am J of Obstet and Gynecol*. 1988. 158:70-74.
22. Impey L, Reynolds M, MacQuillan K, Gates S, Murphy J, Sheil O. Admission cardiotocography: A randomised controlled trial. *Lancet Lond Engl*. 2003. 361(9356):465–70.
23. Bix E, Reiner LM, Klovning A, Oian P. Prognostic value of the labour admission test and its effectiveness compared with auscultation only: A systematic review. *BJOG Int J Obstet Gynaecol*. 2005. 112(12):1595–604.
24. Gourounti K, Sandall J. Admission cardiotocography versus intermittent auscultation of fetal heart rate: Effects on neonatal Apgar score, on the rate of caesarean

sections and on the rate of instrumental delivery: A systematic review. *Int J Nurs Stud.* 2007. 44(6):1029–35.

25. Wiberg-Itzel E, Lipponer C, Norman M, et al. Determination of pH or lactate in fetal scalp blood in management of intrapartum fetal distress: Randomised controlled multicentre trial. *BMJ.* 2008. 336:1284e7.
26. Chandraharan E. Should national guidelines continue to recommend fetal scalp blood sampling during labor? *J Matern Fetal Neonatal Med.* 2016. 29:3682.
27. Arulkumaran S, Ingemarsson I, Ratnam SS. Fetal heart rate response to scalp stimulation as a test of fetal wellbeing in labour. *Asia Oceania J Obstet Gvnaecol.* 1987. 13:131-135.
28. Ingemarsson I, Arulkumaran, S Reactive FHR response to sound stimulation in fetuses with low scalp blood pH. *Br J Obstet Gynaecol.* 1989. 96:562-565.
29. Amer-Wahlin I, Hellsten C, Noren H, et al. Cardiotocography only versus cardiotocography plus ST analysis of fetal electrocardiogram for intrapartum fetal monitoring: A Swedish randomized controlled trial. *Lancet.* 2001. 358: 534e8.
30. Noren H, Carlsson A. Reduced prevalence of metabolic acidosis at birth: An analysis of established STAN usage in the total population of deliveries in a Swedish district hospital. *Am J Obstet Gynecol.* 2010; 202: 546. e1e7.
31. Neilson JP. Fetal electrocardiogram (ECG) for fetal monitoring during labour. *Cochrane Database of Systematic Reviews.* 2015. Issue 12. Art. No.: CD000116.
32. Royal College of Obstetricians and Gynaecologists. Each Baby Counts: 2020 Final Progress Report. London: RCOG. 2021. https://www.rcog.org.uk/media/a4eg2xnm/ebc-2020-final-progress-report.pdf.
33. Lutomski JE, Meaney S, Greene RA, et al. Expert systems for fetal assessment in labour. *Cochrane Database Syst Rev.* 2015. Issue 4. Art. no.:CD010708.

CHAPTER 9

Labour Analgesia

M SUBRAHMANYAM, SAILAJA K

INTRODUCTION

The birth of a baby is one of the most joyous events in a woman's life. However, labour is also one of the most painful experiences a woman can face. Labour pain is rated among the most severe kinds of pain known and ranks higher than cancer pain and only below the pain of amputation [1]. The only difference between labour and other pain is that labour pain ceases immediately with the birth of the baby. In modern obstetric care, the pain of labour and methods to relieve it are areas of concern for both the woman and the medical personnel involved in her care.

Summarising pain relief during childbirth, the American College of Obstetricians and Gynecologists (ACOG) [2] has expressed concern for the fact that 'in no other circumstance is it considered acceptable for a person to experience severe pain, amenable to safe intervention, while under a physician's care'. The ACOG strongly recommends that the labouring woman's request for pain relief is sufficient justification for providing it. Thus, it is imperative that healthcare providers offer pain relief to labouring women in a facility that provides care for labouring women.

Key Point

The maximum amount of abuse faced by labouring women is in response to their desperate cry for pain relief. Globally, women are ignored, scolded, and physically and emotionally abused when they request help and alleviation of the pain they are experiencing.

HISTORY OF LABOUR ANALGESIA

A new chapter in the history of labour analgesia began in the nineteenth century with the use of chloroform by an obstetrician, James Young Simpson, from Edinburgh. In 1902, an Austrian physician Richard von Steinbuchel used morphine and scopolamine for labour analgesia for the first time. This was called 'twilight sleep'; however, this method was found to result in the intoxication of the mother and respiratory distress of the newborn.

Despite other methods of pain relief being available, lumbar epidural anesthesia is still the most effective method of pain relief in labour and is considered the 'gold standard' of labour analgesia [3]. Drug concentrations, doses, volumes, and the equipment used to administer epidural have undergone serial changes over the years.

CAUSES OF LABOUR PAIN

Labour is a painful experience involving both physiological and psychological mechanisms. It has two components, which are explained below:

- **Visceral pain** occurs during the first and second stages of childbirth. It is described as severe cramping in the uterus and may radiate to the abdominal wall, lower back, gluteal areas, and thighs. It involves the **spinal roots T10–L1**. It is caused by both the distension of the uterus and ischemia of cervical and uterine tissues (Fig. 9.1) [4].
- **Somatic pain** occurs during the late first stage and the second stage. This is caused

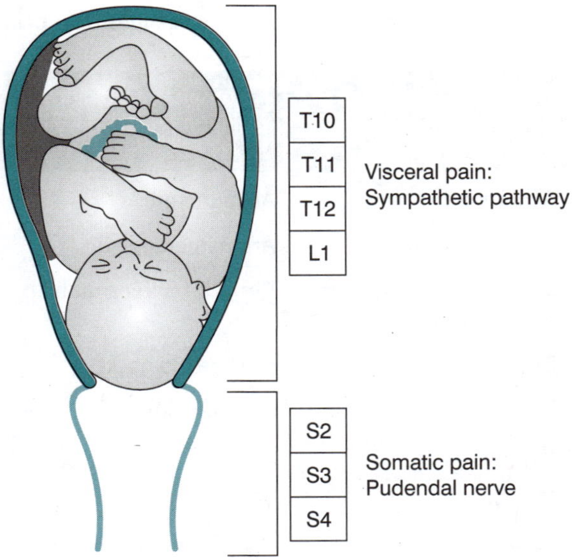

Fig. 9.1 Pain pathways in labour

by the distension of the vagina, perineum, and the pelvic floor as the fetal head passes through the pelvis. It is mediated by the **S2–S4 spinal segments** [4].

The distinction of labour into various stages is important to anesthetists because pain impulses follow different pathways during each stage of labour.

> **Key Point**
>
> Labour pain has two components—visceral pain and somatic pain. The pain of labour in the first stage is mediated by T10 to L1 spinal segments, whereas that in the second stage is carried by the S2 to S4 spinal segments.

Factors Affecting Labour Pain

Pregnant women are most concerned about the pain they will experience in labour and how it will be managed. Labour can be daunting, especially in the first pregnancy, when the woman is not sure what to expect. Some women opt for cesarean section electively because of the fear of pain. Antenatal preparation classes are an excellent opportunity to inform and educate women about various non-pharmacological and pharmacological methods of pain relief. This allows the woman to understand the information when she is pain-free and make an informed choice when in labour.

Every woman's experience during labour is different. Hence, a multidimensional understanding of labour pain provides the basis for a woman-centred approach to its management.

> **Key Point**
>
> One of the important aims of antenatal classes is to provide the woman and her birth companion with a realistic understanding of the quality of pain and to assure her that labour pain can be managed in both non-pharmacological and pharmacological ways.

Many factors can impact the level of pain experienced during delivery and childbirth. These include the following:

- Physical and mental health
- Pain tolerance
- Pelvic size
- Fetal size
- Fetal position
- Intensity of contractions

Effect of Labour Pain on the Mother and the Fetus

Unrelieved pain during labour is emotionally traumatic for most women. It has been linked to postpartum depression [5].

In some women, labour pain is associated with hyperventilation, which may cause a further reduction in maternal carbon dioxide levels. In rare cases, this can lead to respiratory alkalemia, which may cause vasoconstriction in the uterine vascular bed and fetal hypoxia [6,7] (Fig. 9.2).

METHODS OF PAIN RELIEF IN LABOUR

Methods of pain relief in labour can broadly be classified as non-pharmacological and pharmacological.

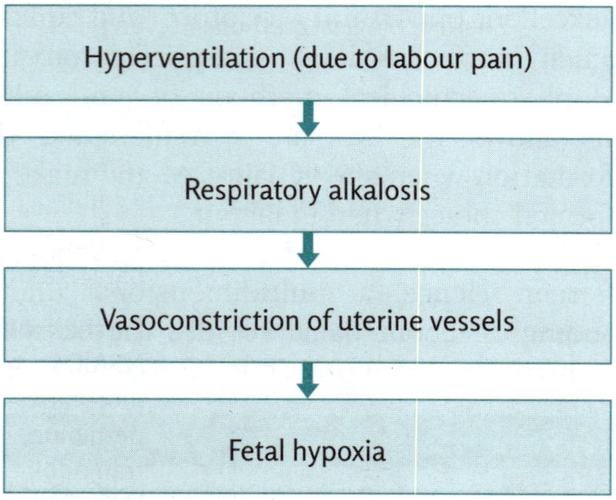

Fig. 9.2 Effect of labour pain on fetal oxygenation

Non-Pharmacological Techniques

Non-pharmacological techniques can further be divided into those requiring devices and those that do not (Table 9.1).

If the woman is lying down, the head end of the bed can be raised to a level that is most comfortable for her.

Various exercises and postures have been described to ease the pain and promote the descent of the baby. Most of these involve the support of the husband and can even be performed with a functioning epidural. Some of the postures include the rocking cat position (with the woman on all fours), supported squat, leaning against the wall, and hip circles on a birthing ball (Fig. 9.3).

Non-pharmacological methods such as relaxation techniques and acupuncture may provide some comfort without any side effects. A systematic review of the Cochrane Database found insufficient evidence to judge whether hypnosis, biofeedback, aromatherapy, and TENS provide satisfactory pain relief [8].

Continuous support during labour

Labour can be very isolating. There is mounting evidence that continuous one-to-one emotional support provided by a midwife or the woman's partner, mother, or female friend is associated with

Table 9.1 Non-pharmacological techniques for pain relief in labour

Non-pharmacological techniques (without devices)	Non-pharmacological techniques (with devices)
Acupressure	Acupuncture
Changing positions	Aromatherapy
Counterpressure on the back	Birthing ball/Peanut ball
Deep breathing	Hot-or-cold packs
Exercises	Hydrotherapy
Hypnosis	Music
Massage	TENS
Movement	Digital entertainment/ distraction in the form of relaxing videos or music
Relaxation techniques	Water immersion

TENS, transcutaneous electrical nerve stimulation

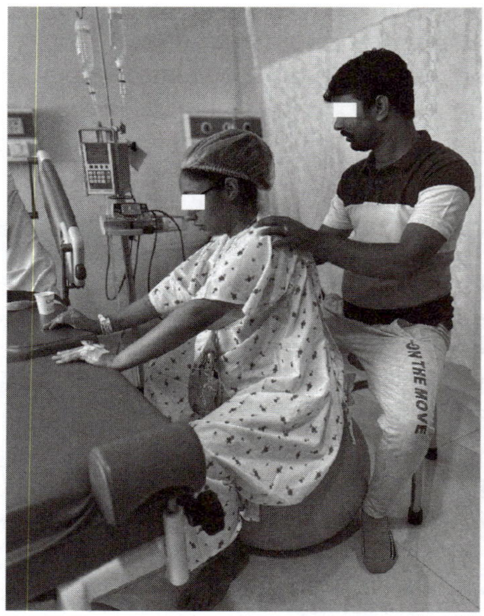

Fig. 9.3 Labouring woman utilising a combination of pain relief techniques—epidural through a continuous infusion, a birthing ball, and her partner's support (*Image courtesy:* Rainbow Hospitals, Hyderabad)

better tolerance of pain and improved outcomes for the woman in labour. This is quite logical since a woman who feels comforted and supported will feel more in control of the birth process [9].

Transcutaneous electrical nerve stimulation (TENS)

Although the exact mechanism is not clear, transcutaneous electrical nerve stimulation may work through the modulation of the pain impulses reaching the substantia gelatinosa and the liberation of endogenous opioids. The electrodes are placed in the T10–T12 area of the back. Though overall not very effective [9], it is probably useful during the early stages of labour, when there is lower back pain [10].

Water birth

Warm water helps relieve tension and shifts the woman's focus onto the warmth of the water rather than the pain of the contraction. It also stimulates the body to produce endorphins which, in turn, promote relaxation.

Breathing techniques

Women often use deep breathing exercises during labour. These exercises stimulate the parasympathetic system and release endorphins; the combination bestows upon the woman a sense of calmness. A recent systematic review and meta-analysis [11] showed that breathing exercises reduce the duration of the second stage of labour, though on their own they do not significantly reduce pain or anxiety.

The ultimate success of the techniques described above predominantly depends upon the woman's motivation. The success of these methods varies widely, and these modes have not been universally accepted.

Pharmacological Methods of Pain Relief

Pharmacological methods of pain relief can be non-opioid or opioid (Table 9.2).

Table 9.2 Pharmacological methods of pain relief

Mode of analgesia	Types of analgesia	Drugs used
Intramuscular medications	Non-opioid and opioid analgesia	NSAIDs, pethidine, tramadol, paracetamol
Intravenous medications	Non-opioid and opioid analgesia	Paracetamol, NSAIDs, morphine, pethidine, tramadol, ketamine
Inhalational analgesia	Gaseous inhalation	Entonox, sevoflurane
Regional blocks	Epidural, combined spinal–epidural, single-shot spinal, continuous intrathecal, quadratus lumborum, erector spinae, pudendal	Bupivacaine, ropivacaine, lignocaine, opioids

Non-opioid systemic analgesics in labour analgesia

Analgesics and sedatives come under this group of labour analgesia (Table 9.3). They improve pain scores moderately and less effectively than parenteral opioids.

Table 9.3 Non-opioid systemic analgesics

Drug	Dosage
Paracetamol	600 mg IM/1 g IV infusion/650–1000 mg orally every 4–6 hours
Ketamine	0.25–0.5 mg/Kg IV as a bolus followed by an infusion of 0.5 mg/Kg/hour

Paracetamol may not control pain adequately. However, in low-resource settings, where narcotics may not be freely available without a narcotics license, several recent studies [12,13] have found that both IM and IV paracetamol provide a moderate reduction in pain scores in labour. Compared to pethidine and tramadol, IV paracetamol has a comparable reduction in pain scores with fewer side effects [14]. Paracetamol may be given as a dose of 600 mg IM or as a 1 g IV infusion. The dose may be repeated after four hours. In the absence of skilled birth attendants, it may also be given orally in doses of 650–1000 mg every 4–6 hours.

Ketamine can cause somnolence and dissociation from the birth when given in regular doses of 2 mg/Kg IV. Ketamine as a bolus of 0.5 mg/Kg followed by an infusion of 0.5 mg/Kg/hr is a reasonable alternative when regional anesthesia is not an option. With this dose, there is a minimal incidence of hallucinations, which are otherwise common with the usual doses of ketamine.

Systemic opioids in labour analgesia

The WHO recommends parenteral opioids such as fentanyl, morphine, and pethidine for healthy pregnant women requesting labour analgesia, depending on the woman's preferences [15].

Morphine, pethidine, fentanyl, and remifentanil are 'pure agonists' on opioid receptors, whereas butorphanol and nalbuphine are 'agonist–antagonists' at the opioid receptors. Tramadol has multiple mechanisms of action.

Parenteral opioids such as pethidine appear to provide relief from labour pain but are associated with drowsiness, nausea, and vomiting. Because of the unpredictability of the time of childbirth, the timing of opioid administration on a need basis may be a challenge. They may depress the baby's breathing if they are given very close to the time of delivery. The measurement of oxygen saturation levels in the baby is therefore essential. Opioids may also interfere with the baby's first feed.

Pethidine by the IM route is the most commonly used opioid in India, especially when there are no other alternatives available. The WHO recommends it for pain relief in labour for healthy pregnant women [15]. The most ideal timing of delivery is within 1 hour of or >4 hours after a dose of pethidine as this drug reaches a maximal concentration in the fetus 2–3 hours after maternal dosing. Delivering the infant within 2–3 hours after the administration of pethidine may result in neonatal respiratory depression. Naloxone may be needed to reverse the effect of opioid analgesics. An estimation of the probable time of delivery should be kept in mind when administering a dose of pethidine.

Tramadol is more potent than paracetamol, but not as potent as other opioids. It is easily available and is not associated with the neonatal depression caused by pethidine. However, there are not enough high-quality studies regarding its efficacy in labour.

Fentanyl administered subcutaneously or as an intranasal spray is as efficacious in relieving labour pain as intramuscular pethidine and was found to result in greater satisfaction and less sedation [16]. However, a scoping review found limited evidence, especially in randomised controlled trials, to evaluate the effectiveness and harms of fentanyl in LMICs [17].

Remifentanil is a very-short-acting potent synthetic opioid. Its onset of action is very quick (<2 minutes) and wears off within a few minutes; hence, it is used as an infusion. Its advantage is that it can be used almost until the baby is born. An open-label, multicentre, randomised controlled trial on IV remifentanil patient-controlled analgesia (PCA) versus IM pethidine for pain relief in labour [18] showed that intravenous remifentanil PCA was superior to pethidine (fewer women asked for an epidural). Remifentanil can cause maternal respiratory depression, nausea, vomiting, and pruritus. It is used in situations where epidural is contraindicated (e.g., coagulopathy, prior surgery at the site of injection).

Various opioids used for labour analgesia and their dosages are listed in Table 9.4.

Inhalational analgesia (Entonox®)

Entonox is an odourless gas which is a mixture of 50% O_2 and 50% nitrous oxide (N_2O). It can be self-administered by the labouring woman through a handheld face mask and takes effect within a minute. It has mild-to-moderate effectiveness in relieving pain. The woman should inhale the gas at least 30 seconds before a contraction. Side effects may include nausea, vomiting, dizziness, and drowsiness. As contractions increase in frequency, the mask has to

Table 9.4 Systemic opioids for labour analgesia

Drug	Dose	Onset by route of administration	Duration
Morphine	2–4 mg IV/IM	3 min IV; 40 min IM	2–4 hrs
Pethidine	1–2 mg/Kg IM or 25–50 mg slow IV	40–45 min IM; 5–10 min IV	2–3 hrs
Fentanyl	0.5–1 mcg/Kg IV or 1–2 mcg/Kg IM	2–3 min IV; 10 min IM; 5–10 min IV;	30–60 min
Tramadol	1–2 mg/Kg IM	10–15 min IM	2–3 hrs
Remifentanil	0.05–0.1 mcg/Kg/min infusion; 0.2-0.5 mcg boluses	1–2 min	2–3 min

be held almost continually and is inconvenient. It is usually used during early labour or when regional analgesia is not an option or not working effectively.

Key Point

Recent studies have shown that N_2O may have potential health effects on medical staff. This has led to several hospitals in the UK withdrawing it for labour analgesia. Being a greenhouse gas, N_2O has also been shown to have a harmful impact on climate change.

Local Infiltration

- **Paracervical block** and **pudendal block** are used in some obstetric units when neuraxial analgesia is not available.
- **Perineal infiltration** with a local anesthetic is commonly used if an episiotomy is to be performed or a perineal tear is to be repaired. Perineal infiltration acts on the terminal nerves in the posterior fourchette and perineum. The commonly used anesthetic agent is a 2% solution of lidocaine. It may be good practice to give the infiltration during a contraction as the mother may experience less discomfort. See **Chapter 7**, *Episiotomy—what does the evidence say?* for further details.

Regional Neuraxial Techniques for Labour Analgesia

Regional techniques for labour have been in use for more than a century.

The neuraxial techniques commonly used are listed below:

- Epidural analgesia (EA)
- Combined spinal–epidural analgesia (CSEA)

The less commonly used ones are as follows:

- Continuous spinalanalgesia (CSA)
- Dural puncture epidural
- Single-shot spinal analgesia (SSSA)
- Bilateral erector spinae block (ultrasound guidance, continuous catheter)
- Bilateral quadratus lumborum block (ultrasound guidance, continuous catheter)

Epidural analgesia

Epidural is the most commonly used neuraxial block for labour analgesia in HICs and among the more advantaged women in LMICs [15]. Due to its cost and requirement for highly trained physicians, its availability within countries not only varies between facilities but also between rural and urban populations [19].

Epidural is one of the safest, most effective, and most widely used form of labour analgesia. With the advent of better techniques, monitoring equipment, and a shift towards lower concentrations of medications, epidural has become the most accepted pain relief method for many labouring women worldwide.

Around 40–50% of women in the UK and Europe opt for epidural analgesia; in the US, the number is closer to 70%. While data from India is not available, utilisation is stated to be about 50–60% in institutions that have an epidural service.

The epidural space is the potential space all around the dura mater extending from the cervical to the sacral segments. Every spinal nerve leaving the spinal cord transverses this space before exiting to supply various dermatomes. Hence, a local anesthetic that spreads in this space has the potential to block the nerve impulses transmitting pain sensations. Depending on the site of injection and the amount of drug injected, specific dermatomal level blocks can be achieved.

Epidural solutions are given by bolus injections or infusion by different techniques. Lower concentrations of local anesthetic given with an opioid allow women to maintain the ability to move around during labour and actively participate in the birthing process.

Timing of epidural

An epidural can be performed any time after the diagnosis of labour has been established and the woman has requested pain relief without waiting for a specific degree of cervical dilation [2]. A systematic review of the Cochrane Database [20] compared early initiation (<4 cm cervical dilatation) with later initiation of epidural analgesia and found no difference in cesarean delivery rate, instrumental delivery, duration of the second stage of labour, and fetal outcomes.

Advanced labour is not a contraindication, as delivery time cannot be accurately predicted. Moreover, an epidural provides analgesia when the woman needs an operative intervention.

Position for epidural analgesia

An epidural can be administered either in the sitting or the lateral position. The authors of this chapter prefer to administer the drug in the sitting position, as this increases the chance of successfully siting epidurals, especially in the obese parturient.

Procedure

After proper positioning and asepsis, a local anesthetic is administered at the intended site of the procedure (L3–L4 or L4–L5 interspace). The epidural needle is inserted towards the epidural space by passing the needle in between the spinous processes (through the skin, subcutaneous tissue, interspinous ligament, and ligamentum flavum; Fig. 9.4). The loss of resistance is assessed either by air or saline. The catheter is threaded into the epidural space until 4–5 cm of the catheter is within the space, and then secured firmly. A bolus dose of the chosen low-dose epidural medication should be given in aliquots of 5–8 mL to rule out intrathecal or intravascular placement.

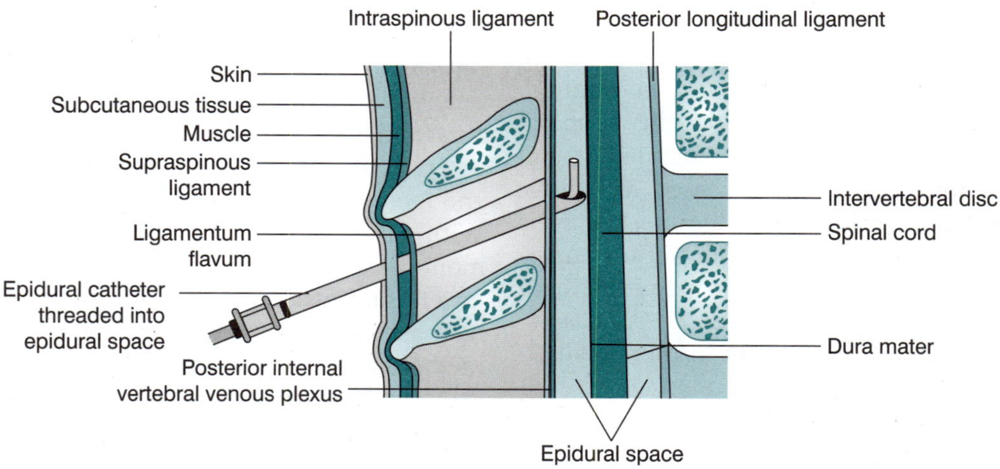

Fig. 9.4 The needle is inserted through the skin, subcutaneous tissue, interspinous ligament, and ligamentum flavum into the epidural space. After checking that the needle is in the right space, the catheter is threaded in

The woman should remain under continuous direct observation by an anesthesia provider, labour nurse, or midwife for at least 30 minutes after the administration of neuraxial medication boluses. During this period, continuous fetal heart rate and maternal oxygen saturation monitoring should be maintained, with the woman's blood pressure measured at least every 5 minutes. In rare cases, severe hypotension can occur acutely from anesthetic drug administration into the intrathecal space (a total spinal), or unintended administration into a blood vessel. Rapid diagnosis and treatment prevent further complications. Similar monitoring is required whenever an additional bolus is administered.

Drugs used for epidural analgesia

The current trend is to use a low concentration of the local anesthetic drug along with an opioid. Typically, bupivacaine is used at concentrations ranging from 0.0625% (ultra-low dose) to 0.125%, with fentanyl 2–3 mcg/mL. A typical starting dose involves giving 10–15 mL of the above mixture as a bolus in two to three aliquots over 3–10 minutes and then, either as an infusion or patient-controlled epidural analgesia (PCEA) as described below.

Maintenance of analgesia

Maintenance of analgesia is done in one of three ways (Table 9.5):

- **Intermittent boluses:** Intermittent boluses are administered by a physician or a nurse when the woman complains of pain. This technique can be utilised in low-resource settings when infusion pumps are not available. Breakthrough pain is more frequent with this method. With each bolus, the woman's hemodynamics are monitored for 15–20 minutes.
- **Continuous infusion**: A syringe pump delivers a continuous infusion of the local anesthetic and opioid mixture at a pre-set rate of 8–10 mL/hour depending on the concentration used.

Table 9.5 Maintenance of epidural analgesia

Maintenance	Description
Intermittent boluses	Manual injection of bolus periodically
Continuous infusions	Through syringe pumps
Patient-controlled epidural analgesia (PCEA)	The woman triggers a pre-set bolus, delivered by an electronic pump
Programmed intermittent boluses	A machine delivers programmed periodic bolus doses
Computerised-integrated background infusions	Programmed to analyse the drug use across the last hour and adjust the background infusion rate according to an algorithm

- **Patient-controlled epidural analgesia (PCEA):** PCEA is a technique in which the woman essentially controls her own analgesia. Many studies have found that the drug usage is lower with PCEA than in a conventional infusion regimen of a fixed volume per hour.

Programmed intermittent epidural bolus (PIEB) and computerised-integrated background infusions are recent techniques for maintaining labour analgesia.

Combined spinal–epidural analgesia (CSEA)

This procedure is usually performed with a CSEA kit involving a needle-through-needle technique (Fig. 9.5) that deposits the opioid in the subarachnoid space followed by a catheter that is threaded into the epidural space to administer a local anesthetic. The remaining steps are similar to those of the epidural technique. A bolus of the intrathecal drug is administered (25 mcg of fentanyl and 0.5 mL bupivacaine). A local anesthetic is given through the epidural if needed as labour progresses.

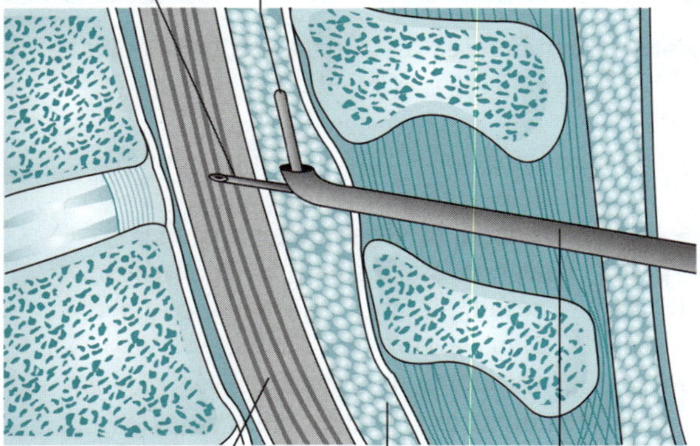

Fig. 9.5 Combined spinal–epidural (CSEA) analgesia: The analgesic agents are given into both the epidural space and the subarachnoid space.

Monitoring the woman receiving epidural analgesia

Whichever technique or drug combination is used, the labouring woman needs to be frequently monitored. The monitoring parameters include BP, pulse, and saturation along with the fetal heart rate. Initial BP monitoring should be every 3 minutes for 20 minutes following a bolus dose and then every 15 minutes till 2 hours post-delivery.

Further, the sensory level of the block should be documented by testing for the loss of cold sensation with ice. The level of the block should be T10 dermatome and below. The woman should also be checked for the presence of a motor block, which should be avoided.

Table 9.6 presents the advantages and disadvantages of the different methods of labour analgesia.

Effects of neuraxial analgesia on maternal and neonatal outcomes

Findings from a recent study in which primigravid women undergoing vaginal delivery with and without neuraxial analgesia were analysed suggest that the use of neuraxial analgesia for vaginal delivery is associated with a decrease in the risk of severe morbidity and mortality. This might be attributable to the sustained intrapartum hemodynamic monitoring of labouring women with neuraxial analgesia, the adequate intravenous access which allows for immediate fluid resuscitation, and the preparedness for acute events which is available with the presence of an anesthetic team. These findings are more relevant in HICs where neuraxial analgesia is available for the majority of labouring women [23].

The most common concerns raised with neuraxial analgesia are the prolongation of labour, the need for instrumental deliveries, and an increase in cesarean delivery rates.

Prolongation of labour

There is a small but insignificant increase in the duration of the second stage (an average of 7.66 minutes), but this does not affect outcomes [21].

Instrumental deliveries

Earlier studies reported that the risk of instrumental vaginal delivery increased with the use of epidural analgesia [22]. However, an analysis of trials conducted after 2005 failed to demonstrate a significant difference and may reflect a lower concentration of local anesthetics used in modern epidurals [2,21].

Cesarean delivery rate

In a systematic review of the Cochrane Database, there was no increase in cesarean delivery rates with epidurals even when initiated early in labour [21].

Key Point

There is no increase in operative or cesarean delivery rates with the use of low-dose epidural analgesia [2,21].

Neonatal outcomes

There is no evidence to show that epidural analgesia has any effect on the fetus or neonate [2].

Table 9.6 Advantages and disadvantages of different methods of labour analgesia

Method of labour analgesia	Advantages	Disadvantages
IV/IM non-narcotic analgesics	Minor analgesia may be provided	Not potent
IV/IM narcotic analgesics	• Moderate analgesia provided • No need for special equipment	• Repeated doses may be needed • Cannot be given too close to the delivery as neonatal respiratory depression may result • Nausea, vomiting, itching, and sedation in the labouring woman
Inhalational analgesia	• Moderate pain relief • Non-invasive	• Needs equipment—cylinder and proper mask unit for inhalation • Cumbersome to hold for long periods
Epidural analgesia	• Gold-standard for labour analgesia • Can be used for anesthesia in case a cesarean section is needed • Titration of medication possible throughout labour • Predictable spread of sensory blockade • Does not require dural puncture	• Side effects present—most of them manageable • Requires knowledgeable healthcare providers to monitor and treat complications • In situ catheter has a potential for errors (e.g., mistaking for an intravenous catheter) if not clearly labelled
Combined spinal–epidural analgesia	• Quick onset and dense initial block and good pain relief compared to epidural • High success rate of epidural catheter placement compared to the epidural technique	• Potentially, higher incidence of fetal bradycardia, but not associated with increased cesarean delivery rate • The epidural cannot be tested until the spinal effect wears off • Has all the disadvantages of epidural (listed above) • There may be increased maternal pruritus as intrathecal opioids are used
Single-shot spinal analgesia	• Does not require extra equipment for infusion • Rapid onset • Does not require ongoing availability of anesthesia providers • Simple procedure	• Re-spinal may be required if the labour is prolonged, due to limited duration • Inadequate analgesia is possible for the second stage of labour • Maternal hypotension is more common depending on the dosage of medications
Continuous spinal analgesia	Usually utilised when an accidental dural puncture occurs	Labelling should be done, and handover should be proper to prevent high doses from being given accidentally

Key Point

One of the most frequently voiced concerns from women about epidural analgesia is the possibility of residual back pain. In a randomised controlled study, Howell et al. [24] found no increase in the risk of post-delivery back pain after epidural analgesia.

Contraindications for neuraxial analgesia

Epidural is safe for the majority of women and has few contraindications. The contraindications are as follows:

- Maternal coagulopathy (inherited or acquired)
- Thrombocytopenia with a platelet count of <70,000/dL
- Increased intracranial pressure
- Infection at the site of injection
- Maternal septicemia
- Maternal hemorrhage
- Prior surgery at the site of injection
- Severe spine deformity

Thrombocytopenia and neuraxial analgesia

The Society for Obstetric Anesthesia and Perinatology (SOAP) task force recommends proceeding with neuraxial anesthesia in most cases if the platelet count is >70,000/dL and there is no evidence of clinical bleeding [25].

Anticoagulation and neuraxial analgesia

The 2018 guidelines from the American Society of Regional Anaesthesia and Pain Medicine (ASRA) [26] and the SOAP Consensus Statement on women receiving thromboprophylaxis both suggest that the use of non-steroidal anti-inflammatory drugs including aspirin does not increase the risk of spinal–epidural hematoma [27]. Table 9.7 lists the anticoagulant medications in use and the timing of the placement and removal of the epidural to prevent epidural hematomas.

The incidence of spinal–epidural hematoma in labouring women is exceedingly low. This may be attributed to the hypercoagulability that exists during pregnancy [25].

Table 9.7 **Management of thromboprophylaxis with epidural analgesia (these guidelines do not address risks with multiple therapies or comorbidities that interfere with coagulation)**

Agent	Interval from the last dose to catheter placement	Time after neuraxial block/catheter removal
Aspirin, NSAIDs	No need to stop	Can give any time
Low-molecular-weight heparin prophylaxis	≥12 hrs	>4 hrs
Low-molecular-weight heparin treatment	24 hrs	>4 hrs
Unfractionated heparin prophylaxis	4–6 hrs	1 hr
Unfractionated heparin treatment	12 hrs	1 hr

Adverse effects of neuraxial techniques

Itching, nausea, vomiting, shivering, and a mild rise in temperature have been noted in some women receiving labour analgesia. Itching has a reported incidence of close to 100% for fentanyl, which is often used for combined spinal–epidural labour analgesia. Nausea and vomiting are caused by epidural opioids. Central neuraxial blockade-related shivering occurs due to vasodilatation caused by sympathetic blockade with redistribution of heat from the core to the periphery.

Maternal hypotension, though rare with the current low-dose mixtures used for epidural analgesia, must be anticipated. It can be prevented by preloading the mother with 500–1000 mL of normal saline IV prior to the epidural. This expands the maternal vascular space. In women with severe preeclampsia, a lower volume of fluid may be given as a preload.

If the BP falls to 20% below the baseline, it can be treated using fluids and vasopressors such as phenylephrine (100 mcg boluses), ephedrine (5 mg boluses), or mephentermine (5–6 mg boluses).

Postdural puncture headache (PDPH) or **spinal headache** may occur if there is an accidental dural puncture, which occurs in 1–2% of epidurals and can be as high as 10% with a spinal. The headache is severe, described as a retro-orbital throbbing and is usually associated with neck stiffness. The headache is positional—it worsens on standing up and is relieved in the supine position. Usually, PDPH appears after 24 hours and disappears in 6–8 days without any treatment. Medical management with drugs such as acetaminophen, NSAIDs, caffeine, and parenteral narcotics, along with good hydration helps in managing it most of the time.

If the headache persists, an **epidural blood patch** (EBP) is administered, which involves injecting 15–20 mL of the mother's blood into the epidural space under strict asepsis. The blood clots and seals the dural puncture made by the epidural needle, thus reducing spinal fluid leakage, and thereby treating the headache. EBP reduces the duration and intensity of postdural puncture headache and usually provides immediate relief.

Urinary retention may occur after an epidural and is managed with intermittent catheterisation or a Foley catheter.

Rare side effects associated with epidurals are breathing difficulty, nerve damage, infection, seizures, hematoma, postpartum nephropathy, epidural abscess, and meningitis.

LABOUR ANALGESIA IN LOW- AND MIDDLE-INCOME COUNTRIES (LMICs) WITH LIMITED RESOURCES

The importance of the **continuous support provided by a birth companion** during labour should not be underestimated in the alleviation of pain. Irrespective of the choice of pain relief offered and accepted, companionship in labour should be offered to all women.

Paracetamol, a non-opioid drug, is easily available in LMICs. Studies have shown that compared to pethidine and tramadol, IV paracetamol has a comparable reduction in pain scores with fewer side effects [14].

Opioid analgesics such as pethidine and tramadol are more cost-effective than epidural analgesia. While parenteral opioids are inexpensive, due to strict laws governing their usage and licensing (NDPS Act), these drugs are not freely available in many centres. The WHO recommends fentanyl for labour analgesia; however, a scoping review found limited evidence, especially from randomised controlled trials, to evaluate the effectiveness and harms of fentanyl in LMICs [17].

Single-shot spinal analgesia may work well for low-resource settings as it does not need the placement of a catheter or the use of an infusion pump, but is limited by the short duration of analgesia.

Epidural analgesia requires skilled healthcare providers and continuous monitoring and is not widely available. However, an epidural with intermittent bolus doses is a viable option provided interdisciplinary support is strong and the staff are well-trained. The World Health Organization recommends epidural analgesia but acknowledges that it requires more resources to implement and to manage its complications [15].

CONCLUSION

Using the available and cost-effective labour analgesia techniques with a minimal possibility of complications in a particular setting is of paramount importance in resource-limited settings. Combining different methods of pharmacological and non-pharmacological analgesia depending on the resources and the ability to manage their complications is essential.

REFERENCES

1. Melzack R. The myth of painless childbirth (the John J. Bonica lecture). *Pain*. 1984. 19(4):321-337.
2. American College of Obstetricians and Gynecologists' Committee on Practice Bulletins—Obstetrics. ACOG Practice Bulletin No. 209: Obstetric Analgesia and Anesthesia. *Obstet Gynecol*. 2019. 133(3):e208-e225.
3. Michalczyk M, Torbé D, Torbé A. A brief historical outline of the development of labor analgesia. *Journal of Education, Health and Sport*. 2018;8(9):827-832.
4. Labor S, Maguire S. The Pain of Labour. *Rev Pain*. 2008. 2(2):15-9.
5. Suhitharan T, Pham TP, Chen H, et al. Investigating analgesic and psychological factors associated with risk of postpartum depression development: A case-control study. *Neuropsychiatr Dis Treat*. 2016. 12:1333-9.
6. Fadl ET, Utting JE. A study of maternal acid-base state during labour. *Br J Anaesth*. 1969. 327-337.
7. Reynolds F. Labour analgesia and the baby: Good news is no news. *Int J Obstet Anesth*. 2011. 20(1):38-50.
8. Jones L, Othman M, Dowswell T, et al. Pain management for women in labour: An overview of systematic reviews. *Cochrane Database Syst Rev*. 2012. 14;2012(3).
9. Bohren MA, Hofmeyr G, Sakala C, Fukuzawa RK, Cuthbert A. 2017. Continuous support for women during childbirth. *Cochrane Database Syst Rev*. Issue 7. Art. no.: CD003766.
10. Dowswell T, Bedwell C, Lavender T, Neilson JP. Transcutaneous electrical nerve stimulation (TENS) for pain management in labour. *Cochrane Database of Systematic Reviews*. 2009. Issue 2. Art. No.: CD007214.
11. Issac A, Nayak SG, T P Balakrishnan D, Halemani K, Mishra P P I, Vr V, Jacob J, Stephen S. Effectiveness of breathing exercise on the duration of labour: A systematic review and meta-analysis. *J Glob Health*. 2023. 13:04023.
12. Kaur Makkar J, Jain K, Bhatia N, Jain V, Mal Mithrawal S. Comparison of analgesic efficacy of paracetamol and tramadol for pain relief in active labor. *J Clin Anesth*. 2015. 27(2):159–163.
13. Elbohoty AE, Abd-Elrazek H, Abd-El-Gawad M, et al. 2012. Intravenous infusion of paracetamol versus intravenous pethidine as an intrapartum analgesic in the first stage of labor. *Int J Gynaecol Obstet*. 118.
14. Aimakhu CO, Saanu OO, Olayemi O. Pain relief in labor: A randomized controlled trial comparing intramuscular tramadol with intramuscular paracetamol at the University College Hospital, Ibadan, Nigeria. *Trop J Obstet Gynaecol*. 2017. 34:91-8.
15. World Health Organization. WHO recommendations: Intrapartum care for a positive childbirth experience. 2018. 1–8. WHO, Geneva.
16. Fleet J, Belan I, Jones MJ, Ullah S, Cyna AM. A comparison of fentanyl with pethidine for pain relief during childbirth: A randomised controlled trial. *BJOG*. 2015. 122: 983–992.
17. Show KL, Ngamjarus C, Kongwattanakul K, Rattanakanokchai S, Duangkum C, Bohren MA, Betrán AP, Somjit M, Win WYH, Lumbiganon P. Fentanyl for labour pain management: A scoping review. *BMC Pregnancy Childbirth*. 2022. 17;22(1):846.
18. Wilson MJA, MacArthur C, Hewitt CA, et al. Intravenous remifentanil patient-controlled analgesia versus intramuscular pethidine for pain relief in labour (RESPITE): An open-label, multicentre, randomised controlled trial. *Lancet*. 2018. 392: 662-672.
19. Huang C, Macario A. Economic considerations related to providing adequate pain relief for women in labour: Comparison of epidural and intravenous analgesia. *Pharmaeconomics*. 2002. 20(5):305–18.
20. Sng BL, Leong WL, Zeng Y, et al. Early versus late initiation of epidural analgesia for labour. *Cochrane Database Syst Rev*. 2014. Issue 10. Art. no.: CD007238.
21. Anim-Somuah M, Smyth RM, Cyna AM, Cuthbert A. Epidural versus non-epidural or no analgesia for pain management in labour. *Cochrane Database Syst Rev*. 2018. Issue 5. Art. No.:CD000331.
22. Cambic CR, Wong CA. Labour analgesia and Obstetric outcomes. *Br J of Anaesth*. 2010. 105; S1; i50-i60C.
23. Guglielminotti J, Landau R, Daw J, Friedman AM, Chihuri S, Li G. Use of labor neuraxial analgesia for vaginal delivery and severe maternal morbidity. *JAMA Netw Open*. 2022. 5(2):e220137.
24. Howell CJ, Dean T, Lucking L, et al. Randomised study of long-term outcomes after epidural versus non-epidural analgesia during labour. *BMJ*. 2002. 325:357.
25. Bauer ME, Arendt K, Beilin Y, et al. The Society for Obstetric Anesthesia and Perinatology interdisciplinary consensus statement on neuraxial procedures in obstetric patients with thrombocytopenia. *Anesth Analg*. 2021. 132:1531–1544.
26. Horlocker TT, Vandermeuelen E, Kopp SL, Gogarten W, Leffert LR, Benzon HT. *Regional Anesthesia in the Patient Receiving Antithrombotic or Thrombolytic Therapy*: American Society of Regional Anesthesia and Pain Medicine Evidence-Based Guidelines (Fourth Edition). *Reg Anesth Pain Med*. 2018. 43(3):263-309. Erratum in: *Reg Anesth Pain Med*. 2018. 43(5):566. Vandermeuelen, Erik [corrected to Vandermeulen, Erik]. PMID: 29561531.
27. Scavone Barbara M, Wong Cynthia A. Neuraxial anesthesia and the ubiquitous platelet count question—How low is too low? *Anesthesia & Analgesia*. 2021. 132(6):p 1527-1530.

CHAPTER 10

Immediate Postpartum Monitoring and Care (Including Postpartum Collapse)

JIJI ELIZABETH MATHEWS, RICHA SASMITA TIRKEY

INTRODUCTION

The immediate postpartum period is the phase during which a large proportion of maternal deaths occur [1,2]. Emphasis on managing this phase optimally can have a major impact on reducing maternal mortality.

The hour following the delivery of the baby and the placenta is an important time to assess for and prevent any complications that could arise. Within this timeframe, the obstetrician safely completes the processes involved with the delivery (including suturing of incisions and tears), especially if it is through the vaginal route. If this time is exceeded, it is a possible sign of complications arising.

The phase after the third stage is sometimes called the **fourth stage of labour**. It starts with the delivery of the placenta and extends over approximately an hour. Importantly, the fourth stage is when there is difficulty in conducting clinical trials, and therefore, management protocols are driven by experience and common sense, with some evidence to support these protocols.

> **Key Point**
>
> The first hour following the birth of the baby is an important one. If the time for the completion of the processes associated with delivery exceeds an hour, it is an indication of complications.

This chapter will deal with care in the immediate postpartum period and the identification of complications in the first 24 hours after delivery, with a focus on postpartum collapse.

SIGNIFICANCE OF THE FIRST HOUR

The first hour after the delivery of the newborn is the time allowed to complete the delivery, which includes the suturing of incisions and tears. Primary postpartum hemorrhage usually occurs in this period. This is the phase when the prevention of blood loss by the administration of uterotonics and uterine massage (if required) is carried out concomitantly (see **Chapter 5,** *Management of the third stage of labour* and **Chapter 13,** *Abnormalities in the third stage of labour: Postpartum hemorrhage and retained placenta*).

Blood Loss

Blood loss must be assessed accurately; it is well known that it is often underestimated.

> **Key Point**
>
> In case of unchecked hemorrhage either from an atonic uterus or due to generalised oozing in the suture area that persists beyond the first hour, the obstetrician should call for help and plan additional interventions.

Disseminated intravascular coagulation (DIC)

It is important to remember that blood loss of more than 2500 mL can trigger disseminated intravascular coagulation (DIC) and intensify generalised oozing from vaginal or uterine tears. If this is suspected, suturing is abandoned, and the vagina is carefully packed to achieve hemostasis for a maximum of 24–48 hours while DIC is investigated and corrected. A total blood loss of 2500 mL or more would need the activation of a massive hemorrhage protocol, requiring transfusions of whole blood, clotting factors and platelets (see **Chapter 13**).

> **Key Point**
>
> Blood loss of more than 2500 mL can trigger disseminated intravascular coagulation (DIC) and warrants the activation of a massive hemorrhage protocol.

POSTPARTUM MONITORING

Shivering Immediately Following Delivery

25–50% of women develop shivering or chills immediately after the birth of the baby [3]. This is usually transient, lasting from 5 minutes to an hour, and usually settles down on its own. The mother should be reassured that shivering is a normal phenomenon. Warm blankets may be useful.

Monitoring After an Uncomplicated Vaginal Delivery

Even when the third and fourth stages are uneventful, the continued monitoring of the mother is important. This necessitates the reallocation of human resources, as postpartum women are generally taken care of by one caregiver. The caregiver could involve family members to share responsibility for the safety of the mother and newborn.

The mother should be comfortable and eager to breastfeed her newborn. Early breastfeeding is known to foster bonding between the mother and newborn and improve lactation (see **Chapter 43**, *Routine care of the newborn*). Any discomfort or hesitancy from the mother to agree to breastfeed the newborn should be taken as a warning sign and must prompt close monitoring and surveillance.

Maternal monitoring in the fourth stage involves the following:

- **Looking for symptoms and signs such as dizziness, restlessness, and fainting episodes:** These could suggest a complication in the mother as these symptoms could be caused by hypotension or hypoxia and call for further evaluation.
- **Assessment of pulse rate and volume:** This is mandatory. Though a rapid pulse is not always alarming, it warrants further hourly monitoring of the pulse and blood pressure till normal values are achieved. A good volume pulse is reassuring.

> **Key Point**
>
> The pulse rate should be checked and recorded hourly for the first 6 hours after a vaginal delivery.

- **Monitoring of blood pressure:** This is critical. Both low blood pressure of <90/60 mmHg (see **Chapter 13**) and high blood pressure >150/100 mmHg (see **Chapter 37**, *The hypertensive woman in labour*) warrant prompt action.

> **Key Point**
>
> Under normal circumstances, the woman's blood pressure is measured soon after delivery and then again after 6 hours, especially if the pulse rate is normal. In the event of excessive bleeding or hypertension complicating delivery, the blood pressure should be recorded more frequently.

- **Examination of the abdomen:** The abdomen should be soft, and the uterus should be firm and below the level of the umbilicus. An enlarged uterus felt above the level of the umbilicus may indicate the collection of blood and clots in the uterine cavity, which would require the evacuation of clots, uterine massage, and the use of therapeutic uterotonic agents.

If the uterus cannot be felt easily due to a palpable bladder, the woman should be asked to empty her bladder at the earliest. A distended bladder is known to cause atonic postpartum hemorrhage.

> **Key Point**
>
> The uterus should be felt below the level of the umbilicus. An enlarged uterus felt above the level of the umbilicus is suggestive of atony and retained clots.

- **Local examination:** It is important to identify any swelling at the suture site. Increased blood loss and the excessive use of sanitary pads should be monitored while being mindful of the underestimation of blood loss.

Frequency of monitoring after vaginal delivery

Following an uncomplicated vaginal delivery in a low-risk woman, the second detailed assessment is ideally performed within 6 hours of the initial postnatal assessment. If any red flags are raised during the hourly pulse rate check or by the birth companion, then an earlier detailed assessment is warranted. The woman can be transferred to the postdelivery area unless any alarming symptoms and signs are identified in the initial assessment by the caregiver or the birth companion. If there is an abnormality in the hourly monitoring of the pulse, it warrants earlier intervention. The woman can be transferred to the ward once she has voided and has initiated breastfeeding.

> **Key Point**
>
> The policy of transferring a woman to an area of low surveillance only after she has voided is a critical strategy for any maternity unit and helps in the early identification of complications.

Inability to void following vaginal delivery

The inability to pass urine following delivery could be due to bladder inertia or vulval hematoma.

Bladder inertia

This is a common cause of retention of urine. In a systematic review of 24 observational studies [4], prolonged labour, instrumental delivery, epidural analgesia, primiparity, and episiotomy were found to be risk factors for postpartum urinary retention.

The inability to void after 6 hours of delivery, along with a distended bladder, should raise suspicion of urinary retention. The woman may be asymptomatic or may have any one or a combination of the following symptoms:

- Small volumes of voided urine
- Urinary frequency or urgency
- A slow or intermittent stream
- Hesitancy
- Bladder pain or discomfort
- Urinary incontinence
- Straining to void
- A sense of incomplete emptying
- No sensation to void

Bladder distension can be confirmed clinically and/or on ultrasound (if readily available). The mother should be reassured that urinary retention typically resolves within one week in most women [4] and that 96–100% of women achieve complete voiding within two to five days of delivery [5].

Management of postpartum urinary retention

Intermittent catheterisation is recommended every 4–6 hours or when the woman has an urge to void but is unable to pass urine [6]. The woman may also be trained in intermittent self-catheterisation if she is motivated enough. Prophylactic antibiotics are not required for intermittent catheterisation.

Continuous bladder drainage for 48–72 hours is also an option, particularly in low-resource areas or when there is a shortage of staff.

Occasionally, a woman is unable to pass urine even after the removal of the catheter. When the post-void residual urine after catheter removal is >150 mL, the woman may be sent home with an indwelling catheter for 2 weeks. She can then be readmitted for a day for the removal of the catheter and to monitor urine output. If she is able to void completely, she can be reassured and sent home.

Vaginal or vulval hematoma

Urinary retention associated with excruciating pain in the vulva should suggest vaginal or vulval hematoma. This diagnosis is confirmed on vaginal examination when an obvious bulge is felt in the vagina and rectum, usually confined to one side (see section on *Genital hematoma* under ***Postpartum Collapse*** below).

> **Key Point**
>
> Severe pain in the perineum and retention of urine should warrant an assessment for genital hematomas.

Monitoring of the Mother After a Cesarean Section

The mother is usually monitored in the recovery room until there is some movement in her legs as she recovers from spinal anesthesia or until she is fully awake after general anesthesia. The monitoring of the mother is continued by the healthcare provider for one to two hours till she is transferred to the ward.

After transfer to the ward, the ward nursing staff takes over the care of the mother. The birth companion from the woman's family is briefed on the important warning symptoms and signs and is instructed to inform the nursing staff if any of them appear.

Monitoring protocol

- **Continuous cardiac monitoring:** The mother is connected to a monitor for continuous cardiac monitoring for two hours, with automatic capture of pulse, blood pressure, and oxygen saturation. Any abnormality in the vital signs warrants calling for additional medical help. After transfer to the ward, hourly monitoring of vital signs by a healthcare provider is recommended for 6 hours.
- **Examination of the abdomen:** This is performed to ensure that the uterus is well contracted (firm) and below the level of the umbilicus. If the uterus is felt above the level of the umbilicus, it may be indicative of the collection of blood in the uterine cavity. However, women who have had a previous cesarean section may present with the uterus at a higher level.
- **Urine output:** The drainage of urine into the urinary catheter and urine collection bag should be checked in order to monitor urine output. A urine output of at least 30 mL/hour is considered normal. Decreased or absent urine output should alert the clinician, and hypotension and hypovolemia should be ruled out and treated. Occasionally, the flow of urine into the collection bag may be blocked by small clots obstructing the catheter. This will require flushing of the catheter with sterile saline with aseptic precautions.
- **Vaginal bleeding:** Regular monitoring of blood loss from the vagina at half-hourly intervals is recommended for the first 4 hours. Any signs of increased hemorrhage may be monitored either by the birth companion or healthcare provider.

> **Key Point**
>
> Severe vital sign abnormalities precede clinical recognition of critical illness. The Maternal Early Warning Criteria (MEWC) and Maternal Early Obstetric Warning system (MEOWS) [7] have been suggested for the early identification of serious complications. However, these criteria cannot replace strict protocols backed by clinical judgement.

Inability to void after catheter removal following cesarean section

Removing the catheter as soon as it is practical minimises infection. The optimal time to do this may be immediately after the closure of the skin and up to 6 hours after [8]. However, removing the catheter after 12–24 hours is acceptable clinical practice. There is no evidence that routine urine culture is useful before the removal of the bladder catheter [9,10].

Although a meta-analysis suggested antibiotic prophylaxis prior to catheter removal to prevent infection [11], the efficacy of this recommendation is not well established, as there were several limitations in the studies included.

Urinary retention following catheter removal that exceeds 6 hours needs prompt medical attention (see section on *Management of postpartum urinary retention* above).

Ambulation

Early ambulation following cesarean delivery is always encouraged to prevent venous thrombosis. It is also helpful for the return of intestinal motility after a cesarean delivery [12]. Following a cesarean delivery, women are encouraged to ambulate as soon as they have recovered from the effects of anesthetic agents or 4 hours following the completion of suturing, whichever is later. However, excellent pain relief must be ensured before the woman is encouraged to ambulate.

Key Point

Early ambulation is important to prevent thrombosis. To ensure early ambulation after a cesarean birth, effective pain relief should be administered and maintained.

PAIN MANAGEMENT IN THE POSTPARTUM PERIOD

Pain management in the postpartum period is indicated in the management of the following:

- Afterpains due to hypertonic uterine contractions elicited by the suckling of the newborn and caused by the release of oxytocin [13]
- Perineal pain following vaginal delivery
- Postoperative pain after cesarean birth

Afterpains and Post-Vaginal Delivery Pain

Mild analgesics such as oral paracetamol and ibuprofen tablets or diclofenac suppositories are effective. Round-the-clock paracetamol is as effective as non-steroidal anti-inflammatory drugs (NSAIDs). These two drugs can be used in combination, when required, for better pain relief [14].

Opioids are unnecessary for afterpains and after vaginal delivery. Excruciating pain that is not relieved with a combination of paracetamol and NSAIDs has to be evaluated for other serious causes of pain.

Key Point

A combination of paracetamol and an NSAID such as ibuprofen is effective for relieving afterpains and post-vaginal delivery pain.

Postoperative Pain Following Cesarean Delivery

Opioids may be used for postoperative pain. Women who have received labour analgesia may have it continued to cover the postpartum period (refer to **Chapter 9**, *Labour analgesia*). Adequate pain relief is vital to encourage both breastfeeding and early ambulation.

Choosing the right opioids requires considerations regarding the safety of the mother and the newborn and the availability of the drug. In the last two to three decades, the practice of administering intrathecal morphine [15] has reduced the routine administration of opioids in the postoperative period after a cesarean section. In the authors' experience at Christian Medical College, Vellore, the practice is to abstain from giving opioids for 12 hours following a cesarean section if intrathecal morphine is administered during regional anesthesia. Morphine is the preferred choice because of its lower excretion in breast milk [16].

Morphine may not be freely available in many institutions for pain relief due to the need for a narcotics license. The following pain relief options are commonly used:

- **Paracetamol** (1 g in a 100 mL vial) is infused intravenously over 15 minutes as the surgery is coming to an end. This is repeated every 6–8 hours for the first 24 hours [17].
- **Opioids**—tramadol is most used in India for postoperative analgesia. It can be given intravenously or orally. This drug is associated with nausea. Promethazine may be administered

as an antiemetic, with close monitoring of the newborn. Opioids may affect newborn alertness and sucking vigor and therefore, the exposure of the newborn to these drugs should be minimised. Tramadol should be used with caution because of its potential sedative effect on the infant [18].

- **NSAIDs**
  - Diclofenac 100 mg suppository can be used at the end of surgery and may be repeated every 8 hours for the first 24 hours.
  - After 24 hours, oral ibuprofen 400 mg in combination with 500 mg/650 mg of paracetamol will provide good pain relief.
  - Ketorolac 10 mg may be given orally after the first 24 hours.
- **Transversus abdominis plane (TAP) block**—using ultrasound guidance, a local anesthetic is injected in the neurovascular plane between the transversus abdominis and internal oblique muscles. TAP block is an effective form of postoperative pain relief and is becoming part of the multimodal approach to postoperative pain relief.

WOMEN WHO NEED SPECIAL CARE IN THE IMMEDIATE POSTPARTUM PERIOD

Women Who Have Had a Successful Vaginal Birth After Cesarean (VBAC)

Women who have had a previous cesarean birth and have successfully undergone a trial of labour and delivered vaginally are at risk of having a small uterine scar dehiscence that may or may not manifest immediately. Therefore, such women require hourly monitoring in a high-dependency area of the labour ward to ensure stable vital signs. The practice of manually assessing the integrity of a scar by the vaginal route following delivery has been discouraged as it was found to be futile. Small defects are usually not sutured when the woman is stable [19,20]. The woman is transferred to the ward after voiding or after 6 hours of monitoring, whichever is later.

Key Point

The practice of manually exploring the uterine cavity to assess the integrity of a uterine scar following VBAC has been discouraged. However, in a facility where close monitoring of the mother and maternal bleeding is not available, a gentle manual exploration of the uterine scar to look for dehiscence (overlying peritoneum intact) or a rupture (peritoneum torn) helps in decision-making and follow-up. Small defects do not require suturing as long as the woman is stable.

Women with Increased Blood Loss and Those with Risk Factors for PPH

Women who have had more-than-usual blood loss and those with risk factors for PPH, e.g., twin pregnancy, need close monitoring with half-hourly monitoring of pulse and hourly monitoring of blood pressure. These women are transferred to the ward when their vitals are stable after 6–8 hours of monitoring.

Women Who Have Had a Difficult Instrumental Delivery

It is known that forceps delivery has the potential to cause injury to the genital tract. Traumatic postpartum hemorrhage, injury to the anal sphincter, vulval or vaginal hematoma, and retention of urine are complications of instrumental delivery. In these cases, prophylactic antibiotics have been shown to decrease wound infection in a randomised controlled trial [21]. However, their use in settings with high episiotomy rates and high instrumental delivery rates has been questioned due to concerns of antibiotic resistance and is, therefore, not yet recommended as a universal guideline. A woman who has had an instrumental delivery can be transferred to the ward after she has voided.

Women Who Have Heart Disease

Women who have heart disease are monitored in the high-dependency area of the labour ward for 24 hours as the chance of them going into failure during this time is very high. Women who are on thromboprophylaxis due to valve replacements and other medical conditions will need additional monitoring (see **Chapter 39**, *Other medical disorders—antiphospholipid syndrome, cardiac disorders, hepatic conditions, and epilepsy*)

Women on Prophylactic or Therapeutic Magnesium Sulfate

Postpartum monitoring of women with preeclampsia or eclampsia (see **Chapter 37**, *The hypertensive woman in labour*) is continued in the high-dependency area for 12–24 hours depending on the severity of the disease.

Monitoring of Postpartum Women with Epidural Analgesia

This is dealt with in **Chapter 9**.

POSTPARTUM COLLAPSE

Definition

Postpartum collapse (PPC) is a state of sudden, unanticipated, complete or partial loss of consciousness following childbirth. The commonest cause for collapse is **vasovagal syncope**, usually precipitated by pain or orthostatic hypotension, in which case, recovery is quick. However, any woman who has a fainting episode must be assessed for evidence of hemorrhage or other causes. **Concealed** or **unnoticed bleeding** is among the serious causes of postpartum collapse.

Postpartum collapse is an unanticipated situation and hence the response must be urgent. The assessment of the woman to look for a potential reversible cause and the treatment of the same go hand in hand. The quicker the response, the better the prognosis for the mother.

> **Key Point**
>
> Postpartum collapse is an unanticipated situation and hence the response has to be urgent. The quicker the response, the better the prognosis for the mother.

Hemorrhagic Causes of Postpartum Collapse

- Undiagnosed rupture of uterus (**Chapter 18**, *Obstructed labour and uterine rupture*)
- Underestimation of blood loss (**Chapter 13**, *Abnormalities in the third stage of labour: Postpartum hemorrhage and retained placenta*)
- Uterine inversion—this is often identified in the third stage of labour and the neurogenic shock due to the pain rather than the hemorrhage is the cause for the collapse (**Chapter 13**)
- Undiagnosed genital hematoma

Genital hematomas

Classification

Hematomas can be infralevator or supralevator. The commonest are the infralevator hematomas, which are further subdivided into vulval, vaginal, and paravaginal.

Infralevator hematoma

This is caused by the laceration of an underlying vessel, which is a branch of the internal pudendal vessels. It may present as a swelling in the vulva. The postpartum woman with a genital hematoma typically presents with excruciating pain in the vulva and the inability to void. This usually occurs after an instrumental delivery, and occasionally after a normal delivery. Failure to identify a bleeding vessel beyond the apex of an episiotomy or a tear may result in a hematoma. Infralevator hematomas are limited by the levator ani muscles superiorly, the perineum medially, and the Colles' fascia and fascia lata laterally. They may also extend laterally into the ischiorectal fossa.

The diagnosis is confirmed by the presence of a large bulge lateral to the vagina on one side, extending posteriorly to compress the rectum. These hematomas have to be surgically evacuated under general anesthesia. Removing the sutures of the completed episiotomy and evacuating the entrapped clots are the initial steps in the surgical management of vulval hematoma. The identification of active bleeding vessels and their ligation, when possible, is important. If there is generalised oozing, the dead space is obliterated to the extent possible. Good exposure with adequate lighting is the key to correct surgical management. Sometimes, the upper limit of the dead space cannot be reached. In such a situation, when an actively bleeding vessel is not identified, the vagina is packed for 24–48 hours. As long as the vaginal pack is removed within 24–48 hours of stabilising the woman, the risk of infection is low.

Supralevator hematoma

These are rare and are often seen in cases of uterine rupture, scar dehiscence, or a cervical tear associated with colporrhexis, following a difficult instrumental delivery.

A supralevator hematoma is more serious than an infralevator hematoma and extends to the broad ligament, the presacral space, and the retroperitoneal space. The branches of the uterine arteries are often involved. This type of hematoma warrants an urgent laparotomy concomitantly with the hemodynamic stabilisation of the woman. The ligation of the anterior branch of the internal iliac artery is performed to stop the progression of the hematoma. A hysterectomy may or may not be performed along with the evacuation of clots during the laparotomy. The concurrent activation of massive transfusion protocol (see **Chapter 13,** *Abnormalities in the third stage of labour: Postpartum hemorrhage and retained placenta*) is vital for the successful management of this type of hematoma as it is often associated with significant hemorrhage.

Hypertensive Causes of Postpartum Collapse

Severe preeclampsia, eclampsia, HELLP syndrome, and intracranial bleeding due to uncontrolled blood pressure are responsible for the PPC.

Cardiac Causes of Postpartum Collapse

Undiagnosed rheumatic heart disease, peripartum cardiomyopathy, arrhythmias, and rarely, myocardial infarction in older women can cause a sudden collapse (**Chapter 39**).

Septic Shock Causing Postpartum Collapse

Septic shock is suspected when a woman with a history of a prolonged period of febrile illness, often due to an unknown infection, presents in labour. The infection can be due to obstetric or medical causes. The obstetric causes for bacterial infection are associated with a prolonged period of ruptured membranes. Undiagnosed and untreated pyelonephritis—which is more common in pregnancy—is a known cause of sepsis. However, sudden collapse without antecedent tachypnea and tachycardia preceding the collapse is unusual in cases of septic shock.

Thromboembolism Causing Postpartum Collapse

Pulmonary embolism, unlike amniotic fluid embolus which occurs within 30 minutes of delivery, can occur at any time during the postpartum phase. Pregnancy is a thrombogenic state, and postpartum women are prone to deep vein thrombosis (DVT). The release of a thrombus from DVT in the leg or pelvis can cause the occlusion of the pulmonary artery, which results in dyspnea and chest pain, followed by collapse. The accompanying hypoxia may result in a state of confusion before the collapse.

Prophylactic anticoagulation is indicated in women at high risk for thromboembolic events. These indications include [22,23]:

- Obesity
- Labour longer than 12 hours
- Grand multiparity
- Age above 35 years
- Immobility
- Preeclampsia

- Sepsis
- Any one major risk factor such as family history of thrombosis, thrombophilia, or antiphospholipid syndrome

The diagnosis of pulmonary embolism is confirmed by lung imaging using ventilation perfusion scan or CT pulmonary angiogram, only if the woman is stable, which is usually not the case.

Amniotic Fluid Embolism (AFE)

AFE is usually responsible for collapse in the intrapartum period, and rarely in the immediate postpartum period. The diagnosis is often made retrospectively after excluding all other causes for collapse. It is often catastrophic and caused by a cytokine storm initiated by an unknown antigen present in the amniotic fluid [24,25].

The clinical presentation is sudden collapse, respiratory distress with hypoxia, and disseminated intravascular coagulopathy. However, all these features may not be seen in every case. Women suspected of having amniotic fluid embolism are managed like all other cases of collapse in an intensive care setting. The subsequent management will need a multidisciplinary approach. The prognosis is often poor.

Uncommon Causes of Postpartum Collapse

Adverse drug reactions or anaphylaxis

This may be seen with magnesium toxicity (**Chapter 37**), local anesthetic toxicity, drug-induced anaphylaxis, and rarely, latex allergy.

Metabolic causes

Hypoglycemia or hyperglycemia, hyponatremia, and diabetic ketoacidosis may be reasons for collapse.

Anesthetic causes

Respiratory depression causing hypoxia and hypotension due to a high block are the usual causes for collapse following regional anesthesia.

Management of Postpartum Collapse

The standard structured approach to adult resuscitation using the **A, B, C of resuscitation** as recommended by the Advance Life Support Group (ALSG) [26] is an effective way of managing postpartum collapse. An organised time-conscious team approach is paramount in improving the survival of the woman.

This approach involves first identifying the cause of the collapse and rectifying it at the earliest. In the postpartum period, one should also be mindful of the physiological factors [28] that may interfere with cardiopulmonary resuscitation. Issues that need special consideration and are a challenge while resuscitating a postpartum woman are as follows:

- A left lateral tilt to avoid aortocaval compression by the postpartum uterus
- Greater oxygen requirement
- Difficulty in identifying the rise and fall of the chest
- Risk of aspiration
- Difficulty in airway maintenance due to left lateral tilt and laryngeal edema

A – Airway

Maintaining the airway with a head tilt, chin lift, or jaw thrust is important to facilitate ventilation, especially in an unconscious woman. There is an increased risk of aspiration due to the hormonal effects of pregnancy causing gastric regurgitation. The use of an Ambu bag is important for bag-and-mask ventilation while help is sought from experienced clinicians. Smaller, cuffed endotracheal tubes should be used because the airway may be narrowed from laryngeal edema.

B – Breathing

The absence of breathing which is identified within 10 seconds warrants the ventilation of the woman. Bag-and-mask ventilation or the insertion of a supraglottic airway should be undertaken till intubation is possible. A rate of **10 breaths per minute and a ratio of 2 breaths per 30 chest compressions should be maintained**. Hypoxemia can develop rapidly in pregnant women due to the increased oxygen demand. Therefore, high-flow oxygen is required. Supplemental oxygen with a **flow rate of 12–15 litres per minute** should be ensured. The anatomical and physiological changes of the elevated diaphragm in pregnancy can pose a challenge to the perception of chest movements during ventilation. Once the woman is intubated, the rate of bagging should be once in 6 minutes. Synchronisation between bagging and chest compressions is not essential.

C – Circulation

Chest compressions are performed slightly above the centre of the sternum in a postpartum woman. A 5 cm compression with adequate recoil will ensure effective chest compressions. Compressions are performed at the **rate of 100–120 compressions per minute** until there is a response on the ECG. There should be no interruptions in the chest compressions, with a change in rescuer every 2 minutes.

D – Drugs

The most important drug recommended for cardiopulmonary resuscitation (CPR) is **adrenaline.** The details of the two most commonly used drugs are presented in Table 10.1.

Mock cardiopulmonary resuscitation drills should be a part of a regular multidisciplinary strategies involving nurse–midwives, obstetricians, and anesthetists for continuous training, preparedness, and capacity building of maternity units.

Fig. 10.1 is a flowchart for adult resuscitation and is adapted from recommendations by the American Heart Association [27].

PERIMORTEM CESAREAN DELIVERY (PMCD)

PMCD is often discussed in the setting of the sudden collapse of a mother with a live baby. It is a rare but potentially life-saving intervention performed for pregnant women who have collapsed due to massive trauma, cardiac arrest, and/or active uterine hemorrhage. It can be a critical component of the maternal resuscitation protocol. Cesarean delivery restores blood flow and respiratory capacity which may otherwise not be possible with a gravid uterus

Table 10.1 Medications recommended for cardiopulmonary resuscitation and their dosage

Medication	Route	Initial dose	Incremental dose	Maximum dose	Type of drug	Adverse effects
Adrenaline	IV/ ETT	1.0 mg (1:10000) IV/IO or 2–2.5 mg (1:1000) through ET tube every 3–5 minutes	0.1–0.5 mg/Kg/ minute infusion	Until there is a response	Catecholamine vasopressor, inotrope	Tachyarrhythmias, severe hypertension, tissue necrosis in case of extravasation
Amiodarone	IV/IO	300 mg	150 mg as a repeat dose, and then infusion of 15 mg/Kg over 24 hours	Until there is a response	Class III antiarrhythmic with effects on sodium, potassium, and calcium channels	Hypotension, bradycardia, heart block, tissue necrosis in case of extravasation

ETT, endotracheal tube; *IO*, intraosseous; *IV*, intravenous

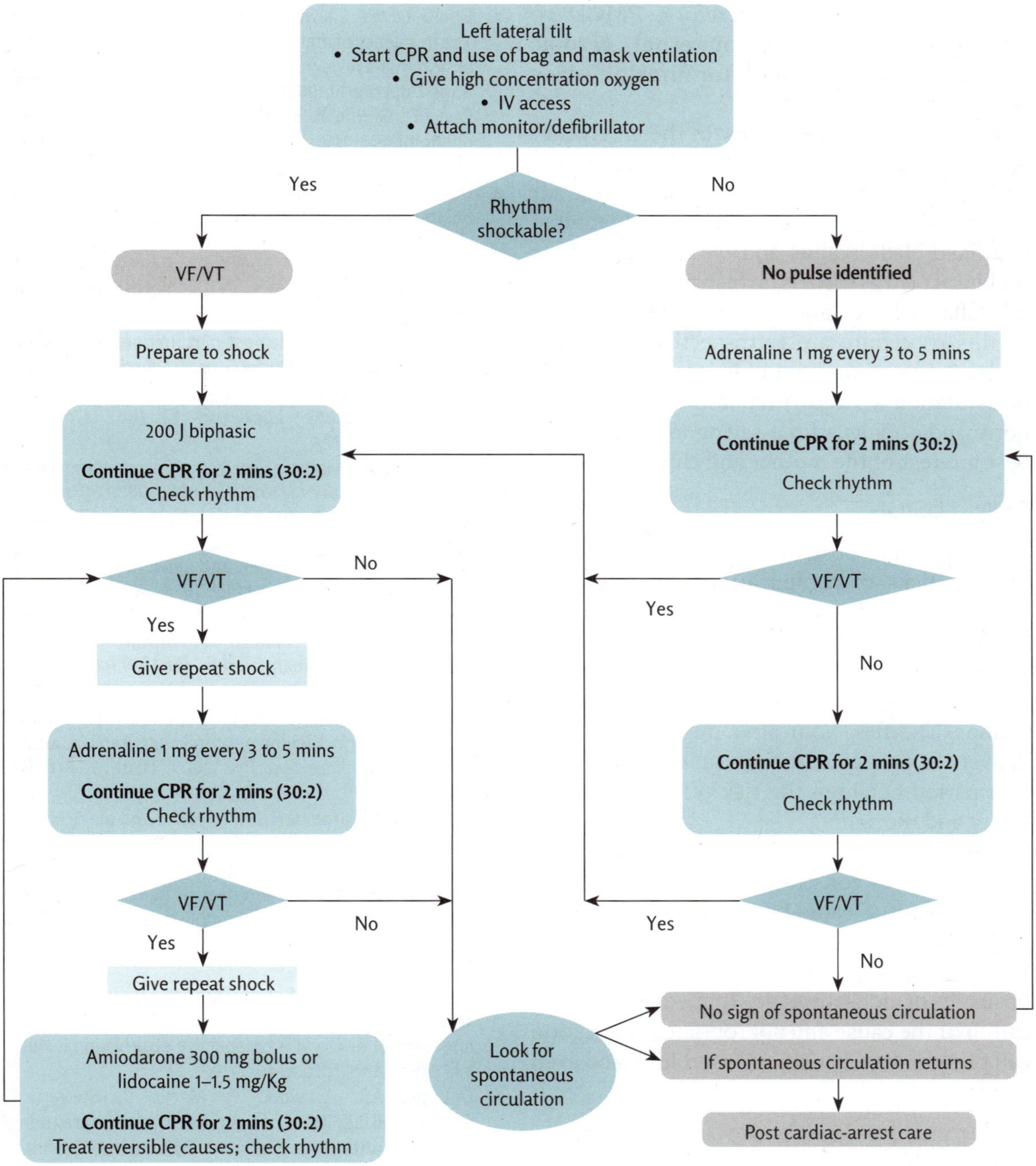

Fig. 10.1 Algorithm for cardiopulmonary resuscitation following postpartum collapse (adapted from the American Heart Association [27])

CPR, cardiopulmonary resuscitation; *VF*, ventricular fibrillation; *VT*, ventricular tachycardia

larger than 24 weeks. Therefore, **PMCD to improve outcomes in maternal cardiac arrest is only indicated for uterine sizes >24 weeks.**

PMCD is performed either in the emergency ward or the labour ward without anesthesia within 4–6 minutes of the cardiac arrest for best results [29]. The only equipment required is a fixed-blade scalpel and two clamps for the umbilical cord as there is no bleeding as a result of the collapsed circulation. Though events leading to this procedure are retrospectively captured in detail after resuscitation is completed, this is one situation where written informed consent is not mandatory as a time-saving measure in the best interest of the mother and child.

CONCLUSION

The immediate postpartum period carries significant risks of complications such as postpartum hemorrhage and sepsis. Postpartum monitoring, which includes taking vital signs and monitoring blood loss, is essential for the early identification and management of complications. The first hour after the completion of delivery is crucial, and abnormalities arising in that period heighten the risk of maternal morbidity and mortality.

Postpartum collapse, which results in the sudden loss of consciousness or reduced consciousness, is a leading cause of maternal morbidity and mortality and requires an urgent, multidisciplinary approach. The causes could be obstetric or non-obstetric. Immediate identification of the cause and appropriate rectification can prevent severe maternal morbidity and even death.

REFERENCES

1. Kassebaum NJ, Bertozzi-Villa A, Coggeshall MS, et al. Global, regional, and national levels and causes of maternal mortality during 1990-2013: A systematic analysis for the Global Burden of Disease Study 2013. *Lancet*. 2014. 384(9947):980-1004. Erratum in: *Lancet*. 2014 Sep 13;384(9947):956.
2. Gon G, Leite A C,alvert C, Woodd S, Graham WJ, Filippi V. The frequency of maternal morbidity: A systematic review of systematic reviews. *Int J Gynecol Obstet*. 2018. 141: 20-38. https://doi.org/10.1002/ijgo.12468.
3. Ravid D, Gidoni Y, Bruchim, I et al. Postpartum chills phenomenon: Is it a feto-maternal transfusion reaction? *Acta Obstet Gynecol Scand*. 2001. 80:149.
4. Mulder FE, Hakvoort RA, Schoffelmeer MA, et al. Postpartum urinary retention: A systematic review of adverse effects and management. *Int Urogynecol J*. 2014. 25:1605.
5. Yip SK, Brieger G, Hin LY, Chung T. Urinary retention in the post-partum period. The relationship between obstetric factors and the post-partum post-void residual bladder volume. *Acta Obstet Gynecol Scand*. 1997. 76:667.
6. Berens P. Overview of the postpartum period: Disorders and complications. Lockwood CJ (Ed), *UpToDate*. 2022. Waltham, MA.
7. Friedman AM. Maternal early warning systems. *Obstet Gynecol Clin North Am*. 2015. 42(2):289-98.
8. Hou D, Jia Y, Han A, Hu Q, Li J, Liang W. Effect of urinary catheter removal at different times after caesarean section: A systematic review and network meta-analysis. *Eur J Obstet Gynecol Reprod Biol*. 2023. 280:160-167.
9. Horowitz E, Yogev Y, Ben-Haroush A, Samra Z, Feldberg D, Kaplan B. Urine culture at removal of indwelling catheter after cesarean section. *Int J Gynaecol Obstet*. 2004. 5(3):276-8.
10. Griffiths R, Fernandez R. Strategies for the removal of short-term indwelling urethral catheters in adults. *Cochrane Database Syst Rev*. 2007. Issue 6. Art. No: CD004011.
11. Marschall J, Carpenter CR, Fowler S, et al. Antibiotic prophylaxis for urinary tract infections after removal of urinary catheter: Meta-analysis. *BMJ*. 2013. 346:f3147.
12. Sahin E, Terzioglu F. The effect of gum chewing, early oral hydration, and early mobilization on intestinal motility after cesarean birth. *Worldviews Evid Based Nurs*. 2015. 12:380.
13. Fang X, Huan Y, Tao Y, Song Y, Du W, Liu Z, Xu Z. Incidence, severity, and determinants of uterine contraction pain after vaginal delivery: A prospective observational study. *Int J Obstet Anesth*. 2021. 46:102961.
14. Deussen AR, Ashwood P, Martis R, Stewart F, Grzeskowiak LE. Relief of pain due to uterine cramping/involution after birth. *Cochrane Database of Systematic Reviews*. 2020. Issue 10. Art. No.: CD004908.
15. Sharpe EE, Molitor RJ, Arendt KW, Torbenson VE, Olsen DA, Johnson RL, et al. Intrathecal morphine versus intrathecal hydromorphone for analgesia following cesarean delivery: A randomized clinical trial. *Anesthesiology*. 2020. 132(6):1382–91.

16. Montgomery A, Hale TW; Academy of Breastfeeding Medicine. ABM clinical protocol #15: Analgesia and anesthesia for the breastfeeding mother, revised 2012. *Breastfeed Med.* 2012. 7(6):547-53.
17. Mitra S, Khandelwal P, Sehgal A. Diclofenac-tramadol vs. diclofenac-acetaminophen combinations for pain relief after caesarean section. *Acta Anaesthesiol Scand.* 2012. 56(6):706-11.
18. American College of Obstetricians and Gynecologists' Committee on Clinical Consensus–Obstetrics. Pharmacologic Stepwise Multimodal Approach for Postpartum Pain Management: ACOG Clinical Consensus No. 1. *Obstet Gynecol.* 2021.138(3):507-517.
19. Scott JR. Vaginal birth after cesarean delivery: A common-sense approach. *Obstet Gynecol.* 2011. 118(2 Pt 1):342-350. [PubMed].
20. ACOG Practice Bulletin No. 205: Vaginal birth after cesarean delivery. *Obstet Gynecol.* 2019 Feb;133(2):e110-e127. [PubMed].
21. Knight M, Chiocchia V, Partlett C, et al. Prophylactic antibiotics in the prevention of infection after operative vaginal delivery (ANODE): A multicentre randomised controlled trial. *Lancet.* 2019. 393:2395.
22. Greer IA. Thrombosis in pregnancy: Maternal and fetal issues. *Lancet.* 1999. 10;353(9160):1258-65.
23. Green-top Guideline No. 37a. Reducing the Risk of Thrombosis and Embolism during Pregnancy and the Puerperium. Available at: https://www.rcog.org.uk/media/qejfhcaj/gtg-37a.pdf.
24. Gilmore DA, Wakim J, Secrest J, Rawson R. Anaphylactoid syndrome of pregnancy: A review of the literature with latest management and outcome data. *AANA J.* 2003. 71:12.
25. Gist RS, Stafford IP, Leibowitz AB, Beilin Y. Amniotic fluid embolism. *Anesth Analg.* 2009. 108:1599.
26. Panchal AR, Bartos JA, Cabañas JG, et al. Adult Basic and Advanced Life Support Writing Group. Part 3: Adult Basic and Advanced Life Support: 2020. American Heart Association Guidelines for Cardiopulmonary Resuscitation and Emergency Cardiovascular Care. Circulation. 2020. 20;142(16_suppl_2):S366-S468.
27. Merchant RM, Topjian AA, Panchal AR, et al. Adult Basic and Advanced Life Support, Pediatric Basic and Advanced Life Support, Neonatal Life Support, Resuscitation Education Science, and Systems of Care Writing Groups. Part 1: Executive Summary: 2020 American Heart Association Guidelines for Cardiopulmonary Resuscitation and Emergency Cardiovascular Care. Circulation. 2020. 142(16_suppl_2):S337-S357. doi: 10.1161/CIR.0000000000000918. Epub 2020.
28. S Nanda, LK Penna. *Postpartum collapse, Obstetrics, Gynaecology & Reproductive Medicine.* Volume 19, Issue 8. 2009. Pages 221-228. ISSN 1751-7214.
29. Tsuei BJ. Assessment of the pregnant trauma patient. *Injury.* 2006. 37:367.

CHAPTER 11

Abnormalities in the Latent Phase and the Active First Stage of Labour

KALAIVANI RAMALINGAM

INTRODUCTION

The sequence of events in normal labour and the management of the first stage of labour have been discussed in **Chapter 4**, *Management of the first and second stages of normal labour*.

This chapter will discuss the management of abnormalities when there is a deviation from the normal course of events in the earlier part of labour. The first stage of labour begins with the onset of regular, often painful, uterine contractions that last for at least 45 seconds. They occur at a frequency of at least 3–4 contractions every 10 minutes or 1 every 2–3 minutes. The first stage of labour is divided into the **latent phase** and the **active phase**.

Respectful Maternity Care

A woman in labour is in a vulnerable position and is dependent on the staff in the maternity ward to support her and enable her to successfully navigate the journey of childbirth. Abnormalities in the latent phase and the first stage of labour may be very frustrating, slow, and confusing from the woman's perspective. The principles of respectful maternity care must be followed at all times. Healthcare providers need to have the patience to treat the labouring woman with dignity and empathy (see **Chapter 3**, *Respectful obstetric care and the role of a birth companion*).

LATENT PHASE

This was first described by Friedman in 1955 [1]. The latent phase of labour commences from the onset of regular painful contractions and lasts until the onset of the active phase of labour. The change from the latent phase to the active phase is marked by progressive cervical effacement and dilatation along with the descent of the presenting part.

The newer definitions of these phases have suggested that the latent phase may last until 5 cm of dilatation of the cervix. This phase may last as long as 20 hours in a primigravida and 14 hours in a multigravida.

Definition

The National Institute of Clinical Excellence (NICE) [2] defines the latent phase as follows: **The latent first stage of labour** is a period of time, not necessarily continuous, when:

- There are painful contractions and
- There are some cervical changes including cervical effacement and dilatation up to 4 cm

Many studies now consider that the latent phase lasts until a cervical dilatation of 5 cm and that the active phase does not commence until 5–6 cm of cervical dilatation [3,4].

Key Point

Contemporary data have confirmed that the latent phase lasts until a cervical dilatation of 5 cm is achieved and that the active phase does not commence until 5–6 cm of cervical dilatation [3,4].

False Labour

The latent phase must be differentiated from false labour. In the latent phase, regular contractions continue until the onset of the active phase of labour. In contrast, in false labour, contractions occur with varying intensity and level of pain and then cease completely after a period of time. This happens in about 10% of women presenting in what is thought to be the latent phase of labour [5]. False labour may be differentiated from true labour only retrospectively.

The potential to progress into active labour and the need to manage expectantly must be explained clearly to the woman. She and her family should have a good understanding of the difference between false and true labour. This may set realistic expectations of false labour, in which case, the woman may be asked to return home to await further events.

There is a school of thought that false labour may be a sign of subsequent dysfunctional labour. An association has been observed between false labour and cases of dysfunctional labour needing interventions in the form of amniotomy, use of oxytocin, and assisted vaginal delivery.

Clinical assessment does not always help in differentiating between true and false labour. The use of ultrasound to measure cervical length has been suggested as an intervention in these women [6]. An arbitrary cervical length below 1.5 cm was chosen as a predictor, and studies were conducted to predict the prospective onset of active labour. The addition of more sonological parameters such as uterocervical angle has also been explored. However, the positive predictive value of cervical shortening on ultrasound imaging varies between 14 and 83% in the studies reported; hence, it is not a reliable predictor of true labour. Moreover, ultrasound imaging is an **unnecessary intervention** in this situation. **It is invasive, observer-dependent, and may not be deliverable universally.**

Management of suspected false labour

It is important to educate the pregnant woman and her family about the nature of these contractions and the likelihood of progress or cessation of contractions. Management includes a careful assessment of the woman and observation for at least two hours to determine whether the contractions are progressive or not.

Key Point

If it is not immediately apparent whether the woman is in false labour or true labour, she may be observed for at least two hours. If the contractions are not progressive and there are no further changes in cervical effacement and dilatation, she may be sent home with instructions to return if contractions resume.

The woman may choose to stay in the hospital for longer if she is anxious, lives in a geographically remote place, or has poor transport facilities. However, if the woman wishes to go home to await the actual onset of labour, she may be reassured and sent home if the following criteria are met:

- Lack of progressive cervical effacement and dilatation
- Intact membranes
- Normal fetal heart rate pattern

Duration of the Latent Phase

The latent phase of labour extends from the initiation of labour to the onset of the active phase. However, since neither the beginning nor the end of the latent phase is precisely identifiable, the duration of the latent phase is often just an estimate.

The duration of the latent phase has been traditionally estimated as 20 hours in a primigravida and 14 hours in a multigravida. These data were originally derived from Friedman's work which projected these durations from the 95th centile of the cohorts they observed [7]. They have been questioned in subsequent studies that have estimated similar but either shorter or longer durations of the latent phase of labour [8]. Contemporary data have produced a smoother labour curve, with the acceleration of cervical dilatation in the active stage starting at 5–6 cm [3]. Labour will progress relatively slowly until a cervical dilatation of 5–6 cm is reached.

> **Key Point**
>
> In the latent phase, labour will progress relatively slowly until a cervical dilatation of 5–6 cm is reached.

PROLONGED LATENT PHASE

If the duration of the latent phase exceeds the upper limit mentioned above, it is said to be prolonged. This happens in 5–6.5% of women in labour [9]. It can cause considerable distress and frustration to the expectant woman.

The factors associated with prolonged latent phase are listed in Box 11.1.

> **Box 11.1 Clinical associations of prolonged latent phase [10]**
>
> - Deficient prelabour cervical remodelling
> - Excessive sedation, analgesia, or anesthesia
> - Maternal obesity
> - Malposition
> - Chorioamnionitis
> - Postterm labour

If the pregnant woman is observed for 2–4 hours with no change in cervical findings, she can be assured that she is in the latent phase. She may be allowed to return home with instructions to return if there are signs of active labour. She can be asked to try the following measures to relieve her discomfort:

- Continue as many routine activities as possible
- Distract herself with activities such as walking, listening to music, and watching television
- Practice breathing and relaxation techniques
- Get a massage or backrub from a partner or another family member
- Use warm water therapy with a bath, shower, or fomentation
- Eat light and drink fluids to stay hydrated
- Try to take a nap
- Be actively aware of fetal movements
- Return if unable to cope with conservative measures

However, if the woman is too distressed and decides to stay in the maternity unit, she may be allowed to choose that option.

Management of Prolonged Latent Phase

Once prolonged latent phase has been diagnosed, a repeat maternal and fetal assessment must be performed along with risk assessment to exclude maternal infection and fetal malposition and to ensure that there is no immediate need to intervene [10]. Management involves the following:

- Supportive measures
- Analgesia
- Intervention

The woman should be given the option to choose **analgesia** (if there is no medical indication to intervene) or **intervention.**

> **Key Point**
>
> A prolonged latent phase is independently associated with an increased incidence of subsequent labour abnormalities [7].

Supportive measures

Initial measures may be supportive, such as massaging, walking, and sleeping. Aromatherapy, yoga, and acupressure are not advised, but if the woman chooses to use these, her wishes must be respected [2].

Key Point

A review of studies [11] has found that there is a profound need for help, support, and empathy, particularly during the latent phase. One-to-one support by labour staff with a suitable birth companion helps the woman feel well-supported and cared for in labour. This also improves the overall birth experience for her.

Analgesia

The woman may be given oral, inhalational, parenteral, or (if needed) epidural analgesia (see **Chapter 9**, *Labour analgesia*).

Oral analgesia

1 g of paracetamol orally may be administered.

Inhalational analgesia

Inhalational analgesia in the form of a combination of nitrous oxide and air (Entonox®) through a mask may be helpful. In this case, the woman needs to be warned about dizziness and nausea.

Parenteral analgesia

Parenteral administration of opioid analgesia given intramuscularly as per the unit guidelines can relieve the pain of prolonged latent phase. The recommended doses are as follows:

- 75–150 mg of pethidine IM or
- 10–15 mg of morphine IM (though morphine has limited application in contemporary obstetric practice owing to its higher rates of maternal and neonatal respiratory depression compared to pethidine)

About 60–85% of these women often wake up after an opioid-induced sleep and progress to labour with cervical dilatation [12]. About 5% may not show any evidence of progress into active labour.

Some concern has been raised about the safety of opioid analgesia and its effect on the oxygenation status and the respiratory drive of the newborn. A study has reported that maternal and fetal outcomes are not adversely affected by using opioid analgesia [13]. However, there is no doubt that fetal heart rate assessment should continue after the administration of opioid analgesia. The parturient is often able to get some restful sleep after a distressing period of non-progressive contractions. This has been termed **therapeutic rest**.

Key Point

Adequate but **not** excessive analgesia must be the aim as a high dose of opioid analgesia is a deterrent to the progression of labour and may prolong the latent phase further.

Epidural analgesia

Traditional obstetric wisdom has long held that epidural analgesia is best considered after a cervical dilatation of 3 cm. This has been questioned more recently. Nulliparous women in labour were randomised to early epidural at 1 cm or delayed epidural after 5 cm dilatation. This trial found no difference in the progression of labour or the rate of cesarean section [13]. Hence, an early epidural remains a viable option for a labouring woman with a prolonged latent phase of labour and should not be withheld. If the woman is extremely distressed and needs more immediate analgesia, combined spinal–epidural analgesia may also be considered.

Key Point

An early epidural (before 3 cm dilatation) remains a viable option for labouring women with a prolonged latent phase of labour and should not be withheld [13].

Intervention

The woman may choose not to use any analgesia at all or may not want any further analgesia at any point during a prolonged latent phase and request an intervention. An intervention is also a good option for women who are well rested and have a prolonged latent phase.

If the cervix is adequately dilated, an amniotomy may be offered as an option to the parturient. This may be followed by oxytocin to augment the contractions. A randomised trial found that these measures worked better together or in tandem than either intervention on its own [14].

Early or delayed intervention?

Earlier intervention in a prolonged latent phase or a delayed intervention after the use of analgesia to allow for spontaneous progress into active labour are both acceptable and safe choices that may be made by the woman in labour after careful consideration of the information provided [2]. No difference in obstetric or neonatal outcomes were seen between these options in a study that compared earlier intervention with conservative management. No significant difference was observed between the rate of cesarean delivery in the two groups. However, cesarean rate was high in both groups (23% with early intervention and 37% with conservative management), suggesting that a prolonged latent phase may be an indicator of poor cervical remodelling with a high association with labour dystocia [7]. More interestingly, there was no difference in the perception of birth experiences in the two groups.

A randomised trial [15] studied the effects of earlier intervention after 8 hours of latent phase as compared to conservative management. Dinoprostone, amniotomy, or oxytocin were used as appropriate. It was found that there was no difference in the rates of cesarean section, which was the primary outcome of the study. However, earlier interventions resulted in quicker delivery and shorter hospitalisation. Intrapartum oxytocin use, epidural analgesia and uterine hyperstimulation, postpartum hemorrhage, patient satisfaction on allocated intervention during labour and delivery, and neonatal outcome were not significantly different between the two groups.

The methods of managing prolonged latent phase are summarised in Box 11.2.

Box 11.2 Management of prolonged latent phase

- Supportive measures
  - Emotional support
  - Sleep
  - Walking
  - Warm water shower/bath/fomentation
  - Inhalational nitrous oxide
  - Oral paracetamol
  - Oral opioid
  - Parenteral opioid
  - Epidural/combined spinal epidural
- Intervention
  - Early
  - Delayed

ABNORMALITIES IN THE ACTIVE PHASE OF THE FIRST STAGE OF LABOUR

The normal progression of labour happens with the traditional concept of the 3 Ps—**power, passage,** and **passenger**.

- The **power** in the first stage of labour is contributed by uterine contractions alone and is augmented in the second stage of labour by the expulsive efforts of the mother as she pushes. Incoordinate or insufficient uterine contractions may delay the progress of labour.
- The **passage** is the bony pelvis, which determines the roominess or capacity for the fetus to fit into the bony cage of the pelvis.
- The **passenger** is the fetus, whose size, lie, and presentation influence the outcome of labour. Asynclitism or extension of the fetal head, occiput posterior or transverse position, or mentum or brow presentation may cause abnormal progress of labour or labour dystocia [16].

Abnormal progress in the active phase of the first stage of labour may be because of any one or a combination of these three, i.e., power, passage, and passenger.

Labour Disorders in the Active Phase of the First Stage

- **Protracted active phase:** Dilatation less than approximately 1–2 cm/hour in women who have reached ≥6 cm dilatation
- **Active phase arrest of dilatation:** If after dilatation of ≥6 cm, in a woman with ruptured membranes, there is:
  - — No cervical change for ≥4 hours despite adequate contractions
  - — No cervical change for ≥6 hours with inadequate contractions
- **Active phase arrest of descent:** The fetal head descends at a rate slower than 1 cm/hour

Protracted active phase of labour

A delay in the first stage during the active phase may happen in as many as 1 in 5 labouring women. This is the main indication for cesarean section in labour in nulliparous women [17]. Unlike other primates, the human fetus experiences a very tight fit in the pelvis in labour due to the assumption of the upright position. This fact has been reintroduced as an explanation for labour disorders [18].

Diagnosis

The diagnosis of a protracted active phase is made in women (nulliparous or multiparous) in the active phase (cervix ≥6 cm) who dilate ≤1 cm over two hours.

Key Point

With protracted active phase dilatation, the risk for subsequent arrest of dilatation or descent may be increased 2.5- to 8-fold, regardless of parity.

Though the progress of labour was originally defined with the help of Friedman's curve, new data have emerged with more recent proposals by Zhang [3,19]. It is interesting to note that if the labour is induced rather than spontaneous, the latent phase may be prolonged; however, there is no difference in the nature of the active phase of the first stage of labour.

A delay in the first stage of labour in its active phase is diagnosed if the following occur:

- Cervical dilatation of <2 cm in 4 hours for first labours
- Cervical dilatation of <2 cm in 4 hours or a slowing in the progress of labour for second or subsequent labours
- Poor descent and rotation of the baby's head
- Changes in the strength, duration, and frequency of uterine contractions in an unfavourable manner

The commonest reason for a delay in the active phase of labour is poor uterine activity [14]. There is still a poor understanding of how and when labour starts and why it progresses differently in different parturients [20].

Fetal and maternal outcomes

If poorly managed, protracted labour may lead to adverse fetal and maternal outcomes.

- **Fetal outcomes:** Protracted labour may lead to poor fetal oxygenation, distress, sepsis, low Apgar scores at 5 minutes, and prolonged hospital stay. There is a higher risk of fetal injury with birth trauma, fetal hypoxia, shoulder dystocia, and brachial plexus injury. In low-resource settings with inadequate monitoring, fetal death may occur in extreme situations.
- **Maternal outcomes**: These include exhaustion, distress, delay in progress to the second stage, interventions in the first and second stages (including operative vaginal delivery), and infection leading to intrapartum sepsis. Without appropriate intervention, it may lead to arrested labour with a pathological Bandl's ring, obstetric fistula formation, or even maternal death. Other associations are increased perineal trauma causing obstetric anal sphincter injuries and increased maternal blood loss due to postpartum hemorrhage [21].

Since a delay in the first stage of labour occurs in 20% of nulliparous women, protracted labour is the commonest indication for primary cesarean section. The increased incidence of placenta accreta and placenta previa in a subsequent pregnancy as a consequence of cesarean delivery contribute to maternal morbidity and mortality [22].

Active phase arrest of dilatation

In the past, secondary arrest of dilatation was diagnosed when there was no change in cervical dilatation for at least 2 hours after the cervix had dilated to 4 cm or more. However, a workshop convened by the United States National Institute of Child Health and Human Development, Society for Maternal–Fetal Medicine, and American College of Obstetricians and Gynecologists [23] concluded that arrest of the active phase of labour is diagnosed if there is cervical dilatation of ≥6 cm in a woman with ruptured membranes but **no further cervical dilatation** [24]:

- After 4 hours of **adequate** contractions with ruptured membranes
- After 6 hours of **inadequate** contractions, with ruptured membranes, despite oxytocin administration

Key Point

Why the change from 2 hours to 4 hours in the diagnosis of arrest in the first stage?

Traditionally, a cesarean would be performed for women who had not progressed with 2 hours of adequate contractions resulting from augmentation with oxytocin. However, it has been found that 91% of multiparas and 74% of nulliparas who had not progressed could go on to achieve a vaginal delivery if given more time [25].

Risk factors for protracted or arrested first stage of labour

A delay or arrest in the active first stage of labour may be due to independent or combined risk factors. These are summarised in Box 11.3.

Box 11.3 Risk factors associated with abnormalities in the active phase of the first stage of labour

- Large fetal size
- Maternal obesity
- Inadequate bony pelvis
- Abnormal position (non-occiput anterior position)
- Nulliparity
- Short stature
- High fetal presenting part at full cervical dilatation
- Infection (chorioamnionitis)
- Postterm pregnancy
- Gestational diabetes
- Hypertensive disorders
- Regional analgesia (combined spinal–epidural or epidural analgesia)

Recognition and Management of an Abnormal Active First Stage of Labour

History

It is prudent to ascertain how the woman is feeling and coping with labour. The lack of regular uterine contractions (at a frequency of at least 3–5 every 10 minutes and lasting at least 45 seconds) is an initial sign of poor progress. In such a situation, one must check when the active phase transition was established and whether it has been diagnosed appropriately beyond 6 cm of cervical dilatation.

Examination

- A general examination helps to estimate maternal hydration, well-being, and the presence of distress.
- An initial **abdominal examination** helps to establish the approximate fetal size, lie, and engagement of the fetal head by palpation.
- A **vaginal examination** helps to ascertain cervical effacement and dilatation, the descent of the fetal head, and progress since the last examination. It is important to keep the number of vaginal examinations to the minimum both to respect the woman's privacy and dignity and to avoid causing discomfort

or introducing infection, particularly in the presence of ruptured membranes.

Assessment of labour

Regular palpation, counting of contractions, and intermittent auscultation with a Pinard's scope, handheld Doppler device, or continuous cardiotocograph help to assess both the adequacy of contractions and fetal well-being.

A tocograph can only record the number of contractions but not how effective they are. The adequacy of contractions can only be assessed in an experimental setting using an intrauterine pressure catheter. Adequate contractions exceed 200–250 Montevideo units [26].

If contractions are between 3 and 5 in number every 10 minutes and last at least 45 seconds, they are efficient contractions that should lead to cervical change and fetal descent in the active phase of the first stage of labour.

The clinical findings may be recorded on a partograph or the WHO labour care guide (see **Chapter 5**, *Monitoring labour: Partograph to labour care guide*) to help guide further management.

Interventions

Further decision-making will depend on the following:

- Parity
- Cervical dilatation and rate of change
- Uterine contractions
- Station and position of the presenting part
- The woman's emotional state

It is imperative to ensure that the woman has received support, hydration, and appropriate and effective pain relief. This helps in the progress of labour with minimal intervention.

Amniotomy (artificial rupture of membranes)

The first step in intervention is to perform an amniotomy or artificial rupture of membranes with a special instrument such as an amnihook or a similar device. There appears to be no increase in any adverse events or any increase in cesarean section, shoulder dystocia, or infection with appropriately performed amniotomy [27]. Amniotomy was noted to reduce the duration of the active phase by at least an hour [28]. A few authors have reported an increased frequency of cardiotocographic abnormalities, particularly variable decelerations, possibly due to the loss of the cushioning effect of the amniotic fluid during contractions in labour.

Use of oxytocin for augmentation of labour

With a diagnosis of delayed active phase in the first stage of labour, the use of oxytocin may be considered when the membranes have been spontaneously or artificially ruptured. Some studies recommend the use of oxytocin 2 hours after an amniotomy if there is no further progress. Several studies on this approach have noted the shortening of the first stage and progress of labour. Hence, oxytocin is recommended as an intervention [29].

An initial detailed examination is required to confirm the diagnosis of delay in the first stage and to exclude contraindications such as fetal distress, pre-existent uterine hyperstimulation, and obstruction before augmenting labour with oxytocin to treat the delay.

Administration of oxytocin

Before starting oxytocin, the woman should have the process explained to her along with the fact that she may require more effective analgesia.

> **Key Point**
>
> Caution needs to be exercised while augmenting labour with oxytocin in a multiparous woman who has a secondary delay or arrest in the active phase. Inadequate contractions are an unusual delaying factor in a woman with a previous successful normal vaginal delivery. Other factors such as a large fetus or infection should be ruled out [2].

There are different regimens for the administration of oxytocin. The key principles are to commence at the smallest therapeutic use and proceed with small increments every 30 minutes in a stepwise fashion. The aim is to establish

4–5 regular contractions every 10 minutes; titration must be done accordingly (see **Chapter 14**, *Induction and augmentation of labour*).

Progress is monitored by a detailed examination after 4 hours. Cervical dilatation of at least 2 cm every 4 hours is expected after augmentation in the presence of adequate uterine contractions. If such progress has been achieved, the labour may continue. A time interval of 6 hours may be considered if contractions are inadequate. If this is not achieved, delivery by cesarean section should be considered for failure to progress despite oxytocin augmentation.

Oxytocin in the first stage of labour is administered continuously as an intravenous infusion, preferably, by means of a variable-speed infusion pump. See **Chapter 14** for more details.

> **Key Point**
>
> In the presence of adequate uterine contractions, a cervical dilatation of at least 2 cm every 4 hours is expected after augmentation with oxytocin. If such progress is not achieved, a cesarean section may be indicated for failure to progress in the active first stage of labour.

Monitoring of maternal and fetal status

The maternal status must be monitored continuously while waiting for vaginal delivery. The diagnosis of arrest in the active phase should be followed with stringent monitoring because, if ignored, it might result in a ruptured uterus. The fetal status must also be monitored carefully for the presence of fetal heart changes (see **Chapter 8**, *Fetal surveillance in labour*).

CONCLUSION

The majority of women will have an uneventful first stage of labour. However, approximately 5% of women will encounter a prolonged latent phase of labour and another 20% will have either a protraction, or arrest of the active stage of labour. Contemporary data have established that labour progresses faster after 5–6 cm of dilatation in nulliparous and multiparous women. The recognition and diagnosis of prolonged, protracted, or arrested labour will enable the initiation of the appropriate interventions to ensure a vaginal birth. Protraction and arrest disorders in the active stage of labour are among the chief indications for cesarean delivery in nulliparous women.

REFERENCES

1. Friedman EA. Primigravid labor: A graphicostatistical analysis. *Obstet Gynecol*. 1955. 6. pp. 567-589.
2. NICE Guideline CG190. Intrapartum care for healthy women and babies. NICE Guideline CG190. 2022.
3. Zhang J, Landy HJ, Branch DW, Burkman R, Haberman S, Gregory KD, et al. Contemporary patterns of spontaneous labor with normal neonatal outcomes. Consortium on Safe Labor. *Obstet Gynecol*. 2010. 116:1281–7.
4. American College of Obstetricians and Gynecologists (ACOG). Safe prevention of the primary cesarean delivery. Obstetric Care Consensus No. 1. *Obstet Gynecol*. 2014 (reaffirmed 2017). 123:693–711.
5. Nelson DB, McIntire DD, Leveno KJ. False labor at term in singleton pregnancies: Discharge after a standardized assessment and perinatal outcomes. *Obstet Gynecol*. 2017. 130, pp. 139-145.
6. Bouzid A, Kehila M, Trabelsi H, et al. Sonographic landmarks to differentiate "false labor" and "early true labor" as a possible new application of ultrasound in labor ward. *J Gynecol Obstet Hum Reprod*. 2017. 46, pp. 363-366.
7. Cohen WR, Friedman EA. *Labor and delivery care: A practical guide*. 2011.
8. Wiley-Blackwell. Oxford, England.Tilden EL, Phillippi JC, Ahlberg M, et al. Describing latent phase duration and associated characteristics among 1281 low-risk women in spontaneous labor. *Birth*. 2019. 46, pp. 592-601.
9. Cohen WR, Friedman EA. The latent phase of labour. *Am J Obstet Gynecol*. 2023.
10. Greulich B, Tarrant B. The latent phase of labor: Diagnosis and management. *J Midwif Wom Health*. 2007. 52(3):190-8.
11. Iliadou M. Supporting women in labour. *Health science journal*. 2012. 6(3):385.
12. Mackeen AD, Fehnel E, Berghella V, Klein T. Morphine sleep in pregnancy. *Am J perinat*. 2014. 31(01):085-90.
13. Wang F, Shen X, Guo X, Peng Y, Gu X, Labor Analgesia Examining Group (LAEG). Epidural analgesia in the latent phase of labor and the risk of cesarean delivery: A five-year randomized controlled trial. *J Am Soc Anesthes*. 2009. 111(4):871-80.

14. Nachum Z, Garmi G, Kadan Y, Zafran N, Shalev E, Salim R. Comparison between amniotomy, oxytocin or both for augmentation of labor in prolonged latent phase: A randomized controlled trial. *Reprod Biol Endoc.* 2010. 8(1):1-8.
15. Sargunam PN, Bak LL, Tan PC, Vallikkannu N, Noor Azmi MA, Zaidi SN, Win ST, Omar SZ. Induction of labor compared to expectant management in term nulliparas with a latent phase of labor of more than 8 hours: A randomized trial. *BMC preg and childbirth.* 2019. 19(1):1-8.
16. Caughey AB, Sharshiner R, Cheng YW. Fetal malposition: Impact and management. *Clin Obstet Gynecol.* 2015. 58(2):241-5.
17. Abalos E, Chamillard M, Díaz V, Pasquale J, Souza JP. Progression of the first stage of spontaneous labour. *Best Pract Res Clin Obstet Gynaecol.* 2020. 67:19-32.
18. Pavličev M, Romero R, Mitteroecker P. Evolution of the human pelvis and obstructed labor: New explanations of an old obstetrical dilemma. *Am J Obstet Gynecol.* 2020. 222(1):3-16.
19. Caughey AB. Is Zhang the new Friedman: How should we evaluate the first stage of labor? *Semin Perinatol.* 2020. 44(2):151215.
20. Kissler K, Hurt KJ. The pathophysiology of labor dystocia: Theme with variations. *Reprod Sci.* 2023. 30(3):729-742.
21. Pospiech K, Czajkowski K. Amniotic fluid lactate level as a diagnostic tool for prolonged labour. *J Mother Child.* 2020. 24(3):3-7.
22. Antoine C, Young BK. Cesarean section one hundred years 1920-2020: The good, the bad and the ugly. *J Perinat Med.* 2020. 49(1):5-16.
23. Spong CY, Berghella V, Wenstrom KD, et al. Preventing the first cesarean delivery: Summary of a joint Eunice Kennedy Shriver National Institute of Child Health and Human Development, Society for Maternal-Fetal Medicine, and American College of Obstetricians and Gynecologists Workshop. *Obstet Gynecol.* 120:1181.
24. Gill P, Henning JM, Carlson K, et al. *Abnormal Labor.* [Updated 2023 Feb 2].
25. Rouse DJ, Owen J, Savage KG, Hauth JC. Active phase labor arrest: Revisiting the 2-hour minimum. *Obstet Gynecol.* 2001. 98:550–4.
26. Cohen WR. Clinical assessment of uterine contractions. *Int J Gynaecol Obstet.* 2017. 139(2):137-142.
27. Casey LM, Judd II EJ. The effect of amniotomy on labor progression. *Spark Repository.* 2019.
28. Hasan NA, Hong JG, Teo IH, Zaidi SN, Hamdan M, Tan PC. Early versus delayed amniotomy with immediate oxytocin after Foley catheter cervical ripening in nulliparous labor induction: A randomized trial. *Int Journal of Gynecol* Obstet. 2022. 159(3):951-60.
29. Alhafez L and Berghella V. Evidence-based labor management: First stage of labor (part 3). *Am J Obstet Gynecol MFM.* 2020. 2(4), p.100185.

CHAPTER 12

Abnormalities in the Second Stage of Labour

MANJIRI KHARE, GAURI KARANDIKAR

INTRODUCTION

The first stage of labour ends with the complete dilatation of the cervix. The second stage of labour begins with the full dilatation of the cervix and ends with the delivery of the fetus. The second stage carries with it the risk of fetal complications such as asphyxia and birth trauma. While the overall risk of problems in childbirth is low, the maximum risk for a baby is on the day of birth [1]. Additionally, there are maternal risks such as perineal trauma and operative vaginal delivery. Therefore, abnormalities in the second stage of labour are likely to contribute to an increased risk of maternal and neonatal morbidity and mortality [2,3].

The role of healthcare professionals caring for women in labour—obstetricians, midwives, and nurses—is vital in ensuring the safe delivery of the baby and reducing risks to the mother and baby. The aim is to optimise the chance of vaginal delivery with recourse to operative interventions when clinically indicated without compromising the safety of the mother and baby. With a global rise in the rates of planned and emergency cesarean deliveries in the first stage of labour, there is also an increase in the challenge of conducting a safe delivery following abnormalities in the second stage of labour due to a lack of training and clinical experience.

This chapter will outline the common problems encountered in the management of the second stage of labour in singleton pregnancies.

SECOND STAGE OF LABOUR

The second stage of labour, as defined by the World Health Organization (WHO), is the period from the full dilatation of the cervix to the birth of the baby and is accompanied by an involuntary maternal urge to bear down as a result of expulsive uterine contractions [4].

Phases of the Second Stage

The second stage can be described to occur in the following two phases [5]:

1. A **latent** or **passive phase**—from the full dilatation of the cervix to the onset of active maternal expulsive efforts
2. An **active phase**—which begins with active maternal expulsive efforts following full dilatation of the cervix to the birth of the baby

The Mechanism of the Second Stage

The second stage chiefly comprises an interplay of three events:

- The descent of the fetus in the vagina
- Maternal expulsive forces
- The cardinal movements of the presenting part when passing through the vaginal canal

The descent of the presenting part in the vaginal canal is affected by the bony pelvis, the pelvic floor muscles and ligaments, and the vascular supply to the pelvis [6]. In the process of human evolution, the anteroposterior diameter of the pelvis reduced due to the prominence of the sacral promontory compared to the previously cylindrical pelvic inlet. This allows the fetal head to enter the pelvis in an oblique and transverse diameter. The presenting part undergoes rotation in the midpelvis and then enters the outlet by a rotation to the anteroposterior diameter. These steps of descent through the bony pelvis are influenced by the pelvic floor muscle or levator ani, the fetal size, the fetal position, and cardinal movements (see **Chapter 2**, *Mechanics, mechanism, and stages of labour*). This process is aided by the intrauterine pressure created by the combination of uterine contractions and maternal expulsive efforts when the woman is bearing down.

A uterine contraction which occurs every 3 minutes and lasts for 1 minute raises the intrauterine pressure near the fetal head from 2.6 to 8.5 kPa, whereas a maternal bearing effort raises it to 19 kPa [7]. Uterine contractions in conjunction with maternal efforts can thus influence the outcome of labour.

Duration of the Second Stage

The normal duration for the second stage in a nulliparous woman is considered to be 2 hours of active pushing without epidural analgesia and 3 hours with analgesia, whereas in multiparous women, the duration is said to be 2 hours and 1 hour, with and without an epidural respectively [8,9]. Since epidural analgesia is known to prolong the duration of the second stage, an additional hour has been added to the duration of active pushing.

Cheng et al. suggested that epidural analgesia significantly affects the duration of the second stage and that the recommendation of an extra hour needs to be reevaluated and recommendations need to be reviewed regarding the optimum duration of the second stage with epidural analgesia [13].

The limits of the duration described in the guidelines diagnose a delay in the second stage in 10–14% of nulliparous and 3–3.5% of multiparous women [10]. The arbitrary fixing of time could lead to unnecessary interventions despite good maternal and fetal status.

Factors influencing the duration of the second stage

The duration of the second stage is influenced by factors that delay or disrupt the progress of events in the second stage. Chiefly, these are described as factors related to the **power** of expulsive forces, the **passage** through the pelvic bones and muscles, the **passenger**, i.e., the fetus, and the **parturient** (Table 12.1).

Women who have a prolonged first stage of labour are more likely to have a prolonged second stage even after other factors such as maternal size, birth weight, and analgesia [11,12] have been taken into consideration.

The station of the fetal head at the time of full cervical dilatation can influence the time required to complete the second stage. The higher the station above the ischial spine, the longer the second stage is likely to be [14].

Maternal exhaustion, obesity, uterine infection, previous cesarean delivery, poor uterine activity, and fetal malpresentation or malposition, all contribute to a prolonged second stage. There are varied reasons for dystocia, some of which overlap. Thus, the approaches to clinical management and the intervention criteria vary. This leaves the clinician with two important decisions—when to deliver and how to deliver.

Table 12.1 Factors influencing the duration of the second stage of labour

Power	Passage	Passenger	Parturient
Uterine activity	Pelvic bones	Position	Age
Maternal expulsive efforts	Soft tissue	Size	History of previous deliveries
	Pelvic shape	Presentation	Comorbidities like hypertension and diabetes
		Gestational age	

Key Point

A prolonged first stage of labour, maternal exhaustion, the shape of the pelvis, abnormal fetal position, and analgesia can all contribute to prolongation of the second stage of labour.

DIAGNOSIS OF PROLONGED SECOND STAGE

There is a lack of consensus among international organisations regarding the following:

- The exact duration of the second stage
- The time span for which pushing can be delayed
- The duration for which the labouring woman should be allowed to push
- The difference in the estimated duration of the second stage after epidural analgesia

According to the ACOG and the SMFM, the second stage can be considered prolonged if there is active pushing for >3 hours in a nullipara and >2 hours in a multipara [15]. The WHO recommendations do not differentiate between a passive and an active second stage and the delay caused by epidural analgesia [16]. Thus, the optimal duration of the second stage beyond which it can be considered prolonged needs further research using objective tools and better predictive models for maternal and neonatal outcomes.

Key Point

While there are time-based definitions for prolonged second stage, clinical experience, and expertise play an important role in management. The healthcare practitioner must balance the need to wait and reduce the chance of a cesarean with the risks to the mother and baby from a prolonged second stage of labour.

Assessment Tools to Aid Management in the Second Stage of Labour

Clinical assessment

The assessment is individualised based on the background history, progress in the first stage, maternal observations, and fetal assessment.

- **Maternal evaluation** should include vital signs and assessment for any associated risk factors from the medical history, e.g., hypertension, cardiac or respiratory diseases, or diabetes. A vaginal examination will provide valuable information about cervical dilatation, effacement, and application of the cervix to the presenting part, along with the station of the presenting part, moulding, caput, and the presentation of the fetus.
- **Fetal evaluation** should be aimed at fetal heart monitoring.
- **Evaluation of the progress of labour** should include the assessment of uterine contractions and the descent of the presenting part by abdominal palpation. A digital vaginal examination helps to evaluate the descent and rotation of the fetal head. A lack of progressive distension of the perineum should alert the clinician.

A diagnosis of delay in the second stage is made by determining the time elapsed since the onset of the active part of the second stage in relation to the parity of the mother. The NICE guidance has recommendations (Table 12.2) based on these two factors and can be used in current clinical practice to manage the delay [8].

The use of a partograph

The use of a partograph helps in the evaluation of progress and identification of delay in labour. Currently, the WHO labour care guide uses a holistic assessment of the progress of labour. This is discussed in detail in **Chapter 6**, *Monitoring labour: Partograph to labour care guide*. The labour care guide has included a section for the follow-up of the second stage of labour.

Key Point

A combination of clinical examination, an assessment of fetal well-being, and a partograph in labour can help to determine the time and mode of intervention for second stage abnormalities.

Table 12.2 NICE guidance for the management of the second stage in nulliparous and multiparous women based on the progress of labour [5]

Progress of the second stage	Nullipara	Multipara	Action to be taken
Completion of the second stage	End of 3 hours	End of 2 hours	Expect birth
Time elapsed since the onset of active labour	2 hours	1 hour	• Suspect delay • Referral or assessment for an imminent operative vaginal delivery should be considered
No progress in terms of descent and rotation of the presenting part	1 hour	30 minutes	Suspect prolonged second stage
The absence of the urge to push without any regional analgesia	1 hour of entering the second stage	1 hour of entering the second stage	Look for factors of dystocia

Ultrasound in labour

The clinical assessment of a woman in labour has traditionally been used to determine the fetal station, position, and cervical dilatation. Ultrasound in labour has been shown to be a helpful tool in the assessment of the progress of labour, especially to determine the fetal position and station in cases with a caput succedaneum and significant moulding. The use of ultrasound has been studied to predict the chances of a successful outcome with operative vaginal birth (see **Chapter 20**, *Role of ultrasound in the labour room*).

Intrapartum fetal heart rate monitoring in the second stage of labour

The assessment of fetal well-being is a very important aspect of the management of a prolonged second stage. If there is a suspicious or pathological CTG trace, delivery should be expedited. This, along with fetal position and station, will dictate the mode of operative delivery (See **Chapter 15**, *Identification and management of fetal distress*).

Uterine activity monitoring

The presence of adequate uterine contractions is a prerequisite for the normal progress of labour. The mechanical efficiency of uterine contractions is measured based on the effective clinical difference in the progress of descent and not by the number and frequency, since both these are associated with wide variations in nulliparous and multiparous women. This must be taken into consideration when making a decision to augment labour [17]. The use of oxytocin in the management of the second stage is recommended for women with inadequate uterine contractions, especially with the use of epidural analgesia.

The use of oxytocin should be monitored—it is advisable to use syringe pumps to monitor the dose administered. In low-resource settings, where pumps are not used for administration, it is extremely important to count the drop rate and correlate it with the frequency of uterine contractions.

MANAGEMENT OF ABNORMALITIES IN THE SECOND STAGE

An abnormal second stage may be related to maternal or fetal factors which could **be physiological**, **pathological,** or **iatrogenic**. Continual risk assessment in the second stage for recognising a delay and responding in a timely manner remains one of the key elements of good clinical practice. In the case of a prolonged non-progressive second stage, there are risks of damage to the fetus from hypoxia, traumatic birth, and infection [18]. Also, the clinical interventions to expedite the delivery in these situations may lead to increased risk to the mother and baby. Appropriate training and skills and timely interventions remain key to preventing complications and reducing the risks to the mother and baby. Some common clinical triggers are listed in Table 12.3. However, there may be others that can be encountered in clinical practice.

A prolonged second stage should be avoided in the presence of the following:

- Persistent fetal heart rate abnormalities, especially with a reduced fetal reserve, e.g., fetal growth restriction
- Maternal cardiac disease with fixed cardiac output
- Maternal arteriovenous (AV) malformations of the brain
- Respiratory conditions with reduced functional lung capacity

Assessment to Expedite Delivery

Nearly 80% of nulliparous and 90% of multiparous women will deliver within 2 hours of full dilatation [19]. In women who have not delivered by this time, an assessment is required to decide on further management. The factors to be assessed are as follows:

- Background medical history, obstetric history, antenatal risk factors, progress in the first stage of labour
- Clinical examination—per abdomen and per vaginum
- Maternal status
- Fetal well-being
- Pain relief
- Instrumental delivery—availability, expertise, and anticipated difficulty
- Maternal preference

Table 12.3 Common clinical triggers for review in the second stage of labour

Maternal	Fetal
Prolonged duration with no progress or descent of the presenting part	Malpositions: Occipitoposterior, occipitotransverse
Maternal exhaustion	Malpresentation: Face, brow, breech (diagnosed in the first stage of labour/late diagnosis in the second stage)
Maternal pyrexia	Fetal heart rate abnormalities
Antepartum hemorrhage	Cord prolapse, hand prolapse, shoulder dystocia
Raised maternal blood pressure	Fetal anomalies causing dystocia

Key Point

The intervention and place of delivery is decided based on maternal status, fetal well-being, and fetal position and station, taking maternal preference into consideration.

Expectant Management

In women with adequate descent and rotation of the fetal head and a reassuring fetal heart trace, a spontaneous delivery can be awaited. If this is not achieved in another hour, birth can be expedited with an instrumental delivery. The role of a supportive member of the team—a nurse, midwife, or birth companion—who has a positive attitude and can encourage the woman to push, can be immensely valuable. For the position and technique for pushing, see **Chapter 4,** *Management of the first and second stages of normallabour*.

Interventions

Several interventions are beneficial in the presence of a prolonged second stage.

Oxytocin

If there is inadequate descent or rotation, the contractions should be assessed. If the contractions are inadequate (<3–4 in 10 minutes), oxytocin can be initiated after ensuring a normal fetal heart trace. If there are adequate contractions, the initiation of oxytocin may be inappropriate. In such a case, an assessment by an experienced obstetrician is important for ruling out **cephalopelvic disproportion** or **malposition**.

Manual rotation

If there are adequate contractions but inadequate descent, then the fetal position should be assessed. If malposition is diagnosed in an average-sized baby, manual rotation can be attempted to help facilitate descent and delivery (for the technique of digital or manual rotation, see **Chapter 4**).

Operative delivery

When the second stage is prolonged and there is less than optimal descent with adequate contractions, a decision for operative delivery is made. The feasibility of an instrumental delivery vs. cesarean section is based on fetal size, station, position, and well-being. This topic is discussed in detail in **Chapter 21**, *Operative vaginal delivery*. Where an instrumental delivery cannot be safely performed, it is prudent to proceed with a cesarean section because the morbidity from a failed instrumental delivery is high.

Interventions of Uncertain or No Benefit

Fundal pressure

There is no evidence to support the practice of fundal pressure to cut short the second stage of labour.

Maternal position

Evidence does not support the use of any one maternal position to reduce the duration of the second stage of labour or facilitate delivery [20,21]. Hence, the FIGO practice guideline recommends that the mother be supported in her decision to deliver in a position of her choice [12].

Pain relief

It is important to ensure adequate pain relief for women with a prolonged second stage. While epidural analgesia has been shown to increase the duration of the second stage, reducing the amount of analgesia or discontinuing epidural analgesia in the second stage does not decrease the chances of an instrumental delivery [22].

Second Stage Cesarean Section

Cesarean section at full dilatation accounts for approximately 10% of all cesarean births. Most of these are undertaken for non-progress due to a macrosomic fetus, a persistent occiput-posterior position, and/or a failure of operative vaginal birth.

Cesarean sections in the second stage, especially with a deeply impacted fetal head, may be technically difficult due to reduced amniotic fluid and space to manoeuvre [23]. See the section on the *Management of an impacted head* in **Chapter 22,** *Cesarean section: Procedure and technique*, for more details.

A cesarean section in the second stage may be associated with a greater risk of complications than one performed in the first stage. There is a significantly higher chance of both maternal and neonatal adverse outcomes [24]. The risks to the mother are bleeding, extension of the cesarean scar, peripartum hysterectomy, and sepsis. Complications in the newborn are brachial plexus injuries, intracranial bleeding, and reduced Apgar scores.

Key Point

Cesarean section in the second stage is associated with an increased risk of maternal and perinatal morbidity.

The decrease in the incidence of operative delivery at full dilatation has been attributed not to the failure of the procedure but to practitioners' reluctance to attempt it and their lower threshold for cesarean section [25]. In privately insured women in a large European centre, the rate of cesarean sections rose from 18% to 25% from 2005 to 2014, whereas there was a sharp decrease in assisted vaginal births from 14% to 11% [26].

Practical points regarding cesarean section in the second stage of labour

- Cesarean section at full dilatation is associated with an increased risk of infection. Hence, proper aseptic techniques in the operation room need to be ensured. Vaginal irrigation with chlorhexidine or betadine prior to the section has been shown to reduce the risk of infection [27].
- A digital vaginal examination on the table, prior to proceeding with the cesarean, is worthwhile as the dynamics of the fetal position rapidly change in the second stage of labour.
- On account of the difficult labour, fetal compromise should be expected, and neonatal back-up must be available.
- The disimpaction and delivery of the fetal head may be difficult. Trained staff should be available to disengage the impacted head through the vagina. An inverted T uterine incision to increase access, uterine relaxants, and a head-down tilt may be considered for the delivery of the baby in this situation. There is an increased chance of uterine tears/ extension of the uterine incision and vaginal tears. The availability of an experienced obstetrician is essential.
- The identification of the lower segment may be difficult as the bladder is pulled up higher when the cervix is fully dilated. The uterovesical reflection of the visceral peritoneum can be used as a landmark. The pathological retraction ring of Bandl may be seen in cases of obstructed labour (see **Chapter 18**, *Obstructed labour and uterine rupture*).
- Since the risk of postpartum hemorrhage is high, blood should be cross-matched and reserved.
- Remaining calm, asking for help or escalation where the assistance of seniors is required, and good communication with team members are important non-clinical skills to practice in these situations.

The increasing incidence of cesarean births at full dilatation and the associated risks highlight the need for education and training with regard to the management of abnormalities in the second stage of labour. The accuracy of the findings on vaginal examination and the correct identification of the fetal head position and asynclitism can help in prompt and proper management. The availability of a skilled senior obstetrician with expertise in operative vaginal birth at an early stage can help in preventing the morbidity associated with this kind of delivery.

DOCUMENTATION

There should be clear and accurate documentation of the operative findings in the maternity records, especially if there is an untoward or unexpected outcome for the mother and/or baby.

IMPLICATIONS FOR FUTURE PREGNANCY FOLLOWING ABNORMALITIES IN THE SECOND STAGE OF LABOUR

A delay in the second stage and an emergency operative delivery can be a traumatic experience for the woman and her birthing partner. It is, therefore, important to debrief the woman postdelivery and, at the review, to discuss the implications for a subsequent pregnancy.

An increased incidence of preterm birth in subsequent pregnancies has been reported following a cesarean section at full dilatation [28]. This could be a result of an intraoperative extension of the uterine incision into the cervix, leading to a potential disruption of the cervical integrity. This has implications for the monitoring cervical length in future pregnancies for the increased risk of preterm delivery [29].

A prolonged second stage, forceps deliveries, and obstetric anal sphincter injuries are intrapartum risk factors for levator avulsions, which, in turn, can lead to pelvic organ prolapse.

CONCLUSION

Abnormalities in the second stage of labour may come to the clinician's attention due to deviations in the progress of labour. Anticipation, recognition, and timely response, along with appropriate skills and expertise are some of the key elements in providing quality care and ensuring a safe delivery.

REFERENCES

1. Walker KF, Cohen AL, Walker SH, et al. The dangers of the day of birth. *BJOG*. 2014. 121(6).
2. Niemczyk NA, Ren D, Stapleton SR. Associations between prolonged second stage of labour and maternal and neonatal outcomes in freestanding birth centres: A retrospective analysis. *BMC Pregnancy and Childbirth*. 2022. 22(1).
3. Clark SL, Garite TJ, Hamilton EF, et al. 'Doing something' about the caesarean delivery rate. *Am J Obstet Gynecol*. 2018. 219(3).
4. World Health Organization. WHO Labour Care Guide User's Manual. WHO, Geneva. 2020.
5. Gill P, Henning JM, Carlson K, et al. *Abnormal Labor* (Nursing). Treasure Island (FL): StatPearls Publishing. 2023 [Updated 2023 Jun 14]. Available from: https://www.ncbi.nlm.nih.gov/books/NBK568801.
6. Posner GD, Dy J, Black AY, Jones GD. *Oxorn–Foote Human Labor and Birth*. Sixth Edition. Vol. 53. McGraw-Hill Education. 2013.
7. Ashton-Miller JA, Delancey JO. On the biomechanics of vaginal birth and common sequelae. *Annu Rev Biomed Eng*. 2009. 11:163-76.
8. National Institute for Health and Care Excellent. Overview Intrapartum care for healthy women and babies. NICE. NHA. 2019.
9. ACOG Practice Bulletin Number 49. Dystocia and augmentation of labor. Vol. 102. *Obstetrics and Gynaecology*. 2003. Nelson DB, McIntire DD, Leveno KJ. Relationship of the length of the first stage of labor to the length of the second stage. *Obstetrics and Gynecology*. 2013;122(1).
10. Cheng YW, Caughey AB. Defining and managing normal and abnormal second stage of labor. *Obstet Gynecol Clin North Am*. 2017. 44(4):547-566.
11. Nelson DB, McIntire DD, Leveno KJ. Relationship of the length of the first stage of labor to the length of the second stage. *Obstet Gynecol*. 2013 Jul;122(1):27-32.
12. Wright A, Nassar AH, Visser G, et al. FIGO Safe Motherhood and Newborn Health Committee. FIGO good clinical practice paper: Management of the second stage of labor. *Int J Gynaecol Obstet*. 2021 Feb;152(2):172-181.
13. Cheng YW, Shaffer BL, Nicholson JM, Caughey AB. Second stage of labor and epidural use: A larger effect than previously suggested. *Obstet Gynecol*. 2014. 123(3):527-535. Erratum in: *Obstet Gynecol*. 2014 May. 123(5):1109.
14. Ludvigsen E, Skjeldestad FE. Station of the fetal head at complete cervical dilation impacts duration of second stage of labor. *Eur J Obstet Gynecol Reprod Biol X*. 2019. 31. 7:100100. doi: 10.1016/j.eurox. 2019.100100.
15. American College of Obstetricians and Gynecologists. Obstetric care consensus no. 1: Safe prevention of the primary cesarean delivery. *Obstetrics and Gynecology*. 2014. 123(3), 693–711.
16. WHO recommendations: Intrapartum care for a positive childbirth experience. 2018. WHO, Geneva. Licence: CC BY-NC-SA 3.0 IGO.
17. Nabhan A, Boulvain M. Augmentation of labour. *Best Pract Res Clin Obstet Gynaecol*. 2020. 67:80-89.
18. Baskett Thomas F, Calder Andew A, Arulkumaran Sabaratnam. *Munro Kerr's Operative obstetrics*. 2014.
19. Cheng YW, Hopkins LM, Caughey AB. How long is too long: Does a prolonged second stage of labor in nulliparous women affect maternal and neonatal outcomes? *Am J Obstet Gynecol*. 2004. 191(3):933-8.
20. Roberts CL, Algert CS, Cameron CA, Torvaldsen S. A meta-analysis of upright positions in the second stage to reduce instrumental deliveries in women with epidural analgesia. *Acta Obstet Gynecol* Scand. 2005. 84(8):794-8.
21. Hofmeyr GJ, Kulier R. Hands/knees posture in late pregnancy or labour for fetal malposition (lateral or posterior). *Cochrane Database Syst Rev*. 2000. Issue 2. Art. no.:CD001063. CD001063. Update in: *Cochrane Database Syst Rev*. 2005. (2):CD001063.
22. Torvaldsen S, Roberts CL, Bell JC, Raynes-Greenow CH. Discontinuation of epidural analgesia late in labour for reducing the adverse delivery outcomes associated with epidural analgesia. *Cochrane Database Syst Rev*. 2004. Issue 4. Art. no.: CD004457.
23. Tempest N, Hart A, Walkinshaw S, Hapangama DK. A re-evaluation of the role of rotational forceps: A retrospective comparison of maternal and perinatal outcomes following different methods of birth for malposition in the second stage of labour. *BJOG*. 2013. 120(10):1277-84.

24. Allen VM, O'Connell CM, Baskett TF. Maternal and perinatal morbidity of caesarean delivery at full cervical dilatation compared with caesarean delivery in the first stage of labour. *BJOG*. 2005. 112(7):986-90.
25. Loudon JA, Groom KM, Hinkson L, et al. Changing trends in operative delivery performed at full dilatation over a 10-year period. *J Obstet Gynaecol*. 2010. 30(4):370-5.
26. Turner MJ, Reynolds CME, McMahon LE, et al. Caesarean section rates in women in the Republic of Ireland who chose to attend their obstetrician privately: A retrospective observational study. *BMC Pregnancy Childbirth*. 2020. 548.
27. Trivedi M, Robinson AM, Islam MR. Effect of vaginal antiseptic prior to caesarean section on the rate of post-caesarean complications: A blinded randomised controlled trial. *Trials*. 2022. 23. 231.
28. Ewington LJ, Quenby S. Full dilatation caesarean section and the risk of preterm delivery in a subsequent pregnancy: A historical cohort study. *J Clin Med*. 2020. 9(12):3998.
29. Vousden N, Cargill Z, Briley A, et al. Caesarean section at full dilatation: Incidence, impact and current management. *The Obstetrician & Gynaecologist*. 2014. 16: 199–205.

CHAPTER 13

Abnormalities in the Third Stage of Labour

Postpartum Hemorrhage and Retained Placenta

SAM ONONGE, ANDREW D WEEKS

POSTPARTUM HEMORRHAGE

INTRODUCTION

Postpartum hemorrhage (PPH) is an obstetric emergency complicating 1–10% of all deliveries globally [1]. It remains the leading obstetric cause of maternal deaths, is responsible for 25% of maternal deaths annually, and affects 14 million women each year, particularly in low- and middle-income countries (LMICs).

Its distribution varies across regions, with the highest prevalence of 5.1–25.7% reported in Africa, followed by North America at 4.3–13% and Asia at 1.9–8%.[2]. In high-income countries, PPH is largely preventable and manageable, with the leading cause of the same being placental abnormalities. In low-resource settings, however, mortality from PPH remains high, and those who survive severe PPH are likely to experience significant iatrogenic morbidity (from blood products, surgical interventions, infections, intensive care admission, and prolonged hospitalisation) [3,4]. The maternal death rate from hemorrhage, more than other causes of maternal death, is closely related to a country's development (Fig. 13.1).

DEFINITION

Postpartum hemorrhage (PPH) is defined as bleeding from the birth canal in the first 24 hours after the birth of the baby and is traditionally defined as blood loss of >500 mL following vaginal or cesarean birth [6].

However, this definition has been criticised as it is neither appropriate to delay treatment to this point nor is it a level that always results in maternal morbidity. Furthermore, the use of 500 mL as a clinical trial outcome has led to the use of treatments that reduce minor bleeds but may not reduce maternal morbidity or mortality [7]. It is, therefore, suggested that clinicians continue their current practice of giving PPH treatment as soon as they are unhappy with the rapidity or volume of blood loss [8,9]. However, clinical trials should use either 1000 mL blood loss or maternal near-miss mortality as the main outcome [9].

> **Key Point**
>
> Since it is not always easy to assess blood loss, it is suggested that clinicians continue their current practice of initiating PPH treatment as soon as they are unhappy with the rapidity or volume of blood loss [8,9].

Clinically, PPH can be defined as any amount of blood loss that results in hemodynamic instability. The American College of Obstetricians and Gynecologists, in 2017 [10], defined PPH as blood loss occurring within 24 hours after birth,

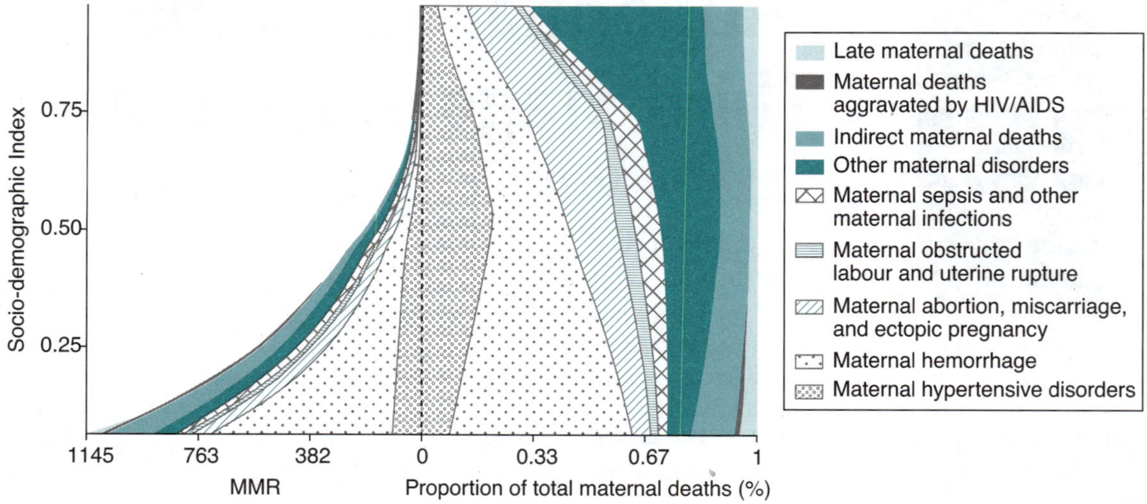

Fig. 13.1 The relationship between cause-specific maternal mortality ratio (*MMR*, the number of maternal deaths during a given time period per 100,000 live births) and socio-demographic index (*SDI*, a representation of social and economic development based on each country's economy, education, and fertility rate) [5]

regardless of the mode of delivery, that results in the following:

- Blood loss of >1000 mL or
- Signs and symptoms of hypovolemia.

A healthy woman without anemia does not develop signs or symptoms of hypovolemia until she has lost 1500 mL. However, it is important to remember that blood volume is related to body weight. Thus, the small, low-weight woman, particularly if she is anemic, may not tolerate even small blood losses. This fact is particularly relevant in LMICs.

> **Key Point**
>
> The small, underweight woman, who is anemic and has a low blood volume to start with may not tolerate even small blood losses, a fact particularly relevant in LMICs.

Classification

PPH is further classified as follows:

- **Primary PPH,** when it occurs within the first 24 hours postpartum and
- **Secondary PPH**, which is defined as excessive bleeding between 24 hours and 6 weeks postnatally.

CAUSES AND RISK FACTORS OF PPH

Primary PPH is commonly due to one or more of the following:

- Uterine atony
- Trauma
- Retained tissue
- Coagulation disorders

Uterine Atony

Uterine atony is the most common cause of PPH (80%) [10] and can be caused by anything that interferes with the ability of the uterus to contract and retract. Although it can occur in low-risk cases, interference with uterine contraction and retraction is most likely in the following clinical situations:

- **Multiparity**
- **Prolonged labour**—particularly if it is associated with chorioamnionitis. The

acidotic and infected uterus is vulnerable to uterine atony and may be unresponsive to oxytocic agents.

- **Precipitate labour**—at the other extreme of uterine action, the very rapid and efficient first and second stages of labour may be followed by uterine atony.
- **Uterine overdistension**—as may occur with multiple pregnancy, macrosomia, and polyhydramnios.
- **Retained blood clots**—may result from a poorly contracting uterus following placental delivery, and oozing from the placental site. As clots accumulate, they interfere with the ability of the uterus to contract and retract, leading to an insidious filling of the uterus with clots and blood and establishing a vicious cycle.
- **Tocolytic drugs**—such as glyceryl trinitrate or terbutaline.
- **Deep general anesthesia**—particularly with fluorinated hydrocarbons.
- **Structural abnormalities of the uterus**—including uterine anomalies and fibroids.
- **Placenta previa**—which limits the ability of the lower uterine segment to contract and retract.
- **Multiparity**—may lead to postpartum hemorrhage, especially in grandmultiparas (women who have had 5 pregnancies).

Trauma

Following vaginal delivery

Traumatic bleeding is the second most common cause of PPH following vaginal birth, accounting for the majority of the remaining 10–15% of cases. It includes the following:

- Lacerations of the perineum, vagina, and cervix
- Episiotomy
- Uterine rupture
- Vulvovaginal and broad ligament hematomas

These are more common after precipitous, uncontrolled deliveries or operative vaginal deliveries where the genital tract undergoes sudden and forced stretching [10].

Following cesarean delivery

In women undergoing a cesarean birth, considerable blood loss may occur from:

- Incisions on a vascular lower segment or
- Lateral extensions from the uterine incision angle

The blood loss may be exacerbated by uterine atony or blood loss from a placental bed that reaches into the relatively non-contractile lower segment.

Retained Tissues

PPH may occur when there is one or more of the following:

- Retained placenta (see section below on *Retained placenta*)
- Adherent placenta
- Retained membranes
- Retained blood clots

Coagulation Disorders

This is a rare cause of primary PPH. Coagulation problems can be divided into the following:

- **Inherited**—such as von Willebrand disease, hemophilia, and idiopathic thrombocytopenic purpura. Most women with inherited coagulation disorders go through childbirth without developing PPH [11], thus demonstrating the efficacy of the physiological uterine muscular ligature. However, underlying coagulation disorders exacerbate blood loss in any woman who develops PPH.
- **Acquired**—such as from the use of anticoagulant therapy [11] and disseminated intravascular coagulopathy (DIC), which may develop secondary to excessive blood loss, complicating severe PPH.

Key Point

DIC may complicate postpartum hemorrhage and placental abruption, severe preeclampsia, intrauterine fetal demise, sepsis, and amniotic fluid embolism [10].

BLOOD LOSS MEASUREMENT

The estimation of blood loss at birth is notoriously inaccurate, with clinicians tending to underestimate blood loss and patients overestimating it. A recent study found that doctors and midwives judge the need to treat PPH not based on blood loss volume, but on intuition based on the speed of the flow and the underlying risk factors in the woman [12]. There were, however, no specific instructions for staff on when to initiate or escalate treatment for PPH. Interviews with maternity staff suggest that blood loss measurement is commonly used 'after the event' to determine the need for monitoring and the place of care.

More recently, two programmes in which blood loss is routinely measured and used in real time to initiate therapy and escalate care have shown great promise.

- In the ObsCymru protocol (pronounced *obs-cum-ree*), routine blood loss is measured by combining the following techniques as opposed to visual estimation for all births:
  - **The volumetric technique**, which measures fluid volume collected in the drapes placed under the woman's buttocks
  - **The gravimetric technique,** which is an indirect measurement of blood loss. Blood loss is calculated by weighing the surgical material contaminated with blood and subtracting the dry weights (1 gram weight = 1 mL blood loss volume).

  This is combined with a strict escalation policy and the use of thromboelastogram (TEG) assessment for blood losses of over 1500 mL. When implemented across Wales, the number of women with blood losses over 2500 mL or those who required a blood transfusion fell by around 25% [13].
- In the E-MOTIVE (Evaluation of blood loss, Massage, Oxytocic, Tranexamic Acid, IV fluids, and Escalation) cluster randomised trial, blood loss in over 200,000 births in four low-income countries was measured using a calibrated blood collection drape, and the treatment bundle was initiated at the point of clinical concern **with a safety limit of a maximum of 500 mL (300 mL if there were additional risk factors)**. The E-MOTIVE intervention resulted in a 60% reduction in severe maternal outcomes and a 20% reduction in death from PPH [14]. See the section below on *Management of PPH* for further details.

> **Key Point**
>
> Studies from both high-resource countries [13] and LMICs [14] suggest that real-time blood loss measurement combined with care bundles can be a highly effective part of improving outcomes of PPH.

PREVENTION OF PPH

While the prevention of PPH has focused for many years on the active management of the third stage of labour, it is now recognised to be a far wider issue than this. Although the use of a bolus of uterotonic at the time of birth does reduce the rate of PPH, there are several modifiable risk factors that also need to be addressed. There are multiple ways in which excessive intervention can result either directly or indirectly in PPH.

The following measures are recommended to help in preventing PPH:

- Reducing the rate of emergency cesarean and operative vaginal birth as both are strongly associated with PPH, especially following prolonged labour.
- Managing induction of labour since PPH is associated with it, although this appears to be due to the underlying reason for induction (and possibly, delays in the induction process) rather than the induction process itself.
- Preventing placenta accreta/previa by reducing cesarean rates.

Public Health Measures

The prevention of morbidity and death from PPH is not only about preventing PPH but also establishing good public health measures to prevent malnourishment and anemia and building health systems that facilitate quality PPH management. The latter includes transport for women with PPH or retained placenta after giving birth at home or in mid-level units, well-organised and staffed maternity units, effective drugs and supplies including blood, and rapid access to expert operative care when needed. All these are necessary to prevent maternal deaths from PPH (Fig. 13.2).

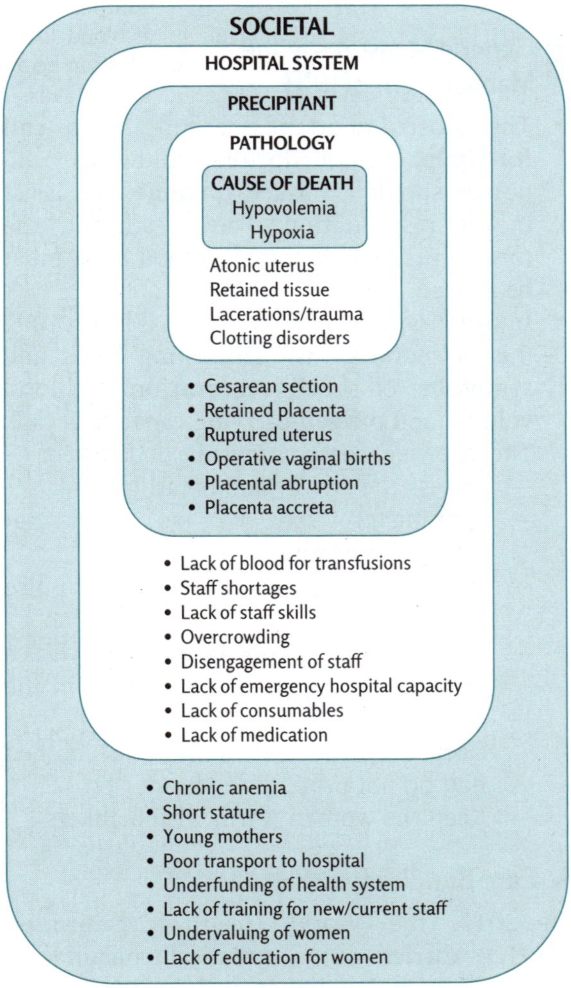

Fig. 13.2 Causes of death from PPH, showing the impact of societal and health service factors

Active Management of the Third Stage of Labour (AMTSL)

Initial descriptions of active management comprised **uterotonics** given at the time of birth, **immediate cord clamping,** and **controlled cord traction**. These three became the classic **'active management triad'**. Large-scale randomised controlled trials have, however, demonstrated that early cord clamping is harmful for the newborn, and that controlled cord traction is largely unnecessary [15]. See **Chapter 5**, *Management of the third stage of labour,* for further details.

Oxytocin

The optimal uterotonic for PPH prophylaxis is widely agreed to be **oxytocin**.

Vaginal birth

- Oxytocin (10 international units [IU] IM) is recommended by the WHO for the prevention of postpartum hemorrhage for all births [16].
- If IV access is already present, IV infusion of 10 IU oxytocin in 500 mL of saline is recommended in preference to IM administration [16].

Cesarean section

- Oxytocin is the recommended uterotonic drug for the prevention of PPH in cesarean section.
- An IV infusion (10–20 IU in 500 mL of saline) is administered, which reduces the need for additional uterotonic agents but does not affect the overall occurrence of major obstetric hemorrhage [16].

Other uterotonics

- **Ergometrine** is a highly effective uterotonic in combination with oxytocin, but may cause hypertension and vomiting and hence is generally reserved as a form of treatment.
- **Misoprostol** is not as effective as oxytocin and frequently causes shivering and an increase in maternal temperature. However, it has the advantages of heat stability and

availability in the tablet form. Hence, it is recommended in settings where high quality oxytocin is unavailable. It can be administered by a community health worker or even self-administered in a low-resource setting. It is given orally as a dose of 400–600 mcg.

- **Carbetocin**, a long-acting analogue of oxytocin, is also heat stable but needs to be administered by injection. Some studies had suggested that it might be more effective than oxytocin, but the large CHAMPION study found no difference between the drugs when given intramuscularly at vaginal birth [17].

A network meta-analysis, in which all randomised trials were compared for a single indication, demonstrated that combining oxytocin with either ergometrine or misoprostol may be a very effective strategy for preventing PPH, albeit with increased side effects [18].

It is important to prevent morbidity in healthy women giving birth. Considering that around 85% of women giving birth will not have a PPH even without prophylaxis, most authorities reserve drugs with side effects for treatment rather than prevention.

Key Point

Combining oxytocin with either ergometrine or misoprostol may be a very effective strategy for preventing PPH, albeit with increased side effects [18].

The dosage of various uterotonics is summarised in Box 13.1.

Box. 13.1 Uterotonics used for the prevention of PPH

The following (in order of preference) are recommended as the most effective uterotonics for the prevention of PPH in all births [10,18]:

1. Oxytocin 10 IU IM/IV infusion
2. Oxytocin 10 IU IM/IV infusion + ergometrine (0.2 mg) IV
3. Oxytocin 10 IU IM/IV infusion + misoprostol 400–600 mcg orally, sublingually, or 800–1000 mcg rectally

MANAGEMENT OF PPH

The management of PPH is complex, consisting of **assessment** (in tandem with **resuscitation** as required), **diagnosis** of the underlying cause, and **treatment**, all of which need to be carried out simultaneously (Fig. 13.3).

Calling for help is a very important first step in management. Multimodal strategies that are implemented to control PPH and that involve multiple interventions points and actors are called **bundles** and consist of a group of interventions [19,20,21].

General Measures in the Management of PPH

- The most important measure is to **call for help.** Senior doctors, midwives, and nurses should be asked to come and assist in the resuscitation. The anesthetist, the theatre personnel, and the blood bank must be alerted.
- In situations when the woman has lost >1000 mL of blood or is manifesting signs and symptoms of shock, **restoration of blood volume and oxygen-carrying capacity** is vital. The following measures must be undertaken:
  - — Assess the airway and breathing
  - — Administer oxygen by mask at 10–15 litres/minute
  - — Monitor the blood pressure and pulse continuously
  - — Establish a second IV access with a large-bore (16–18 gauge) cannula in the opposite arm
  - — Keep the head end of the table or bed flat; do not prop up the head
  - — Keep the woman warm with blankets

Care Bundles for PPH

In 2017, the World Health Organization (WHO) carried out a technical consultation among international maternal health experts to evaluate the development of care bundles for PPH [21].

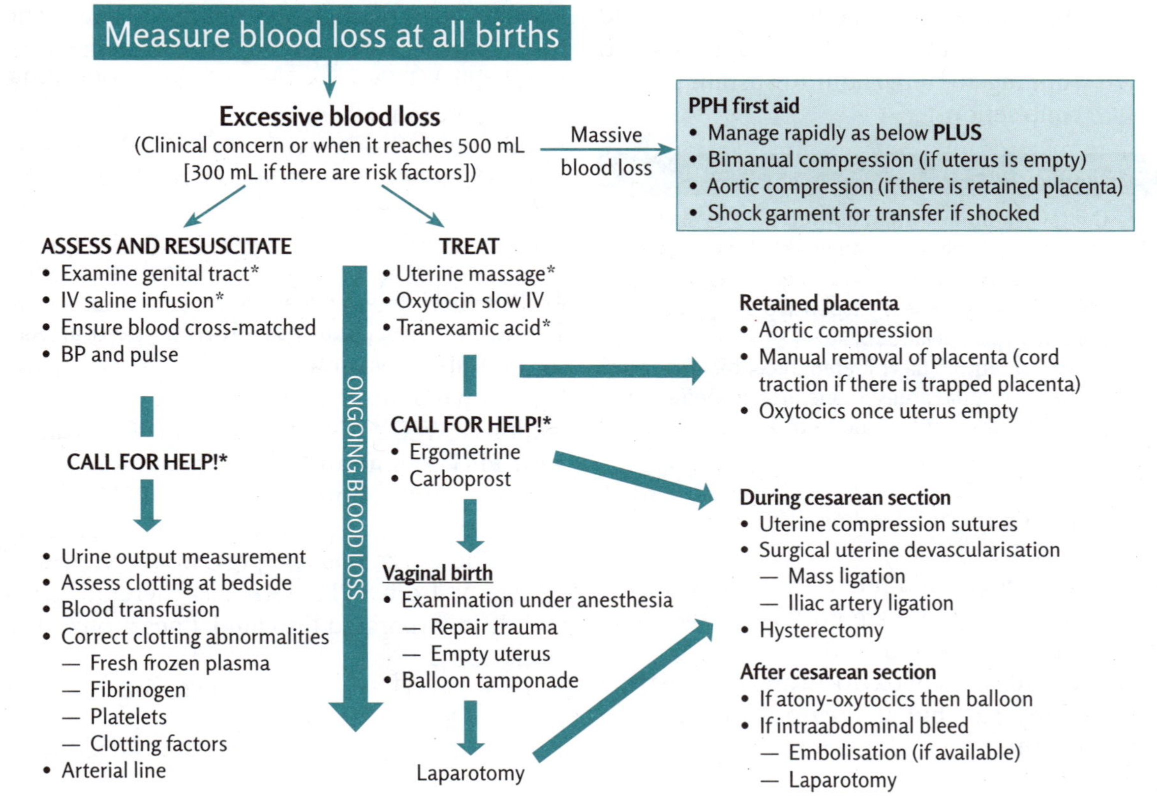

Fig. 13.3 Schemata for the management of PPH (*elements of the E-MOTIVE initial response bundle for PPH)

The consultation led to a definition of two care bundles:

- **First-response PPH bundle**, comprising the following:
  - — Administration of uterotonic drugs
  - — Infusion of isotonic crystalloids
  - — Tranexamic acid injection
  - — Uterine massage
- **Response to refractory PPH bundle**, comprising the following:
  - — Bimanual uterine compression or abdominal aortic compression
  - — Uterine balloon tamponade
  - — Application of non-pneumatic anti-shock garment (NASG)

A large-cluster randomised trial reported in 2023 demonstrated that implementing the first-response bundle after early identification with a calibrated blood-collecting drape reduced severe PPH by 60% [14].

First-response PPH care bundle

The following measures are carried out simultaneously to control PPH.

Uterotonic drugs

The recommended uterotonic drugs for the treatment of PPH include **oxytocin**, **ergometrine**, **misoprostol**, and **carboprost tromethamine** (15-methyl prostaglandin $F_{2\alpha}$).

The following sequence of uterotonic drugs is commonly recommended:

- **Intravenous oxytocin**
  - — 5–10 IU are given as an IV bolus **slowly** over 1–5 minutes if an IV line is available (**may cause sudden hypotension**).

— An infusion is established with 20–40 IU of oxytocin in 500 mL crystalloid running at 10 IU/hour to sustain uterine contractions.

Key Points

- Oxytocin administration down-regulates oxytocin receptors. If labour is augmented by oxytocin during the first and second stages of labour, the receptors may be less responsive to oxytocin in the third stage of labour.
- The myometrium has different receptors for each of the uterotonic drugs. If one drug is ineffective, the clinician should move quickly to the next choice.

- **Ergometrine** (if bleeding is not controlled with oxytocin)
  - 0.2 mg is administered **slowly** by IV (provided there are no contraindications such as hypertension).

The above doses of oxytocin and ergometrine can be repeated, but if they are found to be ineffective, there should be no delay in moving to carboprost.

- **Carboprost tromethamine (15-methyl prostaglandin $F_{2\alpha}$)**
  - 0.25 mg can be given by deep IM injection in the gluteal region using a long needle. **This can be repeated up to 8 times if necessary.** An alternative is an infusion of 0.25 mg in 500 mL crystalloid solution.
- **Misoprostol** has no additional benefit if oxytocin has already been given [22] but can be used if other oxytocics are not available.
  - The preferred route is sublingual or oral 800 mcg [23]. Around 50% of women will have a raised temperature and shivering 1–2 hours post administration. This is transient and self-limiting and does not require antibiotic use.

Intravenous isotonic crystalloid infusion

The urgency and measures taken to resuscitate the woman depend on the amount of blood loss and the presence or absence of shock. The following measures should be instituted:

- Establish IV access with a large bore (16–18 gauge) cannula
- Initiate infusion with crystalloid solution (preferably lactated Ringer's solution)

See the section below on *Resuscitation and the role of transfusion therapy in PPH*.

Tranexamic acid (TXA)

Tranexamic acid is an anti-fibrinolytic that acts by inhibiting plasminogen, thus blocking the breakdown of fibrin and stabilising clots. In the landmark WOMAN study of 20,000 women with PPH, significantly fewer laparotomies for bleeding and significantly fewer PPH deaths were noted among those treated with TXA [24]. The effect was the prevention of 20% of all deaths from PPH. TXA has therefore been rapidly incorporated into guidelines around the world [25].

TXA should be administered as follows [25]:

- 1 g IV bolus over 10 minutes
- Within 3 hours of giving birth to be most effective
- A second IV dose of 1 g if bleeding continues after 30 minutes or if bleeding restarts within 24 hours of birth

Key Point

Tranexamic acid should be administered early, irrespective of the underlying cause of bleeding [25].

Uterine massage

Massaging the uterine fundus to stimulate a uterine contraction is part of the first-response PPH bundle. Though its effectiveness in reducing mortality is controversial, the WHO and FIGO guidelines recommend it [6,20].

Additional supportive measures

These include the following:

- Emptying the bladder to enable the uterus to contract

- Examination of the genital tract to exclude tears
- Emptying the uterine cavity of any retained placental tissue or blood clots
- Reassuring the woman and explaining the procedures carried out to her or her birth companion
- Assigning a member of the staff to specifically keep the woman calm and to explain what is going on

Response to refractory PPH bundle

The WHO response bundle for refractory PPH [21] comprises the following:

- Bimanual uterine compression
- Abdominal aortic compression
- Insertion of uterine balloon tamponade
- Application of non-pneumatic anti-shock garment

Key Point

Additional supportive measures for the response to refractory PPH includes blood transfusion, referral to higher facilities, and surgery to control the bleeding. Continuous infusion with crystalloids, uterotonics, and tranexamic acid may be repeated during this phase.

Bimanual uterine compression

While preparations are being made for surgical intervention, **bimanual uterine compression** may be undertaken as a stop-gap measure. The vaginal hand forms a fist in the anterior fornix while the abdominal hand cups the posterofundal aspect of the uterus, pulling it down against the vaginal fist. The vaginal hand also elevates the uterus. In this way, the uterine vessels may be attenuated and compressed to reduce the bleeding (Fig. 13.4). This method may be very uncomfortable and invasive for the woman.

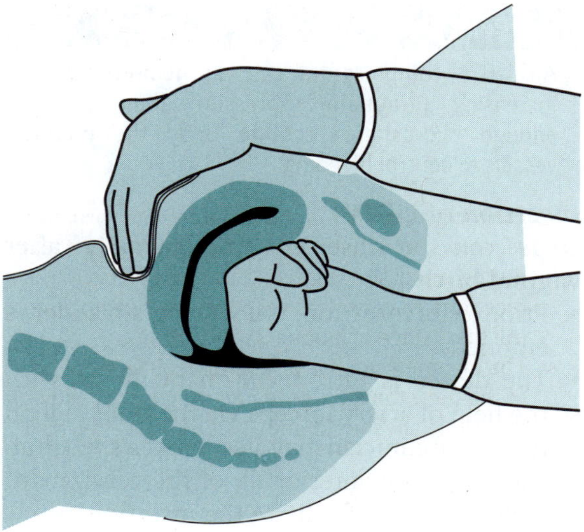

Fig. 13.4 Bimanual compression

Abdominal aortic compression

If the placenta is retained, or while awaiting the mobilisation of surgical instruments, **external aortic compression** can be performed. This involves applying the fist directly in the midline, just above the umbilicus and uterus, with the heel of the hand pressing down on the aorta. This is made feasible by the stretched abdominal muscles and the separation of the rectus muscles in pregnancy. The other hand palpates the femoral artery to check that the applied pressure is adequate to occlude the pulse. **Pressure can safely be continued for an hour if necessary.**

Uterine balloon tamponade (UBT)

Uterine balloon tamponade is one of the non-surgical interventions available for the management of atonic postpartum hemorrhage refractory to uterotonics. There are different varieties of UBTs designed for uterine atony, including Bakri, EBB, BT-Cath, Foley catheter, Sengstaken–Blakemore gastroesophageal tube, Rusch balloon, condom balloon, and Ellavi.

Multiple Foley balloons and condom catheters have been used in low-resource areas. However, a recent study from LMICs [26] concluded that condom catheters in these settings did not improve maternal outcomes.

Key Point

All UBTs compress the site of hemorrhage by increasing intrauterine pressure, thus exerting enough hydrostatic pressure upon the uterine vessels to control bleeding.

Insertion of UBTs

UBTs can be inserted transvaginally after **vaginal birth** [27].

- Prior to its insertion, the woman's bladder is emptied.
- The device is introduced manually or with the help of artery forceps via the transvaginal route; the clinician may also insert a speculum and grasp the anterior lip of the cervix with wide forceps to facilitate the insertion.
- The balloon is gently passed through the cervix until resistance is felt at the uterine fundus.
- At this point, the forceps are released and withdrawn, with care taken not to displace the device from the uterine cavity.

The placement of UBTs **after cesarean delivery** is through the uterine incision. A UBT is generally used to treat a bleeding lower segment after placenta previa in cases that are unsuitable for uterine compression sutures. In such cases:

- The catheter is passed through the cesarean incision.
- The balloon end is slipped upwards into the uterus and the port end downwards through the cervix.
- An assistant pulls the port end through the vaginal canal until the deflated balloon base comes in contact with the internal cervical os.
- The balloon should be inflated after closing the uterine incision to avoid balloon puncture, but before abdominal closure in case of treatment failure.

Inflating the balloon: After either vaginal or cesarean birth, the balloon should initially be filled with 200 mL of saline solution or sterile water. If the bleeding persists, the balloon should be filled with an additional 50 mL, and the bleeding should be re-evaluated. The tamponade is considered to have failed if the bleeding has not subsided even after the balloon has been filled with 500 mL of saline (maximum recommended volume). Surgical management is then considered.

The balloon can be left inside the uterine cavity for 6–24 hours. Although the balloon can be immediately deflated, many gradually deflate the device in 2–3 installments over 2 hours by removing 50–100 mL each time. If bleeding resumes during the process, the balloon can be rapidly re-inflated.

Key Point

The balloon tamponade is considered to have failed if the bleeding has not subsided even after the balloon has been filled with 500 mL of saline (maximum recommended volume).

Prophylactic antibiotics: These are commonly used, though there is only low-quality evidence for their use in preventing infection after inserting UBTs [28].

Follow-up: Women undergoing uterine tamponade require continuous monitoring for vital signs, uterine tone, estimation of vaginal blood loss, and urinary output.

Non-pneumatic anti-shock garment

The non-pneumatic anti-shock garment (NASG) is a temporising technology that aims to increase survival rates in women with hypovolemic shock by extending the available time to perform definitive surgical interventions or for referral to a specialised centre. NASG is a low-cost suit composed of articulated segments which wrap around the lower body—ankles, calves, thighs, pelvis, and abdomen (Fig. 13.5).

Key Point

The NASG is reusable and can be adjusted for women of different heights and abdominal girths. It can be safely used for up to 48 hours until the cause of hemorrhage is resolved and the woman is hemodynamically stable.

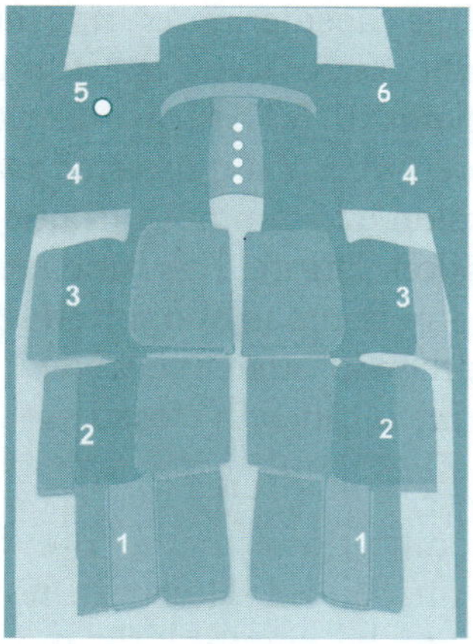

Fig. 13.5 Schematic diagram of the non-pneumatic anti-shock garment (NASG): This figure shows an opened NASG—the articulated leg segments (1, 2, 3) are attached to the pelvic segment (4), and the abdominal segments (5, 6) contain a foam ball for extra pressure

The abdominal segments include a compression ball that is placed over the uterus. The compression over the abdomen diminishes blood flow to the inferior portions of the body, including the pelvis, which results in decreased uterine bleeding. At the same time, the NASG compresses the skin and subcutaneous tissues, thus reducing the circulating blood volume and increasing venous return. This increases cardiac output, which in turn, results in improved upper body tissue perfusion.

Key Point

The woman's vital signs must be monitored carefully. If she develops signs of respiratory distress, the abdominal segment can be gently released without fully removing it.

Surgical Measures for PPH

When all the above techniques for managing PPH have failed, surgical intervention may be life-saving. It is important **not to delay** surgical intervention until the woman is moribund. Delaying control of bleeding may culminate in the lethal triad of hypovolemic shock—coagulopathy, hypothermia, and acidosis.

The surgical options for controlling PPH are as follows:

- Uterine compression sutures
  - B-Lynch suture
  - Other modifications
- Arterial ligation
  - Uterine artery ligation and stepwise devascularisation
  - Internal iliac artery ligation
- Hysterectomy

Uterine compression sutures

The B-Lynch suture, also known as the 'brace suture', was described in 1997 as an alternative conservative surgical management for controlling PPH due to uterine atony [29]. It is a fairly simple, safe, and life-saving procedure. It also preserves the woman's fertility. In atonic PPH, the suture has a success rates above 90% and controls bleeding by compressing the uterine body's anterior wall against its posterior wall. The technique is illustrated in Fig. 13.6.

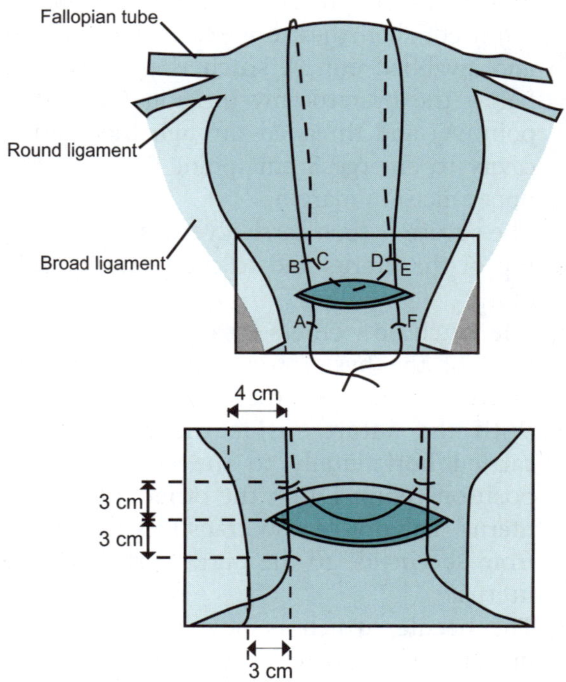

Fig. 13.6 B-Lynch compression suture technique

Procedure

- Under general anesthesia, the woman is catheterised and placed in the lithotomy position to allow an objective vaginal assessment of the control of bleeding.
- The abdomen is opened by a low transverse incision (Pfannenstiel) if the woman has had a vaginal delivery, or the cesarean incision is re-opened if the PPH is postoperative.
- The uterus is exteriorised and rechecked to identify any bleeding points. It is essential to first try bimanual compression to test for the potential efficacy of the B-Lynch suture before performing the procedure. If the bleeding stops on applying bimanual compression, there is a good chance that the application of the B-Lynch suture will also effectively stop the bleeding
- The uterovesical fold of the peritoneum is incised transversely, and the bladder is pushed down gently.
- A lower segment transverse incision is made or sutures of a recent cesarean section are removed. Then, the uterine cavity is examined and swabbed out. A stitch is placed 3 cm below the hysterotomy incision (Fig. 13.6, point A) and threaded through the uterine cavity to emerge 3 cm (point B) above the upper incision margin.
- The suture is then carried vertically over the top of the uterus and to the posterior side of it.
- The stitch now enters into the cavity at the level of the hysterotomy incision and the uterosacral ligament (point C).
- With the suture inside the cavity, it is carried horizontally to the corresponding position (point D) on the other side of the uterus. The needle now transfixes the uterus from the inside to the outer surface of the uterus.
- The needle, which is now outside of the uterine cavity posteriorly, is taken through the same suture steps (point E) but in reverse sequence.
- Finally, the needle picks up the anterior wall at the same level as the initial entry point (point F). The two lengths of the suture are pulled taut, assisted by bimanual compression to minimise trauma and aid compression. During this time, the vagina is checked for the control of bleeding. The two ends are then knotted.
- The uterine incision is closed.

Other compression sutures

Various modifications of the B-Lynch suture have been introduced. However, no technique has proven to be significantly more effective than the other [30].

Transverse and vertical sutures are placed in the **Pereira technique** and multiple vertical sutures are used in the **Hayman technique**. The **Cho technique** uses multiple 'square' sutures, eliminating the spaces inside the uterine cavity and joining the anterior and posterior walls. These sutures do not require the opening of the uterus and may be more suitable for women who have PPH following a vaginal birth.

Uterine artery and internal iliac artery ligation

The uterine arteries are responsible for nearly 90% of the blood supply to the uterine body. Hence, **uterine artery ligation** may be a successful procedure for controlling bleeding in this area. However, **it is not effective in controlling bleeding from the lower uterine segment** or **the cervix.**

- **Bilateral uterine artery ligation** (also known as **O'Leary suture** or 'mass ligation') is a simple, fast, and safe procedure to stop bleeding from the uterine body. The technique consists of a suture 2–3 cm below and lateral to the segmental region of the hysterotomy. It is important to ensure that the bladder is away from the placement of the suture to avoid ureteric or bladder injury. The suture should encompass both the uterine artery and vein.
- **Internal iliac artery ligation** is also indicated with intractable hemorrhage, but is

used less often than the other procedures as it requires more surgical skills. It also needs more time to perform, prevents the further use of embolisation therapy (by closing the main access to the pelvic branches), and is not more effective than other conservative procedures. The failure rate is high, and hysterectomy has been reported in a third of women who had internal iliac ligation [31].

Procedure: The uterus is externalised and the infundibulopelvic ligament is transected, the broad ligament is opened, and the common iliac vessel is identified. The internal iliac artery is located and the anterior division is ligated. The ureter should be clearly identified before placing the ligature.

Uterine artery embolisation

In well-resourced settings, with an appropriately equipped operating room, hemodynamically stable women with persistent bleeding can be offered uterine artery embolisation as an alternative treatment. Various embolisation agents can be used, including gelatin sponge particles, polyvinyl alcohol particles, gelfoam, N-butyl cyanoacrylate, or microcoil. The success rate of this method is reported to be as high as 90% [32].

Hysterectomy

Postpartum hysterectomy is a life-saving procedure when indicated, and should not be postponed. It constitutes the final step after all conservative measures (pharmacological, mechanical, or other more conservative surgical strategies) have failed. In most instances, **subtotal hysterectomy** (STH) is preferred to **total hysterectomy** (TH) as it is quicker, simpler, less bloody, and less likely to cause damage to the ureters and pelvic floor. It must be kept in mind that if the origin of the hemorrhage is from the lower uterine segment, cervix, or vaginal fornices, effective control of bleeding will not be achieved with an STH since the arterial circulation of the cervix has a high blood flow rate and bleeding could persist. In such cases, a TH should be performed. See **Chapter 24**, *Peripartum hysterectomy*, for further details.

RETAINED PLACENTA

INTRODUCTION

The third stage of labour, defined as the period between childbirth and the expulsion of the placenta, is a critical time for both the mother and the healthcare provider. While this is the shortest of the three stages of labour, it carries the greatest risk to the mother (see **Chapter 5**).

Before the delivery of the placenta, there is blood flow to the placental bed of around 500 mL per minute. If the uterus does not contract as the placenta detaches, this flow will continue and the mother can exsanguinate within minutes. Placental expulsion is essential for the uterus to contract and thus reduce blood loss in the third stage of labour.

80% of women receiving physiologic management of the third stage (without oxytocic drugs) will expel the placenta within 30 minutes. However, **in women receiving active management of the third stage of labour (oxytocic drugs, uterine massage, or controlled cord traction), the delivery of the placenta is usually a rapid event, complete within 5 minutes in 50% of deliveries and within 10 minutes in approximately 89%** [33].

Available evidence shows that a prolonged third stage of labour is associated with an increased risk of PPH, with the maximum blood loss in the first 10–20 minutes [34].

NORMAL THIRD STAGE OF LABOUR

In the third stage, **placental separation** is brought about by uterine contraction and retraction greatly reducing the size of the placental implantation site. The placenta is thus sheared from the uterine wall. When the placenta is completely separated from the implantation site, the contractions force its descent to the lower uterine segment, through the cervix, and into the vagina.

Clinical Signs of Placental Separation

See **Chapter 5** for details.

EPIDEMIOLOGY OF RETAINED PLACENTA

A retained placenta is classically defined as the failure of the delivery of the placenta within 30 minutes of the delivery of the baby. The incidence of retained placenta is between 0.3 and 3% [35].

The impact of a retained placenta varies between countries. In low-resource countries, though it affects only about 0.1% of deliveries, a retained placenta has up to 10% case fatality rate. In high-resource countries, retained placenta is more common (about 3% of vaginal deliveries) but is very rarely associated with mortality [35]. The higher incidence in high-resource countries is thought to be a result of interventions such as abortions, labour induction, and the use of oxytocin, all of which are more common in those countries [36].

In addition to primary PPH, retained placenta is associated with an increased risk of endometritis and secondary PPH. Evidence of endometritis has been demonstrated after manual or surgical removal of retained placenta [37].

PATHOPHYSIOLOGY OF RETAINED PLACENTA

A retained placenta is generally attributed to one of the following abnormal processes:

- **Uterine atony** (inadequate contraction of the myometrium behind the placenta) may prevent normal separation and contractile expulsion of the placenta [38].
- **Closure of the cervix** before the delivery of the placenta may lead to a **trapped** or **incarcerated** placenta.
- **Abnormally adherent and invasive placenta** (placenta accreta spectrum) may prevent the normal separation from the uterine wall.

Risk Factors for Retained Placenta

The following are some of the risk factors for retained placenta [39,40]:

- Previous history of retained placenta
- Factors leading to uterine hypocontractility
  - — High parity
  - — Labour dystocia
  - — Prolonged induction/augmentation of labour with oxytocin
  - — Ergometrine use for PPH prophylaxis (leading to a trapped placenta)
- Factors leading to placenta accreta spectrum
  - — History of uterine surgery (myomectomy, curettage, or cesarean section)
  - — Pregnancy following in vitro fertilisation (IVF)
- Preterm delivery
- Congenital uterine anomaly

DIAGNOSIS OF RETAINED PLACENTA

A retained placenta is clinically diagnosed when the placenta fails to spontaneously separate 30 minutes after childbirth. The thirty-minute cut-off was adopted following a 1991 study by Combs et al. that showed that only 3.3% of deliveries had a third stage of labour >30 minutes. They also found that the incidence of PPH with retained placenta did not increase until after 30 minutes [41].

MANAGEMENT OF RETAINED PLACENTA

General Measures

Women with a retained placenta are at a high risk of bleeding. The following steps should be undertaken:

- IV access is established with a large-bore cannula (16–18 gauge)
- A blood sample is obtained for cross-matching
- Availability of blood products is ensured
- Prophylactic IV antibiotics are administered to prevent infection (endometritis) associated with a retained placenta and its management

Key Point

The quantity of intravenous fluids and blood to be transfused depends on the hemodynamic stability of the mother.

Timing of Intervention

The timing of the intervention (manual removal of placenta) depends on whether there is active bleeding or not.

Expectant management

In women presenting with retained placenta **with no active bleeding**, expectant management up to 60 minutes from childbirth is considered reasonable.

- During this period, commencing an oxytocin infusion may enable the uterus to contract and expel the placenta and control bleeding.
- Delaying the intervention has been found to lead to spontaneous delivery of the placenta in 40% of women [42].
- However, some authors have advocated intervening after 15–20 minutes of delivery, even if there is no bleeding. Their recommendation is based on the fact that when the third stage of labour lasts ≥15 minutes, there is a significantly greater risk of blood loss >500 mL [43,44].
- The decision on whether to intervene or wait also depends on the surgical facilities and resources available.

Immediate intervention

In women with **significant bleeding**, immediate intervention with manual removal of the placenta should be initiated.

Technique of Manual Removal of the Placenta

The onset of vaginal bleeding in a woman with a retained placenta may indicate separation of the placenta. In such a case, it is advisable to attempt controlled cord traction to deliver the placenta. When this is not successful, it is best to proceed the manual removal of the placenta.

Anesthesia

The procedure is performed in the surgical operating theatre under aseptic conditions.

Either **general anesthesia** or **regional anesthesia** may be used. General anesthesia has the advantage of speed and also provides uterine relaxation.

Key Point

Just before inducing anesthesia, a pelvic examination should be done. This is recommended because the placenta will deliver spontaneously in a number of cases while the resources for anesthesia are being mobilised.

Prophylactic antibiotic

The WHO [45] recommends a single dose of antibiotic (ampicillin or a first-generation cephalosporin) if manual removal of the placenta is being performed. There is no quality evidence for this recommendation, which was reached by consensus (see **Chapter 19**, *Antibiotic prophylaxis in labour and delivery*, for further details).

Procedure

- With the woman in the dorsal lithotomy position and with appropriate asepsis, one hand is placed on the abdomen to steady the fundus and push the uterus downwards. Throughout the procedure, the external hand steadies the fundus to facilitate internal manipulations.
- Uterine relaxation either by general anesthesia or nitroglycerine may be necessary to allow the exploring hand into the upper part of the uterine cavity.
- The exploring hand follows the cord into the vagina and through the cervix. The lower uterine segment can be very thin and ballooned out. Above it, there is often a thick contraction ring at the junction of

the upper and lower uterine segments. For the unwary operator, this ballooned out lower uterine segment may be mistaken for the uterine cavity proper and the hand may be pushed through the thinned-out lower uterine segment. The fingers of the internal hand should be brought together to form a cone and slowly but firmly pushed upwards through the contraction ring.

- The fingers and thumb of the uterine hand should be kept extended and used as one unit to advance along the umbilical cord to the lower margin of the placenta. This is recognised by the different feel of the membrane surface (smooth and slippery) and the decidual layer (spongy and rough).
- With the correct layer identified, the placenta is detached by sweeping the hand from side to side within the plane of cleavage between the placenta and uterine wall. Once completely separated, the placenta is grasped and removed slowly in one piece. The uterus is re-explored to ensure that there are no placental fragments remaining and that the uterine wall is intact.
- After manual removal, the cervix and vagina are examined, and any lacerations are sutured. Uterotonics are continued for a few hours.

Adherent areas of placenta

Sometimes adherent areas of placenta may be encountered. Small pieces can be removed piecemeal with the fingers and should not interfere with the contraction and retraction of the uterus. An experienced operator may use a large, sharp obstetric curette (at least the size of a teaspoon) to remove any residual placental fragments. However, extreme caution should be used as it is very easy to perforate the uterus in this situation or to strip off the decidua and cause subsequent Asherman's syndrome.

Unexpected Placenta Accreta

Occasionally, a manual attempt to remove a retained placenta after a vaginal delivery may reveal a focal or complete placenta accreta (involving the entire placental surface). In these cases, there is no plane of cleavage between the myometrium and the placenta. Life-threatening hemorrhage may occur if the accreta is not recognised and if the operator continues to try and separate the placenta.

Immediate resuscitative measures with fluids and blood transfusion should be initiated rapidly, and the mother should be prepared for a laparotomy and a life-saving hysterectomy.

See **Chapter 5** and **Chapter 24** for further management of the placenta accreta spectrum.

RESUSCITATION AND THE ROLE OF TRANSFUSION THERAPY IN PPH

In postpartum hemorrhage, maternal vital signs typically do not change severely until significant blood loss has occurred [10].

- Pallor, delayed capillary refill, and diaphoresis can indicate compromised blood volume without change in BP or heart rate.
- Decreased BP and tachycardia may be late signs of compromise.
- Hemoglobin levels will fall by approximately 1 g/dL for every 500 mL of blood loss. However, in PPH, the initial blood counts may not reflect this accurately.

If the obstetric team is not alert and fails to initiate adequate early resuscitation, the resulting hypoperfusion may lead to metabolic complications that can trigger **irreversible coagulopathy, prolongation of the hemorrhage, systemic inflammatory response syndrome (SIRS), and ultimately, multiple organ dysfunction and death** [46].

Shock Index

Shock index (SI) is defined as the heart rate (HR) divided by systolic blood pressure (SBP). It has been found to be useful in predicting outcomes in PPH [20]. In a recent study, SI >1 was associated with the need for operative intervention, SI >1.3 was associated with ICU admission, massive blood transfusion, and increased morbidity; SI >1.6 was associated with mortality [47].

Fluid Resuscitation Measures

The administration of crystalloids (**Ringer's lactate rather than saline solutions**) is the first and most important step in resuscitating a woman with severe PPH.

Aggressive fluid resuscitation

Traditionally, hemorrhagic shock was treated with the administration of large amounts of crystalloids with the goal of restoring the effective circulating blood volume and rapidly normalising the blood pressure.

Data in recent years have shown that **aggressive fluid resuscitation may worsen coagulopathy and hemorrhage** by increasing intravascular hydrostatic pressures, diluting coagulation factors, and inducing more hypothermia, which may rapidly increase the risk of death [48]. Excessive rise in blood pressure could also result in higher red blood cell loss, leading to more hypoxia and acidosis in tissues.

Key Point

The administration of large amounts of crystalloids leads to fluid extravasation which may cause cerebral, cardiac, and pulmonary edema. There is a real risk of third spacing, which may lead to cardiac dysfunction, hemodynamic instability, and decreased renal perfusion [48,49].

Hypotensive resuscitation

The aim of hypotensive resuscitation (also called **permissive hypotension**) is to achieve an adequate, but lower-than-normal systolic or mean blood pressure until definitive hemostasis is performed. This allows adequate tissue perfusion and hemostasis while avoiding further worsening of the coagulopathy. In a cohort study aimed to compare volumes for fluid resuscitation, **women with the lowest fluid administration showed fewer signs of shock and required less administration of blood products** [48].

This approach is based on the following concepts:

- Small crystalloid volumes are less likely to create dilutional coagulopathy
- Lower blood pressure is less likely to break or fragment the already-formed clots

Target blood pressure

Crystalloid infusion in small boluses of 500 mL is recommended to maintain permissive hypotension with a **systolic blood pressure target of 80–90 mmHg** (mean arterial pressure [MAP] of 50–60 mmHg) until major bleeding has been controlled [20].

Hemostatic Resuscitation

Earlier, resuscitation in obstetric hemorrhage consisted mainly of the administration of fluids and **packed red blood cells (PRBC)**. The use of blood products (**fresh frozen plasma [FFP], platelets [PLT]**, and **cryoprecipitate**) was initiated only when coagulopathy was demonstrated.

In contrast, hemostatic resuscitation **limits the use of crystalloids** and **promotes the early administration of blood products** (not only PRBC), making massive transfusion protocols the cornerstone of resuscitation [20,49,50].

Massive transfusion protocols

Massive transfusion protocols involve the early utilisation of blood products and limiting resuscitation with large volumes of crystalloids.

Massive transfusion is defined as transfusion requirements of [10,20]:

- 4 PRBC units within 1 hour when the ongoing need for more blood is anticipated **or**
- 10 PRBC units within 24 hours **or**
- Replacement of total blood volume within 24 hours **or**
- Replacement of 50% of blood volume within 3 hours.

The evidence to support the early use of blood products comes from the PROPPR study which showed that a greater proportion of women in the 1:1:1 group achieved hemostasis and suffered fewer deaths due to exsanguination at 24 hours [51]. Similarly, the PROMMTT study demonstrated that the early administration of plasma (within the first 3 hours and within the first 3–6 units after transfused blood components) decreased mortality at 24 hours and 30 days [52].

Blood products and transfusion ratios

In hemostatic resuscitation, PRBC, FFP, and PLT are administered in a 1:1:1 ratio due to their resemblance to whole blood [10]. Whole blood can be used if PRBC is not available in case of massive hemorrhage. **The additional administration of cryoprecipitate is recommended in women with suspected disseminated intravascular coagulation.**

Key Point

In hemostatic resuscitation, PRBC, FFP, and PLT are administered in a 1:1:1 ratio. In addition, cryoprecipitate is recommended in women with suspected disseminated intravascular coagulation.

Damage Control Resuscitation (DCR)

FIGO recommends DCR for massive PPH. This is a combination of hypotensive resuscitation and hemostatic resuscitation [20]. When combined with damage control surgery (DCS), these techniques have proven to be effective in controlling refractory PPH and bring about an overall decreased mortality among critically ill women [49].

CONCLUSION

Postpartum hemorrhage is a clinically significant cause of maternal complications and death worldwide. To decrease maternal mortality, every unit providing obstetric care should lay down management protocols and algorithms with clearly defined trigger and target values. Management should include non-surgical and surgical techniques and manoeuvres, which should be used in a predefined and step-wise fashion. Evidence-based use of massive transfusion protocol should be utilised according to the resources available. Damage control resuscitation along with damage control surgery are particularly important in saving women's lives.

Retained placenta after vaginal delivery is diagnosed when a placenta does not spontaneously deliver within a designated amount of time. It can occur in the setting of significant uterine atony, abnormally adherent placenta, such as the placenta accreta spectrum (PAS), or closure of the cervix prior to placental expulsion. When it is associated with significant hemorrhage, deployment of a massive transfusion protocol may be necessary.

REFERENCES

1. Borovac-Pinheiro A, et al. Postpartum hemorrhage: New insights for definition and diagnosis. *Am J Obstet Gynecol.* 2018. 219(2): p. 162-168.
2. Calvert C, et al. Identifying regional variation in the prevalence of postpartum haemorrhage: A systematic review and meta-analysis. *PLoS One.* 2012. 7(7): p. e41114.
3. Zelop CM. Postpartum hemorrhage: Becoming more evidence-based. *Obstet Gynecol.* 2011. 117(1): p. 3-5.
4. Theunissen F, et al. Cost of hospital care of women with postpartum haemorrhage in India, Kenya, Nigeria and Uganda: A financial case for improved prevention. *Reprod Health.* 2021. 18(1): p. 18.
5. GBD 2015 Maternal Mortality Collaborators. Global, regional, and national levels of maternal mortality, 1990-2015: A systematic analysis for the Global Burden of Disease Study 2015. *Lancet.* 2016. 388(10053):1775-1812. Erratum in: *Lancet.* 389(10064):e1.
6. World Health Organization Recommendations for the Prevention and Treatment of Postpartum Haemorrhage. 2012. WHO, Geneva.
7. Weeks AD, JP Neilson. Rethinking our approach to postpartum haemorrhage and uterotonics. *BMJ.* 2015. 351: p. h3251.
8. Hancock A, AD Weeks, DT Lavender. Is accurate and reliable blood loss estimation the 'crucial step' in early detection of postpartum haemorrhage: An integrative review of the literature. *BMC Pregnancy Childbirth.* 2015. 15: p. 230.
9. Kerr RS, AD Weeks. Postpartum haemorrhage: A single definition is no longer enough. *BJOG.* 2017. 124(5): p. 723-726.
10. American College of Obstetricians and Gynecologists. 2017. Postpartum hemorrhage. *Obstet Gynecol.* 130:e168–86.
11. Bannow BS, BA Konkle. Inherited bleeding disorders in the obstetric patient. *Transfus Med Rev.* 2018. 32(4): p. 237-243.

12. Hancock A, Weeks AD, Furber C, et al. The Recognition of Excessive blood loss At Childbirth (REACT) Study: A two-phase exploratory, sequential mixed methods inquiry using focus groups, interviews and a pilot, randomised crossover study. *BJOG*. 2021. 128(11):1843-1854.
13. Bell SF, Collis RE, Pallmann P, et al. Reduction in massive postpartum haemorrhage and red blood cell transfusion during a national quality improvement project, Obstetric Bleeding Strategy for Wales, OBS Cymru: An observational study. *BMC Pregnancy Childbirth*. 2021. 21, 377.
14. Gallos I, Devall A, Martin J, et al. Randomized trial of early detection and treatment of postpartum hemorrhage. *N Engl J Med*. 2023.
15. Gülmezoglu AM, Lumbiganon P, Landoulsi S, et al. Active management of the third stage of labour with and without controlled cord traction: A randomised, controlled, non-inferiority trial. *Lancet*. 2012. 379(9827), 1721–1727.
16. World Health Organization recommendation on routes of oxytocin administration for the prevention of postpartum haemorrhage after vaginal birth. 2020. WHO, Geneva.
17. Widmer M, Piaggio G, Nguyen TMH, et al. Heat-stable carbetocin versus oxytocin to prevent hemorrhage after vaginal birth. *N Engl J Med*. 2018. 379(8):743–752.
18. Gallos ID, Papadopoulou A, Man R, et al. Uterotonic agents for preventing postpartum haemorrhage: A network meta-analysis. *Cochrane Database Syst Rev*. 2018. Issue 12. Art. no.: CD011689.
19. Main EK, et al. National Partnership for Maternal Safety: Consensus Bundle on Obstetric Hemorrhage. *Obstet Gynecol*. 2015. 126(1): p. 155-62.
20. Escobar MF, Nassar AH, Theron G, et al. FIGO recommendations on the management of postpartum hemorrhage 2022. *Int J Gynecol Obstet*. 2022. 157(Suppl. 1): 3–50.
21. Althabe F, Therrien MNS, Pingray V, et al. Postpartum hemorrhage care bundles to improve adherence to guidelines: A WHO technical consultation. *Int Journal of gynaecology and Obstetrics*. 2020. 148(3), 290–299.
22. Widmer M, Blum J, Hofmeyr GJ, et al. Misoprostol as an adjunct to standard uterotonics for treatment of post-partum haemorrhage: A multicentre, double-blind randomised trial. *Lancet*. 2010. 375(9728): p. 1808-13.
23. Starrs A, B Winikoff. Misoprostol for postpartum hemorrhage: Moving from evidence to practice. *Int J Gynaecol Obstet*. 2012. 116(1): p. 1-3.
24. WOMAN Trial Collaborators. Effect of early tranexamic acid administration on mortality, hysterectomy, and other morbidities in women with post-partum haemorrhage (WOMAN): An international, randomised, double-blind, placebo-controlled trial. *Lancet*. 2017. 389(10084):2105-2116.
25. World Health Organization recommendation on tranexamic acid for the treatment of postpartum haemorrhage. 2017. WHO, Geneva.
26. Anger HA, Dabash R, Durocher J, et al. The effectiveness and safety of introducing condom catheter uterine balloon tamponade for postpartum haemorrhage at secondary level hospitals in Uganda, Egypt and Senegal: A stepped wedge, cluster-randomised trial. *BJOG*. 2019. 126:1612.
27. Georgiou C. A review of current practice in using balloon tamponade technology in the management of postpartum haemorrhage. *Hypertension Research in Pregnancy*. 2014. 2(1): p. 1-10.
28. Wong MS, Dellapiana G, Greene N, et al. Antibiotics during intrauterine balloon tamponade is associated with a reduction in endometritis. *Am J Perinatol*. 2019. 36:1211.
29. B-Lynch C, Coker A, Lawal AH, et al. The B-Lynch surgical technique for the control of massive postpartum haemorrhage: an alternative to hysterectomy? Five cases reported. *Br J Obstet Gynaecol*. 1997. 104(3):372-5.
30. Kayem G, Kurinczuk JJ, Alfirevic Z, et al. Uterine compression sutures for the management of severe postpartum hemorrhage. *Obstet Gynecol*. 2011. 117:14.
31. Joshi VM, et al. Internal iliac artery ligation for arresting postpartum haemorrhage. *BJOG*. 2007. 114(3): p. 356-61.
32. Zhang XQ, Chen XT, Zhang YT, Mai CX. The emergent pelvic artery embolization in the management of postpartum hemorrhage: A systematic review and meta-analysis. *Obstet Gynecol Surv*. 2021. 76(4):234-244.
33. Magann EF, Doherty DA, Briery CM, et al. Obstetric characteristics for a prolonged third stage of labor and risk for postpartum hemorrhage. *Gynecol Obstet Invest*. 2008. 65(3):201-5.
34. Frolova AI, Stout MJ, Tuuli MG, et al. Duration of the third stage of labor and risk of postpartum hemorrhage. *Obstet Gynecol*. 2016. 27(5):951-956.
35. Weeks AD. The retained placenta. *Best Pract Res Clin Obstet Gynaecol*. 2008. 22(6):1103-17.
36. Urner F, R Zimmermann, A Krafft, Manual removal of the placenta after vaginal delivery: An unsolved problem in obstetrics. *J Pregnancy*. 2014. p. 274651.
37. Ely JW, et al. The association between manual removal of the placenta and postpartum endometritis following vaginal delivery. *Obstet Gynecol*. 1995. 86(6): p. 1002-6.
38. Greenbaum S, et al. Underlying mechanisms of retained placenta: Evidence from a population based cohort study. *Eur J Obstet Gynecol Reprod Biol*. 2017. 216: p. 12-17.
39. Perlman NC and Carusi DA. Retained placenta after vaginal delivery: Risk factors and management. *Int J Womens Health*. 2019. 11: p. 527-534.

40. Endler M, et al. Retained placenta is associated with pre-eclampsia, stillbirth, giving birth to a small-for-gestational-age infant, and spontaneous preterm birth: A national register-based study. *BJOG*. 2014. 121(12): p. 1462-70.
41. Combs CA, EL Murphy, RK Laros Jr. Factors associated with postpartum hemorrhage with vaginal birth. *Obstet Gynecol*. 1991. 77(1): p. 69-76.
42. Weeks AD, Alia G, Vernon G, et al. Umbilical vein oxytocin for the treatment of retained placenta (Release Study): A double-blind, randomised controlled trial. *Lancet* (London, England). 2010. 375(9709). 141–147.
43. Cummings K, Doherty DA, Magann EF, et al. Timing of manual placenta removal to prevent postpartum hemorrhage: Is it time to act? *J Matern Fetal Neonatal Med*. 2016. 29:3930.
44. Rabie NZ, Ounpraseuth S, Hughes D, et al. Association of the length of the third stage of labor and blood loss following vaginal delivery. *South Med J*. 2018. 111:178.
45. World Health Organization recommendation or prevention and treatment of maternal peripartum infections. 2015. WHO, Geneva.
46. Cannon JW. Hemorrhagic shock. *New Eng Journal of Medicine*. 2018. 378, 370–379.
47. Agarwal V, Suri J, Agarwal P, et al. Shock index as a predictor of maternal outcome in postpartum hemorrhage. *J South Asian Feder Obst Gynae*. 2021. 13(3):131–136.
48. Gillissen A, van den Akker T, Caram-Deelder C, et al. Association between fluid management and dilutional coagulopathy in severe postpartum haemorrhage: A nationwide retrospective cohort study. *BMC Preg Childbirth*. 2018. 18(1):398.
49. Javier A Carvajal, Isabella Ramos, Juan P Kusanovic. Damage-control resuscitation in obstetrics. *Journal of Maternal-Fetal & Neonatal Medicine*. 2020.
50. Pacheco LD, Saade GR, Costantine MM, et al. An update on the use of massive transfusion protocols in obstetrics. *Am J Obstet Gynecol*. 2016. 214(3):340-4.
51. Holcomb JB, Tilley BC, Baraniuk S, et al. Transfusion of plasma, platelets, and red blood cells in a 1:1:1 vs a 1:1:2 ratio and mortality in patients with severe trauma: The PROPPR randomized clinical trial. *JAMA*. 2015. 313(5):471–482.
52. Holcomb JB, del Junco DJ, Fox EE, et al. The prospective, observational, multicenter, major trauma transfusion (PROMMTT) study: Comparative effectiveness of a time-varying treatment with competing risks. *JAMA Surg*. 2013. SS148(2):127–136.

CHAPTER 14

Induction and Augmentation of Labour

SHOBANA MAHADEVAN, AMRITHA KARTHIK

INTRODUCTION

Induction of labour is defined as the process of artificially stimulating the uterus to initiate labour with the aim of achieving a vaginal delivery. It commonly involves the administration of oxytocin or prostaglandins and may also include amniotomy.

Induction is generally indicated when the outcomes for the mother and the fetus are expected to be better if the fetus is delivered without awaiting the spontaneous onset of labour. In recent years, there has been a rise in the induction rate in both high-income [1,2] and low- and middle-income countries (LMICs) [3]. In an analysis of the World Health Organization Global Survey on Maternal and Neonatal Health, Vogel et al. [4] found a higher incidence of induction of labour in India and Sri Lanka as compared to other Asian countries. This could lead to increased risks to the mother and the fetus due to inducing agents [5] as well as an increased burden on resources [4].

Induction and Cesarean Section

Concerns have been raised about higher cesarean section rates and lower maternal satisfaction in routinely induced labours before 41 weeks. However, this notion has been challenged by recent evidence. When performed with strict adherence to clear medical indications and with proper ripening protocols in place, induction of labour between 34 and 39 weeks does not increase the incidence of cesarean section [6].

Grobman et al. [7], in the ARRIVE trial, found that elective induction of labour at 39 weeks in low-risk nulliparous women resulted in a significantly lower frequency of cesarean delivery.

DEFINITIONS

- **Cervical ripening** is a prelude to the onset of labour, where the cervix changes from being long and closed to being thinned out and short (effaced) and opened out (dilated) [8]. It occurs either naturally or as a result of physical or pharmacological agents. Induction of labour includes cervical ripening of an unripe cervix.
- **Induction of labour** is the artificial initiation of uterine contractions before the spontaneous onset of labour. However, it is also a commonly used collective term that includes cervical ripening, artificial rupture of membranes, and the initiation and augmentation of contractions.
- **Augmentation of labour** refers to the process of stimulating the uterus to increase the frequency, duration, and intensity of inadequate contractions after the onset of spontaneous labour.

INDICATIONS

Induction is indicated for maternal, fetal, or other situations in pregnancy when the benefits to either mother or fetus outweigh the risks of continuation of pregnancy. There is a considerable overlap between maternal and fetal indications for the induction of labour.

Maternal Indications

The maternal indications for induction of labour include the following:

- Postterm/postdated pregnancy—induction of pregnancies beyond 40 weeks in the absence of any other maternal or fetal indication is the most common indication (see **Chapter 31**, *Late-term and postterm pregnancy*)
- Hypertensive disorders
- Diabetes in pregnancy (pregestational/gestational)
- Premature rupture of membranes
- Intra-amniotic infection
- Hypercoagulable disorder (history of venous thromboembolism, acquired or inherited thrombophilia, sickle cell disease), where elective induction allows time for discontinuing anticoagulant therapy before delivery
- Maternal request

Fetal Indications

Fetal indications for induction of labour include the following:

- Suspected fetal macrosomia—the benefits and risks of induction of labour in comparison to expectant management are not clearly understood (see **Chapter 34**, *Management of labour with fetal macrosomia*)
- Intrauterine fetal death
- Twin pregnancy
- Rh alloisoimmunisation
- Fetal growth restriction (see **Chapter 33**, *Management of labour with a growth-restricted fetus*)

CONTRAINDICATIONS

Induction should be avoided if there are any contraindications to labour and vaginal delivery. These include:

- Increased risk of uterine rupture
  - Prior classical or inverted T uterine incision
  - Prior uterine surgery such as full thickness myomectomy, transfundal uterine surgery
  - Previous uterine rupture
- Previous pelvic surgeries like vesicovaginal fistula/pelvic floor repair, particularly fourth-degree perineal tear repair
- Placenta previa and vasa previa
- Umbilical cord presentation/prolapse
- Abnormal fetal presentations such as transverse lie, brow or face presentation
- Severe fetal growth restriction with Doppler abnormalities
- Active genital herpes
- Invasive cervical carcinoma
- Mobile head and suspected cephalopelvic disproportion are relative contraindications

Key Point

Induction should only be offered when there are no contraindications to labour and vaginal birth.

PRE-INDUCTION COUNSELLING

Women should be provided with adequate information about induction to help them make an informed decision. This includes:

- A clear explanation of the indication for induction
- The benefits and risks of induction
- An outline of the process of induction and its impact on labour and length of hospital stay
- Risks of refusing the induction and consideration of possible alternate options

CHECKLIST FOR INDUCTION

To ensure maternal and fetal safety during induction, it is advisable to have a checklist that will confirm that all prerequisites are met (Box 14.1).

PREDICTION OF SUCCESSFUL INDUCTION

The probability that induction will result in successful vaginal delivery depends on both maternal characteristics and cervical favourability (Bishop's score).

Box 14.1 Checklist for induction of labour

- Informed consent obtained
- Maternal history and risk factors reviewed
- Indications reviewed and any contraindications ruled out
- Maternal pulse rate, blood pressure, temperature, and findings on abdominal palpation documented
- Gestational age, presentation, fetal weight, and placental localisation assessed and documented
- Maternal pelvis assessed clinically for adequacy
- Cervix assessed for favourability by Bishop's score
- Baseline fetal rate pattern recorded and documented by CTG

Maternal and Fetal Factors

The following factors are associated with a higher likelihood of successful induction [9]:

- Previous vaginal delivery
- Higher gestational age (term or close to term)
- Multiparity
- Body mass index (BMI) closer to normal
- The woman's height on the higher side
- Lower estimated fetal weight (<3500 g)
- Ruptured membranes
- Absence of associated comorbidities such as preeclampsia and fetal growth restriction

Bishop's Score

A favourable cervix is associated with a shorter duration of induction and a greater chance of vaginal birth. However, an unfavourable cervix does not rule out labour induction entirely. In 1964, Edward Bishop [10] set forth criteria to be assessed prior to the induction of labour.

The modified Bishop's score is a cervical assessment system that predicts the success of induction and helps in selecting the appropriate inducing agents. It is based on the station of the presenting part and four cervical characteristics—dilatation (cm), length of the cervix (effacement), consistency, and position of the os (Table 14.1). Using this system of scoring, a score of ≥6 is considered favourable for a successful induction. The score should be documented when the decision for induction of labour is made.

Key Point

The modified Bishop's score is the most reliable predictor of the success of induction. In a meta-analysis, Crane [9] concluded that the Bishop's score is equal to, and may even be better than, ultrasound measurement of cervical length in the prediction of successful induction.

SETTING FOR THE INDUCTION OF LABOUR

Induction should be performed in a facility that has the capacity to adequately monitor the well-being of the mother and the baby, as well as being equipped to perform an emergency cesarean section.

RIPENING OF AN UNFAVOURABLE CERVIX

The process of cervical ripening is a complex biochemical process that results in physical softening and distensibility of the cervix. When the Bishop's score is unfavourable (<6), cervical ripening is done to facilitate the process of softening, thinning, and dilating of the cervix, thereby reducing both the rate of failed induction and the time from induction to delivery.

Table 14.1 **Modified Bishop's score**

Parameters	0	1	2	3
Cervical dilatation	<1 cm	1–2 cm	2–4 cm	>4 cm
Length of cervix/effacement	>4 cm/0–30%	2–4 cm/40–50%	1–2 cm/60–70%	<1 cm/80%
Station (cm from ischial spines)	–3	–2	–1/0	+1/+2
Consistency	Firm	Average	Soft	–
Position	Posterior	Mid-position	Anterior	–

The available agents for cervical ripening are listed in Table 14.2.

Table 14.2 Available methods of cervical ripening

Mechanical methods	Pharmacological agents
• Sweeping of membranes • Balloon catheters (including Foley) • Osmotic dilators	• Prostaglandin E1 (oral and vaginal) • Prostaglandin E2 (intracervical gel, sustained release vaginal insert, vaginal tablets)

Mechanical Methods

Membrane sweeping

Membrane sweeping or stripping of membranes is performed by passing a gloved finger through the cervix during vaginal examination, into the space between the membranes and the lower uterine segment (Fig. 14.1a) and rotating it through 360 degrees while keeping the finger close to the uterine wall (Fig. 14.1b). The cervix should be dilated enough to allow the insertion of a finger to sweep the membranes. Separating the chorionic membrane from the decidua stimulates local prostaglandin F2α production.

- Sweeping of membranes reduces the need for formal induction of labour [11].
- It improves the rate of establishment of labour but does not improve maternal or neonatal outcomes.
- It is suitable for non-urgent indications for induction such as term low-risk pregnancy, since the interval between membrane stripping and initiation of labour may be longer than it is with other methods of cervical ripening.
- Sweeping can be repeated if labour does not start spontaneously. However, there are no data on how many times sweeping can be repeated [11].
- The disadvantages of membrane sweeping include maternal discomfort, vaginal bleeding, and an increased risk of membrane rupture. Women should be counselled about these.

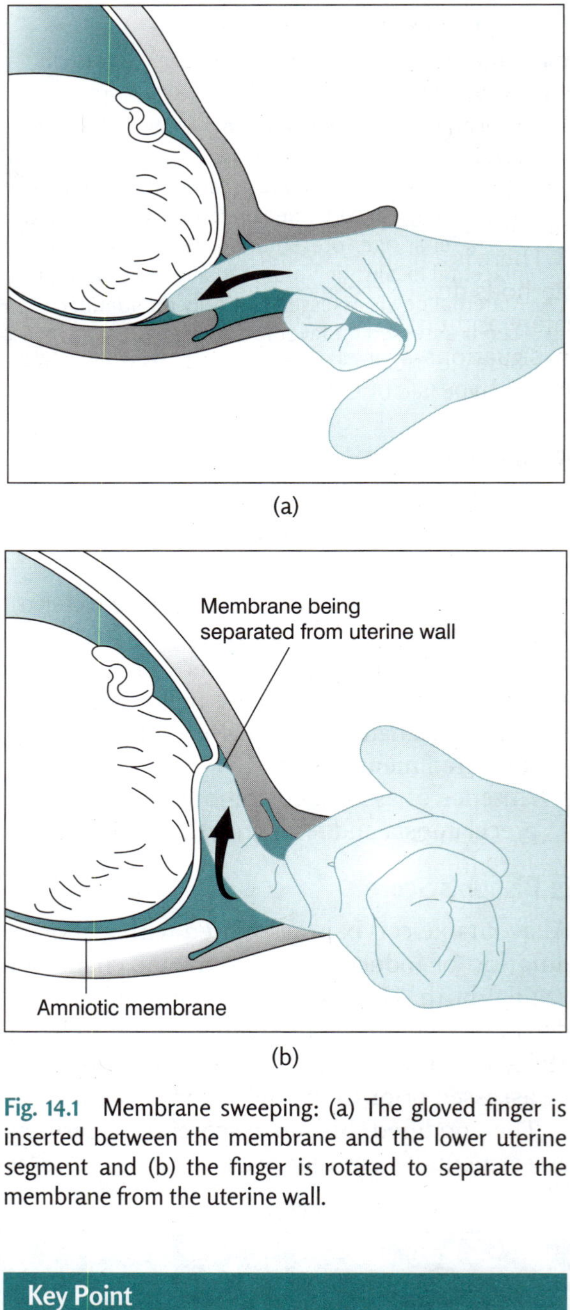

Fig. 14.1 Membrane sweeping: (a) The gloved finger is inserted between the membrane and the lower uterine segment and (b) the finger is rotated to separate the membrane from the uterine wall.

> **Key Point**
>
> Membrane sweeping is a relatively simple intervention that reduces the need for formal induction of labour and may be offered to women after 39 weeks. Verbal consent may be obtained before the procedure [8].

Mechanical devices

In the mechanical methods, ripening is achieved chiefly by applying direct physical pressure on the internal os and stretching the cervix, which leads to the release of prostaglandins. These are usually followed by amniotomy and oxytocin infusion for the completion of delivery.

There is a resurgence in the use of mechanical methods due to recent evidence regarding their safety and efficacy. They are particularly useful in situations where it would be beneficial to avoid hyperstimulation or when the use of prostaglandins is contraindicated, such as in a scarred uterus.

Two types of mechanical devices are used:

- Transcervical balloon catheters (Foley, double balloon)
- Osmotic dilators
  - Natural (Laminaria)
  - Synthetic (Dilapan)

Balloon catheter devices

A **Foley catheter** is safe, economical, easy to store, and readily available (Fig. 14.2). Both low- and high-volume Foley bulb inflation have been used. The achievement of a favourable cervix is likely with the use of high-volume catheters, and results in a higher rate of delivery within 24 hours. However, there is no difference in the cesarean section rate [12].

Double balloon catheters (Fig. 14.3) have also been used and are expensive, but studies show no significant differences in induction–delivery intervals or modes of birth with the single balloon catheter and the double balloon catheter [13,14].

Insertion technique

Under aseptic precautions, a 16F Foley catheter is inserted into the cervix. Once it passes the internal os, the balloon is distended with 30–50 mL of saline and gently retracted so that it rests against the internal os. A small degree of traction is exerted on the catheter by taping it on the medial aspect of the woman's thigh. It is left in place until it falls out spontaneously or is removed after 12 hours.

Hygroscopic dilators

There are two types of hygroscopic dilators. Laminaria tents are made from **natural seaweed** and are currently being replaced by a more commonly available synthetic product (**Dilapan**).

Hygroscopic dilators absorb moisture and thus gradually expand within the cervical canal. They disrupt the chorioamniotic decidual interface, causing lysosomal destruction and prostaglandin release. The passive mechanical stretching provided by the dilator also triggers changes in cervical tissue, resulting in

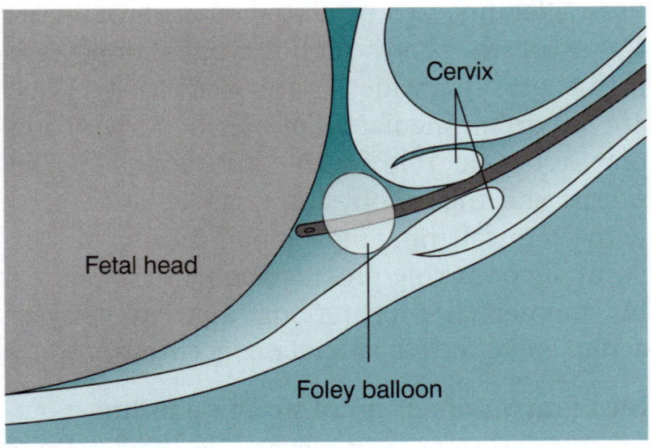

Fig. 14.2 Intracervical Foley catheter

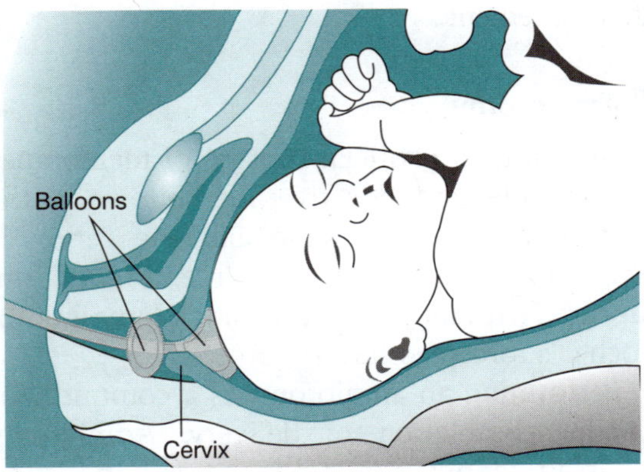

Fig. 14.3 Double balloon catheter

ripening. Oxytocin, with or without amniotomy, is usually administered following ripening with hygroscopic dilators.

Though they were used more commonly in the past for medical termination of pregnancy (MTP), hygroscopic dilators are proving to be as safe and effective as other cervical ripening agents in term pregnancies. A recent study [15] showed that the synthetic hygroscopic dilator was not inferior to the Foley catheter in bringing about cervical ripening. Women were also more satisfied with the hygroscopic dilator because, unlike the catheter, it does not protrude from the introitus and is, therefore, more comfortable.

Procedure for hygroscopic dilator placement

Under aseptic conditions, the anterior lip of the cervix is held with a non-traumatic clamp. The tip of the dilator is dipped into sterile lubricant to make the insertion easier. As many dilators as possible are gently inserted into the endocervical canal. The number of dilators inserted must be documented. Care must be taken not to exert undue force. A moistened roller gauze is then gently placed in the vagina to keep the dilators in place. Some women may complain of cramping during the procedure.

Synthetic dilators are removed after 6–8 hours. Laminaria tents are removed 12–24 hours after placement.

Amniotomy

Amniotomy or artificial rupture of membranes is a simple and effective method when the membranes are accessible and the cervix is favourable. The accessible membranes are ruptured with the use a plastic hook (amnihook), Kocher's forceps or artery forceps.

Performing an amniotomy is a commitment to the completion of delivery. Amniotomy by itself is not recommended for induction of labour and is usually performed before induction with oxytocin.

The amount and colour of liquor are observed. The fetal heart is monitored after the procedure.

Amniotomy with an unengaged vertex

Amniotomy is usually avoided in such cases. If performed, it should be done with great care, and the fingers in the vagina should not be removed until the vertex rests against the cervix. The flow of amniotic fluid should be controlled with the vaginal fingers, allowing the liquor to be drained slowly to avoid sudden decompression of the uterus.

> **Key Point**
>
> Performing an amniotomy with an unengaged presenting part can result in cord prolapse. The sudden release of liquor when amniotomy is performed in cases of polyhydramnios can cause placental abruption.

Pharmacological Methods

Pharmacological methods used for ripening may lead to the onset of contractions as a continuum. Though they are used for cervical ripening, 50% of women will go into labour and may not require oxytocin [16]. The pharmacological agents that are used for induction are **prostaglandins** and **oxytocin**.

Prostaglandins

Prostaglandins are produced by almost every tissue of the body and serve as important messengers in a wide variety of functions. They are important mediators of uterine activity and play a pivotal role in the contraction of the uterus and the biophysical changes associated with cervical ripening. Modification of the naturally occurring prostaglandins has resulted in commercial preparations that are longer-acting and effective at lower concentrations.

Mechanism of action of prostaglandins

Prostaglandins promote several biochemical and biophysical changes, leading to cervical ripening and an increase in myometrial contractility.

Types of prostaglandins used for cervical ripening

The two types of prostaglandins used for cervical ripening are presented in Table 14.3.

Prostaglandin E2 (Dinoprostone)

Prostaglandin E2 is available in different formulations, which determine the site of administration.

- **Intracervical PGE2 gel:** The gel is best refrigerated at 2–8°C. It is available as a 2.5 mg preloaded syringe containing 0.5 mg of dinoprostone. With the woman in the dorsolithotomy position, the vagina and the cervix are cleaned with an antiseptic solution. The cervix is exposed with a speculum and the anterior lip of the cervix is held with sponge-holding forceps. The tip of the cannula, which is attached to the prefilled syringe, is inserted gently through the external os into the cervical canal. It is important to release the gel into the cervical canal, just below the internal os (Fig. 14.4).

Table 14.3 Types of prostaglandins used for cervical ripening

Prostaglandin E2 (Dinoprostone)	Misoprostol (Prostaglandin E1)
• Intracervical gel • Controlled–release vaginal insert • Vaginal tablets	• Oral • Vaginal

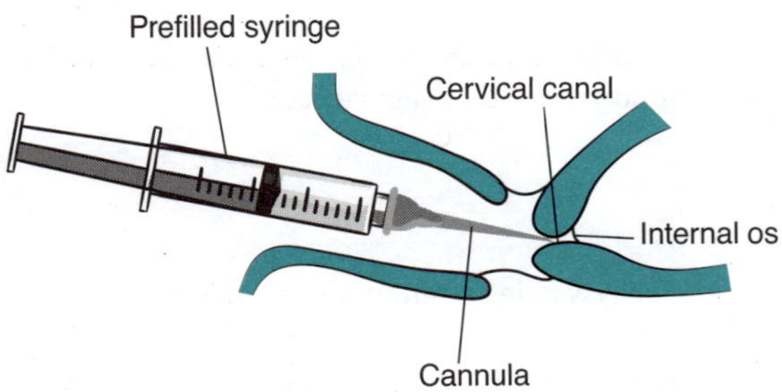

Fig. 14.4 Intracervical PGE2 gel administration

Key Point

PGE2 gel is effective only if applied intracervically. Inserting the gel into the vagina without visualising the cervix is not acceptable clinical practice.

One must also be careful not to deposit the gel above the internal os. High deposition may release the drug into the extra-amniotic space and can lead to excessive stimulation of the uterus. The woman can be allowed to ambulate after 30 minutes of insertion. The 0.5 mg gel can be repeated in 6 hours, going up to a maximum of three doses in a 24-hour period.

- **PGE2 sustained release vaginal insert:** The dinoprostone pessary contains 10 mg of the medication embedded in a mesh with an attached tape. It is placed transversely in the posterior fornix, behind the cervix. It releases PGE2 at a constant rate of 0.3 mg/hour over the 12-hour dosing period. The woman can ambulate 30 minutes after insertion. Monitoring at frequent intervals for uterine contractions and fetal heart rate should begin after the administration of the drug.

  The attached tape enables easy removal. The pessary is removed after 12 hours or once active labour sets in. One of the advantages of the pessary is that it need not be removed if the membrane ruptures and induction can continue. It, however, limits the number of pelvic examinations.

  The advantages of the pessary are easy administration and quick reversal on removal in case of hyperstimulation. The pessary should be stored in a freezer at –10 to –25°C, which makes good cold chain maintenance a prerequisite. This requirement makes it less useful in low-resource areas.
- **Dinoprostone vaginal tablets:** They are available in doses of 2 and 3 mg. The tablets are inserted into the posterior fornix and repeated every 6 hours for a maximum of 4 doses. **PGE2 vaginal tablets are not available in India.**

Prostaglandin E1 (Misoprostol)

Misoprostol is an orally-active synthetic PGE1 analogue, widely used in the termination of pregnancy in the first and second trimesters. In term pregnancies, it is used at a much lower dose, either vaginally or orally, for the induction of labour. It is cheap and stable at room temperature and has proved useful in developing countries.

Misoprostol is available as a 25 mcg or 100 mcg tablet. The 100 mcg tablet can be broken into four equal sizes for cervical ripening. The tablets are administered by the oral and sublingual routes and are rapidly absorbed, peaking approximately at 30 minutes versus 70–80 minutes when given vaginally.

Oral misoprostol has a half-life of 20–40 minutes, resulting in a shorter duration of action of 2 hours, compared to a duration of action of 4 hours by vaginal administration.

The prostaglandin regimens for cervical ripening in an unscarred uterus are presented in Table 14.4.

INDUCTION OF LABOUR WITH A FAVOURABLE CERVIX

For successful induction of labour, the cervix should be favourable. Methods of ripening for an unfavourable cervix have been described above. Prostaglandins used for ripening the cervix may also stimulate uterine contraction, and labour may follow. If labour does not set in, then once cervical ripening is achieved with mechanical methods or prostaglandin, induction is continued with oxytocin.

With a favourable cervix, labour is usually induced with **oxytocin**, with or without **amniotomy**. Amniotomy, in itself, may be ineffective without the use of oxytocin. In any case, it cannot be performed unless the cervix is dilated enough to allow the passage of an instrument (see section on *Amniotomy* above).

Oxytocin

Intravenous oxytocin is the most commonly used method of induction for women with a favourable cervix. It is most effective with a ripe cervix or when the membranes have ruptured.

A systematic review of the Cochrane Database [17] looked at the best and most cost-effective method for induction of labour. Oxytocin infusion, along with amniotomy, and vaginal misoprostol were found to be the most effective in resulting in a vaginal delivery within 24 hours.

Synthetic oxytocin is among the most potent uterotonic agents known. It is administered as

Table 14.4 Prostaglandin regimens for cervical ripening in an unscarred uterus

Drug	Route/dose	Caution
Dinoprostone gel (PGE2)	0.5 mg intracervically every 6 hours for a maximum of 3 doses	To avoid hyperstimulation oxytocin should be started ≥6 hours after the final dose of PGE2
Dinoprostone (PGE2) intravaginal insert	• 10 mg • Placed high in the posterior fornix for a maximum of 12 hours • Easy to remove in case of tachysystole	Uterine tachysystole (hyperstimulation) most common with PGE2 vaginal insert
Misoprostol (PGE1)	• Vaginal: 25 mcg tablet every 3–6 hours • Oral: 50 mcg every 4 hours **or** 25 mcg every 2 hours for a maximum of 6 doses	• Tachysystole common with a vaginal dose of >25 mcg • Interval of 4 hours before oxytocin is started for augmentation

an intravenous infusion. The uterus responds to oxytocin with increasing sensitivity with advancing gestational age due to an increase in myometrial oxytocin binding sites.

Each obstetric unit should adopt an evidence-based protocol for oxytocin administration, and this protocol should be readily available in the labour ward. An infusion pump should be used to control the rate of infusion precisely. In the absence of an infusion pump, the drops per minute have to be titrated and monitored accurately.

Oxytocin should be used with caution in women with a previous cesarean delivery and in grand multiparous women. It is administered intravenously as an infusion to achieve a continuous effect and to have precise control of the dose administered.

Initiating oxytocin after cervical ripening

The timing of initiation of oxytocin administration in women who have undergone cervical ripening is presented in Table 14.5.

Preparation, administration, and monitoring of oxytocin infusion

Preparation

Each ampoule of 1 mL contains 5 units of oxytocin. 5 units of oxytocin are added to 500 mL of Ringer's lactate or normal saline solution. The infusion is preferably given through an infusion pump. If an infusion pump is not available, a regular intravenous set may be used, with close monitoring.

Table 14.5 Timing of initiation of oxytocin after different methods of cervical ripening

Agent used for cervical ripening	Timing of initiating oxytocin
Dinoprostone gel	6–12 hours after the final dose
Dinoprostone insert	30 minutes after removal of insert
Misoprostol	4 hours after the final dose
Foley catheter	Immediately after removing the catheter

Administration

Infusion of oxytocin should be documented in **mU/minute**, **mL/minute** (with an infusion pump) or **drops/minute**. The uterine response starts gradually and reaches a steady state in 20–40 minutes. Since the half-life of oxytocin is 15–20 minutes, the rate of infusion is increased every 20 minutes until **good uterine contractions—each lasting for 40–45 seconds with a minimum of 3 contractions in 10 minutes—are established.** Increasing the drip rate before 20 minutes have elapsed has the potential to cause a cumulative effect resulting in hyperstimulation. The upper limit of the oxytocin infusion during labour is 32 mU/minute.

Monitoring of effect

The **frequency, intensity (strength),** and **duration** of uterine contractions should be assessed every 20–30 minutes and with each increase in the oxytocin infusion rate. It should also be noted whether the uterus relaxes between contractions and for how long. **Cervical status** and **the station of the presenting part** should be assessed before administering oxytocin; these should be assessed again after 2–4 hours of moderate contractions.

Maternal monitoring

During oxytocin administration, maternal blood pressure and pulse rate should be assessed every hour. Intake and output should be assessed every 4 hours. Fetal heart monitoring by intermittent auscultation or continuous cardiotocography is recommended (see **Chapter 8**, *Fetal surveillance in labour*).

Dosage of oxytocin

Two regimens are described for the administration of intravenous oxytocin—low-dose and high-dose regimens (Table 14.6).

Table 14.6 **Low- and high-dose regimens for oxytocin administration**

Regimen	Starting dose (mU/min)	Incremental dose (mU/min)	Dosage interval
Low-dose	0.5–2	1–2	20–40 minutes
High-dose	6	3–6	20–40 minutes

- **Low-dose regimen**: The regimen of low doses of oxytocin and less frequent increases in dosage mimics endogenous maternal physiology. This method is advantageous because it is associated with a lower incidence of uterine tachysystole and associated FHR changes.
- **High-dose regimen:** High doses of oxytocin and more frequent increases in dosage are associated with shorter labour and lower rates of cesarean delivery for dystocia. However, this regimen is associated with higher rates of uterine tachysystole with associated FHR changes [18].

Key Point

Less frequent increases in dosage are associated with a decreased risk of uterine tachysystole with associated FHR changes. Though increasing the dose of oxytocin at 20-minute intervals may be associated with tachysystole, it results in a significant reduction of cesarean sections for dystocia. Increasing the dose at 40-minute intervals seems to offer no clear advantage over the 20-minute intervals.

Incremental administration of oxytocin

When 5 units of oxytocin are added to 500 mL of Ringer's lactate or normal saline, the concentration achieved is 10 mU/mL. A flow rate of 15 mL/hour will deliver the drug at the rate of 2 mU/min (Table 14.7). The maximum rate of 32 mU/min is rarely required.

Terminology used to describe contractions during labour induction

The best way to monitor the efficacy of oxytocin is to monitor contractions. It is important to quantify uterine contractions in terms of the following:

- Frequency
- Duration
- Intensity
- Relaxation time between contractions

Based on these indicators, the following definitions are used:

- **Normal frequency**: 3–5 contractions in 10 minutes
- **Tachysystole**: >5 contractions in 10 minutes, over a 30-minute window; tachysystole may or may not be associated with FHR decelerations
- **Uterine hypertonus**: A single contraction lasting more than 2 minutes
- **Uterine hyperstimulation:** Denotes increased rate or strength of contractions associated with abnormal fetal heart rate patterns

Table 14.7 **Dosage of oxytocin for induction of labour in mU, drops/minute and mL/hour (using 5 units in 500 mL of normal saline)**

mU of oxytocin	Drops/minute (manual)	mL/hour (infusion pump)
2	4	15
4	8	30
6	12	45
8	16	60
10	20	75
14	24	90
16	28	105
18	32	120
20	36	135
24	40	150
28	44	165
30	48	180
32	52	195

Role of amniotomy in induction with oxytocin

Early amniotomy is recommended to increase the success of induction with oxytocin. The combination of early amniotomy and oxytocin administration during induction appears to shorten the time to vaginal delivery. In a randomised trial of nulliparous women undergoing labour induction, Macones et al. [19] found that routine early amniotomy (defined as being performed at a cervical dilatation of ≤4 cm) shortened the time to delivery by approximately 2 hours and increased the number of deliveries that occurred within 24 hours of starting induction. Early amniotomy also provides the opportunity to assess the amniotic fluid for the presence of meconium.

Complications of induction with oxytocin

Uterine hyperstimulation

Hyperstimulation may appear as **tachysystole** (defined as >5 contractions in 10 minutes) or **hypertonus** (a single contraction lasting more than two minutes). The incidence of uterine tachysystole is 5% with oxytocin but may be as high as 15% if dinoprostone and oxytocin are used concurrently. Hyperstimulation may be associated with fetal heart rate abnormalities.

Excessive uterine activity leads to increased perinatal morbidity when associated with abnormal fetal heart rate changes, particularly changes such as the **absence of baseline variability, recurrent variable** or **late decelerations,** and **prolonged bradycardia.**

Management of hyperstimulation

Hyperstimulation is managed by intrauterine resuscitation, which involves the following:

- Immediate cessation of administration of any uterotonic agents/removal of vaginal PG
- Turning the woman to the left lateral position
- Administration of crystalloids

Tocolysis should be considered if these measures are not effective in correcting the abnormal fetal heart pattern. The tocolytic agent used most often for this purpose is subcutaneous terbutaline in a dose of 250 mcg.

Uterine rupture

The absolute risk of uterine rupture is very low if labour induction is supervised and if the uterus is unscarred. Rupture is suspected when there is suprapubic tenderness and loss of station of the presenting part on vaginal exam. An abnormal CTG pattern is one of the earliest features of an imminent rupture. If rupture is suspected, cesarean section should be performed immediately (see **Chapter 18**, *Obstructed labour and uterine rupture*).

Failed induction

A successful induction is one that results in a vaginal delivery in 24–48 hours [20]. The criteria for failed induction are not uniform but can be defined as failure to progress from the latent phase to the active phase of labour by any chosen method of induction, irrespective of the outcome.

A failed induction necessitates a cesarean section. It is important to discuss the available options with the woman and take her preference into account while deciding between further induction and cesarean section.

Enough time should be allowed to pass before the induction is considered to have failed. Grobman et al. [7] suggest that cesarean delivery should not be undertaken during the latent phase unless at least 15 hours have passed after initiating oxytocin and rupture of membranes has occurred.

Failure to achieve vaginal delivery should not be considered a failure of induction as there can be other indications for cesarean section such as arrest of labour in the first stage or arrest of descent after full dilatation.

Other side effects

- Hyponatremia and fluid overload result when oxytocin is diluted in large volumes of solutions, particularly in hypotonic solutions. Large doses result in hypotension with reflex tachycardia.
- The risk of amniotic fluid embolism is increased in induced labours as compared to spontaneous labour.

Key Point

The induction of labour should be undertaken in the presence of facilities for assessing maternal and fetal well-being. Women receiving oxytocin or prostaglandins should never be left unattended. The centre should be equipped to proceed with an emergency cesarean section if required.

PAIN RELIEF IN INDUCED LABOUR

Women should be informed that induced labour is likely to last longer and be more painful than spontaneous labour [8]. The usual methods of pain relief including epidural analgesia are recommended. These are discussed in detail in **Chapter 9**, *Labour analgesia*.

SPECIAL SITUATIONS

Previous Cesarean Section

Induction of labour in women attempting vaginal birth after cesarean (VBAC) is associated with less success of vaginal delivery as compared to those with spontaneous onset of labour. It is also associated with an increased risk of serious maternal morbidity [21].

A recent systematic review of the Cochrane Database regarding methods of term labour induction for women with a previous cesarean section [22] was unable to recommend the optimal method for induction of labour in women with a prior cesarean birth because of a lack of robust data.

Mechanical methods of cervical ripening are recommended over pharmacological methods because balloon catheter induction is not reported to be associated with scar dehiscence [23]. Misoprostol, when administered to those with previous cesarean births, was found to increase the risk of uterine rupture [24,25] and hence, should **not** be used in this situation. Macones and colleagues [26] found an increased incidence of rupture with the sequential use of PGs and oxytocin.

Postterm Pregnancy

The chief goals in the management of postterm pregnancies are reduction in perinatal mortality rate, and choosing the ideal time for intervention to achieve this goal without increasing the cesarean section rate. A systematic review of the Cochrane Database [27] concluded that elective labour induction at 40 or 41 weeks' gestation is associated with fewer perinatal deaths and fewer cesarean sections than expectant management.

Preterm Prelabour Rupture of Membranes (PPROM)

In preterm PROM, expectant management up to 34 weeks is recommended to attain fetal maturity. Expectant management can be followed in the absence of maternal or fetal infection. In the presence of a favourable cervix, labour can be induced at 34 weeks with oxytocin. Both vaginal PGE2 and misoprostol can be used if the cervix is unfavourable [28].

Prelabour Rupture of Membranes (PROM) at Term

Women with term PROM should be induced promptly. A systematic review of the Cochrane Database [29] comparing induction and expectant management showed that induction resulted in a shorter time to delivery with no increase in cesarean delivery. There was also a decrease in the incidence of maternal infection. Oxytocin is regarded as the first option, though prostaglandins may be considered if the Bishop's score is low.

WOMEN'S PREFERENCES

It is of utmost importance to take into consideration the woman's preferences and circumstances and involve her in the decision-making process. As far as methods of induction are concerned, it is evident from various studies that the oral route and mechanical methods are generally preferred by women as they have fewer side effects, allow mobility, and do not require repeated vaginal exams.

CONCLUSION

Labour induction has undergone rigorous research and has become an increasingly safe and effective practice. Some of the available evidence is resource- and area-specific. For this reason, every obstetric unit should identify what is locally applicable and develop its own evidence-based protocol.

There is scope for future development in the areas of prediction of successful induction so that women can be counselled appropriately. Women with a previous cesarean section are an important group in whom more trials are needed. Finally, with so many induction methods in our armamentarium, failed induction should be as minimal as possible, and failure should be reduced by choosing and individualising the most effective method among those available.

REFERENCES

1. Martin J, Brady M, Hamilton E, Osterman M, Driscoll A, Drake P. Births: Final Data for 2016. National Vital Statistics Reports. 2018. 67(1).
2. Zeitlin J, Mohangoo AD, Delnord M, et al. The second European Perinatal Health Report: Documenting changes over 6 years in the health of mothers and babies in Europe. *J Epidemiol Community Health.* 2013. 67:983-985.
3. Shah A, Faundes A, Machoki MI, Bataglia V, Amokrane F, Donner A, Mugerwa K, Carroli G, Fawole B, Langer A, Wolomby JJ. Methodological considerations in implementing the WHO global survey for monitoring maternal and perinatal health. Bulletin of the World Health Organization. 2008. 86:126-31.
4. Vogel JP, Souza JP, Gülmezoglu AM. Patterns and outcomes of induction of labour in Africa and Asia: A secondary analysis of the WHO Global Survey on Maternal and Neonatal Health. *PLoS One.* 2013. 8(6):e65612.
5. Rygh AB, Skjeldestad FE, Korner H, Eggebo TM. Assessing the association of oxytocin augmentation with obstetric anal sphincter injury in nulliparous women: A population-based, case-control study. *BMJ Open.* 2014. 4(7):e004592.
6. Danilack VA, Dore DD, Triche EW, Muri JH, Phipps MG, Savitz DA. The effect of labour induction on the risk of caesarean delivery: Using propensity scores to control confounding by indication. *BJOG.* 2016. 123:1521.
7. Grobman WA, Rice MM, Reddy UM, et al. Labor Induction versus expectant management in low-risk nulliparous women. *N Engl J Med.* 2018. 379:513-23.
8. Inducing labour. NICE guidance (NG 207). 2021.
9. Crane JM. Factors predicting labor induction success: A critical analysis. *Clin Obstet Gynecol.* 2006. 49:573.
10. Bishop EH. Pelvic scoring for elective induction. *Obstet Gynecol.* 1964. 24:266-8. PMID:14199536.
11. Finucane EM, Murphy DJ, Biesty LM, Gyte GML, Cotter AM, Ryan EM, Boulvain M, Devane D. Membrane sweeping for induction of labour. *Cochrane Database of Systematic Reviews.* 2020. Issue 2. Art. No.: CD000451.
12. Gu N, Ru T, Wang Z, Dai Y, Zheng M, Xu B, Hu Y. Foley catheter for induction of labor at Term: An open-label, randomized controlled trial. *PLoS One.* 2015. 10(8): e0136856.
13. Liu X, Wang Y, Zhang F, Zhong X, Ou R, Luo X, Qi H. Double- versus single-balloon catheters for labour induction and cervical ripening: A meta-analysis. *BMC Pregnancy Childbirth.* 2019. 16;19(1).
14. de los Reyes SX, Sheffield JS, Eke AC. Single versus double-balloon transcervical catheter for labor induction: A systematic review and meta-analysis. *Am J Perinatol.* 2018. 36(08):790–7.
15. Saad A, Villarreal J, Eid J, et al. A randomized controlled trial of Dilapan-S vs Foley balloon for preinduction cervical ripening (DILAFOL trial). *Am J Obstet Gynecol.* 2019. 220:275.e1.
16. Thomas J, Fairclough A, Kavanagh J, Kelly AJ. Vaginal prostaglandin (PGE2 and PGF2a) for induction of labour at term. *Cochrane Database Syst Rev.* 2014. Issue 6. Art. no.:CD003101.
17. Alfirevic Z, Keeney E, Dowswell T, et al. Methods to induce labour: A systematic review, network meta-analysis and cost-effectiveness analysis. *BJOG.* 2016. 123:1462.
18. Budden A, Chen LJ, Henry A. High-dose versus low-dose oxytocin infusion regimens for induction of labour at term. *Cochrane Database Syst Rev.* 2014. Issue 10. Art. No.: CD009701.
19. Macones GA, Cahill A, Stamilio DM, Odibo AO. The efficacy of early amniotomy in nulliparous labor induction: A randomized controlled trial. *Am J Obstet Gynecol.* 2012. 207:403.e1.
20. Shantha S, Dr K, Malhotra J. Good Clinical Practice Recommendations FOGSI-ICOG. 2018. Induction of

Labor: Good Clinical Practice Recommendations Chairperson, ICOG President. *FOGSI.*

21. Sims EJ, Newman RB, Hulsey TC. 2001. Vaginal birth after cesarean: To induce or not to induce. *Am J Obstet Gynecol.* 184:1122–4
22. West HM, Jozwiak M, Dodd JM. Methods of term labour induction for women with a previous caesarean section. *Cochrane Database Syst Rev.* 2017. Issue 6. Art no.:CD009792.
23. de Vaan MD, Ten Eikelder ML, Jozwiak M, et al. Mechanical methods for induction of labour. *Cochrane Database Syst Rev.* 2019. Issue 10. Art. No.: CD001233.
24. Bennett BB. Uterine rupture during induction of labor at term with intravaginal misoprostol. *Obstet Gynecol.* 1997. 89(5 Pt 2):832-833.
25. Aslan H, Unlu E, Agar M, Ceylan Y. Uterine rupture associated with misoprostol labor induction in women with previous cesarean delivery. *Eur J Obstet Gynecol Reprod.* 2004.113(1):45–48.
26. Macones GA, Peipert J, Nelson DB, Odibo A, Stevens EJ, Stamilio DM, Pare E, Elovitz M, Sciscione A, Sammel MD, Ratcliffe SJ. Maternal complications with vaginal birth after cesarean delivery: A multicenter study. *Am J Obstet Gynecol.*2005. 193(5):1656–1662
27. Middleton P, Shepherd E, Crowther CA. 2018. Induction of labour for improving birth outcomes for women at or beyond term. *Cochrane Database Syst Rev.* Issue 7. Art. no.: CD004945.
28. Zhang Y, Wang J, Yu Y, et al. 2015. Misoprostol versus prostaglandin E2 gel for labor induction in premature rupture of membranes after 34 weeks of pregnancy. *Int J Gynaecol Obstet.* 130:214.
29. Middleton P, Shepherd E, Flenady V, McBain RD, Crowther CA. Planned early birth versus expectant management (waiting) for prelabour rupture of membranes at term (37 weeks or more). *Cochrane Database of Systematic Rev.* 2017, Issue 1. Art. No.: CD005302.

CHAPTER 15

Identification and Management of Fetal Distress

SABARATNAM ARULKUMARAN

INTRODUCTION

The phenomenon of 'too little, too late or too much, too soon' as regards emergency cesarean section for fetal distress is well known. Though external fetal monitoring is the most widely used screening tool for fetal distress during labour in women with high-risk pregnancies, it has not lived up to early expectations and is a poor predictor of fetal acidosis.

Early interventions for presumed fetal distress are associated with a significant increase in cesarean rates. Late interventions lead to stillbirths, early neonatal deaths, and neurological injuries including cerebral palsy. This is reflected in the global increase of cesarean rates without any decline in the incidence of cerebral palsy. This paradox is partly due to the imprecise nature of the manual interpretation of the cardiotocograph (CTG), failure to incorporate the clinical picture, delay in taking action, and fear of litigation.

In 2018, the Royal College of Obstetricians and Gynaecologists (RCOG) conducted a four-year study, 'Each baby counts' [1], with the intention of reducing asphyxia-related morbidity and mortality. The study consisted of 1145 cases of intrapartum-related fetal deaths, early neonatal deaths, and neurological injuries. Of these cases, 11% ended in stillbirths, 14% in early neonatal deaths, and 75% in severe brain injuries [1]. The study identified five factors that were associated with poor outcomes. They were as follows:

1. Poor or delayed recognition of clinical risk factors
2. Improper interpretation of CTG and fetal blood sampling
3. Education and training issues
4. Poor team communication
5. Individual human factors

One or more of the above factors were involved in each of these cases, i.e., a combination of factors resulted in a poor outcome.

If we can improve on these five factors, i.e., correctly identify a distressed fetus and institute timely intervention, it may be possible to reduce stillbirths, early neonatal deaths, and catastrophic neurological injuries. In addition, this should help to reduce the rising cesarean rates and escalating medicolegal costs related to poor outcomes. A staggering £10.2 million per day is paid out in the UK towards birth-related injuries [2].

This chapter will deal with a few of the identified issues associated with poor outcomes:

- The **clinical risk factors** that are likely to increase the risk of acidosis compared with an appropriately grown fetus at term with no clinical risk factors
- The **speed of onset of acidosis** with certain cardiotocography patterns to guide how quickly one should intervene
- Patterns that are **misunderstood**

The chapter will conclude with recommendations to avoid medicolegal issues related to fetal surveillance with CTGs.

CLINICAL RISK FACTORS

In addition to maternal high-risk factors such as preeclampsia and diabetes, some specific pre-existing fetal risk factors reduce the physiological reserve of the fetus while other such factors develop during labour [3].

- **Fetus at risk with reduced physiological reserve**
  - Preterm
  - Postterm
  - Fetal growth restriction (FGR)
  - Thick meconium with scanty fluid
  - Intrauterine infection
  - Intrapartum bleeding
- **Fetus at relative risk with a chance of hypoxia developing during labour due to**
  - Injudicious use of oxytocin
  - Epidural in cases of suspected fetal compromise
  - Difficult instrumental delivery/macrosomia/malpresentation
  - Acute events—cord prolapse, scar rupture, placental abruption
  - Suspicious/abnormal admission test detected by auscultation or electronic fetal monitoring (EFM)

The RCOG in the UK is working on the **ABC programme** (Avoiding Birth Injuries in Childbirth) to identify clinical risk factors that may lead to fetal compromise, including the management of a deeply impacted fetal head [4].

THE RATE OF DEVELOPMENT OF ACIDOSIS WITH SPECIFIC CTG PATTERNS AND RECOMMENDATIONS FOR TIMELY INTERVENTION

Though different classifications for CTG trace readings have been described (see **Chapter 8,** *Fetal surveillance in labour*), a comparison of these classifications shows that they all demonstrate poor specificity of pathological tracings in the prediction of fetal acidemia and neurological damage [5].

The approach to the interpretation of intrapartum CTG has undergone a change in the last few years. This approach addresses fetal physiology and relies on the timing and velocity of the onset of the hypoxic insult and not only on the recognition of the CTG pattern. This has led to the description of the following subtypes of fetal hypoxia which may occur prior to or during labour: **acute, subacute, gradually evolving, and chronic antepartum hypoxia.**

The different CTG patterns that suggest the rate of decline of fetal pH, leading to poor outcomes if not for timely intervention, are described below:

- **Acute hypoxia** is indicated by prolonged deceleration (bradycardia). The rate of decline of fetal pH is approximately 0.01/minute [6,7]. Delivery should be expedited and should be carried out within 15–30 minutes.
- **Subacute hypoxia** is recognised by repetitive prolonged decelerations lasting 90–120 seconds with very short inter-deceleration intervals. The rate of progression of acidosis is approximately 0.01 over 2–3 minutes [8,9]. The baby should be delivered within 30–45 minutes to avoid poor fetal outcomes.
- **Gradually developing hypoxia** is characterised by a progressive increase in the depth and duration of decelerations, shortening of inter-deceleration intervals, rise in the baseline rate, and reduction in baseline variability. It takes hours for acidosis to set in and is reflected by a trace with absent variability and late/atypical variable decelerations for >1 hour [10,11]. Delivery should be expedited and should be carried out within one hour after the onset of absent variability with repeated late decelerations.
- **Chronic** or **pre-existing** or **long-standing hypoxia** is usually characterised by absent variability and shallow late decelerations. Clinical signs of compromise such as absent fetal movements, and thick meconium may be present. The fetal pH may be at acidotic or pre-acidotic levels [12].

Acute Hypoxia

Acute hypoxia is usually reflected by prolonged deceleration (bradycardia). Prolonged FHR deceleration of **<80 bpm for <3 minutes is termed suspicious**, and that for **>3 minutes is considered abnormal** (see **Chapter 8,** *Fetal surveillance in labour*). Some consider prolonged deceleration to be a drop to **<100 bpm**. The pH declines at a rate of 0.01/minute on an average [5,6]. The lower the heart rate and the longer the FHR remains low, the greater the chance of acidosis (e.g., a rate of 50 bpm for 10 minutes provides only 500 blood circulations and, therefore, less oxygenation as compared to a rate of 80 bpm, which provides 800 circulations).

Key Point

The lower the heart rate and the longer the FHR remains low, the greater the chance of acidosis.

Irreversible or reversible causes

Prolonged deceleration may be due to an irreversible or a reversible cause.

Irreversible causes: Prolonged deceleration due to cord prolapse, placental abruption, or scar dehiscence (Fig. 15.1) warrants immediate delivery within 15–30 minutes. It has been shown that a delay of >18 minutes in cases of scar rupture increases the incidence of severe perinatal morbidity [13]. This may be due to the interruption of uterine blood flow due to scar rupture in addition to the prolonged deceleration. Placental abruption should be suspected in a woman who presents with continuous abdominal pain, vaginal bleeding, a tender, tense or irritable uterus, and prolonged deceleration. Such cases warrant immediate delivery (see **Chapter 29,** *Antepartum hemorrhage*).

Reversible causes: If the prolonged deceleration is due to reversible causes such as an epidural top-up, vaginal examination, or

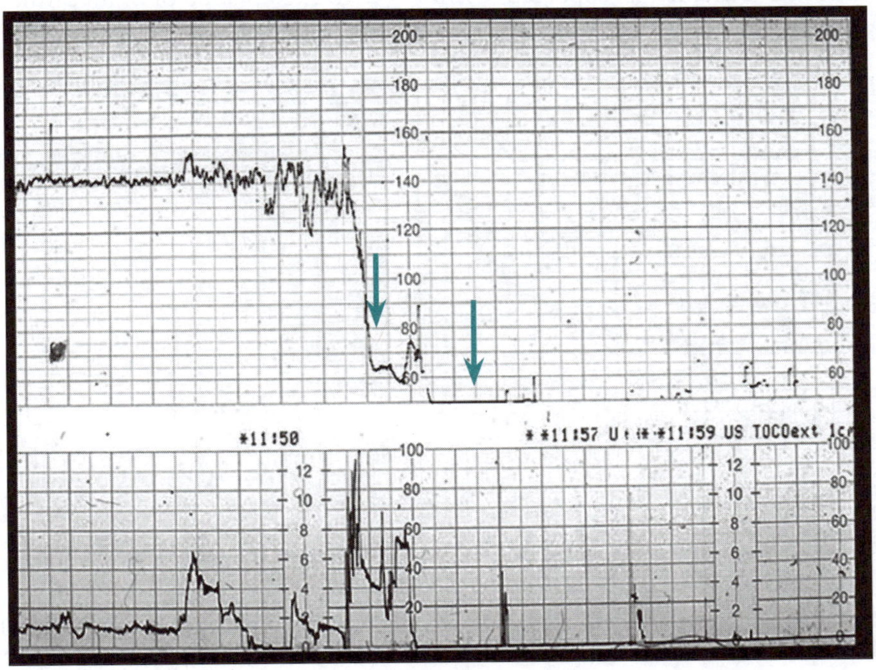

Fig. 15.1 Irreversible prolonged deceleration following cesarean scar rupture (*Image courtesy:* Prof. Sabaratnam Arulkumaran)

uterine hyperstimulation (Figs. 15.2a and b), the following measures should restore the FHR to normal:

- Adjusting the maternal position
- Correcting hypotension
- Stopping the oxytocin infusion
- Administering acute tocolysis

Key Point

In the presence of uterine hyperstimulation due to oxytocics/prostaglandins, a bolus dose of a tocolytic drug such as terbutaline or atosiban may help abolish uterine contractions and improve the chances of delivering a less compromised neonate.

Fetuses at lower risk of acidosis

If the clinical picture does not suggest abruption, scar dehiscence, or cord prolapse, and if the fetus is appropriately grown at term with clear amniotic fluid and a reactive FHR pattern before the episode of bradycardia, recovery of the FHR towards the baseline is expected within 9 minutes. The recovery of the FHR towards the normal baseline rate within 6 minutes with good baseline variability is reassuring.

Key Point

Reactivity (accelerations) and cycling (quiet and active sleep cycles) are indicative of a non-hypoxic fetus and are reassuring signs.

Fetuses at higher risk of acidosis

Fetuses that have a greater risk of non-recovery or delayed recovery back to the baseline FHR and of developing hypoxia may have one or more of the following features:

- Postterm
- Growth restriction
- Oligohydramnios or no amniotic fluid (anhydramnios)
- Thick meconium-stained fluid at rupture of membranes
- An abnormal or suspicious FHR trace prior to the episode of bradycardia

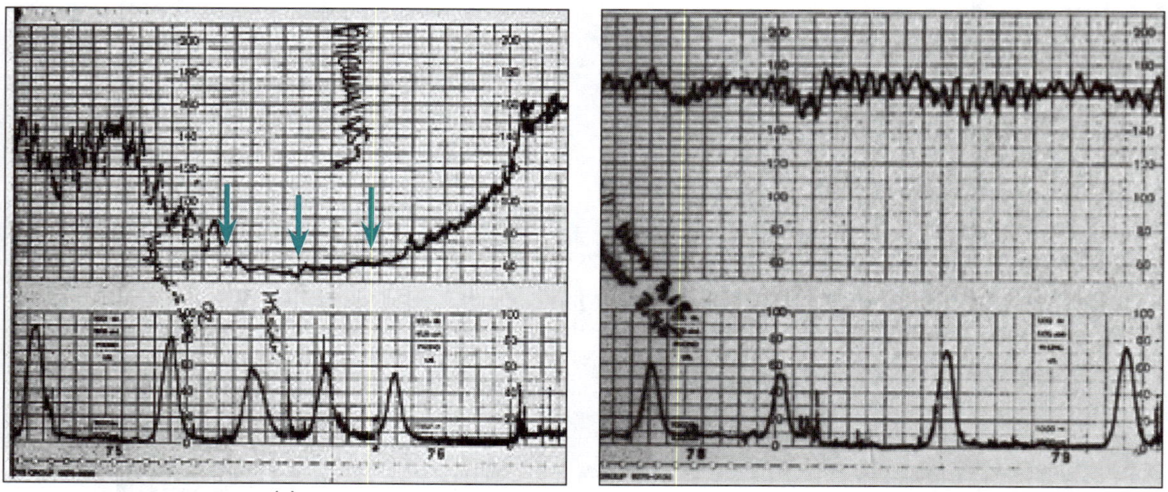

(a) (b)

Fig. 15.2 (a) Reversible prolonged deceleration due to uterine hyperstimulation is seen (arrows) and (b) recovery to normal FHR is seen after stopping oxytocin and administering acute tocolysis (in this case, scalp pH done for research purposes showed acidosis immediately after deceleration which reverted to normal once the FHR was at the normal baseline for several minutes). (*Image courtesy:* Prof. Sabaratnam Arulkumaran)

In these situations, it may be better to act early if the FHR fails to show signs of recovery to normal.

Management of acute hypoxia

Abruption, cord prolapse, or scar rupture warrant immediate intervention. Fetal scalp blood sampling is of no value as the decision to act is based on whether the deceleration is due to a reversible or irreversible pathology, and if it is reversible, whether the FHR is returning to the normal rate.

> **Key Point**
>
> Abruption, cord prolapse, or scar rupture warrant immediate intervention. Fetal scalp blood sampling (FBS) is inappropriate in such situations.

If there are no signs of recovery towards the baseline rate within 6 minutes, action should be taken to:

- Determine the cause
- Determine cervical dilatation
- Consider delivery
  - If the cervix is fully dilated and the head is low, a forceps or ventouse delivery should be carried out.
  - A cesarean should be performed if the cervix is not fully dilated or if the head is high. Such a cesarean is considered a **category 1** or **immediate cesarean** and is performed as an emergency when there is an immediate threat to the life of the woman or fetus [14]. Category 1 cesarean should have a specific code or term assigned, such as 'Code Red' or 'immediate' cesarean. This helps in mobilising all the staff members (obstetricians, anesthetists, additional midwifery/nursing staff, theatre staff, operating department assistants, and pediatricians) needed to accomplish delivery within 15–30 minutes of the onset of the prolonged deceleration.

> **Key Point**
>
> Obstetric units should have the facilities to perform Category 1 cesarean section. Since Category 1 cesarean is performed as an emergency procedure, it should have a specific code or term assigned, such as 'Code Red' or 'immediate' cesarean, in order to mobilise all the staff on an urgent basis.

Ensuring early action

Early action is possible if the midwife/nurse and the doctor in the room push the bed into the theatre while the supervisory midwife/nurse in charge of the ward calls for the anesthetist, neonatologist, and OT staff. The couple should have the reason for the cesarean explained to them and they should be reassured. Early entry into the theatre makes it possible for more people to help with the various tasks to be performed, such as setting up an IV line, sending blood for Hb and type and cross-match, and bladder catheterisation.

Recommended actions for the management of prolonged deceleration

Table 15.1 outlines the timeline for the management of acute hypoxia with prolonged deceleration.

Table 15.1 Management of prolonged deceleration on CTG [15, 16]

Time	Action points
3 minutes	• Review clinical picture • Review risk factors • Determine whether the insult is reversible or irreversible • Review CTG prior to deceleration
6 minutes	Expect recovery towards the baseline if it was due to reversible or unknown cause
9 minutes	If no recovery, prepare for operative delivery
12 minutes	Make every attempt to start operative procedure
15 minutes	The baby should have been delivered by this time or within 30 minutes at the most

CTG, cardiotocograph

Subacute Hypoxia

Subacute hypoxia presents with prolonged decelerations. The FHR decelerates and is below the baseline rate for a longer duration (e.g., >60–90 seconds) and spends a shorter duration at the baseline rate (<30 seconds). With such FHR, there is less than optimal circulation through the placenta, and the fetus becomes compromised with a progression of acidosis of approximately 0.01 every two to three minutes in some cases [8,9] (Figs. 15.3a–e). Due to the rapid onset of hypoxia, the variability in between decelerations can exhibit saltatory variability [17] (Fig. 15.3b). With progressive acidosis, the baseline FHR declines, resulting in terminal bradycardia, severe metabolic acidosis and poor fetal/neonatal outcome.

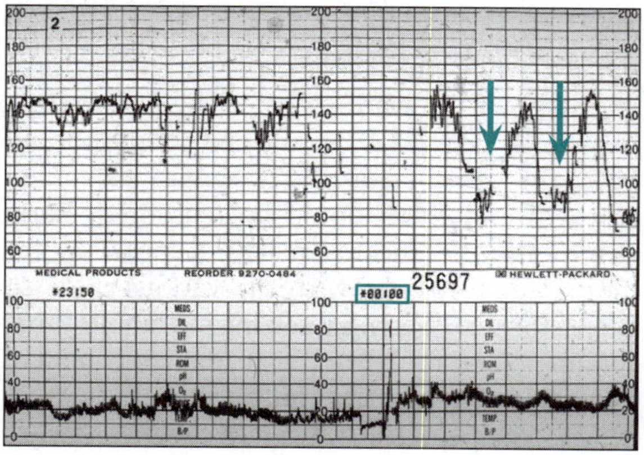

Fig. 15.3 (a) The early decelerations before 00.00 hrs evolve to show deep prolonged variable decelerations (arrows) (*Image courtesy:* Prof. Sabaratnam Arulkumaran)

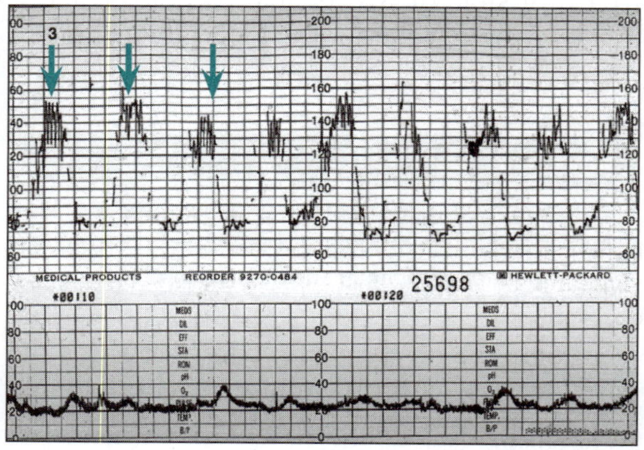

Fig. 15.3 (b) Decelerations lasting for 2 minutes each with inter-deceleration intervals of 30 seconds and exhibiting saltatory variability (arrows) (*Image courtesy:* Prof. Sabaratnam Arulkumaran)

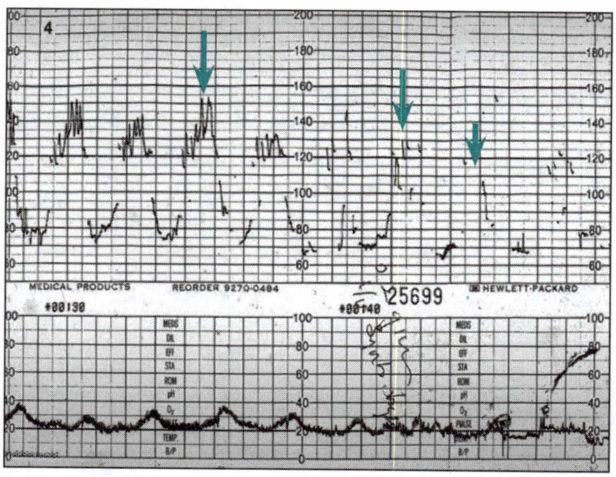

Fig. 15.3 (c) The baseline FHR (arrows) gradually drops to a lower rate after each deceleration (*Image courtesy:* Prof. Sabaratnam Arulkumaran)

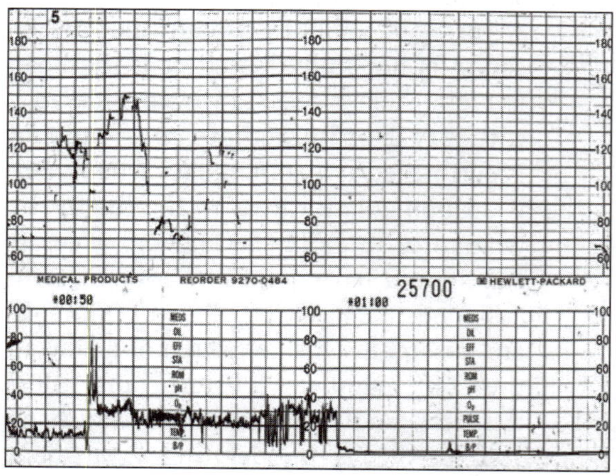

Fig. 15.3 (d) The prolonged decelerations and decline of baseline FHR end in terminal deceleration (*Image courtesy:* Prof. Sabaratnam Arulkumaran)

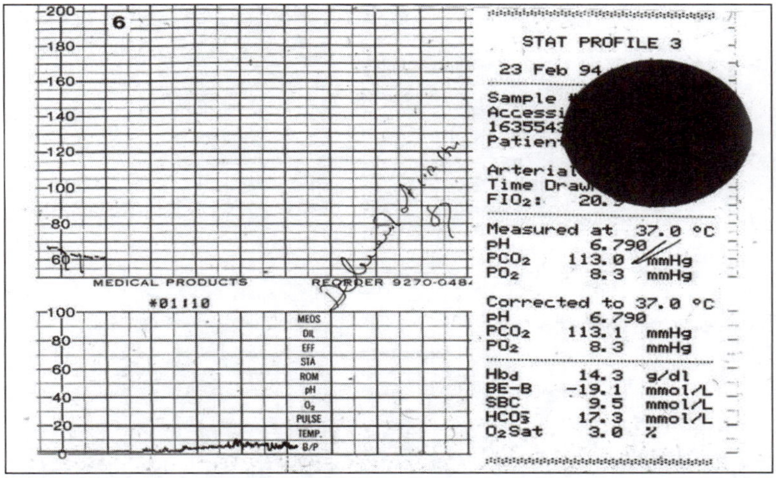

Fig. 15.3 (e) 60 minutes of prolonged decelerations and 10 minutes of terminal bradycardia resulted in severe fetal metabolic acidosis of pH 6.79 and base excess (BE) of –19.1 mmol/L. The Apgar score of the newborn was 0 at 1 and 5 minutes, and 6 at 10 minutes. Delivery of the fetus within 30 to 45 minutes from the onset of the prolonged FHR decelerations may have resulted in a better neonatal outcome. (*Image courtesy:* Prof. Sabaratnam Arulkumaran)

Key Point

Considering the clinical picture in planning management is essential. Injudicious use of oxytocin, epidural analgesia, and difficult operative delivery can compromise the fetus when the CTG is pathological.

Gradually Developing Hypoxia

With gradually developing hypoxia, a normal FHR starts to show decelerations with the following characteristics:

- An increase in depth and duration with time
- Reduction in the intervals between decelerations
- A rise in the baseline rate and reduction in baseline variability with increasing hypoxia before proceeding to a rapid, stepwise drop of the baseline rate prior to terminal bradycardia

Figs. 15.4a–j show FHR traces from early labour to delivery in a woman with sickle cell disease and a growth-restricted fetus. The variable decelerations show an increase in depth and duration with an increase in FHR from 140 to 160 bpm within 4 hours. There was reduced baseline variability for one to two hours with absent accelerations. The baseline FHR then declined in a short period to terminal bradycardia and resulted in a stillbirth. If the baby had been delivered within 4 hours of onset of labour, when there was normal baseline variability, the baby would not have been acidotic. **Tachycardia with loss of variability and late or variable decelerations results in fetal acidosis if it persists for 1–2 hours [10,11].**

'Chronic' or Pre-existing Hypoxia

Some fetuses get compromised very slowly (chronic or longstanding) in the antenatal period and are on the verge of acute compromise with uterine contractions in labour. The CTGs show shallow decelerations as they are unable to generate decelerations due to the 'blunted response' by the hypoxic brain.

The CTG of a fetus with chronic hypoxia has the following characteristics:

- A higher baseline rate in the normal range, or tachycardia, but there are no accelerations
- A silent pattern of baseline variability
- Subtle, shallow late decelerations

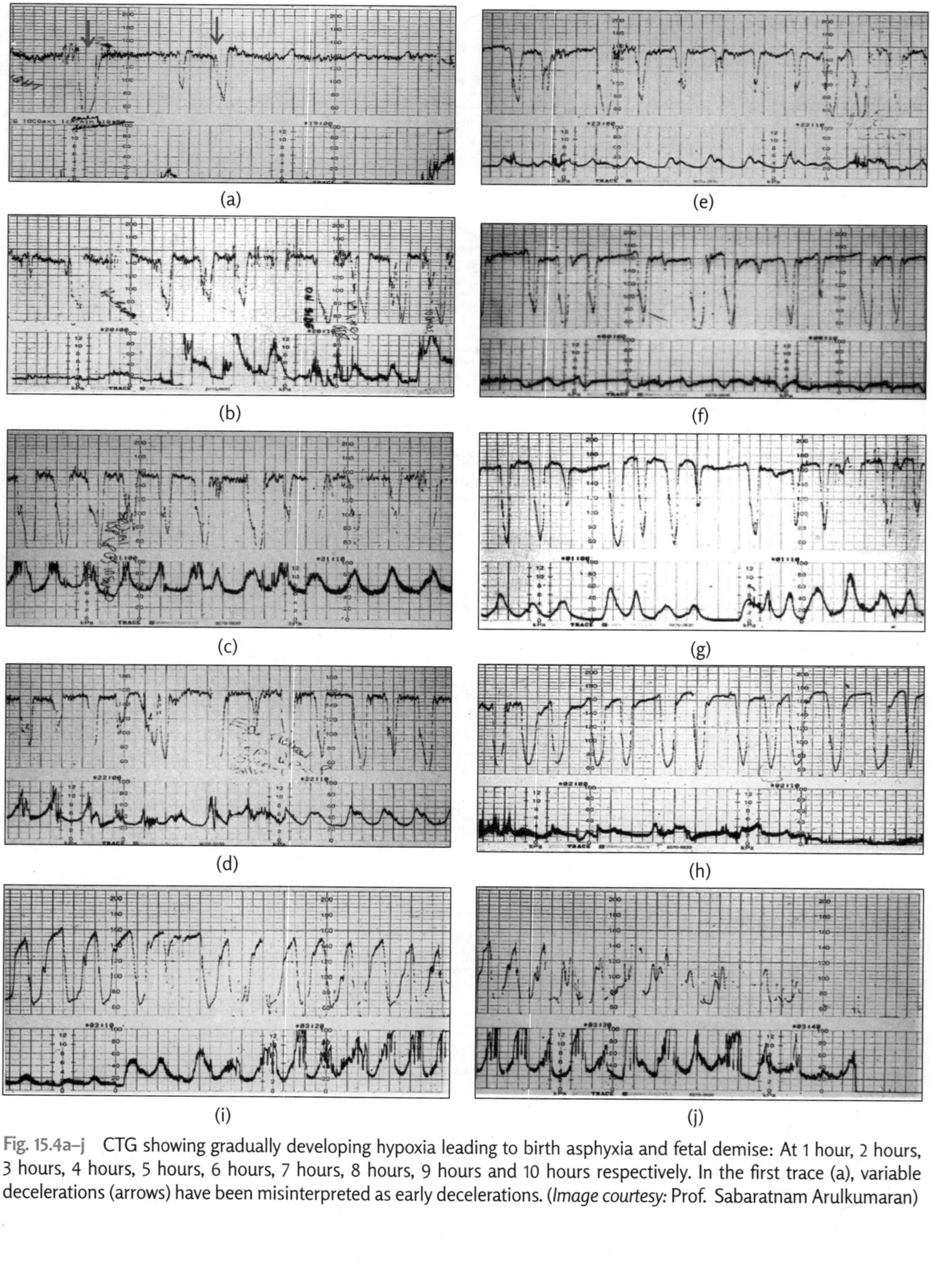

Fig. 15.4a–j CTG showing gradually developing hypoxia leading to birth asphyxia and fetal demise: At 1 hour, 2 hours, 3 hours, 4 hours, 5 hours, 6 hours, 7 hours, 8 hours, 9 hours and 10 hours respectively. In the first trace (a), variable decelerations (arrows) have been misinterpreted as early decelerations. (*Image courtesy*: Prof. Sabaratnam Arulkumaran)

This type of trace is often not recognised. This is an **ominous CTG** and should be acted on if:

- The features of the CTG do not improve in 40 to 60 minutes or
- There are clinical symptoms or signs of fetal compromise such as:
  - — Absent fetal movements
  - — Fetal growth restriction
  - — Intrauterine infection
  - — Bleeding
  - — Postterm pregnancy
  - — Scanty fluid with thick meconium

These babies tend to have chronic hypoxia with pre-acidosis or acidosis and need to be delivered as the CTG can deteriorate suddenly due to increasing metabolic acidosis with subsequent contractions (Figs. 15.5a–f).

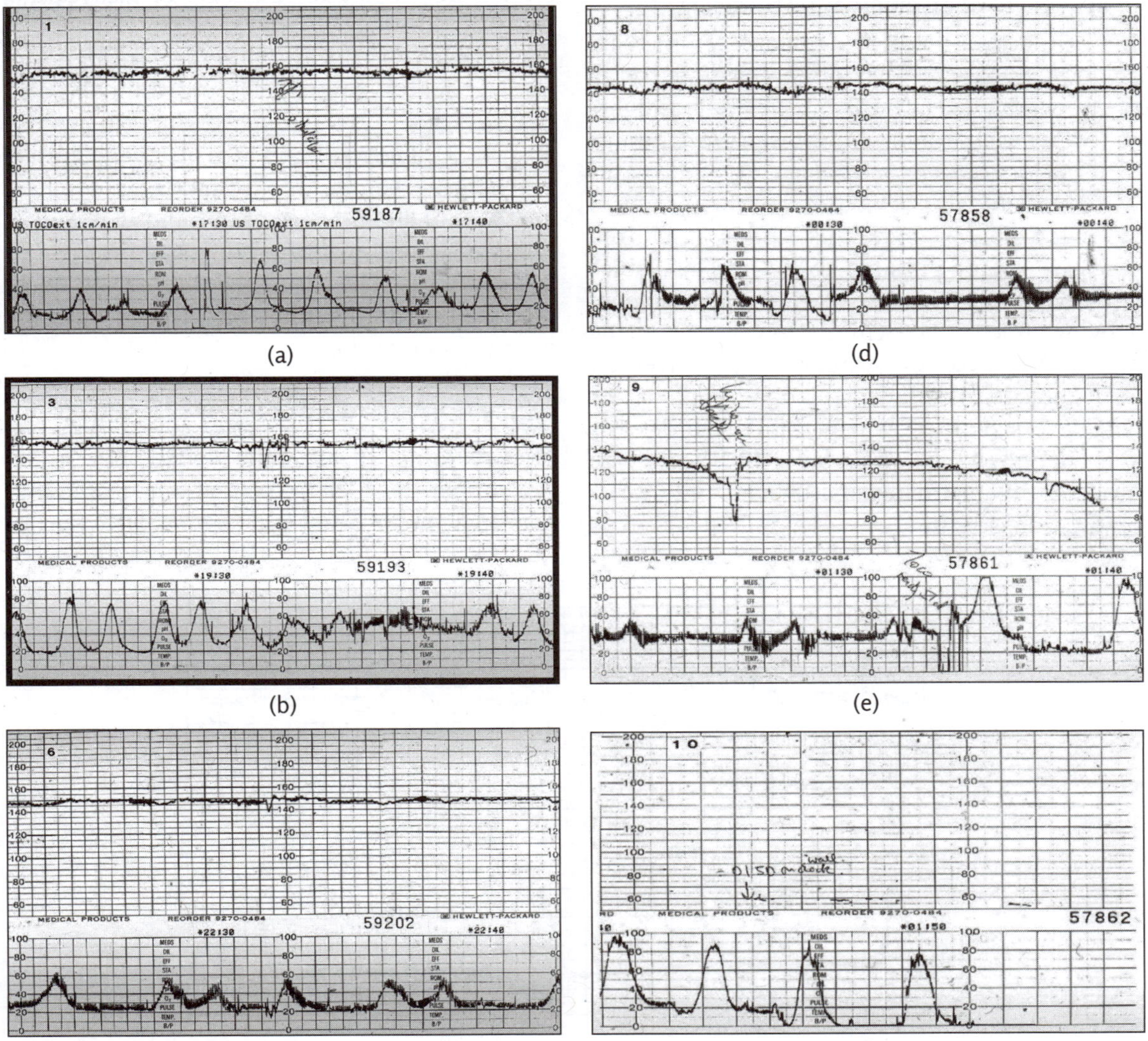

Fig. 15.5 (a) Absent variability and shallow decelerations suggest pre-existing hypoxia. The chronically hypoxic fetus is unable to compensate with an increase in the baseline rate. The shallow decelerations are due to the blunted response of the CNS. Each contraction makes the hypoxia and metabolic acidosis worse (b-d), leading to terminal collapse (e and f) without any change in the CTG trace. (*Image courtesy:* Prof. Sabaratnam Arulkumaran)

Key Point

Prompt action should be considered in the presence of FGR, preterm and postterm pregnancy, intrauterine infection, intrapartum bleeding, and thick meconium with scanty fluid. A non-reactive trace with baseline variability <5 bpm and shallow late decelerations (<15 beats) that last for >90 minutes suggests the possibility of hypoxia.

Management of an ominous CTG tracing

An ominous tracing demands immediate delivery. Such cases are often associated with prelabour hypoxia (Fig. 15.6). This highlights the value of the admission test (see **Chapter 8**, *Fetal surveillance in labour*) for all cases when possible and if not, whenever there is a suspicion of fetal compromise and in un-booked cases. It is not possible to deliver all babies with ominous traces with the expectation of a living, undamaged child. However, it is the responsibility of the caregiver to deliver all such babies. It is difficult to know which babies will have a poor prognosis, but the prognosis will definitely be poor if the healthcare provider procrastinates and delivers only when bradycardia sets in.

PRE-TERMINAL FHR PATTERNS

Interventions for a fetus with a previously normal reactive trace within a reasonable period of a sentinel event such as an abruption is likely to result in a good outcome, assuming a reasonable gestational age. Intervening when the main feature is tachycardia suggests some ability of the fetus to survive. Once terminal deceleration develops after a period of tachycardia, the situation may be irremediable (Fig. 15.7). An undulatory pattern without a steady baseline variability suggests the possibility of central nervous system damage due to hypoxia (Fig. 15.8). The challenge is to intervene in such pregnancies before this situation is reached. However, it should be kept in mind that central nervous system malformations can give rise to such patterns. The expectant parents should be informed of the likelihood of a poor outcome despite intervention.

MISINTERPRETATION OF CTG TRACINGS

The maternal heart rate (MHR) recording can mimic the FHR recording and result in a maternal heart rate artefact (MHRA). The

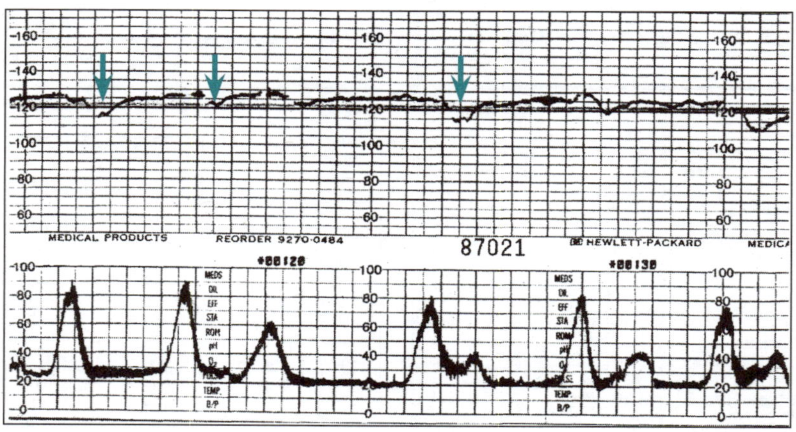

Fig. 15.6 Ominous trace with absent baseline variability and shallow late decelerations (arrows) despite the baseline rate being within the normal range. Accelerations and normal baseline variability, which are the hallmarks of fetal health, are absent. A normal baseline rate alone does not imply good fetal health. (*Image courtesy*: Prof. Sabaratnam Arulkumaran)

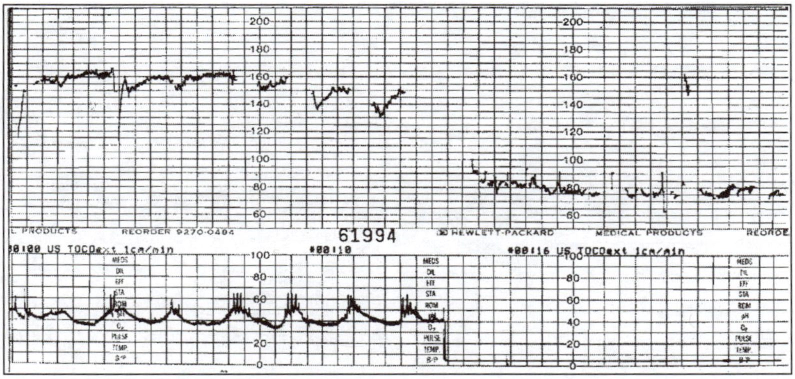

Fig. 15.7 Terminal prolonged deceleration following a period of tachycardia, reduced variability, and late decelerations (*Image courtesy:* Prof. Sabaratnam Arulkumaran)

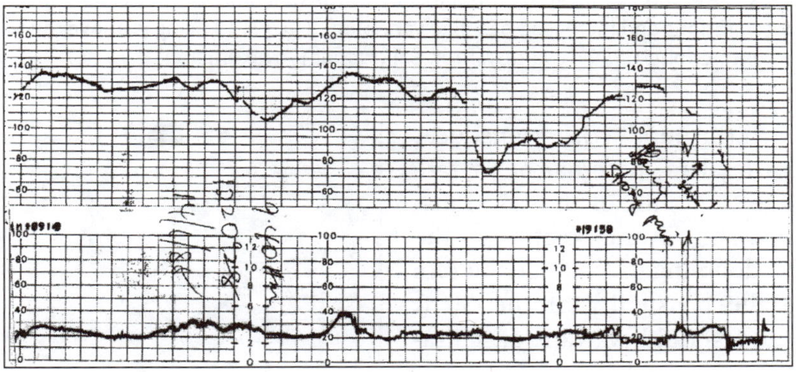

Fig. 15.8 Terminal hypoxic central nervous system damage reflected by the inability to maintain a steady baseline rate and absent variability (*Image courtesy:* Prof. Sabaratnam Arulkumaran)

misinterpretation of FHR tracings due to MHRA is not uncommon. In fact, this has been described as one of the five most common FHR monitoring errors [18].

Key Point

Sometimes, it is difficult to distinguish whether the heart rate recording is that of the mother or the fetus as the maternal heart rate also shows baseline variability and accelerations (Fig. 15.9).

Misinterpretation due to MHRA may arise in many situations. Following the advice of the Medical Devices Agency, i.e., to auscultate the FHR before applying the ultrasound transducer to the maternal abdomen, helps in avoiding this mistake. Comparing with the maternal pulse may lead to errors as the ultrasound transducer can pick up the maternal pulse and double it or increase it by 50%.

Key Point

When the monitor/recorder is attached, it is crucial to make sure that the heart rate recording is that of the fetus. This is done by auscultating the fetal heart prior to application.

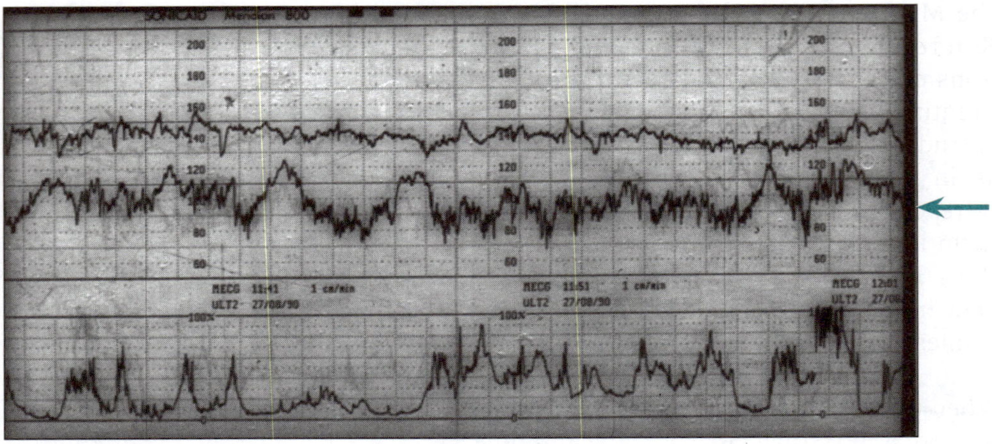

Fig. 15.9 The maternal heart rate (MHR) is recorded by a precordial electrocardiograph (ECG) lead on the anterior aspect of the mother's chest and is indicated automatically by the machine as 'MECG' (arrow). The MHR recording shows features of accelerations and increased baseline variability. The FHR tracing is above the MHR, and the lowest tracing is of uterine contractions. (*Image courtesy:* Prof. Sabaratnam Arulkumaran)

At times, the ultrasound (US) transducer may switch from fetal to maternal heart rate during labour due to a shift of the US transducer. Any sudden shift in the position in the baseline rate or a doubling of the baseline rate should indicate the possibility of the MHR being recorded and should warrant auscultation of the FHR.

An unsatisfactory recording with an US transducer warrants the use of a fetal scalp electrode unless there is a contraindication to the use of a scalp electrode. Poor quality CTG is more common in the late first and second stages of labour when the head moves down, when the mother is restless, or when there are too-frequent contractions with too many decelerations.

In the second stage of labour, the FHR should show decelerations with head compression. If the trace shows accelerations with contractions, the recording is likely to be that of the maternal heart rate (Fig. 15.10) [19]. Maternal heart rate accelerations result from increased maternal venous return during a contraction, the exertion of pushing, and maternal anxiety and pain.

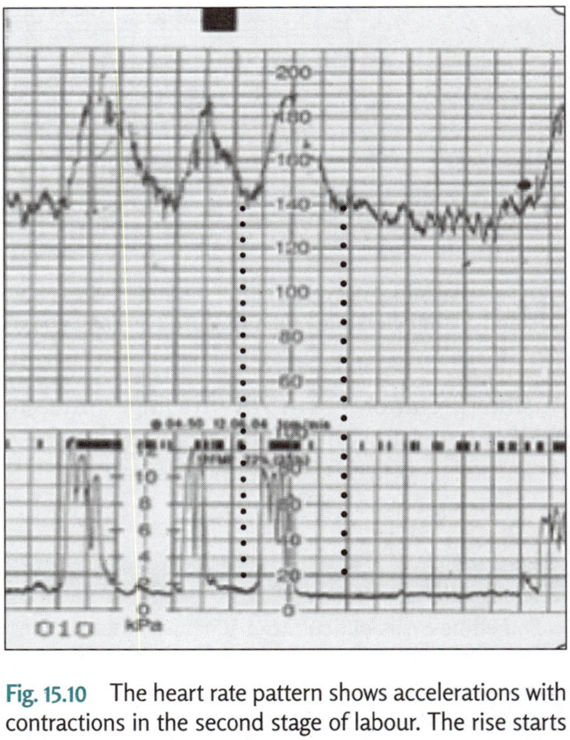

Fig. 15.10 The heart rate pattern shows accelerations with contractions in the second stage of labour. The rise starts with the onset of the contractions and returns to its baseline rate with the offset of the contractions (see dotted lines). This suggests that it is the maternal heart rate that is being recorded. (*Image courtesy:* Prof. Sabaratnam Arulkumaran)

The MHR recording is very similar to the FHR. It requires close observation of the accelerations corresponding to the contractions to differentiate between the two. Sherman et al. [20] studied the characteristics of MHR patterns in labour. Such studies have increasingly reported the unintentional recording of MHR in labour. It has been shown that accelerations of the MHR with contractions are present in most cases and may not be identified unless one carefully observes the tracing (Fig. 15.11).

When the FHR is recorded by the US transducer and is less than 80 bpm, the machine can double the count and give two tracings, giving the impression that the higher rate is that of the fetus and the lower rate is that of the mother (Fig. 15.12). This tends to happen in the late first and second stages of labour due to the hyperstimulation of the uterus by oxytocin, which is further enhanced by the Ferguson reflex. Non-recognition of this 'doubling' of the FHR may result in delayed intervention and a poor neonatal outcome.

There are several examples of misinterpretation of the CTG, and the reader is encouraged to read specific books devoted to intrapartum fetal surveillance for the same.

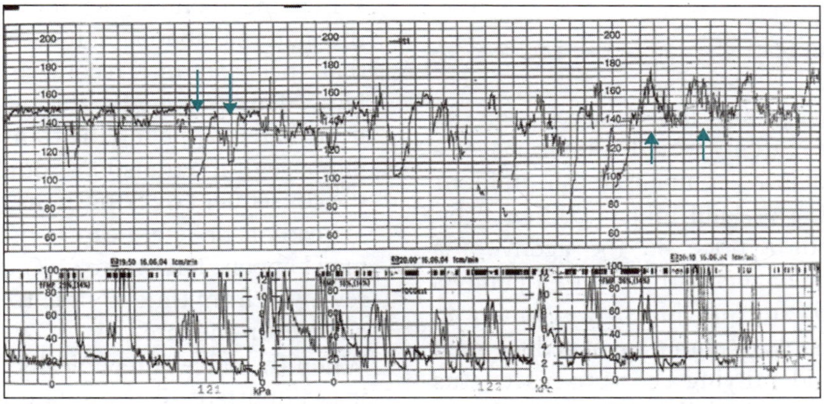

Fig. 15.11 The FHR decelerates with head compression in the earlier part of the trace (downward pointing arrows), whereas the last five minutes show accelerations as the MHR was being recorded (upward arrows). The non-recognition of this condition for one hour resulted in a fresh stillbirth. (*Image courtesy:* Prof. Sabaratnam Arulkumaran)

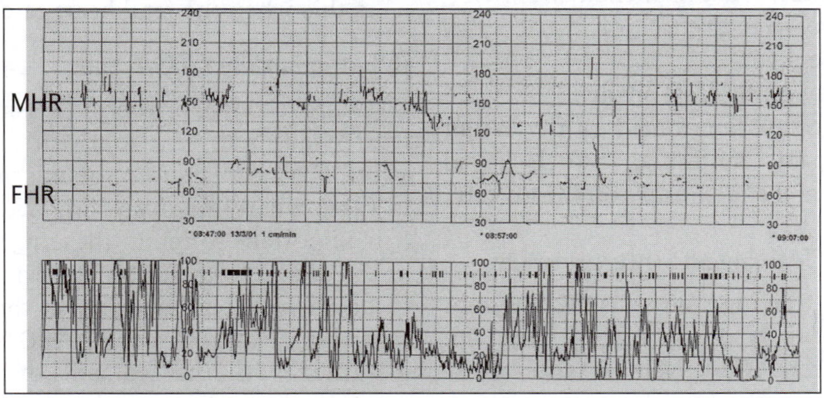

Fig. 15.12 Trace showing fetal bradycardia of 70–75 bpm and doubling of the rate to 140–150 bpm, thus giving two heart rates. (*Image courtesy:* Prof. Sabaratnam Arulkumaran)
FHR, fetal heart rate; *MHR*, maternal heart rate

Key Point

Special attention needs to be paid during a twin delivery after the first baby is born. The second twin will move down in the pelvis, and it is important to ensure that its heart rate is identified and recorded.

MEDICOLEGAL ISSUES

Litigation in obstetrics is on the increase. Medicolegal cases related to CTG arise from the following factors:

- Failure to incorporate clinical risk factors
- Inability to interpret traces
- Inappropriate action or delay in taking action
- Technical aspects
- Poor communication, teamwork, and record-keeping

Obstetric litigation is distressing to all involved. Any parent would rather have a healthy child than be compensated in millions for a debilitating or fatal injury to their baby. One cannot put a price on the agony of a child's suffering or the disruption of a family's life. As healthcare providers, we must do everything possible to eliminate or reduce such occurrences by identifying a compromised fetus and performing timely delivery.

The majority of litigations result from parents demanding the following:

- Wanting to know what happened and why
- Prevention of recurrence of what they perceive as negligence
- Accountability of the staff involved
- Recovery of costs determined by the extent of injury, pain, suffering, actual losses experienced, and expenditure on future care

Emphasis on Training and Interpretation

Education and training, supervision, incident reporting, auditing, and risk management can help reduce errors. Caregivers in the labour room may not have the knowledge to interpret the CTG tracing due to inadequate training and failure to maintain standards. Ongoing education with refresher courses that comprise appropriate training material helps in this regard.

There is a constant influx of new doctors and midwives in any labour ward. Some are there soon after they qualify; others may be there after working in a non-labour ward setting. Immediate attention is needed to evaluate the trace if it looks pathological and to take action. The availability of a senior doctor with adequate knowledge of CTG is useful to allay anxiety, to educate, to take appropriate action, and to avoid unnecessary operative delivery.

Precautions During CTG Monitoring

- When the monitor/recorder is attached to the maternal abdomen, it is crucial to ensure that the heart rate recording is that of the fetus. This is done by auscultating the fetal heart before applying the transducer.
- Slippage of the transducer during labour and the consequent tracking of the maternal pulse instead of the fetal heart is not common but may happen. The entire CTG trace should be reviewed from time to time to detect sudden changes in the rate.
- When the trace is technically unsatisfactory, it is important to auscultate the fetal heart and record the findings in the notes or on the CTG paper. Often, uterine contractions are not recorded. Attention should be paid to this when the fetal heart rate is abnormal.

Safeguarding CTG Traces

CTGs are recorded on thermosensitive paper and tend to fade in three to four years. Despite every effort, CTG traces tend to go missing, especially in cases where there was an adverse outcome. It is important to retain these particular traces in the digital form and safeguard them. Failure to do so may be damaging in the case that a medicolegal suit ensues. The CTG should be identified with the woman's name, place of recording, recording speed, date, and time.

CTG traces need to be conserved for twenty-five years for medicolegal purposes. The CTG and archival should be available for download in magneto-optic disks or from cloud storage.

Incident Reporting of Adverse Outcomes and Audit of Poor Outcomes

Incident reporting of adverse outcomes and audit of poor outcome (poor Apgar scores, low cord arterial pH, need for assisted ventilation, admission for neonatal intensive care, and hypoxic–ischemic encephalopathy) are essential to find out whether there is a failure in education and training, induction of personnel, supervision, inadequate staffing, or system failure. All potential litigation cases need to be thoroughly evaluated by the risk management team and findings disseminated to prevent further recurrence.

CONCLUSION

Fetal distress is a combination of respiratory and circulatory insufficiency caused by intrauterine fetal hypoxia during labour and is closely associated with changes in fetal heart rate patterns. Fetal distress may cause hypoxic–ischemic encephalopathy, eventually leading to cerebral palsy or perinatal death. Early detection and diagnosis of fetal distress are essential in preventing damage. Education and training, supervision, incident reporting, auditing, and risk management can help reduce errors.

REFERENCES

1. Royal College of Obstetricians and Gynaecologists, UK. Each baby counts. 2020. Final progress report. https://www.rcog.org.uk/media/a4eg2xnm/ebc-2020-final-progress-report.pdf. Accessed 30.07.2023.
2. NHS Resolution. Annual report and accounts 2021/ 2022. chrome-extension://efaidnbmnnnibpcajpcglclefindmkaj/https://assets.publishing.service.gov.uk/government/uploads/system/uploads/attachment_data/file/1092946/nhs-resolution-annual-report-and-accounts-2021-2022-print-version.pdf.
3. Perrine Lorain, Alexandra Bower, Elsa Gottardi, et al. Risk factors for hypoxic–ischemic encephalopathy in cases of severe acidosis: A case–control study. *Acta Obstet Gynecol Scand*. 2022. 101:471-478.
4. Royal College of Obstetricians and Gynaecologists, UK. Avoiding brain injury in childbirth (ABC) programme. 2022. https://www.rcog.org.uk/about-us/quality-improvement-clinical-audit-and-research-projects/avoiding-brain-injury-in-childbirth-abc/ Accessed 30.07.2023.
5. Santo S, Ayres-de-Campos D, Costa-Santos C, Schnettler W, Ugwumadu A, Da Graça LM. For the FM—Compare Collaboration. Agreement and accuracy using the FIGO, ACOG, and NICE cardiotocography interpretation guidelines. *Acta Obstet Gynecol Scand*. 2017. 96: 166–175.
6. Ingemarsson I, Arulkumaran S, Ratnam SS. Single injection of terbutaline in term labor: I. Effect on fetal pH in cases with prolonged bradycardia. *Am J Obstet Gynecol* [Internet]. 1985. 153(8):859–65.
7. Leung TY, Chung PW, Rogers MS, Sahota DS, Lao TT-H, Chung TKH. Urgent cesarean delivery for fetal bradycardia. *Obstet Gynecol* [Internet]. 2009. 114(5).
8. Cahill AG, Caughey AB, Roehl KA, Odibo AO, Macones GA. Terminal fetal heart decelerations and neonatal outcomes. *Obstet Gynecol* [Internet]. 2013. 122(5):1070–1076. Available from: https://journals.lww.com/greenjournal/FullText/2013/11000/Terminal_Fetal_Heart_Decelerations_and_Neonatal.20.aspx
9. Cahill AG, Roehl KA, Odibo AO, Macones GA. Association and prediction of neonatal acidemia. Am J Obstet Gynecol [Internet]. 2012. 207(3):206.e1-206.e8. Available from: https://www.ajog.org/article/S0002-9378(12)00660-6/abstract.
10. Williams KP, Galerneau F. Intrapartum fetal heart rate patterns in the prediction of neonatal acidemia. *Am J Obstet Gynecol* [Internet]. 2003. 188(3):820–3.
11. ACOG Practice Bulletin No. 106: Intrapartum fetal heart rate monitoring: Nomenclature, interpretation, and general management principles. *Obstet Gynecol* [Internet]. 2009. 114(1):192–202. Available from: insights.ovid.com.
12. Phelan JP, Ahn MO. Perinatal observations in forty-eight neurologically impaired term infants. *Am J Obstet Gynecol*. 1994. 171:424-31.
13. Anna S Leung, Eleanor K Leung, Richard Paul. Uterine rupture after previous caesarean delivery: Maternal and fetal consequences. *Am J Obstet Gynecol*.1993. 169:945-50.
14. NICE guidelines NG 192. Caesarean Births. Published 21.10.21. Updated 2023. https://www.nice.org.uk/guidance/ng192/chapter/Recommendations#factors-affecting-the-likelihood-of-emergency-caesarean-birth-during-intrapartum-care. Accessed 02.08.2023.

15. Fetal monitoring in labour. NICE guideline: 229. 2022. https://www.nice.org.uk/guidance/ng229/chapter/Recommendations
16. Gibb D, Arulkumaran S. Chapter 12. Cardiotocographic interpretation: Additional clinical scenarios. *Fetal Monitoring in Practice*. Fifth Edition. Oxford: Elsevier Ltd. 2023. p.130-140.
17. Gracia-Perez-Bonfils Anna, Cuadras Daniel, Whelehan Virginia, Archer Abigail, Río Maria, Chandraharan Edwin. Saltatory pattern vs zigzag pattern on the CTG, and perinatal outcomes. *European Journal of Obstetrics & Gynecology and Reproductive Biology*. 2019. 234. e55. 10.1016/j.ejogrb.2018.08.276.
18. Nageotte Michael P. Avoiding 5 common mistakes in FHR monitoring. *Contemporary OB/GYN*. 2007. 52.5.
19. Murray ML. Maternal or fetal heart rate? Avoiding intrapartum misidentification. *J Obstet Gynecol Neonatal Nurs*. 2004;33:93–104.
20. Dan J Sherman, Eugenia Frenkel, Yaffa Kurzweil, Anna Padua, Shlomo Arieli, and Murat Bahar. Characteristics of maternal heart rate patterns during labour and delivery. *Obstet Gynecol*. 2002. 99:542-7.

CHAPTER 16

Meconium-Stained Amniotic Fluid

Assessment and Management

N HEPHZIBAH KIRUBAMANI

INTRODUCTION

The passage of fetal colonic contents into the amniotic fluid during the antenatal period or in labour results in **meconium-stained amniotic fluid (MSAF)**. There is no confirmatory test to diagnose meconium-stained amniotic fluid; it is only a clinical diagnosis and relies on the visual observation of greenish discolouration of the amniotic fluid.

The passage of meconium in the neonate usually occurs within 24 to 48 hours after birth [1]. Meconium in the amniotic fluid is seen in 10–20% of deliveries. Perinatal morbidity and mortality are increased when there is meconium in the amniotic fluid [2].

The occurrence of MSAF is usually after 37 weeks of gestation and is a sign of the maturation of the fetal gut. **Fetal hypoxia** causes increased peristalsis and relaxation of the anal sphincters and results in the passage of meconium in utero. Clinicians must differentiate pathological causes, namely hypoxia or infection, from physiological causes of MSAF. Meconium in the amniotic fluid may be a sign of fetal distress [5], and when associated with fetal heart rate abnormalities, may require immediate delivery.

The aspiration of meconium can result in respiratory distress and **meconium aspiration syndrome** (MAS). In severe cases, it can be life-threatening. In recent times, the incidence of meconium aspiration syndrome has decreased because of reduced postterm deliveries and timely management of abnormal fetal heart rate patterns, which in turn, reduces the number of infants with low Apgar scores. Significant reductions in the incidence of MAS and perinatal deaths are attributed to elective induction of pregnancies at or beyond 41 weeks [6,7].

Key Point

Elective induction of pregnancies at or beyond 41 weeks has brought about a significant reduction in the incidence of MAS and perinatal deaths [6,7].

MECONIUM

Composition of Meconium

Meconium is a thick, green or brown, germ-free, viscous substance formed in the fetal intestine at 11–14 weeks of gestation. It is made up primarily of water (70–80%). It is stored in the fetal colon throughout gestation. Its green colour is due to bile pigments [8]. The composition of meconium is detailed in Box 16.1.

Box 16.1 Composition of meconium

- 70–80% water
- Desquamated cells from the intestine and skin
- Gastrointestinal mucin
- Fatty material from the vernix caseosa
- Intestinal secretions
- Lanugo hair
- Bile acids and salts
- Lipids and proteases

There is evidence that inflammatory modulators like IL8 and phospholipase A2 present in the meconium may be the cause of meconium aspiration syndrome.

Fetal Maturation and Meconium

With increasing gestational age, the occurrence of meconium-stained amniotic fluid increases [3,4]. MSAF occurs in 5% of births before 37 weeks of gestation, in 25% of births at term, and in up to 52% of postterm births [9]. The passage of meconium by newborn infants normally occurs within the first 24–48 hours after birth and is a developmentally programmed incident.

The passage of meconium is thought to be caused by **motilin**, a polypeptide that is responsible for peristalsis. Umbilical cord blood in term infants with MSAF has been shown to have higher levels of motilin [8].

The passage of meconium, although a relatively rare event in the preterm fetus, is associated with a particularly high rate of perinatal morbidity and mortality. See the section below on *Preterm meconium staining of the amniotic fluid* for further details.

Key Point

As the maturation of the fetal intestinal myelination and innervation of the parasympathetic system increase with increasing gestational age, the incidence of the passage of meconium also increases. The parasympathetic autonomic nervous system controls fetal bowel movements and sphincter relaxation. When the colon gets filled up, the parasympathetic nervous system gets activated, resulting in the passage of meconium.

EFFECT OF MECONIUM ON THE FETUS

Meconium in the amniotic fluid is hazardous for the fetus. It can cause tissue inflammation in the neonatal lung and placental tissues. In the presence of meconium, the umbilical cord demonstrates vasospasm. It also causes severe ulceration of the umbilical cord [10].

Skin damage can occur due to the corrosive nature of the bile salts and pigments and epithelial cells in MSAF. This damage and desquamation of the skin are collectively called **erythema toxicum neonatorum**.

GRADING AND CLASSIFICATION OF MECONIUM-STAINED AMNIOTIC FLUID

It is difficult to correlate the thickness of meconium with worsening of perinatal outcome due to the subjectivity of assessing meconium thickness. Inter- and intra-observer agreement on the visual grading of MSAF thickness is poor, and it is difficult to compare studies [10]. Many obstetricians consider thick meconium a more ominous sign than thin. Quality evidence is limited regarding the use of a system to grade meconium and its impact on neonatal outcomes.

There is, however, a significant linear association between meconium thickness and the following outcomes:

- Abnormal fetal heart rate patterns during labour
- Low Apgar scores
- The risk of cesarean section delivery
- NICU admission

Grading System for Meconium

A system of grading meconium is summarised in Table 16.1.

Classification of MSAF

The National Institute for Health and Care Excellence [11] classifies MSAF as follows:

- **Non-significant MSAF:** The amniotic fluid is thin, yellow-tinged, or greenish, and contains non-particulate meconium.

Table 16.1 Grading system for meconium

Grade	Description
Grade I—thin	Light green
Grade II	Green, light yellow, or brown; thin, uniform staining of the amniotic fluid
Grade III—thick	Dark green or brown; thick, uniform staining of the amniotic fluid

- **Significant MSAF:** The amniotic fluid is dark green or black, and is thick or tenacious. It may contain lumps of meconium.

MATERNAL RISK FACTORS FOR MSAF

Antenatal and intrapartum factors associated with the presence of MSAF are listed in Table 16.2. MSAF occurs in up to 52% of **postterm pregnancies**[9]. Postterm is the commonest cause of meconium aspiration syndrome. When associated with oligohydramnios and fetal heart rate irregularities due to cord compression, it is associated with increased perinatal morbidity and mortality.

Table 16.2 **Antenatal and intrapartum risk factors for MSAF**

Antenatal risk factors	Intrapartum risk factors
• Postterm pregnancy • Preeclampsia • Advanced maternal age • Fetal growth restriction • Oligohydramnios • Cholestasis of pregnancy • Anemia • Maternal drug abuse (tobacco and cocaine use)	• Fetal heart rate abnormalities • Poor biophysical profile • Oligohydramnios • Induced labour • Prolonged labour (first and second stages) • Malpresentation • Obstructed labour • Chorioamnionitis

Key Point

Postterm pregnancy is the commonest cause of MSAF and associated meconium aspiration syndrome.

There is a strong correlation between **intra-amniotic infection** (chorioamnionitis and endometritis) and the in utero passage of meconium. It is not clear whether the presence of meconium in the amniotic fluid inactivates neutrophil phagocytosis and promotes bacterial growth or whether ingested infected amniotic fluid causes fetal bowel irritation and peristalsis.

Key Points

- Meconium inhibits phagocytosis and reduces neutrophilic oxidative bursts, thus permitting bacterial growth, and changing the antibacterial properties of the amniotic fluid.
- Labour complicated by MSAF has higher rates of chorioamnionitis and endometritis.

There is a higher incidence of meconium-stained amniotic fluid in **obstetric cholestasis** because of the independent association between maternal serum bile acid levels and MSAF.

MSAF AND HYPOXIA

Several theories have been put forward for an association between meconium-stained amniotic fluid and fetal hypoxia and acidosis. Studies conducted in fetal rabbits demonstrated that fetal swallowing and defecation and the normal processes of meconium clearing in fetuses are impaired in hypoxic conditions.

Frequently, when umbilical vein oxygen saturations are below 30%, the passage of meconium occurs. In response to hypoxia, fetal circulation shunts blood away from the bowel and directs it to the brain and heart, resulting in intestinal ischemia. This results in the relaxation of the fetal anal sphincter and increased gastrointestinal peristalsis. As a result, meconium is passed from the fetal gastrointestinal tract.

Key Point

Umbilical cord compression and hypoxic insult stimulate the parasympathetic nervous system which is responsible for fetal bowel movements. This, in turn, causes peristalsis of the bowel and relaxation of the anal sphincter, leading to the passage of meconium into the amniotic cavity.

In a hypoxic situation, erythropoietin is produced but does not cross the placenta. Studies have shown that in fetuses with MSAF secondary to hypoxia, erythropoietin levels were significantly increased. In the rat model, it has been shown that the corticotrophin-releasing factor is a mediator of colonic motility and has been implicated in the pathogenesis of hypoxia-induced meconium-stained amniotic fluid [12].

MSAF and Fetal Distress

The exact correlation between MSAF and fetal distress is still not completely understood, and hence more research is required. Since there is no proper maternal or fetal indicator for MSAF, it is difficult to predict which neonate will require immediate intervention, which one will have adverse outcomes, and which one will develop a cardiorespiratory compromise when born through MSAF. Hence, in the presence of significant MSAF, the neonatal team should be available prior to delivery to provide the full range of newborn resuscitation, from simple stabilisation to full resuscitation, including intubation/ventilation and cardiopulmonary resuscitation (CPR).

> **Key Point**
>
> Fetal hypoxia and infection can be ruled out if the CTG tracing shows reassuring features—stable baseline fetal heart rate with good variability, the presence of accelerations, and the absence of decelerations. In this case, labour can be allowed to continue with vigilant monitoring of the progress of labour. If there is slow progress in labour, oxytocin can be used judiciously.

Preterm Meconium Staining of the Amniotic Fluid

Data on MSAF in preterm pregnancies is limited. Its incidence is approximately 5%. Meconium usually appears as the fetus matures, so its appearance in a preterm fetus suggests that MSAF in this case is a gestational age-independent risk factor. In these neonates, the outcome is poorer than that of neonates with similar gestation and clear amniotic fluid [13].

The greater colonic distance over which the meconium has to travel in the preterm fetus implies that greater severity or duration of stress is required for the passage of meconium. This is the reason for increased perinatal morbidity and mortality in preterm infants born through MSAF.

Meconium passage is a risk factor for microbial invasion, chorioamnionitis, and preterm delivery. It is not clear whether meconium-stained amniotic fluid is a sign of illness or whether it predicts an adverse outcome.

DIAGNOSIS OF MSAF

The diagnosis of MSAF is only made by clinical visualisation after the rupture of membranes; no practical confirmatory test is available [14].

Transcervical amnioscopy has been used to visualise the colour of the membranes and to predict the presence of MSAF, but this procedure is **no longer performed in a clinical setting**.

There is some evidence to show that **echogenic amniotic fluid seen during ultrasound examination** is associated with an increased incidence of MSAF but the **sensitivity of this method is poor**.

> **Key Point**
>
> No practical test is available to predict or diagnose MSAF prior to the rupture of membranes.

MANAGEMENT OF A WOMAN IN LABOUR WITH MSAF

Clinical Assessment

- In women in labour with MSAF, an initial assessment is performed by abdominal palpation to confirm presentation and rule out breech presentation. The presence of meconium is common with breech presentation and is not significant. Fetal growth restriction should also be ruled out.
- A vaginal examination is performed to assess the stage of labour.
- The fetal heart rate is assessed by auscultation or by cardiotocography to rule out fetal distress.

Principles of Intrapartum Management

- The presence or absence of **significant MSAF** should be documented. In the presence of non-significant MSAF, if there are no other risk factors, intermittent fetal heart monitoring should be continued [15].
  - — **Significant MSAF:** Continuous CTG for any woman with significant MSAF is ideal but may not always be available in low-resource facilities. The obstetric staff should be well-trained in recognising changes in the fetal heart rate using intermittent auscultation. The emphasis should be on listening to the fetal heart immediately after a contraction.
  - — **Non-significant MSAF:** Continuous CTG or careful intermittent auscultation is recommended for a woman with non-significant MSAF depending on risk assessment including the stage of labour, the volume of liquor, parity, and the fetal heart rate pattern.
- The value of intrapartum fetal monitoring in preventing meconium aspiration syndrome (MAS) has not been proven. Nevertheless, fetal heart monitoring alerts the clinician to the presence of fetal hypoxia and allows for the rapid initiation of interventions to reduce the risk of MAS.
- The overall clinical picture, namely parity, the presence of chronic uteroplacental insufficiency or fetal growth restriction, the progress of labour and the need for augmentation of labour should be taken into consideration.
- Induction or augmentation with oxytocin should be undertaken with caution (see section below on *Oxytocin in the presence of MSAF*).
- A neonatologist trained in neonatal resuscitation must be available at the time of delivery.

Indicators of Fetal Distress with MSAF

The presence of **fetal heart rate abnormalities** is a better predictor of fetal hypoxia than the presence of meconium-stained liquor alone (see **Chapter 8**, *Fetal surveillance in labour*). The absence of fetal heart rate abnormalities in the presence of meconium passage is reassuring and is associated with higher Apgar scores.

Key Points

- Hypoxia should be suspected if the CTG tracing shows prolonged fetal bradycardia, persistent fetal tachycardia, loss of accelerations, or deep variable decelerations (see **Chapter 8,** *Fetal surveillance in labour*).
- In such a situation, if spontaneous or operative vaginal birth is not imminent, an emergency cesarean section is indicated.

With MSAF and the absence of fetal heart rate abnormalities, reduced Apgar scores and increased perinatal morbidity and mortality are likely to be due to meconium aspiration at the birth of an otherwise healthy fetus.

Recommendations to Minimise Risk of Fetal Hypoxia in MSAF

Key Point

Every effort should be made to conduct careful intrapartum monitoring in cases of labour with MSAF since it is not possible to avoid antenatal meconium passage.

The role of fetal scalp blood sampling

A difficult test to perform, both technically and in terms of laboratory support, fetal scalp blood sampling never became widely available in India.

Its use has been questioned since it has not been shown to reduce emergency cesarean sections or operative vaginal births or improve long-term perinatal outcomes [16,17]. Fetal scalp blood sampling is now rarely performed, even in high-income countries [18].

Prelabour Rupture of Membranes with Meconium-Stained Amniotic Fluid

In a woman admitted with PROM and MSAF, continuous electronic fetal monitoring (if available) should be carried out. A senior obstetrician should review the woman, and a decision for induction of labour should be taken only after ascertaining all the clinical data. If the meconium is thick and tenacious (significant MSAF), an emergency cesarean delivery is a safe option.

Where Should a Woman with MSAF Deliver?

- **Non-significant MSAF:** A woman with non-significant MSAF and good fetal heart rate and without other risk factors can be retained and managed at the low-risk obstetric unit (primary health centre). She should be monitored as per the guidelines for a low-risk pregnant woman in labour.
- **Significant MSAF:** If meconium is significant, depending on the stage of labour, parity, and current fetal well-being, the woman should be transferred in an ambulance with health personnel to a tertiary obstetric care unit with a neonatal intensive care unit.

Oxytocin in the Presence of MSAF

Before starting oxytocin, the overall clinical picture should be considered. In the presence of thin, non-significant meconium, and if the clinical condition is suitable for oxytocin, vigilant monitoring should be continued.

If the woman is in the early stage of labour, the clinician should weigh the benefits of oxytocin over the risk of hypoxic injury. When fetal heart monitoring shows a non-reassuring trace, the oxytocin should be stopped immediately and, if necessary, a tocolytic should be administered. If these measures fail to improve the fetal condition, the baby should be delivered immediately, with a neonatal team trained in neonatal resuscitation standing by.

In the presence of chronic hypoxia, e.g., postterm pregnancy, and in the presence of an infection, the risks of oxytocin administration may outweigh its benefits.

Key Point

Oxytocin augmentation in arrest disorders, in the presence of thick meconium, may be associated with a higher risk of meconium aspiration.

Amnioinfusion

Amnioinfusion has been proposed as a method of reducing the risk of meconium aspiration syndrome in pregnancies with MSAF. It is suggested that normal saline be infused at body temperature into the amniotic cavity through the cervix. The potential mechanisms for preventing meconium aspiration syndrome and improving fetal outcomes are as follows:

- Dilution of meconium, which reduces mechanical and inflammatory effects
- Relief of oligohydramnios to provide a cushioning effect on the umbilical cord, which corrects recurrent umbilical cord compression that may result in variable fetal heart rate decelerations and fetal acidemia

An earlier systematic review [19] stated that amnioinfusion is associated with significant improvements in perinatal outcomes only in settings that have limited facilities for perinatal surveillance. However, a recent systematic review and meta-analysis [20] found that amnioinfusion appears to decrease the risk of meconium aspiration syndrome in the setting of significant (moderate to thick) amniotic-stained fluid.

Risks of amnioinfusion

Amnioinfusion is associated with the risk of uterine overdistension, hypertonus, infection and amniotic fluid embolism.

The intrapartum management of MSAF is summarised in Fig. 16.1.

Key Point

It is still not clear whether amnioinfusion is the accepted clinical intervention to prevent meconium aspiration syndrome in the presence of moderate to thick meconium. Though a recent meta-analysis [20] states that there is a significant decrease in MAS with amnioinfusion, it has not been adopted as a recommendation in clinical guidelines.

DELIVERY ROOM MANAGEMENT OF THE INFANT BORN THROUGH MSAF

Deliveries with meconium-stained amniotic fluid should be attended by appropriately

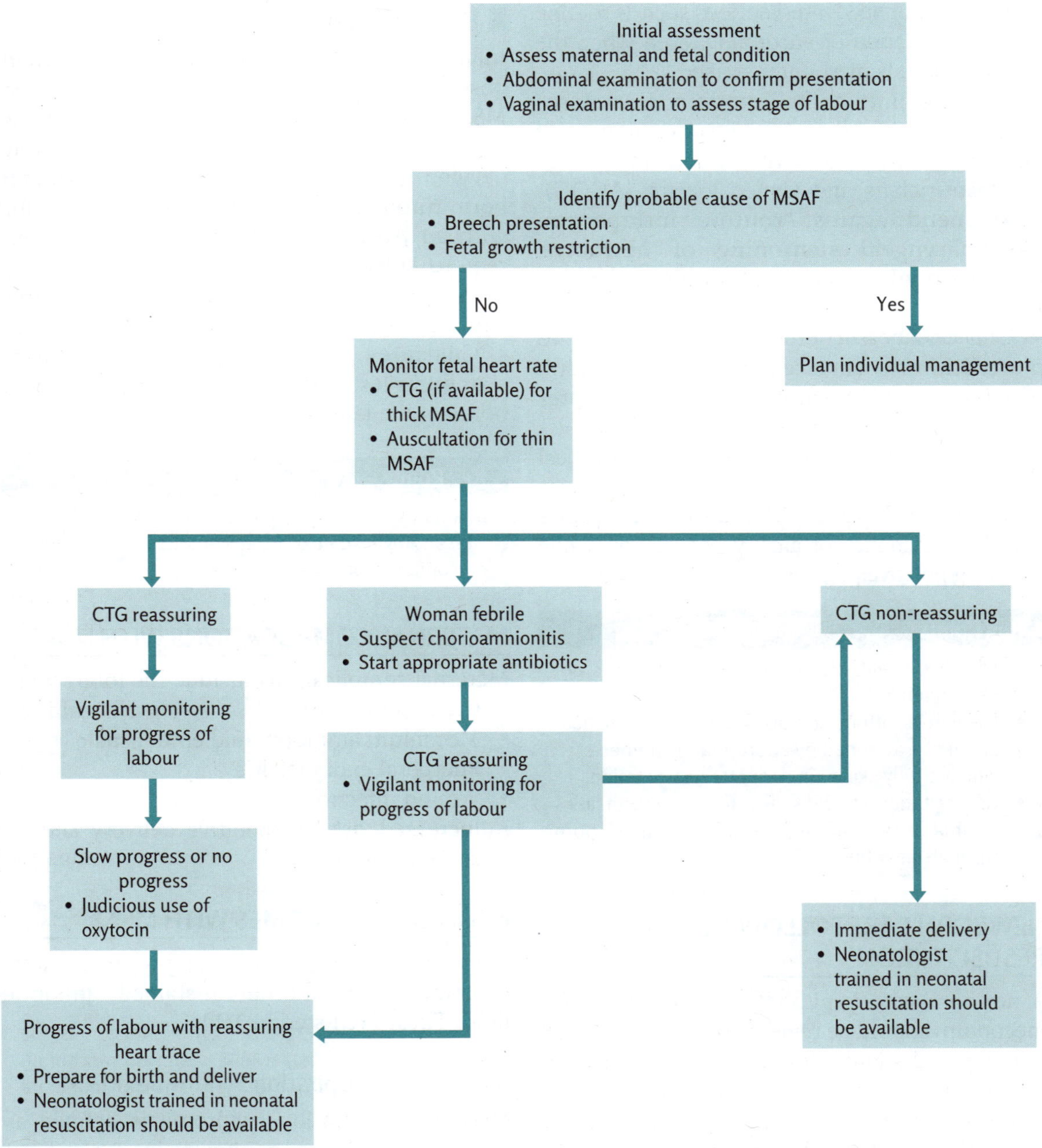

Fig. 16.1 Intrapartum management of meconium-stained amniotic fluid

trained staff fully skilled in neonatal resuscitation. Equipment to monitor the condition of the infant and to support ventilation should be immediately available.

Oropharyngeal Suction on the Perineum

Babies who are breathing well and/or crying are provided skin-to-skin contact with their mothers and should not need interventions such as routine tactile stimulation or suctioning, even when the amniotic fluid is meconium-stained [21].

The guidelines of the American Heart Association (AHA), the American Academy of Pediatrics (AAP), and the American College of Obstetricians and Gynecologists (ACOG), **recommend against routine intrapartum nasopharyngeal suctioning of newborns born through meconium-stained amniotic fluid** [22].

Unnecessary suctioning is best avoided to prevent the risk of induced bradycardia as a result of suctioning of the airway [23]. See **Chapter 44**, *Neonatal resuscitation,* for more details.

Direct laryngoscopy and endotracheal suctioning are not routinely required for babies born through MSAF but can be beneficial to babies who have evidence of airway obstruction while receiving positive pressure ventilation [21,23].

Key Points

- Oropharyngeal suction on the perineum is **not recommended.**
- Deliveries with meconium-stained amniotic fluid should be attended by appropriately trained staff who are fully skilled in neonatal resuscitation.
- Resuscitation should follow the same principles for infants born through MSAF as for those born through clear fluid.

NEWBORN CARE FOLLOWING RESUSCITATION

A newborn who is pink after resuscitation for meconium should be reviewed clinically after 15 minutes and should be assessed for admission to the NICU. Admission to the NICU should be considered if there is a need for respiratory support, ongoing respiratory distress, evidence of encephalopathy or other clinical factors requiring admission. If there are no further problems, the newborn can be observed in the regular nursery and transferred back to the mother when stable.

Postnatal Ward Care

Infants born through MSAF need further observation. Only 5% of infants born through MSAF develop meconium aspiration syndrome (MAS). Newborns presenting with MAS develop it within 15 minutes of birth. Infants born through significant meconium staining with an Apgar score >8 at 5 minutes rarely require subsequent respiratory support [24]. They should be observed at 1 and 2 hours of life and then every 2 hours until 12 hours of life.

Guidance for non-significant meconium staining is less clear but monitoring at 1 and 2 hours of life is recommended [25].

Key Point

Infants born through significant meconium staining with an Apgar score of >8 at 5 minutes rarely develop meconium aspiration syndrome.

MATERNAL COMPLICATIONS WITH MSAF

Maternal complications include the following:

- Chorioamnionitis
- Meconium amniotic fluid embolism
- Puerperal endometritis
- Wound infection
- Increased risk of operative delivery and its complications

NEONATAL OUTCOMES WITH MSAF

There are short-term and long-term neonatal outcomes with meconium-stained amniotic fluid. These are listed in Table 16.3.

Meconium Aspiration Syndrome (MAS)

Meconium aspiration syndrome is defined as respiratory distress occurring in a newborn born through MSAF due to the aspiration of meconium into the tracheobronchial airways prior to, during, or immediately after birth, with radiological findings not attributable to any other cause [24].

Table 16.3 Neonatal outcomes with MSAF

Short-term outcomes	Long-term outcomes
• Low Apgar score • Increased need for neonatal resuscitation • Respiratory distress • Admission to the neonatal intensive care unit • Meconium aspiration syndrome • Neonatal sepsis • Pulmonary disease	• Intellectual disability • Cerebral palsy

Earlier, it was thought that the aspiration of meconium-stained amniotic fluid occurred only during the first few breaths after delivery. However, meconium has been found distally as far as the alveoli in some stillborn infants. Studies with radio-opaque contrast and Cr51-labelled erythrocytes injected into the amniotic fluid have demonstrated that amniotic fluid enters the fetal lungs in the non-asphyxiated human fetus, suggesting in utero aspiration of meconium. Animal experiments have shown that intrauterine gasping results in greater aspiration of meconium in fetuses when they are exposed to hypoxia.

Key Point

Intrauterine gasping in the presence of hypoxia results in greater aspiration of meconium in fetuses. There is no way of predicting which fetus will develop meconium aspiration from intrauterine gasping and which one will develop it by inhalation at birth.

MAS develops in approximately 5–10% of infants born through MSAF. Persistent pulmonary hypertension develops in 5–6%. Mortality varies from 5–10% despite appropriate treatment [25]. Neonatal seizures and chronic seizure disorders are also associated with MAS [26].

The commonest cause of severe respiratory distress in term neonates is MAS which can result in significant neonatal morbidity and mortality. MAS is most commonly associated with postterm delivery and oligohydramnios [27]. Oligohydramnios can lead to cord compression and meconium passage, which results in thicker meconium-stained liquor and hence, leads to MAS.

Diagnosis of MAS

The diagnosis of MAS in the neonate is based on clinical and radiological findings.

Clinical findings

- Low Apgar score (<8)
- Rapid, laboured, or absent breathing
- Barrel-shaped chest with an increased anterior–posterior diameter caused by overinflation
- Nasal flaring, and in-drawing of intercostal spaces
- Cyanosis
- Rales and rhonchi on auscultation
- Signs of postmaturity such as peeling of the skin

Radiological findings

Radiological findings in moderate to severe disease may include the following:

- Hyperinflated lung fields
- Widespread patchy infiltrations alternating with areas of expansion
- Small pleural effusion in 20–30% of cases

Pathophysiology of MAS

The mechanism of MAS is multifactorial and complex, resulting in neonatal hypoxia. The pathophysiology of MAS involves the intrauterine passage of meconium, aspiration, and pulmonary disease resulting in hypoxemia, acidosis, and potentially, pulmonary hypertension (Fig. 16.2).

The aspirated meconium interferes with normal lung function leading to pulmonary disease resulting from the following mechanisms [28]:

- Airway obstruction
- Chemical irritation and inflammation

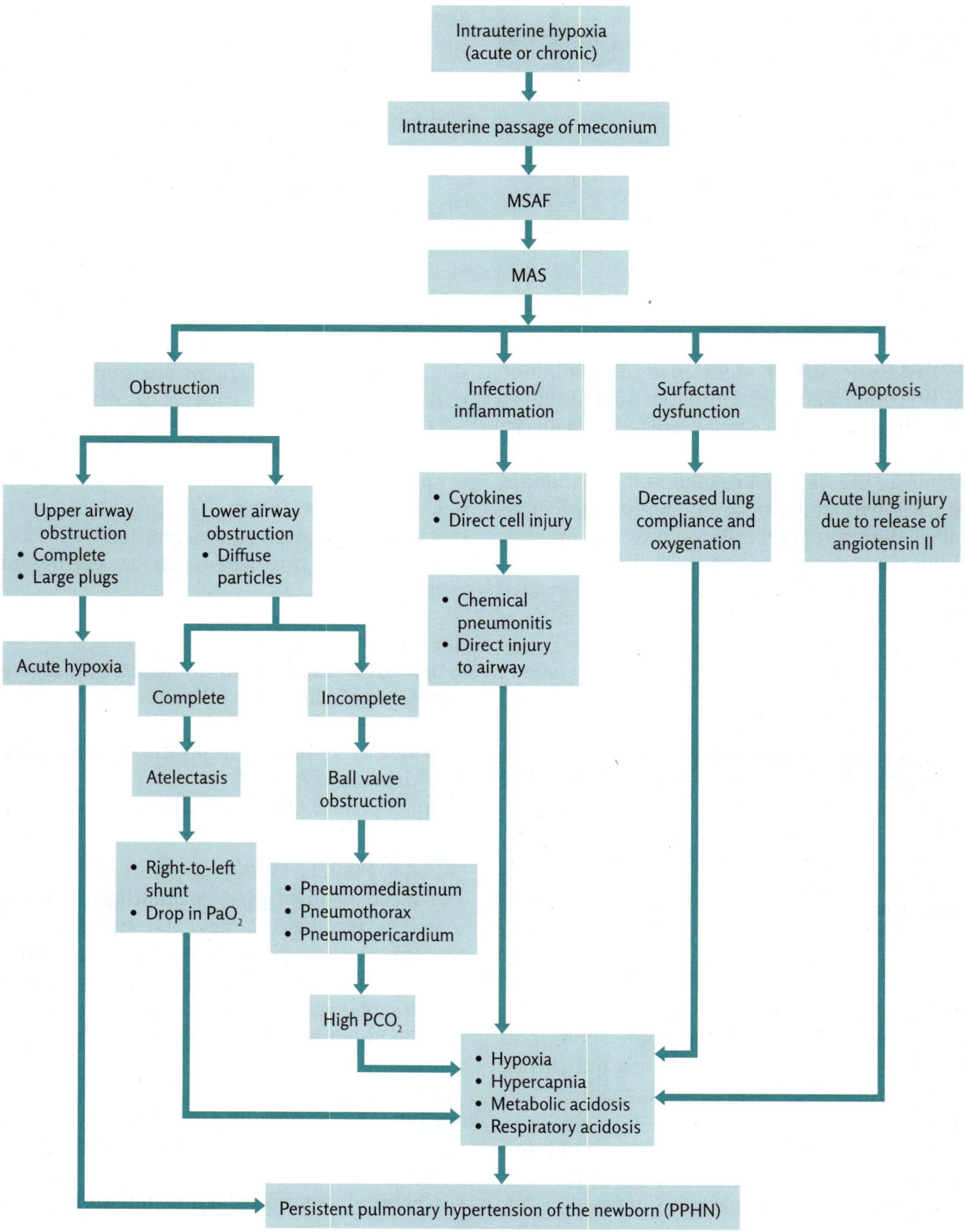

Fig. 16.2 Pathophysiology of meconium aspiration syndrome

- Inactivation and reduced production of surfactant
- Apoptosis

Key Point

Common findings in severe or fatal meconium aspiration syndrome are hypoxia, acidosis, and hypercarbia leading to pulmonary vasoconstriction, which may result in **persistent pulmonary hypertension (PPHN).**

Airway obstruction

Airway obstruction can be partial or complete. Pulmonary air trapping and hyperinflation of the lungs occur when small amounts of meconium migrate to the distal airways. The gas is trapped, rupturing into the pleura and resulting in pneumomediastinum or pneumothorax. Alternately, there is rupture into the pericardium, resulting in pneumopericardium. Atelectasis is caused by an obstruction of the smaller airways with meconium.

Pneumonitis

This is caused by the direct toxic effect of meconium contents and the infiltration of large numbers of polymorphonuclear leukocytes and macrophages into the airway. This inflammatory response of the lung parenchyma results in direct tissue injury and pulmonary vasoconstriction. Chemical pneumonitis is caused by enzymes, bile salts, and free fatty acids which are present in the meconium and irritate the airways. This may occur within a few hours of aspiration.

Surfactant inactivation

Meconium inhibits surfactant synthesis. Surfactant is affected by meconium which lowers the surface tension, thereby decreasing lung compliance and oxygenation. Studies showed that surfactant treatment of infants with MAS did not significantly affect mortality but it reduced the infant's need for extracorporeal membrane oxygenation (ECMO).

Apoptosis

Meconium exposure leads to an angiotensin II-induced apoptosis in lung cells leading to acute lung injury.

Management of MAS in the Labour Room

Delivery room management

Infants who develop MAS generally exhibit signs of respiratory distress immediately after birth [24]. Prompt identification and care of affected neonates decreases morbidity and mortality, especially in those with severe disease. Coordination between the obstetric and neonatal teams is essential in initiating efficient management of infants with MAS.

CONCLUSION

Meconium staining of the amniotic fluid due to the passage of meconium is unpredictable and generally unpreventable. Clinicians should understand the pathogenesis of MSAF and its effect on the fetal respiratory system and be prepared to manage MAS. Thorough evaluation of the woman and monitoring with continuous or periodic FHR monitoring are recommended in cases of labour with significant meconium-stained amniotic fluid.

The combination of a non-reassuring FHR tracing and significant (thick) meconium in the amniotic fluid has been associated with an increased risk of MAS. However, the value of intrapartum fetal monitoring in preventing MAS has not been proven [22]. Nevertheless, fetal heart monitoring alerts the clinician to the presence of fetal hypoxia and allows for the rapid initiation of interventions to reduce the risk of MAS.

REFERENCES

1. Qadir S, Jan S, Chachoo JA, Parveen S. Perinatal and neonatal outcome in meconium-stained amniotic fluid. *Int J Reprod, Contracept, Obstet & Gynecol.* 2016. 5(5):1400-1405.
2. Khatun MHA, Arzu J, Haque E, Kamal M, Al Mamun MA, Khan MFH, et al. Fetal outcome in deliveries with

meconium-stained liquor. *Bangladesh J Child Health.* 2009. Vol 33 (2): 41-45.

3. Kashikar S, Kotpalliwar M, Uttarwar P. Meconium-stained liquor and its impact on maternal and neonatal outcome. *Int J Reprod, Contracept, Obstet & Gynecol.* 2021. 10. 1629. 10.18203/2320-1770.ijrcog20211149.
4. Addisu D, Asres A, Gedefaw G, et al. Prevalence of meconium-stained amniotic fluid and its associated factors among women who gave birth at term in Felege Hiwot comprehensive specialized referral hospital, North-West Ethiopia: A facility based cross-sectional study. *BMC Pregnancy Childbirth.* 2018. 18, 429.
5. Begum Nasrin, Sharmeen Mahmood, Salma Akthter, Munmun M, Haque S, Nahar KN, Chowdhury SB. Perinatal outcome associated with meconium-stained amniotic fluid in pregnancy. *Journal of Paediatric Surgeons of Bangladesh.* 2013. Vol. 4 (2): 44-49.
6. Swarnam K, Soraisham AS, Sivanandan S. Advances in the management of meconium aspiration syndrome. *Int J Pediatr.* 2012. 359571.
7. Arwa Abbas Hussain, Mohammad Yawar Yakoob, Aamer Imdad, Zulfiqar A Bhutta. Elective induction for pregnancies at or beyond 41 weeks of gestation and its impact on stillbirths: A systematic review with meta-analysis. *BMC Public Health.* 2011. 11(Suppl 3). S5, 2-12.
8. Rahman S, Unsworth J, and Vause S. Meconium in Labour. *Obstetrics, Gynaecology & Reproductive Medicine.* 2013. 23, 247-252.
9. Silassie R, Gebretsadik W, Degefa N, Getahun D, Kassie N. Determinants of meconium-stained amniotic fluid at Hadiya Zone Hospitals, Southern Ethiopia. Unmatched case-control study. *Int J Women's Health.* 2022.14:1351-1360.
10. Sian Mitchell, Edwin Chandraharan. Meconium-stained amniotic fluid. *Obstetrics, Gynaecology & Reproductive Medicine.* 2018. Vol 28. Issue 4, Pages 120-124.
11. National Institute for Health and Care Excellence (NICE) guidance (CG190). Intrapartum care for healthy women and babies. 2014.
12. Jayaraman Lakshmanan, Sureshbabu N Ahanya, Virender Rehan, Noboru Oyachi, Michael G Ross. Elevated plasma corticotrophin release factor levels and *in utero* **meconium passage.** *International Pediatric Research Foundation, Inc.* 2007 Vol. 61, No. 2-176 -179.
13. Scott H, Walker M, Gruslin A. Significance of meconium-stained amniotic fluid in the preterm population. *J Perinatol.* 2001. 21:174–7.
14. Karamustafaoglu Balci B, Goynumer G. Incidence of echogenic amniotic fluid at term pregnancy and its association with meconium. *Arch Gynecol Obstet.* 2018. (4) 297:915.
15. National Institute for Health and Care Excellence (NICE) guidance. 2017. Meconium-stained liquor. Guidelines for the management of labour.
16. Chandraharan E. Should national guidelines continue to recommend fetal scalp blood sampling during labor? *J Matern Fetal Neonatal Med.* 2016. 29:368.
17. Carbonne B, Pons K, Maisonneuve E. Foetal scalp blood sampling during labour for pH and lactate measurements. *Best Pract Res Clin Obstet Gynaecol.* 2016. 30:62.
18. Miller DA. Prenatal care: Intrapartum fetal heart rate monitoring. Berghella V (Ed). *UpToDate.* 2022. Waltham, MA.
19. Hofmeyr GJ, Xu H, Eke AC. Amnioinfusion for meconium-stained liquor in labour. *Cochrane Database of Systematic Reviews.* 2014. Issue 1. Art. No.: CD000014.
20. Davis JD, Sanchez-Ramos L, McKinney JA, et al. Intrapartum amnioinfusion reduces meconium aspiration syndrome and improves neonatal outcomes in patients with meconium-stained fluid: A systematic review and meta-analysis. *Am J Obstet Gynecol.* 2023. 228:S1179.
21. Wyckoff MH, Wyllie J, Aziz K, et al. On behalf of the Neonatal Life Support Collaborators. Neonatal life support: 2020 International Consensus on Cardiopulmonary Resuscitation and Emergency Cardiovascular Care Science with Treatment Recommendations. *Circulation.* 2020. 142 (suppl 1): S185–S221.
22. Garcia-Prats JA. Meconium aspiration syndrome: Prevention and management. Martin R. (Ed). *UpToDate.* 2023. Waltham, MA.
23. Aziz K, Lee HC, Escobedo MB, et al. Part 5: Neonatal resuscitation: 2020 American Heart Association Guidelines for Cardiopulmonary Resuscitation and Emergency Cardiovascular Care. *Circulation.* 2020. 142(suppl 2):S524–S550.
24. van Ierland Y, de Boer M, de Beaufort AJ. Meconium-stained amniotic fluid: Discharge vigorous newborns. *Arch Dis Child Fetal Neonatal Ed.* 2010. 95(1):F69-71.
25. Swarnam K, Soraisham AS, Sivanandan S. Advances in the management of meconium aspiration syndrome. *Int J Pediatr.* 2012. 359571.
26. Iliodromiti Z, Grigoriadis C, Vrachnis N, Siristatidis C, Varras M, Creatsas G. Association of meconium-stained amniotic fluid with fetal and neonatal brain injury. *Neonatal Care.* InTech. 2012.
27. Fleischer A, Anyaegbunam A, Guidetti D, Randolph G, Merkatz IR. A persistent clinical problem: profile of the term infant with significant respiratory complications. *Obstet Gynecol.* 1992 Feb;79(2):185-90.
28. Garcia-Prats JA. Meconium aspiration syndrome: Pathophysiology, clinical manifestations, and diagnosis. Martin R. (Ed). *UpToDate.* 2023. Waltham, MA.

CHAPTER 17

Management of Labour in Multiple Pregnancy

NASHWA ELTAWEEL, HELENA BLAKEWAY, ASMA KHALIL

INTRODUCTION

Multiple pregnancies are at an increased risk of preterm birth, preeclampsia, low birth weight, stillbirth, and intrapartum complications. This results in increased perinatal morbidity and mortality as compared to singleton births. Admission to the neonatal unit, perinatal death, and cerebral palsy are more common in multiple pregnancies as compared to singletons [1]. Additionally, chorionicity independently impacts perinatal mortality and morbidity with higher perinatal complications reported even in uncomplicated monochorionic (MC) pregnancies when compared to dichorionic (DC) and singleton pregnancies [2,3].

Twin pregnancies have a higher rate of preterm birth when compared to singletons and account for almost 20% of all preterm births [4]. Chorionicity affects this risk—it is higher among MC twins when compared to DC twins [5]. Both iatrogenic and spontaneous preterm birth are more common in MC compared to DC twins.

This chapter will summarise the evidence on the management of labour in multiple pregnancies, including the mode and timing of delivery in complicated and uncomplicated twin births.

Key Point

There is a higher incidence of preterm birth (spontaneous or iatrogenic) and of cesarean birth, both elective and emergency, in multiple pregnancy.

NOMENCLATURE DURING LABOUR

Twins are labelled during the first-trimester scan as Twin A and B or Twin 1 and 2. This depends on the position (lower and upper; left and right) of the twins. Labelling is important in the management of all twin pregnancies to ensure that biometric measurements from longitudinal growth scans are consistently allocated to the same twin at each visit.

This nomenclature should be followed by everyone involved in the management of the pregnancy to ensure the correct identification of the twins as Twin A or B even if they change position, which can happen during pregnancy or around birth. Labelling may be easier in dichorionic diamniotic (DCDA) twins with discordant sex or different placental locations. In monochorionic monoamniotic (MCMA) twins, a discordant anomaly or obvious weight discordance can be helpful in identifying the twins.

In same-sex twins, identification is based on the orientation of one twin relative to the other—left or right lateral for twins positioned next to each other and top (fundal) or bottom (cervical) for twins positioned vertically (Fig. 17.1a and b). While the presenting twin in laterally-oriented twins may change as the pregnancy or labour progresses, the bottom twin of vertically-oriented twins is likely to remain the presenting twin throughout pregnancy.

It is important to maintain the nomenclature of twins during labour too. Twin A or Twin 1 does not necessarily mean the presenting twin.

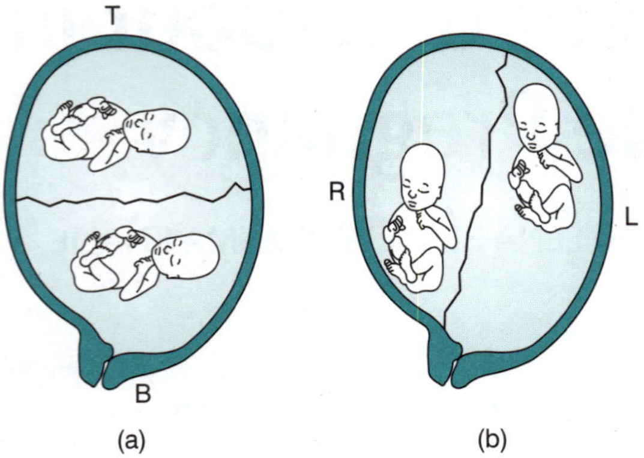

Fig. 17.1 Diagrammatic representation of twin orientation relative to the longitudinal axis of the uterus: (a) The twins may be vertically oriented (top/bottom [T/B]) or (b) laterally oriented (right/left [R/L])

Twin B or Twin 2 may become the presenting twin and can be delivered first. A careful review of the antenatal reports can help to determine which twin is which.

Key Point

Twin labelling is defined differently by obstetricians and sonographers during the pregnancy than it is by pediatricians at birth. Pediatricians label the first-born twin as Twin 1.

ADVERSE OUTCOMES IN MULTIPLE PREGNANCY

There are often concerns surrounding labour and delivery in twin pregnancy due to the difficulty in monitoring both twins during labour.

With the reducing incidence of vaginal breech delivery, fewer obstetricians have the skill to manage a breech delivery or perform internal podalic version if it is required. This must be taken into account when making decisions regarding delivery.

Research has shown that it is particularly difficult to monitor the second twin; often, substandard monitoring takes place [6].

The risks to the second twin in labour include the following:

- Cord prolapse
- Malposition
- Abnormal CTG
- Placental abruption
- Prolonged latency between both deliveries

Key Point

An experienced obstetrician should be present during labour in cases of multiple pregnancies as there is a fair chance of interventions being required.

Preterm Birth and Vaginal Delivery

- **32–36+6 weeks:** A decade ago, the twin birth study [7] did not show any differences in composite fetal and neonatal outcomes between elective cesarean and vaginal delivery in uncomplicated DC twins between 32 and 36+6 weeks, with the first twin being cephalic.
- **Late preterm (37–39 weeks):** A secondary analysis of the same data revealed that elective cesarean can be protective against poor neonatal outcomes after 37 weeks but not for deliveries between 32 and 37 weeks [8].
- **Extremely preterm birth (<28 weeks):** An individualised care plan should be put in place regarding the mode of delivery. This should include a multidisciplinary discussion including the risks and benefits of both cesarean and vaginal delivery. The chances of survival should be considered depending on gestational age, estimated fetal weight, and the neonatal care available. The impact of cesarean birth on future obstetric outcomes should also be kept in mind.

PLACE OF DELIVERY

When planning a twin birth, it is important that the place of delivery has the following (Fig. 17.2):

- A labour room big enough to accommodate the larger number of personnel needed at the time of delivery
- Experienced obstetrician and midwives/nurses
- Ultrasound equipment to locate the fetal heart of both twins and determine fetal position and presentation
- Facility for continuous fetal heart monitoring of both twins during labour

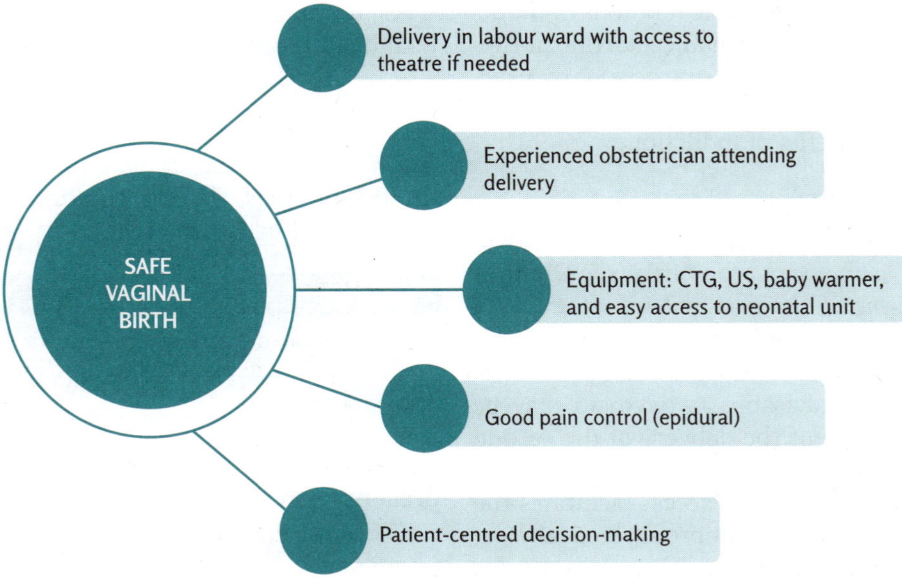

Fig. 17.2 Requirements for a safe twin vaginal birth
CTG, cardiotocography; *US*, ultrasound scan

- Pediatrician/neonatologist, resuscitation equipment, and easy access to the neonatal ICU
- Anesthetist who can provide epidural analgesia (if feasible)
- Immediate access to the theatre if an urgent cesarean section is required
- Measures for prevention and management of postpartum hemorrhage
- Access to blood bank

Key Point

Ultrasound imaging may be used to locate the fetal heart of each twin while establishing CTG monitoring.

MODE OF DELIVERY

The choice of route of delivery depends on:
- Amnionicity
- Fetal presentation at the onset of labour (80% of first twins are cephalic)
- Gestational age
- The obstetrician's familiarity with internal podalic version, breech extraction, and external cephalic version

Vaginal Delivery and Trial of Labour

- **Cephalic–cephalic diamniotic twins:** In the absence of any obstetric indication for cesarean birth, vaginal delivery is recommended.
- **Cephalic–non-cephalic diamniotic twins:** Trial of labour and breech extraction of the second twin is recommended if the obstetrician has experience with internal podalic version. Non-cephalic second twins have comparable, if not higher, rates of vaginal delivery than second twins in cephalic presentation [9].

The majority of twins are cephalic–cephalic at the onset of labour [10]. However, 30% of non-cephalic second twins are known to become cephalic after the birth of the first twin [9].

Induction of labour

In the presence of an obstetric indication, neither induction nor augmentation of labour is contraindicated. A standard protocol of labour induction for singleton gestations would apply for twins with overall favourable intrapartum outcomes [11]. The available methods of induction (prostaglandins, mechanical, artificial rupture of membranes, and oxytocin) are used. Women should be counselled antenatally about the risks and benefits of induction.

Delivery of the first twin

The procedure for the delivery of the first twin is the same as in a singleton birth (see **Chapter 4**, *Management of the first and second stages of normal labour*). The indications for episiotomy or operative delivery follow the same principles.

IV access is advisable as oxytocin may be required to augment the delivery of the second twin. Women with multiple pregnancy are at a higher risk of PPH, and IV access facilitates the administration of oxytocics prophylactically.

Delayed cord clamping is appropriate for DC twins but not for MC twins.

> **Key Point**
>
> It is good practice to use a single clamp to help identify the cord of the first twin, and two clamps for the cord of the second twin.

Delivery of the second twin

After clamping the cord of the first twin, uterotonics are avoided. The membranes should not be artificially ruptured till the presentation of the second twin is confirmed, and a decision has been made about the mode of delivery.

Interval between the delivery of the first and second twin

The interval between the births of the two twins can be variable. Though 30 minutes is often said to be the maximum time that should be allowed between the birth of the two babies, as long as the second twin can be monitored and its well-being can be confirmed, there are no specific recommendations on how soon after the birth of the first twin the second twin can be delivered.

It is essential to continuously monitor the fetal heart rate of the second twin. Continuous CTG (if available) is strongly recommended for fetal heart monitoring during labour [6].

Confirming presentation

It is important to check the presentation of the second twin because, as mentioned earlier, in up to 30% of cases, the presentation may change from what it had been earlier.

> **Key Point**
>
> Following the delivery of the first twin, ultrasound is useful in determining the presentation of the second twin.

Options for vaginal delivery based on presentation

- **Second twin in cephalic presentation and engaged:** If contractions decrease or stop, labour is augmented with oxytocin. Artificial rupture of membranes is performed once the head is engaged.
- **Second twin in cephalic presentation and unengaged:**
  - Controlled amniotomy till the head drops into the pelvis, followed by augmentation and delivery

    or
  - Internal podalic version by grasping the feet and performing breech extraction
- **Second twin in non-cephalic presentation:**
  - External cephalic version followed by delivery (see **Chapter 27**, *Breech delivery [including external cephalic version]*)
  - Internal podalic version followed by breech extraction

Internal podalic version (IPV)

This procedure is ideally performed in a relaxed uterus with adequate analgesia. Oxytocin is stopped if it is being infused for augmentation. If ultrasound is available, it can help in the visualisation of the fetal lie, particularly to identify which side the fetal back is on. It is important to identify the foot by feeling the heel so that a fetal hand is not mistakenly pulled down.

The operator grasps both feet at the ankles, with the middle finger inserted between the ankles (Fig. 17.3) and, with gentle traction, brings the feet down into the vagina. The membranes are not ruptured until the feet are in the vagina. However, the membranes may rupture during the process of manipulation. Delivery is then completed by breech extraction.

A Danish study did not show increased benefits of cesarean when compared to IPV with respect to fetal outcomes or reduction of adverse perinatal outcomes [12]. However, IPV is not a procedure that all obstetricians are trained to perform. If the attending obstetrician is not trained to perform IPV and vaginal breech delivery, cesarean section may be a safer option.

Cesarean section for the second twin

The reported incidence of an unplanned cesarean for the second twin is 3–10% of twin labours. The reasons for this include the following:

- Change in the cephalic presentation of the second twin
- Fetal distress
- Cord prolapse
- Maternal complications
- Non-progress of labour

An unplanned section for the second twin increases neonatal morbidity.

Cesarean Delivery

The indications for cesarean delivery for a twin pregnancy are as follows:

- All monoamniotic twins
- Diamniotic twins with a non-cephalic presenting twin
- Other obstetrical indications such as placenta previa
- Twin-to-twin transfusion syndrome
- Second twin with an estimated fetal weight of <1500 g
- Gestational age <28 weeks

TIMING OF DELIVERY

Uncomplicated Twin Pregnancy

The timing of delivery is dictated by chorionicity and amnionicity. However, it is not always possible to schedule a delivery as 50% of twin pregnancies will deliver preterm, either spontaneously or for an obstetric indication [13].

There are many factors that must be considered when deciding on delivery, in

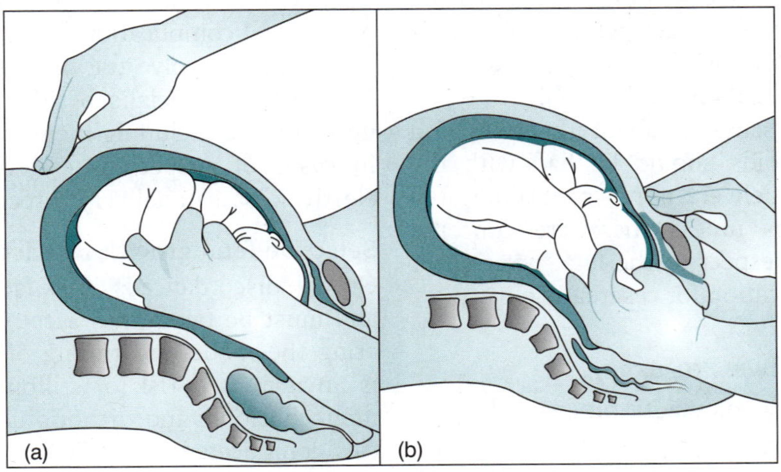

Fig. 17.3 Internal podalic version: (a) The fetal feet are identified and grasped at the ankles, with the operator's middle finger inserted between the ankles and (b) as downward traction is exerted on the feet, the suprapubic hand applies upward pressure on the head, and a breech extraction is carried out

particular, the increased risks associated with twin pregnancy. This includes the increased risk of preeclampsia, selective fetal growth restriction (sFGR), as well as monochorionic-related risks, mainly twin-twin transfusion syndrome (TTTS), leading to spontaneous or iatrogenic preterm birth.

Dichorionic diamniotic (DCDA) pregnancy

A systematic review and meta-analysis [14] assessed the prospective risk of stillbirths and neonatal complications in uncomplicated DCDA pregnancies and recommended **delivery at 37+0 to 37+6 weeks.**

Monochorionic diamniotic (MCDA) pregnancy

Monochorionic twins are at a higher risk of stillbirth near term even without identified pregnancy complications. The stillbirth rate is reported to be three times higher as compared to dichorionic twins. This could be due to undiagnosed twin anemia polycythemia sequence (TAPS), acute fetal transfusion, or selective fetal growth restriction (sFGR) [15].

The NICE guideline for twins and triplet pregnancy [16] recommends that delivery should be offered **from 36 weeks** onwards. ACOG and SMFM recommend a wider gestational age for uncomplicated MC twins and suggest delivery **between 34 and 37+6 weeks** [17].

A detailed discussion about the risks and benefits of steroids should be had with the couple. Vaginal delivery is not contraindicated in MCDA twins unless there are concerns identified with respect to the fetal position or an obstetric indication for cesarean delivery.

Complicated Twin Pregnancy

Monochorionic monoamniotic pregnancy

For monochorionic monoamniotic pregnancies, planned delivery is recommended **between 32 and 34 weeks** of gestation due to the increased risk of intrauterine fetal death in the third trimester. Evidence shows double the risk of intrauterine fetal demise (IUFD) between 32 and 34 weeks.

Antenatal hospital admission is recommended, with a reported 3% rate of IUFD among the inpatient group, whereas the rate was 7% among the women managed as outpatients in the MONOMONO study [18]. The study showed an overall perinatal mortality of 10.8% with a non-significant statistical difference in fetal mortality between the inpatient and outpatient groups.

In MCMA twin pregnancies, **cesarean section** is the recommended mode of delivery [19].

1 in 5 women scheduled for delivery at 32 weeks will deliver before that date; 1 in 3 women will deliver before their planned delivery at 34 weeks [20]. An individualised plan is recommended, taking into account the full clinical picture, maternal risks, course of pregnancy, and chronic complications associated with pregnancy.

Complicated monochorionic diamniotic (MCDA) pregnancy

When complications occur, especially among monochorionic twins, the risks and benefits of early delivery to prevent stillbirth versus the risk of neonatal complications should be discussed. This should involve the neonatologist and the fetal medicine specialist besides the obstetrician, updating and including the woman at all times. In cases of suspected fetal compromise, an elective cesarean delivery is recommended.

Selective fetal growth restriction

Growth discordance is a risk factor for stillbirth and must be taken into account when considering the mode and timing of delivery. There is an increased risk of stillbirth among both monochorionic and dichorionic twin pregnancies complicated with sFGR. The risk of stillbirth is higher from 37 weeks onwards than it is between 36 and 37 weeks [15]. Therefore, delivery is recommended **before 36 weeks**. The decision about delivery must be individualised to balance neonatal mortality and morbidity with stillbirth risk. There is no evidence to support vaginal birth among cases of selective growth restriction.

Twin-to-twin transfusion syndrome (TTTS)
Fetal laser surgery (FLS) is the most successful treatment for twin-to-twin transfusion syndrome. If delivery is indicated as a treatment of acute TTTS or late-onset TTTS, cesarean section should be considered as the most suitable mode of delivery. A history of FLS alone is not considered an indication for cesarean delivery.

The recommended timing of delivery for uncomplicated and complicated twin pregnancy is summarised in Fig. 17.4.

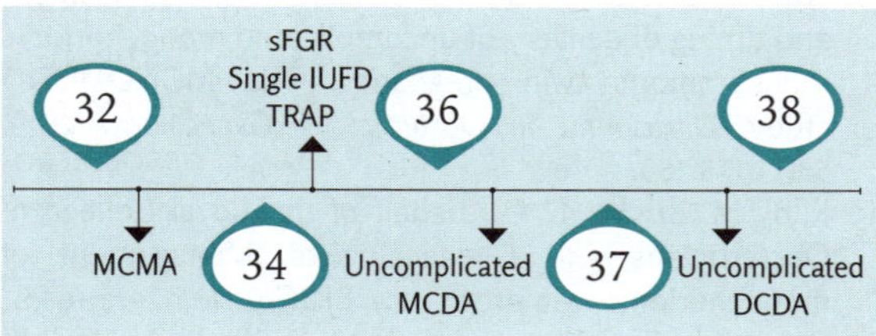

Fig. 17.4 Recommended gestational age for the delivery of complicated and uncomplicated twin pregnancies
DCDA, dichorionic diamniotic twin; *IUFD*, intrauterine fetal demise; *MCDA*, monochorionic diamniotic twin; *MCMA*, monochorionic monoamniotic twin; *sFGR*, selective fetal growth restriction; *TRAP*, twin reversed arterial perfusion

THIRD STAGE OF LABOUR

PPH: Women with multiple pregnancies are at increased risk of **atonic PPH** due to an overdistended uterus and prolonged delivery. Active management of the third stage of labour is recommended. It is good practice to have access to the PPH box in the room during labour (uterotonics, urinary catheter, and IV fluids) anticipating PPH.

Cord clamping: Delayed cord clamping is considered safe for the first twin if there are no CTG concerns for the second twin. If there are any concerns with the second twin, immediate cord clamping is advisable to enable managing the second twin.

Placenta: Delivery of the placenta of the first twin and the administration of uterotonics should be postponed until the delivery of the second twin to avoid placental separation.

> **Key Point**
>
> Active management of the third stage of labour is recommended in anticipation of PPH. The placenta should not be delivered until both twins are delivered, even in DCDA twins.

CONCLUSION

Multiple pregnancy is associated with an increased risk of maternal and perinatal morbidity and mortality. Management of labour depends on the presentation of the first twin, the chorionicity and amnionicity of the twins and the presence of complications specific to twin pregnancy. The mode and timing of delivery should be discussed early in the third trimester and decisions should be made taking the woman's preferences into consideration. An experienced obstetric and neonatal team should be available at the time of labour. The risk of postpartum hemorrhage is increased with a twin pregnancy, and hence, preparations should be made in anticipation.

REFERENCES

1. Gezer A, Rashidova M, Güralp O, Öçer F. Perinatal mortality and morbidity in twin pregnancies: The relation between chorionicity and gestational age at birth. Archives of *Gynecology and Obstetrics*. 2012. 285:353–60.
2. Hack KE, Derks J, Elias S, Franx A, Roos E, Voerman S, et al. Increased perinatal mortality and morbidity in monochorionic versus dichorionic twin pregnancies: Clinical implications of a large Dutch cohort study. *BJOG*. 2008. 115(1):58-67.
3. Sung J-H, Kim SH, Kim Y-M, Kim J-H, Kim M-N, Lee HR, et al. Neonatal outcomes of twin pregnancies delivered at late-preterm versus term gestation based on chorionicity and indication for delivery. *Journal of Perinatal Medicine*. 2016. 44(8):903-11.

4. Martin JA, Hamilton BE, Osterman MJ. Births in the United States, 2013. NCHS Data Brief. 2014.
5. Litwinska E, Syngelaki A, Cimpoca B, Frei L, Nicolaides KH. Outcome of twin pregnancy with two live fetuses at 11-13 weeks' gestation. *Ultrasound Obstet Gynecol.* 2020. 55(1):32–38.
6. Bakker P, Colenbrander G, Verstraeten A, Van Geijn H. Quality of intrapartum cardiotocography in twin deliveries. *American Journal of Obstetrics and Gynecology.* 2004. 191(6):2114-9.
7. Barrett JF, Hannah ME, Hutton EK, Willan AR, Allen AC, Armson BA, et al. A randomized trial of planned cesarean or vaginal delivery for twin pregnancy. *New England Journal of Medicine.* 2013. 369(14):1295-305.
8. Zafarmand M, Goossens S, Tajik P, Bossuyt P, Asztalos E, Gardener G, et al. Planned cesarean or planned vaginal delivery for twins: Secondary analysis of randomized controlled trial. *Ultrasound in Obstetrics & Gynecology.* 2021. 57(4):582-91.
9. Easter SR, Lieberman E, Carusi D. Fetal presentation and successful twin vaginal delivery. *Am J Obstet Gynecol.* 2016. 214(1):116.e1-116.e10.
10. Chasen ST, Spiro SJ, Kalish RB, Chervenak FA. Changes in fetal presentation in twin pregnancies. *J Matern Fetal Neonatal Med.* 2005. 17(1):45-8.
11. Wolfe MD, de la Torre L, Moore LE, et al. Is the protocol for induction of labor in singletons applicable to twin gestations? *J Reprod Med.* 2013. 58:137.
12. Jonsdottir F, Henriksen L, Secher NJ, Maaløe N. Does internal podalic version of the non-vertex second twin still have a place in obstetrics? A Danish national retrospective cohort study. *Acta obstetricia et gynecologica Scandinavica.* 2015. 94(1):59-64.
13. Kogan MD, Alexander GR, Kotelchuck M, et al. Trends in twin birth outcomes and prenatal care utilization in the United States, 1981-1997. *JAMA.* 2000. 284:335.
14. Cheong-See F, Schuit E, Arroyo-Manzano D, et al. Prospective risk of stillbirth and neonatal complications in twin pregnancies: Systematic review and meta-analysis. *BMJ.* 2016. 354:i4353.
15. Koch AK, Burger RJ, Schuit E, Mateus JF, Goya M, Carreras E, et al. Timing of delivery for twins with growth discordance and growth restriction: An individual participant data meta-analysis. *Obstetrics and Gynecology.* 2022. 139(6):1155.
16. NICE Guidance. Twin and triplet pregnancy. 2019. Available at www.nice.org.uk/guidance/ng137
17. Multifetal gestations: Twin, triplet, and higher-order multifetal pregnancies. ACOG Practice Bulletin, number 231. *Obstet Gynecol.* 2021. 1;137(6):e145-e162.
18. Group MW, Saccone G, Berghella V, Locci M, Ghi T, Frusca T, et al. Inpatient vs outpatient management and timing of delivery of uncomplicated monochorionic monoamniotic twin pregnancy: The MONOMONO study. *Ultrasound in Obstetrics & Gynecology.* 2019. 53(2):175-183.
19. Kilby M, Bricker L. On behalf of the Royal College of Obstetricians and Gynaecologists. Management of monochorionic twin pregnancy. *BJOG.* 2016. 124:e1-e45.
20. D'Antonio F, Odibo A, Berghella V, Khalil A, Hack K, Saccone G, et al. Perinatal mortality, timing of delivery and prenatal management of monoamniotic twin pregnancy: Systematic review and meta-analysis. *Ultrasound Obstet Gynecol.* 2019. 53(2):166-174.

CHAPTER 18

Obstructed Labour and Uterine Rupture

KANIKA CHOPRA, MANJU PURI

INTRODUCTION

Complications during labour and childbirth are responsible for more than one-third of maternal deaths, half the number of stillbirths, and one-fourth of neonatal deaths [1]. The majority of these deaths occur in low- and middle-income countries (LMICs). Obstructed labour is one of the five major causes of maternal and perinatal morbidity and mortality in LMICs.

Magnitude of the Problem and Impact

Obstructed labour is the most common cause of uterine rupture in LMICs and has been reported to occur in 2–8% of deliveries [2]. The rates of maternal mortality due to obstructed labour and uterine rupture range from 4–70% [3]. In a meta-analysis of the burden of obstructed labour in Ethiopia, the reported prevalence of obstructed labour was found to be 11.79% [4]. These figures may not be a true reflection of the actual burden as they are derived from tertiary-level hospitals and referral centres.

The causes of maternal mortality in obstructed labour are usually as follows:

- **Multigravidas:** Uterine rupture and related hemorrhage
- **Primigravidas:** Uterine inertia with resultant hemorrhage, prolonged rupture of membranes, chorioamnionitis, and sepsis

Key Point

The consequences of obstructed labour are uterine rupture in a multigravida and uterine inertia in a primigravida.

Long-term complications from obstructed labour include vesicovaginal and rectovaginal fistulae, vaginal stenosis, and psychological morbidity. Perinatal mortality is increased, and results from birth asphyxia.

Non-availability of adequately equipped healthcare facilities coupled with a poor transport and referral system contributes significantly to obstructed labour and its consequences.

Thorough knowledge about normal and abnormal labour processes, timely diagnosis, and interventions can help reduce maternal and perinatal mortality and morbidity related to obstructed labour and uterine rupture.

DEFINITIONS

- **Obstructed labour** is defined as labour in which the presenting part of the fetus cannot pass through the birth canal due to mechanical reasons despite strong uterine contractions.
- **Uterine rupture** is defined as a full thickness tear of the uterine wall including the uterine serosa.

PATHOPHYSIOLOGY

Obstructed labour generally arises in the second stage of labour. The obstruction most often occurs at the level of the pelvic brim but may occur in the midpelvis or the outlet. In obstructed labour, because of the disparity in the size of the presenting part and the passage, the presenting part is not well applied to the cervix. The following consequences may be seen:

- There may be early rupture of the membranes and slow dilatation of the cervix.

Subsequently, as a result of continuous pushing by the mother, the cervix becomes thick and edematous.

- In vertex presentation, there is formation of caput succedaneum and moulding.
- The head presses the bladder and urethra against the pubic bone. If this is prolonged, it can result in ischemic necrosis and vesicovaginal fistula.
- The head becomes elongated and may be visible at the introitus even when the largest diameter of the presenting part is above the brim (unengaged).

As labour continues, the upper segment continues to contract and retract in an attempt to push the fetus down through the passage. This results in the stretching, distension, and thinning of the lower uterine segment, ultimately leading to rupture. The upper segment is tonically contracted over the fetus. The junction of the contracted upper segment and the thinned-out, distended lower uterine segment **(Bandl's ring)** becomes prominent and visible on the abdomen. It rises gradually upwards with progressive distension of the lower segment, and ultimately ruptures.

Uterine rupture most often follows obstructed labour but may sometimes occur due to direct blunt trauma to the abdomen in advanced pregnancy or due to external or internal manipulation of the fetus.

OBSTRUCTED LABOUR

ETIOLOGY

Any degree of mismatch between the maternal pelvis and fetal size can cause obstructed labour. This could be due to bony or soft tissue abnormalities. The various causes of obstructed labour are as follows:

- **Contracted pelvis**: Women of short stature and women with deformities due to rickets (less common in the modern era), polio, pelvic trauma
- **Malpresentation:** Face (mentoposterior), brow, and shoulder presentation, persistent occipitoposterior position, occipitotransverse position (see **Chapter 35,** *Malpositions and malpresentations [other than breech]*)
- **Asynclitism:** Moderate to severe
- **Fetal macrosomia**: Especially in women with diabetes mellitus or women with a high BMI
- **Fetal malformations**: Hydrocephalus, fetal ascites, locked twins, conjoined twins
- **Abnormalities of the reproductive tract:** Tumours such as large ovarian cysts impacted in the pouch of Douglas or fibroids arising from the lower uterine segment or cervix, a large bladder calculus, cervical or vaginal stenosis

RISK FACTORS

- **Age <17 years**: Pregnancies in women aged <17 years are associated with a higher chance of contracted pelvis and obstructed labour due to an inadequately developed pelvis and poor nutrition. This is a concern especially in LMICs, where child marriages and adolescent pregnancies are not uncommon [5].
- **Malnutrition:** Poor socio-economic status along with malnutrition is associated with short stature (maternal height <145 cm) [6]. The cut-off maternal height as a risk factor may vary with the population under study owing to genetic diversity. Malnutrition may also be associated with diseases affecting the pelvis and include rickets in childhood and osteomalacia in adolescence.
- **Poliomyelitis:** In many LMICs, polio is still endemic. The affected individual may suffer from deformities of the spine, pelvis, and lower limbs, resulting in a contracted pelvis. However, the prevalence of polio has decreased over the years due to robust vaccination programmes.
- **Grand multigravida:** Progressive increase in the birth weight with increasing parity, subluxation of sacroiliac joints with a resultant decrease in the anteroposterior diameter of the pelvis, and an increase in the incidence of

malpresentations in multigravidas (due to a lax abdominal wall) contribute to an increase in obstructed labour in grand multigravidas.

- **Community-related factors:** These result from delays in seeking care, in reaching an appropriate facility, and in receiving care at the facility [7]. Community related factors include the following:
  - Lack of autonomy and economic opportunity, which compels many women to have home births assisted by untrained birth attendants
  - Inadequate health infrastructure and dearth of trained healthcare providers, and consequently, poor quality of antenatal and intrapartum care
  - Inadequate transport facilities with resultant delay in transfer of women with prolonged labour in need of assisted vaginal delivery or cesarean section from primary- to secondary- or tertiary-level health centres

CLINICAL DIAGNOSIS

- **History:** A detailed history is important in a case of obstructed labour. This includes demographic profile (age, socio-economic status, education status), obstetric history (gravida, parity, abortions, and number of living children), current pregnancy (period of gestation, supervised or unsupervised pregnancy, duration of labour, duration of leaking per vaginum), any history of lower limb or spine surgery or malformation due to poliomyelitis.
- **Examination:** The examination findings can be divided into two stages of obstruction—early and late.

Findings in the Early Stages of Obstruction

The salient findings are as described below:

- **General physical examination**: The woman is found to be mildly dehydrated.
- **Abdominal examination:** Strong, frequent uterine contractions are present with inadequate relaxation in between. The presenting part is palpable on pelvic grip and may not be engaged in the pelvis. Fetal distress may be detected. The liquor is often reduced.
- **Vaginal examination:** The cervix is partially or fully dilated, thick, edematous, and not well applied to the presenting part. The presenting part is usually above 0 station. In vertex presentation, a large caput succedaneum along with grade 2/3 moulding is present along more than one suture line.

In neglected cases, the caput may be visible at the introitus even with an unengaged head. Other presentations may be noted such as shoulder presentation with or without arm prolapse, face presentation (mentoposterior), or brow. Minimal or no liquor can be present at this stage. Significant (thick) meconium may be present.

Findings in the Late Stages of Obstruction

If the diagnosis is missed in the early stage, the following findings can be appreciated:

- **General physical examination**: The woman is exhausted and dehydrated.
- **Vitals**: The woman may be febrile with tachycardia and tachypnea.
- **Abdominal examination**: The uterus is usually tender on palpation. The upper uterine segment feels hard. The lower segment of the uterus is distended and stretched. The contractions may or may not be appreciated. Bandl's ring may be present on inspection of the abdomen (Fig. 18.1a and b). The ring is formed at the junction of the thick upper uterine segment and thin lower uterine segment. The ring gradually ascends towards the umbilicus in advanced cases of obstruction. The uterus appears to be filled with the fetus, with no liquor. The fetal heart rate is usually very slow or absent. The maternal intestines and bladder may be distended.

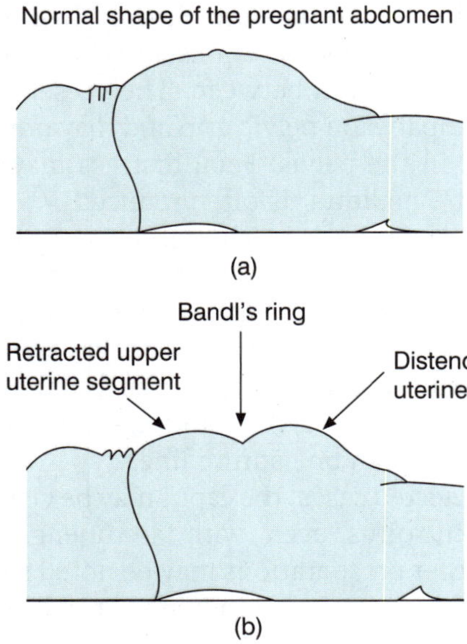

Fig. 18.1 Bandl's ring seen in the abdomen of a woman with obstructed labour

- **Perineal examination:** The vulva is swollen and edematous. In transverse lie with shoulder presentation, the prolapsed arm may be swollen and lying outside the introitus.
- **Vaginal examination:** The vagina appears hot and dry. The liquor may be foul-smelling or meconium-stained. The cervix is partially or fully dilated, edematous, and not well-applied to the presenting part, which is unengaged. Membranes are absent. In cases of vertex presentation, a large caput succedaneum along with grade 3 moulding is felt.

Key Point

A woman in the late stage of obstruction is dehydrated, febrile, has a Bandl's ring, and a moribund or dead fetus.

MANAGEMENT

The principles of management include fluid resuscitation and stabilisation, antibiotics, and delivery of the baby.

Initial Management

An intravenous line is set up with a wide-bore cannula. Fluid resuscitation is initiated, and dehydration and acidosis are corrected with dextrose saline and Ringer's lactate solution.

The woman is catheterised, and an intake and output chart maintained. Urinary catheterisation at this stage may be difficult due to the impacted fetal head pressing on the bladder neck. Digital vaginal examination is used to push the fetal head upwards so that it is no longer pressing on the bladder neck, and the catheter is introduced. Drained urine is scanty, concentrated, and may be hemorrhagic.

Antibiotics

If the membranes have been ruptured for >18 hours or if there are signs of infection (chorioamnionitis), **intravenous broad-spectrum antibiotics** are started to cover gram-positive and gram-negative organisms after collecting relevant samples for culture and sensitivity.

- Injection ampicillin 2 g IV stat is given followed by 1 g IV every 6 hours till delivery.
- Injection gentamicin 5 mg/Kg IV is given every 24 hours (in 100 mL of saline, as an infusion).
- Alternatively, second- or third-generation cephalosporins may be used instead of ampicillin and gentamicin.

Antibiotics are discontinued when the mother has been afebrile for 48 hours. Appropriate antibiotics may be started if the woman is in a state of sepsis or septic shock.

Investigations

Blood samples are collected for baseline investigations. The investigations include complete blood count with peripheral smear, blood grouping, and Rh typing, serum electrolytes, arterial blood–gas analysis, and renal and liver function tests. Relevant samples are collected for cultures such as a vaginal swab, urine, and blood. Urine is examined for ketones.

Abdominal ultrasonography may be performed in selected cases to rule out any malformation in the fetus. Blood is sent for cross-matching and at least 4 units of blood are reserved.

Delivery

Immediate cesarean section is recommended for all women in obstructed labour, irrespective of the presentation, cervical dilatation, or condition of the fetus.

Craniotomy followed by vaginal delivery is an option if the cervix is fully dilated, the vertex is at or below the level of the ischial spines, and the fetus is dead. This must be performed in the operating theatre by an experienced obstetrician. Destructive operations have a limited role in modern obstetrics but can be offered in select cases with appropriate consent to avoid a uterine scar and a complicated postoperative period [8].

Cesarean section in obstructed labour

During cesarean section, the parietal peritoneum is opened at a higher level to avoid injury to the bladder. The uterine incision is placed high to avoid a cervical incision as the lower uterine segment is markedly distended and stretched out. A liberal uterine incision is made to avoid extension of the incision while delivering the baby, as the lower segment is thinned out. An assistant can help disengage the presenting part through the vagina. After delivering the fetus, the uterine incision is explored for downward or lateral extensions. The placental membranes are sent for culture and sensitivity.

> **Key Point**
>
> There is **no recommendation** for irrigation of the peritoneal cavity at cesarean delivery as there is no evidence that irrigating with saline, antiseptic solutions, or antibiotics reduces surgical site infection [9].

Postoperative care

Postoperatively, the woman is kept well hydrated. Antibiotics are continued as clinically indicated and modified as per culture reports. They are discontinued when the woman has been afebrile for 48 hours. Ryle's tube may be indicated in the presence of acute gastric dilatation or paralytic ileus. The indwelling urinary catheter is left in place for continuous drainage of the bladder for 14–21 days to prevent the formation of a vesicovaginal fistula. Electrolytes must be monitored and corrected if there is electrolyte imbalance.

The woman can have a difficult postpartum period, and is at risk of bladder dysfunction, infection, and thromboembolism. Appropriate preventive steps and management need to be initiated. If the pregnancy resulted in a stillbirth, the woman should receive empathetic support from all staff members.

At discharge, the woman is given advice regarding contraception and future childbirth.

UTERINE RUPTURE

Uterine rupture is defined as a full thickness tear of the uterine wall, including the serosa. It is associated with catastrophic maternal and fetal complications. It may result in protrusion of the fetus, with or without the placenta, into the abdominal cavity, leading to intrauterine fetal demise, significant hemoperitoneum, and a need for emergency laparotomy, hysterectomy, or uterine repair (individualised to the woman), and multiple blood transfusions.

> **Key Point**
>
> Uterine rupture in resource-limited settings usually results from obstructed labour while that in resource-rich settings occurs due to trial of labour after cesarean section (TOLAC). Uterine rupture in an unscarred uterus is rare and is associated with higher maternal and neonatal morbidity and mortality as compared to that occurring in a scarred uterus.

UTERINE RUPTURE IN A SCARRED UTERUS

The incidence of uterine rupture in a scarred uterus is 0.2–1% [10]. Most studies describing uterine rupture following trial of labour after cesarean (TOLAC) do not differentiate between complete (rupture) and partial separation (dehiscence). Catastrophic rupture is most commonly associated with maternal morbidity and mortality (see **Chapter 26,** *Vaginal delivery after previous cesarean section*).

Uterine dehiscence is the tearing or separation of a pre-existing uterine scar without involving the overlying visceral peritoneum. In uterine dehiscence, the fetus and placenta remain inside the uterine cavity. It is rarely associated with any signs and symptoms and is detected incidentally during cesarean section. It is not associated with significant maternal or fetal complications.

Risk Factors

There are certain risk factors that are associated with uterine rupture in women with a previous cesarean section. The rupture could occur both antepartum and intrapartum.

- **Antepartum**: The following antepartum factors are associated with an increased risk of uterine rupture [11,12,13,14,15,16]:
  - — Maternal age >40 years
  - — Maternal obesity, i.e., body mass index (BMI) >30 Kg/m^2
  - — Inter-delivery interval of <18 months, and particularly <6 months, is associated with a higher chance of scar rupture
  - — More than one previous cesarean section
  - — A previous classical cesarean section is associated with uterine rupture in 1–12%; a previous transfundal or T-type uterine incision increases the risk of rupture
  - — Single layer uterine closure in previous cesarean section, especially when locked
  - — Previous preterm cesarean section
  - — Postterm pregnancy
  - — Macrosomia with fetal weight >4 Kg
  - — Previous uterine surgeries like myomectomy, adenomyomectomy, or uterine septal resection
- **Intrapartum:** The following factors are associated with an increased risk of uterine rupture in labour [11,12,13,17]:
  - — A low pre-labour Bishop's score
  - — Induction of labour with oxytocin as compared to the spontaneous onset of labour
  - — Women with labour dystocia in the active phase of labour with longer time for progression after cervical dilatation of >7 cm
  - — Prolonged second stage of labour
  - — Prostaglandins
    - ▪ PGE1 (misoprostol) is contraindicated in women with a previous cesarean section. The risk of uterine rupture with misoprostol is approximately 5–10%.
    - ▪ Medical induction of labour with prostaglandin E2 (dinoprostone) is associated with an increased risk of uterine rupture and hence, its use is not recommended in trial of labour after cesarean.

UTERINE RUPTURE IN AN UNSCARRED UTERUS

The incidence of uterine rupture in an unscarred uterus has increased over recent decades. In a study conducted over a period of 40 years in Norway, it was found that incidence rates per 10,000 maternities in the first, second, third, and fourth decades were 1.2, 0.9, 1.7, and 6.1 respectively [18]. Obstetric interventions may be the contributory factor behind the increased rate. The rate of serious maternal and neonatal morbidity is higher in cases of rupture in an unscarred uterus as compared to that in a scarred uterus [19]. Rupture of the unscarred uterus is more frequently a consequence of prolonged obstructed labour in resource-limited settings where access to cesarean or operative vaginal births may not be immediately available [20]. Higher parity, longer labours, and a higher frequency of contracted pelvis also contribute to the higher rate of uterine rupture in an unscarred uterus in LMICs.

Etiology

The etiology of rupture in the unscarred uterus includes the following:

- Weakening of the uterine myometrium due to:
  - Prolonged and obstructed labour
  - The injudicious use of uterotonic drugs
  - Congenital weakening in women with Ehlers Danlos syndrome
- Trauma due to:
  - Obstetric manoeuvres such as external cephalic version or internal podalic version
  - Road traffic accident

Risk Factors

- **Antepartum:** The following antepartum factors are associated with an increased risk of uterine rupture [18,19,21]:
  - Advanced maternal age
  - High parity
  - Shorter interpregnancy interval
  - Multiple gestation
  - Macrosomia
  - Uterine anomaly
- **Intrapartum:** Factors during labour that may increase the risk of uterine rupture include the following [21]:
  - Use of oxytocin and prostaglandins for induction or augmentation of labour
  - Undiagnosed cephalopelvic disproportion in unsupervised labour or in the presence of untrained birth attendants
  - Internal podalic version

CLINICAL DIAGNOSIS

- **History:** When a woman is admitted with a suspicion of uterine rupture, a detailed history should be obtained as she is being examined and resuscitated. The most common complaint is the sudden onset of acute, continuous abdominal pain and the cessation of uterine contractions. Women with neuraxial analgesia for labour may complain of excessive abdominal pain despite effective analgesia. There can be fresh vaginal bleeding, which is an important sign of possible uterine rupture.
- **Examination:** The following findings may be present in women with uterine rupture:
  - *General condition:* The woman may look anxious, dehydrated, and pale.
  - *Vitals:* She may have tachypnea, tachycardia, and hypotension and may be in shock.
  - *Abdominal examination:* The uterine contour is distorted or lost. The abdomen is tender, and there is muscle guarding. The fetal parts are felt easily and superficially. The flanks are dull on percussion, indicating the presence of free fluid in the abdomen.
  - *FHR:* Fetal heart rate may be slow or absent. The most common FHR abnormality in uterine rupture is prolonged fetal bradycardia, which may be sudden or preceded by significant variable or prolonged decelerations.
  - *Vaginal bleeding:* Fresh vaginal bleeding may be seen. On catheterisation of the bladder, hematuria may be present, suggesting the extension of uterine rupture into the bladder.
- **Vaginal examination**: This may reveal loss of station of the presenting part as compared to previous examination findings. The cervix is not applied to the presenting part.

MANAGEMENT

Management decisions are based on the following:

- Hemodynamic stability of the mother
- Fetal condition as indicated by fetal heart rate monitoring

Principles of management include resuscitation and stabilisation of the mother, calling for help from a senior obstetrician, and informing the blood bank, anesthetist, and neonatologist. The woman is mobilised for an urgent laparotomy for definitive treatment, which could be uterine repair or a hysterectomy.

The surgical decision is based on the following factors:

- Hemodynamic stability of the woman intraoperatively
- Type and extent of uterine rupture
- The mother's desire for future fertility
- Skills of the surgeon
- Hemostasis

Uterine Repair

Uterine repair is undertaken if the woman is hemodynamically stable, the rent is clean and easily repairable, a cesarean scar has given way, and the woman is young and wishes to have more children.

The goals of conservative surgery are to repair the uterine defect, achieve hemostasis, and identify and repair the other organs involved, e.g., the bladder. After extracting the fetus and placenta from the abdominal cavity and/or uterus, a primary double-layer closure with a delayed absorbable suture is performed to achieve hemostasis.

Hysterectomy

A hysterectomy is usually considered for women who are hemodynamically unstable or have completed their family. It may also be the only option in the following circumstances:

- Rupture of an unscarred uterus
- Ragged or spiral tears
- Rupture involving the upper uterine segment
- Colporrhexis

See the section on *Hysterectomy for uterine rupture* in **Chapter 24,** *Peripartum hysterectomy*, for further details.

Postoperative Care

The principles of postoperative care are the same as for any major surgical procedure. Antibiotics are prescribed as indicated.

PREGNANCY AFTER PRIOR UTERINE RUPTURE

There is an increased risk of recurrent rupture in a future pregnancy. If the rupture was surgically repaired, the couple should be counselled against another pregnancy. However, if the couple has lost the previous child and wants to attempt a pregnancy, the pregnancy should be followed in a fully-equipped tertiary-care facility [22]. A study spanning 25 years [23] found that longitudinal ruptures (in an unscarred uterus) and short intervals (less than 2 years) between rupture and subsequent pregnancy predispose to the recurrence of uterine rupture.

The risk of repeat rupture ranges from 0–40% [23], the range being so wide because of its dependency on the availability of resources. Delivery should be scheduled before the onset of labour. Delivery by elective cesarean section is indicated between 36+0 and 37+0 weeks of gestation [12]. In certain cases, cesarean section may be indicated before 36+0 weeks, depending upon the extent of damage. In cases of previous scar dehiscence, repeat elective cesarean section is planned between 37+0 and 38+0 weeks of gestation [24].

Consequences of Obstructed Labour and Uterine Rupture

Obstructed labour and uterine rupture are associated with catastrophic consequences for the mother and the fetus. Obstructed labour is often complicated by chorioamnionitis, atonic postpartum hemorrhage, uterine rupture, and puerperal sepsis. Prolonged obstructed labour results in ischemic injury to the bladder base, rectum, and vagina with resultant vesicovaginal and rectovaginal fistulae and vaginal stenosis due to the impaction of the hard fetal head against the pelvic bones. Women with these fistulae suffer from extreme physical and psychological morbidity.

Uterine rupture may result in laparotomies with cesarean hysterectomy or repair of the uterus and bladder. There is high maternal morbidity and mortality due to related complications. There is a higher incidence of blood transfusion, ICU or HDU admission, and prolonged hospitalisation. Postoperative complications like paralytic ileus, surgical site infections, prolonged catheterisation, and puerperal sepsis are common.

The fetal consequences include stillbirth, birth asphyxia, birth injuries, neonatal sepsis, NICU admission, and neonatal death. The survivors may have delayed milestones due to prolonged asphyxia.

PREVENTION

Strategies to prevent obstructed labour, early diagnosis, and timely management to prevent complications and related morbidity are discussed below.

Antenatal Interventions

Antenatal diagnosis of risk factors associated with obstructed labour such as contracted pelvis, anticipated cephalopelvic disproportion, or malpresentations should receive timely referral to an appropriate facility.

Intrapartum Interventions

All births should ideally be conducted by skilled birth attendants. The progress of labour should be monitored objectively, and there should be timely referral to a facility adequately equipped for performing an operative vaginal delivery or cesarean section. Early diagnosis of prolonged labour and appropriate management can minimise related mortality and morbidity.

The judicious use of oxytocic agents such as oxytocin and prostaglandins for induction and/or augmentation of labour is essential to prevent hyperstimulation and consequent uterine rupture. Oxytocics must be used with caution in grand multigravidas and those with previous uterine scars. Experienced obstetricians must manage complicated cases to optimise outcomes.

CONCLUSION

Obstructed labour is a preventable obstetric complication. It is, however, an important cause of maternal morbidity and mortality and of adverse perinatal outcomes in resource-limited countries. The major causes of obstructed labour are known to be cephalopelvic disproportion and malpresentation. The complications of obstructed labour are sepsis, stillbirth, postpartum hemorrhage, uterine rupture, and maternal death. In LMICs, the inability to access appropriate care due to economic hardship, lack of transportation, or lack of tertiary units leads to maternal mortality.

Uterine rupture may occur in a scarred uterus (following a previous cesarean) or in an unscarred uterus. When rupture occurs in an unscarred uterus, the maternal mortality is high.

REFERENCES

1. Lawn JE, Blencowe H, Waiswa P, Amouzou A, Mathers C, Hogan D, et al. Stillbirths: Rates, risk factors and accelerations towards 2013. *Lancet.* 2016. 387(10018): 587-603.
2. Kabakyenga JK, Ostergren PO, Turyakiru E, Mukasa PK, Pettersson KO. Individual and health facility factors and risk for obstructed labour and its adverse outcomes in South-Western Uganda. *BMC Pregnancy Childbirth.* 2011. 11: 73.
3. World Health Organization. Maternal Health and safe motherhood programme. World Health organization. Partograph is management of labour. *Lancet.* 1994. 343: 1399-404.
4. Addisu D, Mekie M, Melkie A, Yeshambel A. Burden of obstructed labour in Ethiopia: A systematic review and meta-analysis. *Midwifery.* 2021. 95:102930.
5. Neilson JP, Lavender T, Quenby S, Wary S. Obstructed labour. British Medical Bulletin. 2003. 67: 191–204.
6. Abdo RA, Halil HM. Magnitude and factors associated with obstructed labour among women delivered at

Halaba Kulito Primary Hospital, Halaba Special district, Southern Ethiopia. *J Women's Health Care*. 2019. 8(1): 453.

7. Melah GS, El-Nafaty AU, Massa AA, Audu BM. Obstructed labour: A public health problem in Gombe, Gombe State, Nigeria. *J Obstet Gynaecol*. 2003. 23 (4): 369-73.
8. Nain S, Suman S, Meena D, Lal P, Kumar M, et al. Revisiting destructive operations to prevent second stage caesarean sections in COVID times: A case series. *Trop Doct*. 2023. 53(1): 154-157.
9. Eke AC, Shukr GH, Chaalan TT, Nashif SK, Eleje GU. Intra-abdominal saline irrigation at caesarean section: a systematic review and meta-analysis. *J Matern Fetal Neonatal Med*. 2016. 29(10): 1588-94.
10. Motomura K, Ganchimeg T, Nagata C, Ota e, Vogel JP, Betran AP, et al. Incidence and outcomes of uterine rupture among women with prior caesarean section: WHO multi-country survey on Maternal and Newborn health. *Sci Rep*. 2017. 10(7): 44093.
11. RCOG Green-top Guideline No. 45. Birth After Previous Caesarean Birth. Available at https://www.rcog.org.uk/
12. ACOG Practice Bulletin No. 184: Vaginal Birth After Cesarean Delivery. *Obstet Gynecol*. 2017. 130(5):e217-e233.
13. Dy J, DeMeester S, Lipworth H, et al. SOGC clinical practice guideline no. 382. Tial of labour after caesarean. 2019. Volume 41, Issue 7, p992-1011.
14. Landon MB, Lynch CD. Optimal timing and mode of delivery after caesarean with previous classical incision or myomectomy: A review of the data. *Semin Perinatol*. 2011. 35: 257.
15. Roberge S, Chaillet N, Boutin A, Moore N, Jastrow N, Brassard R, et al. Single versus double layer closure of the hysterotomy incision during caesarean and risk of uterine rupture. *Int J Gynecol Obstet*. 2011. 115:5.
16. Tanos V, Toney ZA. Uterine scar rupture—prediction, prevention, diagnosis, and management. *Best Practice & Research Clinical Obstetrics and Gynaecology*. 2019. 59: 115-131.
17. Harper LM, Cahill AG, Roehl KA, Odibo AO, Stamilio DM, Macones GA. The pattern of labour preceding uterine rupture. *Am J Obstet Gynecol*. 2012. 207 (3): 210 e1-e6.
18. Al Zirqi I, Stray-Pederson B, Forsen L, Daltveit AK, Vangen S. Uterine rupture: Trends over 40 years. *BJOG*. 2016. 123(5):780-7.
19. Gibbins KJ, Weber T, Holmgren CM, Porter TF, Varner MW, Manuck TA. Maternal and fetal morbidity associated with uterine rupture of the unscarred uterus. *Am J Obstet Gynecol*. 2015. 213(3): 382.e1-6.
20. Batra K, Gaikwad HS, Gutgutia I, Prateek S, Bajaj B. Determinants of rupture of the unscarred uterus and the related fetomaternal outcome: Current scenario in a low-income country. *Trop Doct*. 2016. 46 (2): 69-73.
21. Smith JF, Wax, JR. DA. Uterine rupture: Unscarred uterus. Caughey AB (Ed). *UpToDate*. 2023. Waltham, MA.
22. Chibber R, El-Saleh E, Al Fadhli R, et al. Uterine rupture and subsequent pregnancy outcome—how safe is it? A 25-year study. *J Matern Fetal Neonatal Med*. 2010. 23:421.
23. Usta IM, Hamdi MA, Musa AA, Nassar AH. Pregnancy outcome in patients with previous uterine rupture. *Acta Obstet Gynecol Scand*. 2007. 86:172.
24. Fox NS. Pregnancy outcomes in patients with prior uterine rupture or dehiscence: A 5-year update. *Obstet Gynecol*. 2020. 135: 211.

CHAPTER 19

Antibiotic Prophylaxis in Labour and Delivery

GITA ARJUN

INTRODUCTION

Antibiotics are prescribed in pregnancy for both **prophylactic** and **therapeutic indications**. The principles underlying the use of prophylactic antibiotics must be clearly distinguished from those governing the administration of therapeutic antibiotics in the presence of established infection.

This chapter addresses antibiotic prophylaxis in labour and delivery.

THE PRINCIPLES OF ANTIBIOTIC PROPHYLAXIS

Prophylactic antibiotics reduce the colony count of microorganisms introduced into the organ or surgical site during the procedure. Though they do not completely sterilise tissues, this decrease in colony count allows the person's immune system to effectively handle the low level of contamination.

Antibiotic prophylaxis is intended for both elective and emergency procedures and is administered:

- Before exposure to contaminating bacteria
- For a limited duration (usually 24 hours)

Key Point

Prophylactic antibiotics **prevent** infection. Therapeutic antibiotics **treat** established infections.

CHARACTERISTICS OF A PROPHYLACTIC ANTIBIOTIC

The ideal prophylactic antibiotic should:

- Reduce surgical site infection and peripartum infections
- Have few maternal and fetal side effects
- Be long-acting
- Be effective against organisms likely to be encountered during the surgical procedure
- Be inexpensive

TIMING OF ANTIBIOTIC PROPHYLAXIS

To be effective, the antibiotic should be administered within 60 minutes before bacterial inoculation [1,2]. The administration of the prophylactic antibiotic should be timed to ensure that serum and tissue levels are adequate before the procedure or before the incision is made. The dose used should be chosen to maintain therapeutic levels of the agent in serum and tissues during surgery and for a few hours after the incision is closed [1,3]. A single dose is usually effective.

INDICATIONS DURING LABOUR AND DELIVERY

In this chapter, antibiotic prophylaxis will be discussed for the following situations:

- Vaginal birth
- Operative vaginal delivery

- Third- and fourth-degree perineal tears during vaginal birth
- Cesarean delivery
- Obstetric complications
- Obstetric procedures
- Prophylaxis for bacterial endocarditis during delivery

Vaginal Birth

The World Health Organization, in its recommendations for the prevention and treatment of maternal peripartum infections, strongly states that spontaneous, uncomplicated vaginal birth is **not** an indication for prophylactic antibiotics [3]. Instead, good standards of hygiene and aseptic techniques are advocated.

Unfortunately, many obstetric facilities in low- and middle-income countries (LMICs) continue to use antibiotics for uncomplicated vaginal deliveries. This practice should be strongly discouraged. In a study from a non-teaching, tertiary care hospital in an Indian city [4], 87% of women undergoing vaginal deliveries received a third-generation cephalosporin. A systematic review of the Cochrane Database on routine antibiotic prophylaxis for a normal vaginal birth with the intention of reducing maternal infectious morbidity [5] concluded that antibiotics in the peripartum period **should not be considered a substitute for infection prevention and control measures** (e.g., hand hygiene and the use of clean equipment).

> **Key Point**
>
> Prophylactic antibiotics are **not** recommended for a spontaneous, uncomplicated vaginal delivery.

Operative Vaginal Delivery

Until recently, routine administration of prophylactic antibiotics was not recommended for operative vaginal delivery because of the potential adverse effects of unnecessarily exposing mothers and fetuses to antibiotics. In 2017, a systematic review of the Cochrane Database found no definitive evidence to recommend prophylactic antibiotics for operative vaginal delivery [6]. However, a recent multicentre randomised controlled trial from the UK [7] showed a 42% decrease in the risk of postpartum infection with the administration of a single dose of antibiotic administered within 6 hours of birth. It must be noted that **approximately 90% of these women had an episiotomy**. Based on this study, the latest systematic review of the Cochrane Database [8] has changed its recommendation in favour of a single dose of prophylactic antibiotic in this scenario. The World Health Organization too changed its recommendation in 2021 [9] and strongly supports the use of prophylactic antibiotics for this indication. The ACOG does not feel this recommendation can be generalised to all women undergoing operative vaginal birth in the United States but recommends the judicious use of a single dose of antibiotic if a third- or fourth-degree tear occurs [10].

The antibiotic, dosage, and timing are as follows:

- A single dose of IV amoxicillin (1 g) and clavulanic acid (200 mg)
- Administered as soon as possible after birth and no more than 6 hours after birth

The feasibility of applying the results of a study from a high-income country to LMICs, in terms of resources and cost, has not been studied.

Third- or Fourth-Degree Perineal Laceration

For the repair of a third- or fourth-degree obstetric anal sphincter injury, though the evidence is not strong and is based on a single study [11], it is currently recommended that a single dose of antibiotic (a second-generation cephalosporin, e.g., cefuroxime or cefoxitin) at the time of repair is reasonable [12,13].

> **Key Point**
>
> Prophylactic antibiotics are not recommended for the repair of episotomy or first- and second-degree tears.

Cesarean Section

The rates of infection after a cesarean section are significantly higher than those with vaginal birth [14]. The single most important risk factor for postpartum maternal infection is cesarean section [15]. For antibiotic prophylaxis for cesarean delivery, the World Health Organization recommends a single dose of a first-generation cephalosporin or penicillin in preference to other classes of antibiotics. [16]. A recent systematic review of the Cochrane Database found no advantage to using third-generation cephalosporins, piperacillin–tazobactam, ticarcillin–clavulanate, and ampicillin–sulbactam over first- or second-generation cephalosporins [17].

Recommended antibiotics

Guidelines have recommended regimens that have become the gold standard globally [1,18]. Recent studies have suggested that the addition of a single dose of azithromycin (500 mg IV infused over 1 hour) to the routine single dose of prophylactic antibiotic in women who undergo a cesarean in labour (emergency cesarean section) or who have ruptured membranes for >4 hours prior to cesarean section significantly decreases the risk of wound infection and endometritis [19]. Additional azithromycin is **not recommended** for elective cesarean sections [1,20]. As a general principle, antibiotics that are used for the treatment of established infection are best avoided as prophylactic antibiotics. The recommended antibiotic regimens are listed in Table 19.1.

Key Point

Co-amoxiclav (amoxicillin and clavulanic acid) **should not be used** because of the increased risk of neonatal necrotising enterocolitis in cases where it is given as prophylaxis before skin incision or cord clamping [21].

Timing of antibiotic

It is recommended that a single dose of antibiotic be administered within 60 minutes before making the skin incision [1,24]. Intravenous antibiotics may be administered at the start of surgery, just before the induction of anesthesia. The evidence in favour of administering the antibiotic **before cord clamping** is robust and of high quality [2].

Table 19.1 Antibiotic regimens for cesarean section

Drug	Time of administration	Number of doses
No penicillin allergy Inj. cefazolin 2 g IV **or** Inj. cefuroxime 1.5 g IV (if cefazolin not available)	Within 60 minutes before skin incision or just before induction of anesthesia	Single dose
Penicillin allergy Clindamycin 900 mg IV **plus** gentamicin 5 mg/Kg IV	Within 60 minutes before skin incision	Single dose
Emergency cesarean *or* ***membranes ruptured >4 hours before cesarean*** Azithromycin (500 mg IV, infused over 1 hour) in addition to routine antibiotic prophylaxis	Within 60 minutes before skin incision	Single dose

Key Point

Why a single dose?

The aim of prophylactic antibiotics is to get the most effective infection prevention with the least amount of exposure to both the mother and the fetus. Studies in general surgical populations have shown no benefit from postoperative antimicrobial prophylaxis; this has been applied to cesareans too.

Antibiotic Prophylaxis for Obstetric Complications

Preterm premature rupture of membranes (PPROM)

Women with preterm premature rupture of membranes at <34 0/7 weeks of gestation, benefit from antibiotic prophylaxis to prolong pregnancy and delay delivery [1,22] (see **Chapter 30**, *Preterm labour and prelabour rupture of membranes*).

Key Point

In PPROM at <34 0/7 weeks, antibiotic prophylaxis is indicated when delivery is not imminent.

A systematic review of the Cochrane Database showed that prophylactic antibiotics in this situation also reduce the incidence of respiratory distress syndrome, necrotising enterocolitis, intraventricular hemorrhage, and early-onset sepsis but do not significantly reduce perinatal mortality [23].

Dosage and duration of antibiotic prophylaxis for PPROM

The recommendations for the antibiotic regimens for PPROM [1,22,24] are based on the largest randomised controlled trial for this condition. The recommendations are summarised in Table 19.2.

Preterm labour

A systematic review of the Cochrane Database [25] showed that antibiotic prophylaxis is **not indicated** for pregnancy prolongation in women with preterm labour and **intact membranes**.

Antibiotic Prophylaxis for Obstetric Procedures

Manual removal of placenta

No data exists to support the administration of prophylactic antibiotics to women who give birth vaginally and for whom a manual removal of the placenta has been performed [26].

However, the WHO [3] recommends a single dose of antibiotics (ampicillin or a first-generation cephalosporin) if manual removal of the placenta is performed. There was no good-quality evidence for this recommendation, which was reached by consensus.

Table 19.2 Antibiotic regimens for PPROM

Drug regimen	Duration
Inj. ampicillin 2 g IV 6 hourly and Inj. erythromycin 250 mg IV 6 hourly	48 hours
Followed by T. amoxicillin 250 mg orally every 8 hours and T. erythromycin 333 mg orally every 8 hours	5 days
Alternative regimen Azithromycin 1 g orally at admission and ampicillin 2 g IV at admission and then every 6 hours	48 hours
Followed by Amoxicillin 500 mg orally every 8 hours	5 days

Prevention of bacterial endocarditis

Infective endocarditis prophylaxis is **not recommended** for women with acquired or congenital structural heart disease for either vaginal or cesarean delivery according to the guidelines issued by the American Heart Association and the American College of Cardiology [27]. The small subset of women who require prophylaxis for bacterial endocarditis are those who have:

- Cyanotic cardiac disease
- Prosthetic valves

DANGERS OF ANTIBIOTIC OVERUSE AND ABUSE

The indiscriminate use of antibiotics, especially in LMICs, is a cause for concern. Too often, antibiotics are prescribed for an uncomplicated vaginal delivery without any indication [4].

Even in high-income countries, the use of pre-delivery antibiotics has been documented in ≥40% of women [28]. This is primarily a result of the implementation of protocols for the prevention of group B *Streptococcus* (GBS) infections in newborns and the routine administration of antibiotics for cesarean births. To put it in perspective, over 100 infants are exposed to antibiotics to protect one small preterm infant from GBS infection. Similarly, 100 women undergoing a cesarean delivery end up receiving prophylactic antibiotics to prevent one maternal infection.

The effect of exposing the mother and the fetus to antibiotics has a significant impact on the development of antibiotic resistance and, more concerningly, on the neonate's oral and gut microbiome.

Antibiotic Resistance

The inappropriate and irresponsible use of antibiotics has resulted in the emergence of pathogens that are multi-drug resistant. In obstetrics, this is reflected in increased neonatal infection and maternal infectious morbidity. What is more worrisome is that the bacterial spectrum causing sepsis is changing. Studies have shown that *Escherichia coli* is now the commonest organism causing sepsis in neonates, particularly after maternal antibiotic administration. New types of highly virulent methicillin-resistant *Staph. aureus* (MRSA) strains in the community are posing concerns for populations at risk, including pregnant women and children. There is currently a shortage of effective therapies along with a lack of successful prevention measures.

Effect on Neonatal Oral and Gut Microbiome

Recent studies have focused attention on the ill effects of early antibiotic exposure on the neonatal oral and gut microbiome, which is essential for immunological development. The aim should be to get the most effective infection prevention with the least exposure.

In the **short term**, newborns at full term **without antibiotic exposure** bear a lower health risk of early-onset sepsis or respiratory distress than preterm or antibiotic-exposed neonates [29]. In the **long term**, antibiotic-induced alterations of the gut microbiota have been shown to affect the maturation of the immune system, thus increasing susceptibility to obesity, diabetes, inflammatory bowel disease, and immune-related diseases such as asthma and allergies [30].

Key Point

Perinatal exposure to antibiotics not only increases the risk of **antibiotic resistance**, but also prevents the neonate from developing a healthy **oral** and **gut microbiome.**

CONCLUSION

Antibiotics are potent drugs used to prevent and treat perinatal infections. Studies around the world are showing a high rate of antibiotic exposure during pregnancy and childbirth. Overuse of antibiotics leads to antibiotic resistance, has potential side effects, and influences the maternal and neonatal microbiome. Hospitals should urgently establish and implement antibiotic stewardship programmes to prevent the harmful effects of perinatal antibiotic exposure.

REFERENCES

1. ACOG Practice Bulletin No. 199. Use of prophylactic antibiotics in labor and delivery. American College of Obstetricians and Gynecologists. *Obstet Gynecol.* 2018 (reaffirmed 2021). 132:e103-19.
2. Bollig C, Nothacker M, Lehane C, et al . Prophylactic antibiotics before cord clamping in cesarean delivery: A systematic review. *Acta Obstet Gynecol Scand.* 2018. 97: 521–535.
3. WHO. WHO recommendations for prevention and treatment of maternal peripartum infections. 2015. World Health Organization, Geneva. https://apps.who.int/iris/handle/10665/186171 (accessed on 25 March 2023).
4. Sharma M, Sanneving L, Mahadik K, et al. Antibiotic prescribing in women during and after delivery in a non-teaching, tertiary care hospital in Ujjain, India: A prospective cross-sectional study. *J Pharm Policy Pract.* 2013. 4;6:9.
5. Bonet M, Ota E, Chibueze CE, Oladapo OT. Routine antibiotic prophylaxis after normal vaginal birth for reducing maternal infectious morbidity. *Cochrane Database Syst Rev.* 2017. Issue 11. Art. No.: CD012137.

6. Liabsuetrakul T, Choobun T, Peeyananjarassri K, Islam QM. Antibiotic prophylaxis for operative vaginal delivery. *Cochrane Database Syst Rev.* 2017. Issue 8. Art. No.: CD004455. *Update in: Cochrane Database Syst Rev.* 2020. Issue 3. Art. no. CD004455.
7. Knight M, Chiocchia V, Partlett C, et al. Prophylactic antibiotics in the prevention of infection after operative vaginal delivery (ANODE): A multicentre randomised controlled trial. *Lancet.* 2019. 393:2395.
8. Liabsuetrakul T, Choobun T, Peeyananjarassri K, Islam QM. Antibiotic prophylaxis for operative vaginal delivery. *Cochrane Database Syst Rev.* 2020. Issue 3. Art. No.: CD004455.
9. WHO. WHO recommendation on routine antibiotic prophylaxis for women undergoing operative vaginal birth. 2021. World Health Organization, Geneva. https://apps.who.int/iris/handle/10665/341862.
10. Operative vaginal birth. ACOG Practice Bulletin No. 219. American College of Obstetricians and Gynecologists. *Obstet Gynecol.* 2020. 135:e149–59.
11. Duggal N, Mercado C, Daniels K, et al. Antibiotic prophylaxis for prevention of postpartum perineal wound complications: A randomized controlled trial. *Obstet Gynecol.* 2008. 111:1268.
12. Royal College of Obstetricians and Gynaecologists. Green-top guideline no. 29: The management of third- and fourth-degree perineal tears. 2007. https://www.rcog.org.uk/en/guidelines-research-services/guidelines/gtg29/. Accessed on March 27 2023.
13. ACOG Practice Bulletin No. 195: Prevention of Infection After Gynecologic Procedures. *Obstet Gynecol.* 2018 (reaffirmed 2022). 131:e172.
14. Declercq E, Barger M, Cabral HJ, Evans SR, Kotelchuck M, Simon C, et al. Maternal outcomes associated with planned primary cesarean births compared with planned vaginal births. *Obstet Gynecol.* 2007. 109:669–77.
15. Smaill FM, Grivell R. 2014. Antibiotic prophylaxis versus no prophylaxis for preventing infection after cesarean section. *Cochrane Database Syst Rev.* 2014. Issue 10. Art. no.: CD007482. Accessed 28 March 2023.
16. WHO. WHO recommendation on prophylactic antibiotics for women undergoing caesarean section. 2021. World Health Organization, Geneva.
17. Williams MJ, Carvalho Ribeiro do Valle C, Gyte GML. Different classes of antibiotics given to women routinely for preventing infection at caesarean section. *Cochrane Database Syst Rev.* 2021. Issue 3. Art. No.: CD008726.
18. Kawakita T, Huang CC, Landy HJ. Choice of prophylactic antibiotics and surgical site infections after cesarean delivery. *Obstet Gynecol.* 2018. 132(4):948-955.
19. Farmer N, Hodgetts-Morton V, Morris RK. Are prophylactic adjunctive macrolides efficacious against caesarean section surgical site infection: A systematic review and meta-analysis. *Eur J Obstet Gynecol Reprod Biol.* 2020. 244:163-171.
20. Berghella V. 2020. Cesarean delivery: Preoperative planning and patient preparation. Lockwood CJ (Ed). *UpToDate.* Waltham, MA.
21. National Institute for Health and Clinical Excellence. Caesarean section (update). Clinical guideline 132. 2011.
22. Kenyon SL, Taylor DJ, Tarnow-Mordi W. Broad-spectrum antibiotics for preterm rupture of the fetal membranes: The ORACLE I Randomised Trial. *Lancet.* 2001. 357:981-90.
23. Kenyon S, Boulvain M, Neilson J. Antibiotics for preterm rupture of membranes. *Cochrane Database Syst Rev.* 2001. Issue 12. Art. no.: CD001058.
24. Yudin MH, van Schalkwyk J, Eyk NV, et al. SOGC Clinical Practice Guideline No. 233. Antibiotic therapy in preterm premature rupture of the membranes. *J Obstet Gynaecol.* 2017. Volume 39, Issue 9. e207–e212.
25. Flenady V, Hawley G, Stock OM, Kenyon S, Badawi N. Prophylactic antibiotics for inhibiting preterm labour with intact membranes. *Cochrane Database Syst Rev.* 2013. Issue 12, Art no.:CD000246. Accessed 29 March 2023.
26. Chongsomchai C, Lumbiganon P, Laopaiboon M. Prophylactic antibiotics for manual removal of retained placenta in vaginal birth. *Cochrane Database Syst Rev.* 2014. Issue 10. Art. No.: CD004904.
27. Nishimura RA, Otto CM, Bonow RO, et al. + AHA/ACC focused update of the 2014 AHA/ACC guideline for the management of patients with valvular heart disease: a report of the American College of Cardiology/American Heart Association Task Force on Clinical Practice Guidelines. Circulation. 2017. 135:e1159–195.
28. Ledger WJ, Blaser MJ. Are we using too many antibiotics during pregnancy? *BJOG.* 2013. 120(12):1450-2.
29. Zhou P, Zhou Y, Liu B, et al. Perinatal antibiotic exposure affects the transmission between maternal and neonatal microbiota and is associated with early-onset sepsis. *mSphere.* 2020. 5(1):e00984-19.
30. Morreale C, Giaroni C, Baj A, et al. Effects of perinatal antibiotic exposure and neonatal gut microbiota. antibiotics (Basel). 2023. 12(2):258.

CHAPTER 20

Role of Ultrasound in the Labour Room

MARIYA KOVALENKO, SANA USMAN, ARWA HANIDU, CHRISTOPH LEES

INTRODUCTION

Ultrasound is being used with increasing frequency by midwives and doctors caring for pregnant women in labour and its use has been proposed to aid in the management of labour.

The use of ultrasound in the labour room can improve awareness and clinical safety at all stages of labour. Some healthcare professionals may consider the use of technology in labour as a precursor to the deskilling of the physical examination findings. However, the overall benefit of ultrasound in objectively demonstrating antenatal, intrapartum, and postpartum parameters outweighs this concern. Ultrasound in the labour room allows immediate confirmation of clinical findings, thereby enhancing and reinforcing the feedback obtained from clinical examinations. Given the current knowledge and experience with this modality in labouring women, ultrasound examination is recommended as an adjunct and not as a substitute for clinically indicated digital vaginal examination [1].

Traditionally, the assessment of the progress of labour is made by clinical examination. This includes the palpation of the maternal abdomen to determine fetal presentation combined with internal digital vaginal examination for fetal head position. More recently, clinical studies have demonstrated that vaginal examinations are subjective and poorly reproducible in the assessment of labour progress and fetal head position [2].

In labour, a curvilinear probe is used for transabdominal and transperineal examination, which are most commonly performed for assessment in labour.

- **Transabdominal ultrasound** may be useful in the delivery room to ascertain the fetal head position and presentation of the presenting part, placental localisation, and amniotic fluid assessment.
- **Transperineal ultrasound** is a non-intrusive form of ultrasound imaging in which the transducer is placed between the labia to obtain sagittal and transverse images of the presenting fetal part, cervix, amniotic membrane, and birth canal. It has been shown to be more acceptable when compared to digital examination in labour [3] and has been gaining popularity over the last decade.
- **Transvaginal examination** is not routinely performed in labour but may be used to assess cervical length in the case of suspected preterm labour. It may also be useful in determining placental location in women in labour who have not had a previous ultrasound examination.

Key Point

Women tend to prefer the use of ultrasound over digital vaginal examination in the labour ward. However, women who have been given regional analgesia are more accepting of digital examination [3].

This chapter describes the basic and advanced uses of ultrasound in the labour room for all clinicians. The International Society of Ultrasound in Obstetrics and Gynecology (ISUOG) [1] and the World Association of Perinatal Medicine (WAPM) [4] have published clinical practice guidelines on intrapartum ultrasound in which imaging parameters are discussed in more detail. At present, there is no consensus on recommended sonographic parameters to be routinely established in regular clinical practice.

Key Point

Currently, ultrasound examination in the labour room is recommended as an adjunct, and not as a substitute for clinically indicated digital vaginal examination [1].

ULTRASOUND EQUIPMENT

The current ultrasound machines are compact, mobile, and easily accessible. Their availability in the labour room has allowed clinicians to identify more objective labour parameters. Devices used in labour must be robust and portable in order to be used in different clinical areas. The battery packs of these devices have a limited capacity; hence, a charging point should be available in close proximity when they are in use.

Handheld point-of-care ultrasound devices are more easily available now and help in delivering easily deployed bedside diagnoses. Their use has been well established in other specialities such as cardiology.

Transducer

A commonly used, low-frequency (<4 MHz), wide-sector, curved transducer can be used both transabdominally and transperineally during antenatal care and labour. A transvaginal ultrasound probe has no role in labour except in the assessment of cervical length for risk stratification in threatened preterm labour.

Sterile ultrasound gel sold in single-use packets is recommended for use in the labour room to avoid cross-contamination between women in labour. If single-use containers are not available, to reduce infection rates, it is best to avoid direct contact between the gel bottle and the skin or the probe.

Before transabdominal scanning, the ultrasound gel is applied over the woman's abdomen. In the transperineal ultrasound method, the ultrasound gel should be first applied on the transducer, which is subsequently covered with a sterile probe cover or a glove. Sterile ultrasound gel is then used between the cover and maternal skin during scanning (Figs. 20.1a–c).

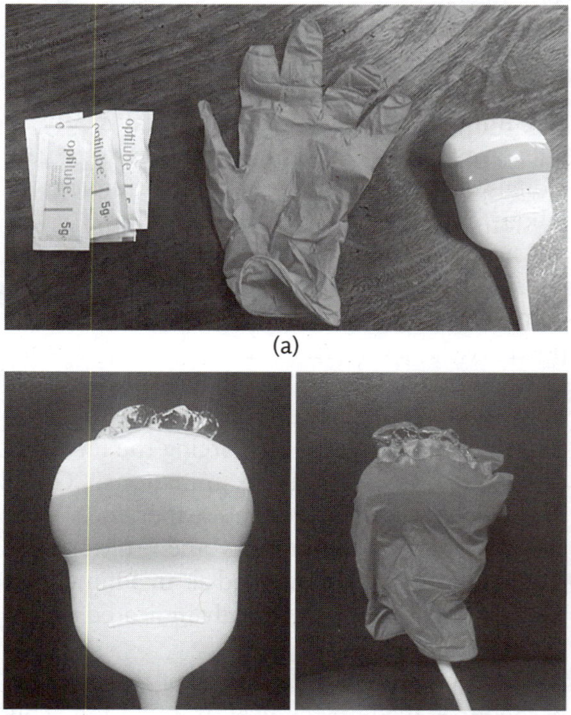

(a) (b) (c)

Fig. 20.1 Assembling the ultrasound transducer for transperineal ultrasound: (a) Sterile ultrasound gel, examination glove, and curvilinear ultrasound probe; (b) preparation of the ultrasound probe with sterile ultrasound gel; and (c) covering the ultrasound probe with a sterile examination glove and applying more ultrasound gel over the glove (*Images courtesy*: Dr Mariya Kovalenko)

TRAINING AND SKILL DEVELOPMENT

Clinicians working in the labour ward should have the basic skills to use ultrasound imaging for the recognition of obstetric emergencies. In low- and middle-income settings where antenatal care may not be universal or complete, an ultrasound assessment in the labour room can aid in identifying antenatal diagnoses missed in the pregnancy [5].

The training required to correctly practice a new skill is resource-dependent and time-consuming. Simulation-based training in ultrasound usage has expanded the opportunities for clinicians to experience sonography without direct patient contact. In a study by Clark et al., [6] 66 novice participants experienced simulation training. A comparison of pre- and post-training ultrasound image scores demonstrated that a novice ultrasound user was able to improve their ultrasound skills by completing such simulation sessions. Ultrasound training through simulation can produce similar results as face-to-face training with pregnant women [7].

Transperineal ultrasound can be taught to those with no prior sonography experience. When midwives in control and training groups were taught to record a transperineal ultrasound image and measure the parameters of the fetal head station [8], the image quality was higher in the training group that had received multimedia teaching. This study demonstrated the benefit of simulation-based ultrasound teaching. However, both groups had comparable measurements of the head–perineum distance (HPD) and the angle of progression (AoP). An AoP measurement requires greater expertise than that required to correctly measure the HPD.

Key Point

Clinicians working in the labour ward should be trained in performing ultrasound. Simulation training is a good option for those who have no prior scanning experience, particularly for transperineal ultrasound.

CLINICAL HISTORY AND PREVIOUS ULTRASOUND SCANS

On admission into the labour room, a history of maternal clinical presentation and relevant background antenatal history is important in any pregnancy. Clinical history is an adjunct to ultrasound examination and interpretation. Together, they provide an integrated understanding of the level of risk and specific attributes of the pregnancy.

Review of Previous Ultrasound Scans

The following information from prior ultrasound imaging is useful in the current pregnancy:

- Calculation of gestational age using the crown–rump length (CRL) or head circumference (HC)
- Singleton or multiple pregnancy
- Mid-trimester (anomaly) ultrasound
- Placental localisation
- Biometry measurements for estimated fetal weight
- Amniotic fluid—single deepest vertical pool (SDVP) or amniotic fluid index (AFI)
- Doppler measurements—umbilical artery Doppler waveform and pulsatility index (PI)

LIMITATIONS OF DIGITAL VAGINAL EXAMINATION

Digital vaginal examination (VE) is widely performed by clinicians to assess cervical dilatation and effacement, establish the fetal station of the presenting part, verify the presence or absence of membranes, and confirm fetal presentation and position.

Assessment of Cervical Changes

The assessment of cervical dilatation can be inaccurate [9] and has been shown to have interobserver variability [10]. Women may also find the examination painful [3], and care should be taken to discuss analgesia options prior to the examination. Repeated examinations increase the risk of chorioamnionitis in labour and should be minimised in the presence of preterm rupture of membranes [11].

Determining Fetal Position

The fetal head position is identified by digital vaginal examination, wherein the anterior and posterior fontanelles and the midline sagittal suture are palpated and the relation of the occiput to the maternal pelvis is determined (see **Chapter 4**, *Management of the first and second stages of normal labour*).

Clinical errors in identifying the fetal head position may occur due to:

- Difficulty in identifying the anterior and posterior fontanelles in the presence of:
  - Caput succedaneum and moulding
  - Fetal asynclitism
  - High fetal head station
  - Cervical dilatation <4 cm

INTRAPARTUM ULTRASOUND

Ultrasound in the labour room can be performed with a conventional 'static' ultrasound machine, a portable laptop machine, or a hand-held ultrasound machine. Currently, intrapartum ultrasound is not widely used clinically, but several studies have established its usefulness in the labour room. Transabdominal and transperineal imaging are used in labour.

Clinical Indications

The indications for the use of ultrasound in the labour room include the following:

- Placental localisation
- Assessment of amniotic fluid volume
- Confirming fetal presentation and lie
- Fetal head position and position of fetal spine
- Progress of labour
- Assisted vaginal birth

Most of these can be achieved by transabdominal ultrasound. Transperineal ultrasound is used for tracking the progress of labour.

Progress of labour

In cases of suspected abnormality in the progress of labour, intrapartum ultrasound can document the following:

- Fetal position and descent (fetal station)
- The presence and extent of caput

For assessing fetal position and station, intrapartum ultrasound appears to be more objective and reproducible than digital examination.

Assisted vaginal birth

Assessment of the fetal position by transabdominal ultrasound and measurement of the fetal head station by transperineal ultrasound help in predicting the outcome of the procedure. The most reliable sonographic parameters to predict the outcome of instrumental delivery are HPD and AoP (see the section below on *Role of ultrasound in assisted vaginal birth*).

TRANSABDOMINAL ULTRASOUND

Transabdominal imaging is performed with the probe placed on the maternal abdomen. It is useful in assessing the following:

- **Placental localisation:** Imaging is used to identify the site of placental implantation in the uterine cavity in relation to the internal os of the cervix.
- **Amniotic fluid volume:** This is assessed by measuring the single deepest pocket or the amniotic fluid index.
- **Lie:** This is the relationship between the longitudinal axis of the fetus and the longitudinal axis of the mother. The lie may be **longitudinal** (the fetal and maternal axes are the same), **transverse** (the fetus is at 90 degrees to the maternal axis), or **oblique** (the fetal axis is at less than 90 degrees to the maternal axis, often 45 degrees). See **Chapter 2**, *Mechanics of labour*, for further details.
- **Presentation:** Imaging allows for the identification of the leading part of the fetal body that is closest to the cervix, which could

be the head (cephalic), buttocks (breech), or umbilical cord.

- **Fetal position:** The location of the occiput and fetal spine are used as anatomic landmarks and related to a clock face to determine the fetal head position.
  - The relation of the **occiput** to the maternal pelvis with reference to a 12-hour clock face helps define fetal position. Occiput anterior is situated between 10:00–02:00 hours; occiput posterior corresponds to 04:00–08:00 hours; left occiput transverse (LOT) corresponds to 02:00–04:00 hours; and right occiput transverse (ROT) corresponds to 08:00-10:00 hours [12] (Fig. 20.2a).
  - The location of the **fetal spine** helps confirm the fetal position. Axial views of the fetal trunk help locate the vertebrae. The relation of the fetal spine in the transverse plane to the maternal abdomen is described with reference to a 12-hour clock face—the 12 o'clock position is anterior, 3 o'clock is the woman's left, 6 o'clock is posterior, and 9 o'clock is the woman's right (Fig. 20.2b).

Placental localisation

An unexpected low-lying placenta or a placenta previa is a life-threatening situation. Identifying a low-lying placenta before the commencement of labour can be life-saving for the woman and the fetus because it allows for interventions to prevent unanticipated massive obstetric hemorrhage and fetal demise. This may be more significant in LMICs, where the labouring woman may not have received adequate antenatal care or had a detailed ultrasound performed during her pregnancy [4].

> **Key Point**
>
> Placental localisation at the time of admission to the labour room may be very relevant in LMICs where the labouring woman may not have had a detailed ultrasound done in her pregnancy [4].

Low-lying placenta

A placenta is defined as low-lying if the leading edge is <20 mm from the internal cervical os after the completion of 16 weeks of pregnancy [13].

Placenta previa

Placenta previa refers to a placenta that covers the internal os during transabdominal or transvaginal imaging. See **Chapter 29,** *Antepartum hemorrhage,* for further details.

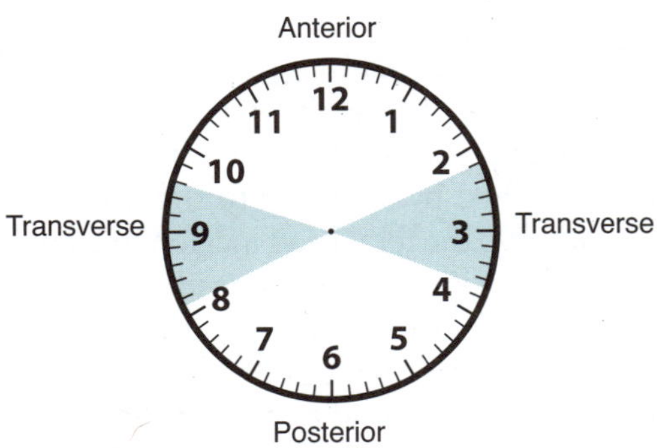

Fig. 20.2(a) Classification of fetal lie, i.e., the relation of the fetal occiput to the maternal pelvis as compared to a twelve-hour clock face

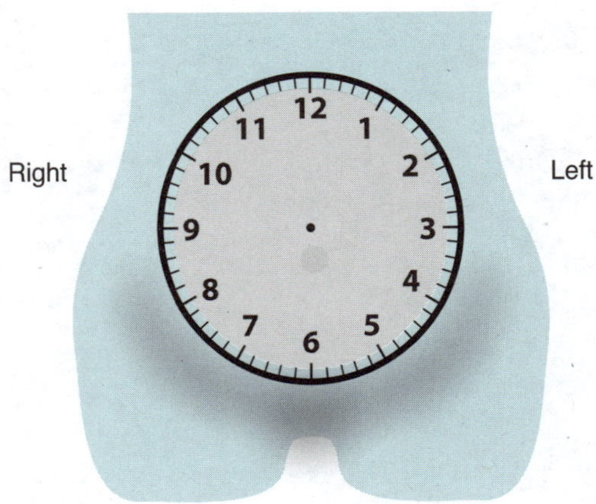

Fig. 20.2(b) Depiction of the twelve-hour clock face for transabdominal ultrasound used to assign the position of the fetal spine

Vasa previa

Vasa previa is said to be present when the fetal arterial or venous vessels lie exposed in the placental membranes without the protection of placental tissue. If the vessels rupture during labour, the perinatal mortality rate can be up to 60% [14]. During ultrasound imaging, vessels can appear as 'bubbles' or fine, tubular lines on grayscale imaging; this can be confirmed by a colour Doppler [15].

Placenta accreta spectrum

When placenta previa is identified, particularly along with a history of a prior cesarean birth, the chance of a coexisting placenta accreta increases. The identification of the placenta accreta spectrum allows time for planning delivery or early referral to specialised maternity units. See **Chapter 29** for more details.

Amniotic fluid

The assessment of the amniotic fluid volume in high-risk women in labour helps in the anticipation of a possible fetal compromise. The ultrasound probe is aligned with the sagittal plane, allowing the amniotic fluid volume to be calculated using a single deepest vertical pool measurement (Fig. 20.3) or a measurement of the four quadrants to obtain an amniotic fluid index (AFI). Care should be taken to place the probe at right angles to the abdominal contour. Normal amniotic fluid volume in the third trimester is represented by a single vertical pool of 2–8 cm or an AFI of 5–25 cm.

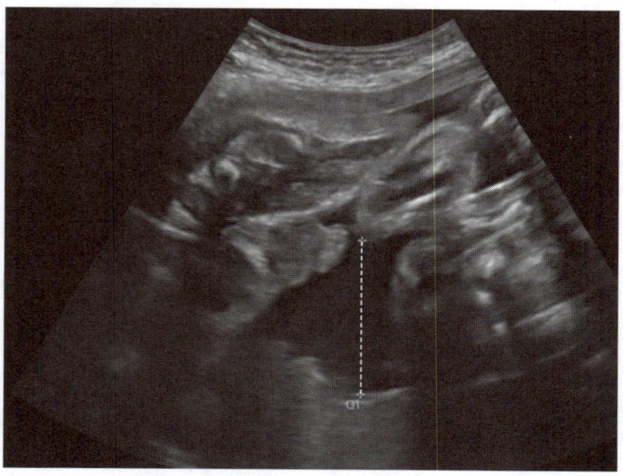

Fig. 20.3 Measurement of the single deepest vertical pocket to assess the amniotic fluid volume (*Image courtesy*: Dr Mariya Kovalenko)

Fetal lie

The fetal lie is initially determined by clinical abdominal palpation. In cases where the fetal axis does not correspond to the maternal axis (longitudinal lie), ultrasound can be used to obtain images of the fetal head and fetal buttocks to aid in determining the orientation of the fetus.

Fetal presentation

Clinical examination using abdominal palpation has low sensitivity for determining malpresentations. Transabdominal ultrasound scanning in the sagittal plane is useful in identifying malpresentations and non-cephalic presentations [16].

The transducer is placed in the midline of the maternal abdomen, at the level of the symphysis pubis [4]. A hyperechoic round shape of the fetal skull denotes a **cephalic presentation.** Confirmation is obtained by rotating the probe from the mid-sagittal plane to the transverse plane to obtain a view of the fetal skull. In **breech presentation**, the fetal buttocks, lower limbs, or feet will be seen (footling, flexed or extended) in the lower pole. Scanning from the left to the right on the maternal abdomen can demonstrate what type of breech presentation it is. Confirmation is obtained by scanning to the uterine fundus to observe the fetal head in a longitudinal lie.

A **cord presentation** may be identified above the internal cervical os on transabdominal ultrasound. This should be confirmed on transvaginal ultrasound and differentiated from vasa previa. Cord presentation can occur in cases of non-engagement of the cephalic presentation or malpresentation with a transverse, oblique, or breech fetus.

Fetal head position

Ultrasound can provide objective and reproducible measurements of the fetal head position and parameters related to labour progression [17]. If it is not possible to accurately diagnose the fetal position by digital vaginal examination, a transabdominal ultrasound is performed in the transverse plane at the level of the symphysis pubis in a cephalic presentation. This method is useful only when the head is not deeply engaged in the pelvis.

The location of the fetal spine and occiput are used as anatomic landmarks and related to a clock face (Fig. 20.2).

Fetal occipital position

The occipital position is determined by using the following as landmarks:

- Fetal midline brain structures, including the thalami, which are most easily seen in the occiput transverse position (Fig. 20.4)
- Fetal cerebellum
- Fetal orbits, which are visualised in the occiput transverse or occipital posterior position (Fig. 20.5)
- Cervical vertebrae, which are most notably seen in the occipital anterior position

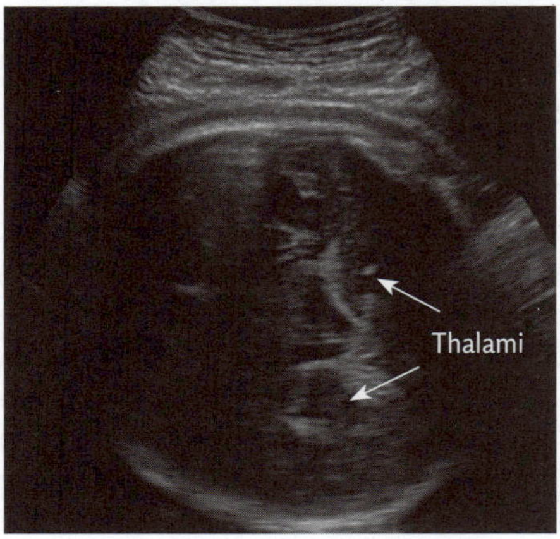

Fig. 20.4 Left occiput transverse position—the occiput can be identified as being on the maternal left, based on the visualisation of the thalami (arrows) (*Image courtesy*: Ms Arwa Hanidu)

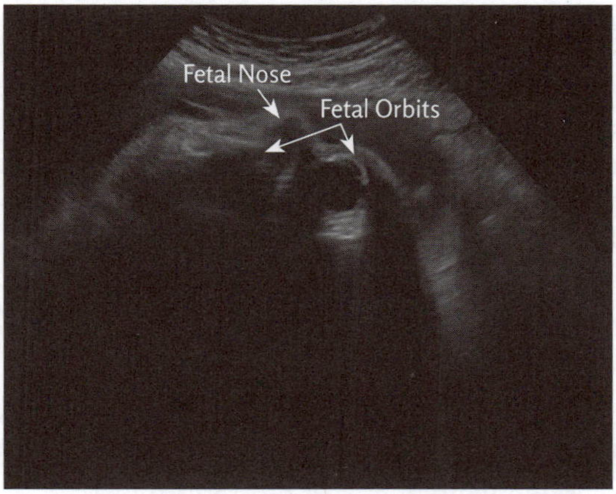

Fig. 20.5 Occiput posterior position with both orbits visualised anteriorly on ultrasound (*Image courtesy:* Dr Mariya Kovalenko)

Fetal spine position

Transabdominal ultrasound with the transducer in the transverse plane is used to evaluate the fetal heart at the level of the fetal thorax. Once this view of the fetal heart is obtained, the fetal spine is visualised distally as a hyperechoic spherical structure (Fig. 20.6).

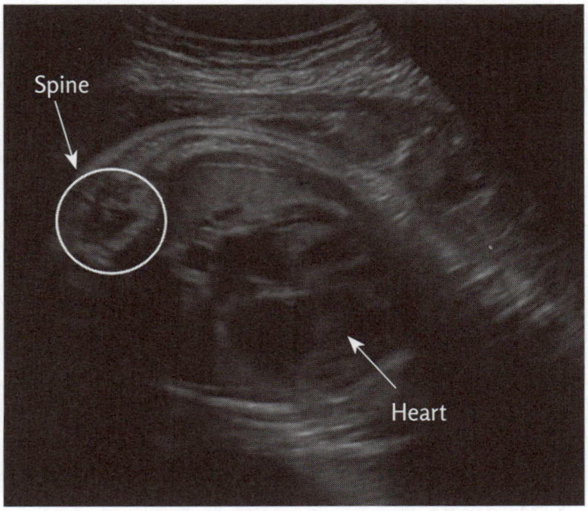

Fig. 20.6 Transabdominal ultrasound assessment to determine the fetal spine position; the spine is visualised at the 10.00 o'clock position (circle) (*Image courtesy:* Dr Mariya Kovalenko)

ULTRASOUND IN MULTIPLE PREGNANCY

Ultrasound is useful in identifying fetal presentation in non-singleton pregnancies. When a woman with a multiple pregnancy presents in the labour room, it is important for the obstetrician to identify the presentation of the first twin, and once the first twin is delivered, the presentation of the second twin [18].

TRANSVAGINAL ULTRASOUND

Transvaginal ultrasound may be useful for assessing women at risk of preterm birth.

Cervical Length Measurement

In women presenting acutely to the labour room with symptoms of preterm birth at 30+0 gestation or more, a transvaginal cervical length assessment can be used to determine the likelihood of birth in the next 48 hours in cases where the membranes are intact. If the cervical length is ≤15 mm, this can be diagnostic of preterm labour. Appropriate management should be offered in such cases [19].

TRANSPERINEAL ULTRASOUND

Transperineal imaging is performed with the probe placed on the outside of the woman's labia majora, with gentle pressure applied on the surrounding soft tissue (Figs. 20.7a and b). It is useful in the labour room for the assessment of the following:

- Cervical dilatation
- Fetal head position
- Fetal head station
    - — Head–perineum distance (HPD)
    - — Angle of progression (AoP)
- Presence of caput succedaneum
- Moulding

Cervical Dilatation

The cervix can be identified in the transverse ultrasound plane by visualising the anterior and posterior rims. It is easily visualised if the cervical dilatation is <4 cm (Fig. 20.8). Visualisation becomes progressively more difficult at greater cervical dilatations [20]. This is particularly useful in preterm gestations where unnecessary internal examinations should be avoided to reduce the risk of ascending infection. This method can also be used in term intrapartum women with vaginismus, those who are in early labour, women who have not received analgesia in labour, and those who decline vaginal examination.

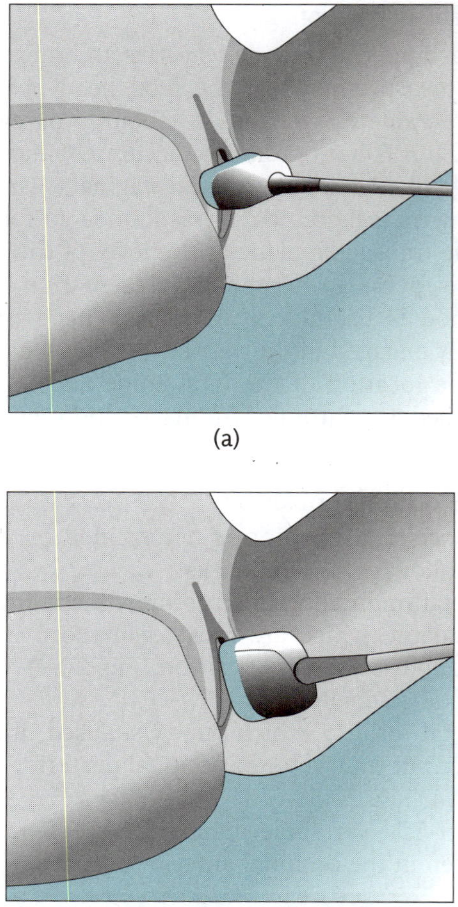

(a)

(b)

Fig. 20.7 Transducer placement for transperineal ultrasound: (a) In the transverse plane and (b) in the sagittal plane

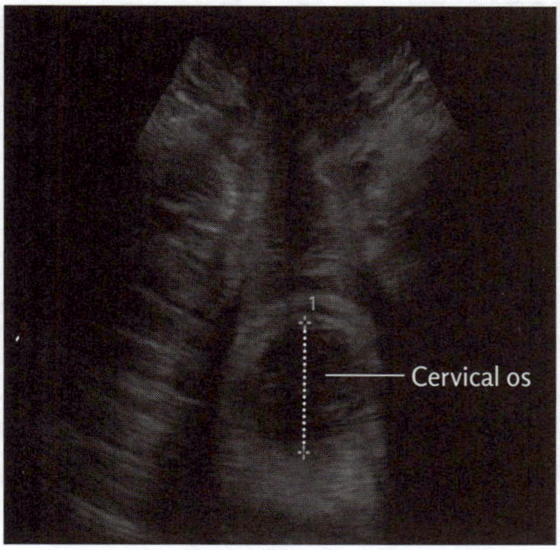

Fig. 20.8 Transperineal ultrasound assessment of cervical dilatation in the transverse plane: The dilatation is 29 mm (*Image courtesy*: Arwa Hanidu)

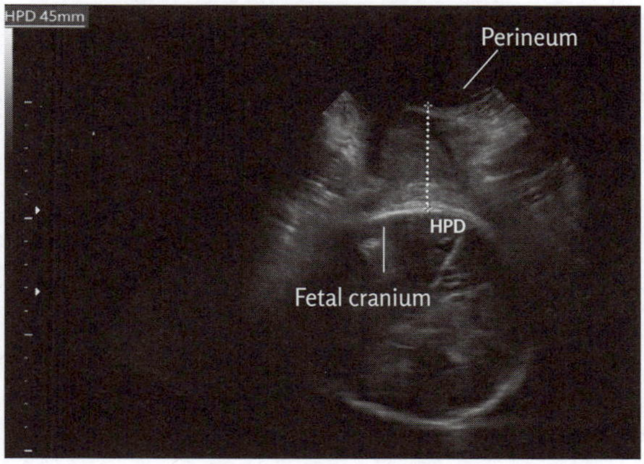

Fig. 20.9 Transperineal ultrasound in the transverse plane to measure the head–perineum distance (HPD) (dotted line) (*Image courtesy*: Dr Mariya Kovalenko)

Fetal Head Station

Traditionally, the fetal head station is assessed by digital vaginal examination in labour. However, a large caput and moulding in labour may be misinterpreted as a low fetal head station. An objective assessment of fetal head descent can be made using either a combination of the head–perineum distance and the angle of progression or either one of those measurements [20]. HPD is easy to measure and is reproducible. AoP (in degrees) is equivalent to the head station expressed in centimetres, from –3 cm to +5 cm (direct conversion is possible) [1].

Head–perineum distance (HPD)

The head–perineum distance is evaluated by placing the transducer in the transverse plane on the outer labia majora. Direct pressure is applied to compress the soft tissues. The fetal cranium can be seen in a cephalic presentation. An image of the same is captured to measure the distance between the leading fetal cranium and the edge of the ultrasound transducer (Fig. 20.9).

Angle of progression (AoP)

The angle of progression is the angle between the long axis of the pubic bone and a line from the lowest edge of the pubis drawn tangential to the deepest bony part of the fetal skull [1]. It is evaluated by placing the transducer in the midsagittal plane on the outer labia majora. Angling and dipping movements of the probe are undertaken to visualise the symphysis pubis anteriorly and the fetal cranium below or adjacent to the symphysis pubis. A still image or a cineloop video recording is captured to proceed. A straight line is drawn through the midline of the long axis of the pubic symphysis to meet another line drawn on the edge of the fetal skull, tangential to it (Fig. 20.10a and b). Table 20.1 lists the clinical conversions of HP and AoP values.

Table 20.1 Clinical conversion table of HPD and AoP measurements for fetal station [1]

Head station (cm)	HPD (mm)	AoP (degrees)
–3	54	84
–2	48	95
–1	42	106
0	36	116
+1	31	127
+2	*	138
+3	*	148

*Further data required

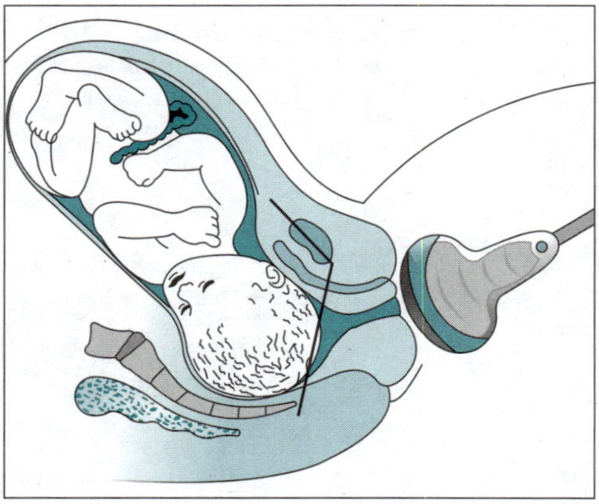

(a)

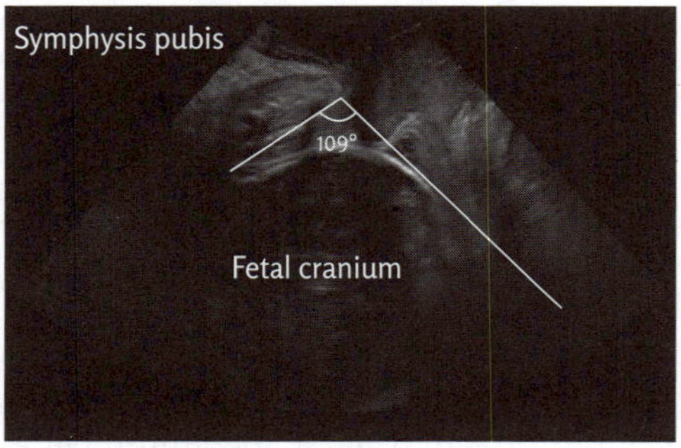

(b)

Fig. 20.10 Transperineal ultrasound in the mid-sagittal plane for the measurement of the angle of progression (AoP): (a) Graphic representation of the measurement and (b) ultrasound image of the measurement of AoP (*Image courtesy:* Dr Mariya Kovalenko)

Caput succedaneum

The caput on the fetal head is a 'boggy' swelling of the soft tissues overlying the fetal cranial bones. On ultrasound imaging, it either has a 'tented' appearance or is seen as a rounded swelling. An objective measurement in mm can be used to quantify the amount of caput by the skin-to-skull distance taken in the mid-sagittal plane (Fig. 20.11).

Cranial moulding

Cranial moulding occurs during the process of labour and results in the overlapping of fetal cranial bones. This can be visualised in the mid-sagittal plane (Fig. 20.11).

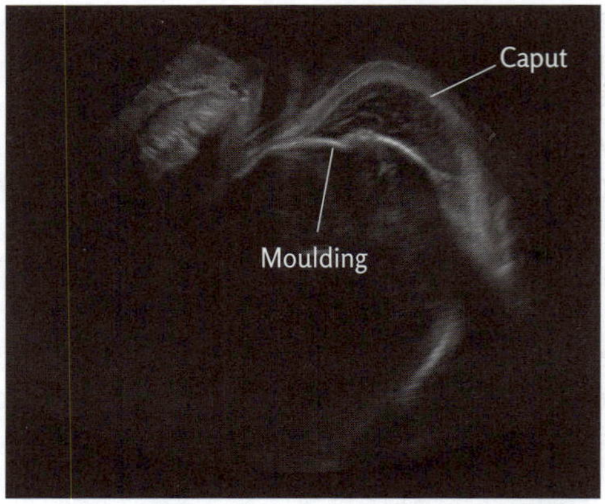

Fig. 20.11 Transperineal ultrasound in the mid-sagittal plane, depicting significant caput and moulding (*Image courtesy:* Dr Mariya Kovalenko)

The various intrapartum measurements useful in the management of labour are summarised in Table 20.2.

Table 20.2 Summary of transabdominal and transperineal ultrasound assessments in the management of labour

Transabdominal ultrasound imaging	Transperineal ultrasound imaging
Placental localisation	Cervical dilatation
Assessment of amniotic fluid volume	Fetal position
Confirming fetal presentation and lie	Fetal head station • Head–perineum distance (HPD) • Angle of progression (AoP)
Fetal position and position of fetal spine	Presence of caput succedaneum and moulding

ROLE OF ULTRASOUND IN ASSISTED VAGINAL BIRTH

Acknowledging the difficulty in ascertaining the fetal head position during labour, the Royal College of Obstetricians and Gynaecologists

(RCOG) recommends ultrasound assessment of the fetal head position in cases of uncertainty prior to undertaking an assisted vaginal birth (AVB) [22].

The accurate assessment of the fetal position and station are important prerequisites to instrumental delivery and a highly important indicator to determine correctly in order to achieve a safe AVB. The presence of significant caput and moulding during labour can prevent the clinician from adequately palpating the suture lines. This can result in a misdiagnosis of the fetal position. Studies have shown that though clinical and ultrasonographic assessments correlated within 45 degrees in 70–80% of cases, occiput posterior and transverse head locations were associated with a significantly higher rate of clinical error [23]. Therefore, even though digital examination is considered the gold standard, it is subjective and prone to error.

In contrast, ultrasound in the labour room can provide objective information when used to image the fetus in labour using both transabdominal and transperineal imaging. The fetal head station can be assessed based on the head–perineum distance (HPD) and the angle of progression (AoP).

A retrospective cohort study of 951 midcavity vacuum-assisted births found that an HPD of >55 mm is associated with a more difficult delivery with a higher chance of failure [24]. The AoP has a high overall accuracy in predicting a complicated assisted vaginal birth [25]. A cut-off level of >120 degrees at rest without a contraction demonstrates the potential of a complicated or failed assisted birth.

Intrapartum ultrasound has been researched as an adjunctive tool in assisted vaginal birth by which the fetal head position can be monitored prior to the commencement of the delivery as well as during the delivery to visualise progressive rotation and the descent of the fetal head [26].

Training in intrapartum ultrasound to monitor labour progress in conjunction with training on AVB skills can give obstetricians the confidence to make the appropriate choice for a successful vaginal delivery. This can help reduce the rising burden of cesarean sections in many parts of the world.

CONCLUSION

The introduction of the ultrasound scan into clinical obstetric practice gave clinicians a whole new perspective into the intrauterine environment. As its clinical applications have expanded over the past few decades, ultrasound imaging may have a greater role to play in the management of labour. Ultrasound in labour uses a transabdominal approach, chiefly to determine head and spine position, or a transperineal approach, which is useful for the assessment of head station and position in the late stages of labour. Though the clinical application of ultrasound imaging in the labour ward is broadening, training for its use in the labour room is not widely available.

Moreover, there is no consensus regarding timing and indications for ultrasound in the labour room and how the sonographic findings should be integrated into clinical practice. With increase in training and clinical use, intrapartum ultrasound has the potential to bring in objectivity in assessment and improve management of the woman in labour.

REFERENCES

1. Ghi T, Eggebo T, Lees C, Kalache K, Rozenberg P, Youssef A, et al. ISUOG Practice Guidelines: Intrapartum ultrasound. *Ultrasound Obstet Gynecol.* 2018. 52(1):128-39.
2. Akmal S, Kametas N, Tsoi E, Hargreaves C, Nicolaides KH. Comparison of transvaginal digital examination with intrapartum sonography to determine fetal head position before instrumental delivery. *Ultrasound in Obstetrics and Gynecology.* 2003. 21(5):437–40.
3. Usman S, Barton H, Wilhelm-Benartzi C, Lees CC. Ultrasound is better tolerated than vaginal examination in and before labour. *Aust N Z J Obstet Gynaecol.* 2019. 59(3):362-6.
4. Rizzo G, Ghi T, Henrich W, Tutschek B, Kamel R, Lees CC, et al. Ultrasound in labor: Clinical practice guideline

and recommendation by the World Association of Perinatal Medicine (WAPM) and the Perinatal Medicine Foundation (PMF). *Journal of Perinatal Medicine*. 2022.

5. Isabirye N, Kisa R, Santos N, Shah S, Mulowooza J, Walker D, et al. Ultrasound at labour triage in eastern Uganda: A mixed methods study of patient perceptions of care and providers' implementation experience. *PLOS ONE*. 2021. 16(11):e0259770.
6. Clark AE, Shaw CJ, Bello F, Chalouhi GE, Lees CC. Quantitating skill acquisition with optical ultrasound simulation. *Australas J Ultrasound Med*. 2020. 23(3):183-93.
7. Rosen H, Windrim R, Lee YM, Gotha L, Perelman V, Ronzoni S. Simulator-based obstetric ultrasound training: A prospective, randomized single-blinded study. *J Obstet Gynaecol Can*. 2017. 39(3):166–73.
8. di Pasquo E, Ramirez Zegarra R, Kiener AJO, Gobbi L, Dall'Asta A, Fieschi L, et al. Usefulness of an intrapartum ultrasound simulator (IUSim) for midwife training: Results from an RCT. *Fetal Diagn Ther*. 2021. 48(2):120–7.
9. Buchmann EJ, Libhaber E. Accuracy of cervical assessment in the active phase of labour. *BJOG*. 2007. 114(7):833–7.
10. Tuffnell DJ, Bryce F, Johnson N, Lilford RJ. Simulation of cervical changes in labour: Reproducibility of expert assessment. *Lancet*. 1989. 2(8671):1089–90.
11. Lewis DF, Major CA, Towers CV, Asrat T, Harding JA, Garite TJ. Effects of digital vaginal examinations on latency period in preterm premature rupture of membranes. *Obstet Gynecol*. 1992. 80(4):630–4.
12. Rane SM, Guirgis RR, Higgins B, Nicolaides KH. The value of ultrasound in the prediction of successful induction of labor. *Ultrasound in Obstetrics and Gynecology*. 2004. 24(5):538-49.
13. Jauniaux E, Alfirevic Z, Bhide A, Belfort M, Burton G, Collins S, et al. Royal College of Obstetricians and Gynaecologists. Placenta praevia and placenta accreta: Diagnosis and management. Green-top Guideline No. 27a. *BJOG*. 2019. 126(1):e1–e48.
14. Jauniaux E, Alfirevic Z, Bhide A, Burton G, Collins S, Silver R. Royal College of Obstetricians and Gynaecologists. Vasa praevia: Diagnosis and management. Green-top Guideline No.27b. *BJOG*. 2019. 126(1):e49–e61.
15. Ranzini AC, Oyelese Y. How to screen for vasa previa. *Ultrasound Obstet Gynecol*. 2021. 57(5):720-5.
16. Bellussi, F, Ghi, T, Youssef, A, Salsi, G, Giorgetta, F, Parma, D, et al. The use of intrapartum ultrasound to diagnose malpositions and cephalic malpresentations. *Am J Obstet Gynecol*. 2017. 217:633–41
17. Hassan WA, Eggebo T, Ferguson M, Gillett A, Studd J, Pasupathy D, et al. The sonopartogram: A novel method for recording progress of labor by ultrasound. *Ultrasound Obstet Gynecol*. 2014. 43(2):189–94.
18. National Institute for Health and Care Excellence. Twin and triplet pregnancy (NG137). 2019. Available from: https://www.nice.org.uk/guidance/ng137.
19. National Institute for Health and Care Excellence. Preterm labour and birth (NG25). 2022. Available from: https://www.nice.org.uk/guidance/ng25.
20. Usman S, Wilkinson M, Barton H, Lees CC. The feasibility and accuracy of ultrasound assessment in the labor room. *J Matern Fetal Neonatal Med*. 2019. 32(20):3442–51.
21. Usman S, Hanidu A, Kovalenko M, Hassan WA, Lees C. The sonopartogram. *American Journal of Obstetrics & Gynecology*. 2023. 228(5):S997-S1016.
22. Murphy D, Strachan B, Bahl R. Royal College of Obstetricians and Gynaecologists. Assisted vaginal birth. Green-top Guideline No. 26. *BJOG*. 2020. 127(9): e70–e112.
23. Dupuis O, Ruimark S, Corinne D, Simone T, André D, René-Charles R. Fetal head position during the second stage of labor: Comparison of digital vaginal examination and transabdominal ultrasonographic examination. *Eur J Obstet Gynecol Reprod Biol*. 2005. 123(2):193–7.
24. Nallet C, Ramirez Zegarra R, Mazellier S, Dall'asta A, Puyraveau M, Lallemant M, et al. Head-to-perineum distance measured transperineally as a predictor of failed midcavity vacuum-assisted delivery. *Am J Obstet Gynecol*. 2023. 5(2):100827.
25. Skinner SM, Giles-Clark HJ, Higgins C, Mol BW, Rolnik DL. Prognostic accuracy of ultrasound measures of fetal head descent to predict outcome of operative vaginal birth: A comparative systematic review and meta-analysis. *Am J Obstet Gynecol*. 2023. 229(1):10–22.e10.
26. Hinkson L, Henrich W, Tutschek B. Intrapartum ultrasound during rotational forceps delivery: A novel tool for safety, quality control, and teaching. *Am J Obstet Gynecol*. 2021. 224(1):93 e1–e7.

CHAPTER 21

Operative Vaginal Delivery

TULIKA SINGH, SAMERA A KHALIL

INTRODUCTION

Operative vaginal delivery, by vacuum extractor (ventouse) or forceps, forms an essential part of obstetrical services. Assisted vaginal delivery using the vacuum cup is one of the most common instrumental procedures in obstetrics.

The ability to perform an operative delivery is a critical skill for those who provide maternity care. It allows the caregiver to accomplish or expedite a safe vaginal delivery for maternal or fetal indications.

The concept of operative vaginal delivery gained popularity in the 18th century [1]. Today, a variety of devices are available to the modern obstetrician. The frequency of operative vaginal deliveries is estimated to be between 10 and 15% of all births [2]. Over the past three decades, there has been a global decline in instrumental delivery rates, while cesarean rates have increased. This is probably because the teaching of instrumental delivery is inadequate, and many obstetricians do not receive sufficient hands-on experience during their training.

Although the terms 'operative vaginal delivery' and 'assisted vaginal birth' have the same meaning, for this chapter, the term 'operative vaginal delivery' will be used to ensure consistency. Additionally, ventouse and vacuum are often used interchangeably in literature. However, to ensure consistency, the term 'vacuum' will be used across this chapter.

TYPES OF INSTRUMENTS

Forceps

All forceps share the same basic design comprising a **handle**, **shank, lock,** and **blades** (Fig. 21.1 a and b). The blades usually have a **pelvic curve** and a **cephalic curve**. Various versions differ from each other in features like blade length, fenestration, type of lock, and the presence or absence of a pelvic curve.

Forceps may be broadly divided into those used for **non-rotational deliveries** (Neville–Barnes, Simpsons, Piper, axis traction, Wrigley, and Naegle) and those used for **rotational deliveries** (Kielland and Tucker–McLane). Rotational forceps such as Kielland forceps have a less pronounced pelvic curve (Fig. 21.1c) and a **sliding (French) lock** to correct asynclitism. In contrast, the Neville–Barnes forceps have a more pronounced pelvic curve and a **fixed (English) lock** (Fig. 21.1d).

> **Key Point**
>
> Forceps may be broadly divided into those used for **non-rotational deliveries** and those used for **rotational deliveries.**

Vacuum Extractor

The vacuum consists of a cup that is applied to the fetal head and connected via a tube to an apparatus that creates a vacuum (Fig. 21.2a). The vacuum allows the operator to provide

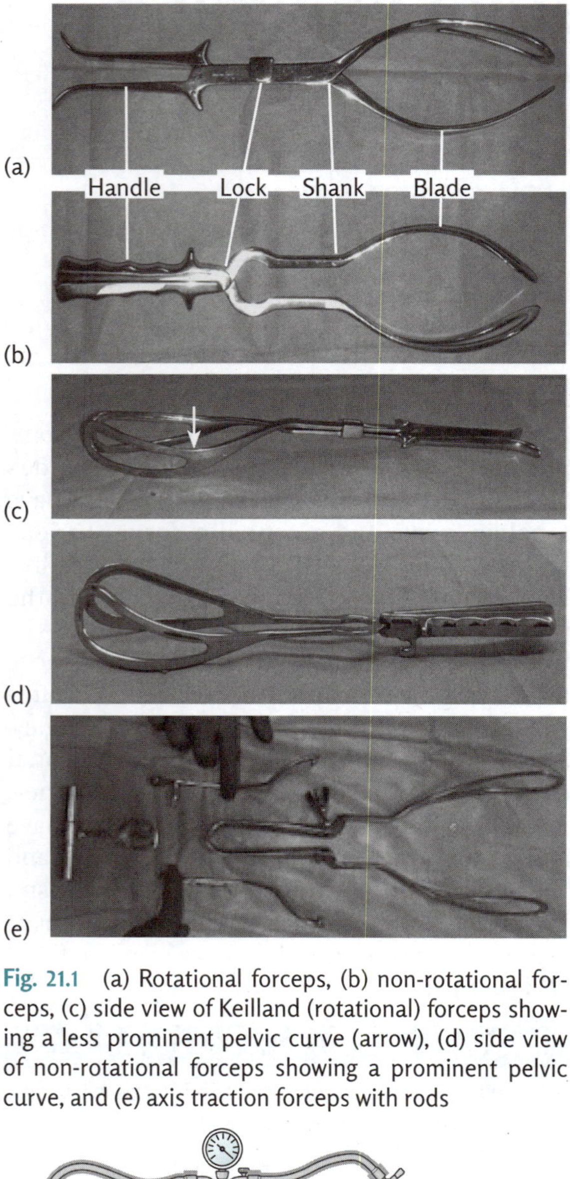

Fig. 21.1 (a) Rotational forceps, (b) non-rotational forceps, (c) side view of Keilland (rotational) forceps showing a less prominent pelvic curve (arrow), (d) side view of non-rotational forceps showing a prominent pelvic curve, and (e) axis traction forceps with rods

traction to the fetal head along the axis of the birth canal, thus facilitating delivery.

Two types of cups are used—the rigid cup and the soft cup.

Rigid cups

The original vacuum device was the Malmström disc-shaped metal cup (Fig. 21.2a). Bird innovatively attached the suction tubing to the side of the cup, allowing it to slide into position in occipitoposterior (OP) fetal positions.

Rigid cups are more likely to achieve vaginal delivery when compared to soft cups [3]. The rigid cup is a better choice for more complicated deliveries such as occipitoposterior, occipitotransverse and difficult occipitoanterior deliveries because it is less likely to get detached from the fetal head.

Though the traditional teaching is that rigid cups are more likely to cause scalp trauma than soft cups, evidence of low certainty suggests that there may be no difference in the rates of overall maternal trauma [3].

Soft cups

The silastic soft cup is a pliable funnel- or bell-shaped cup made of silicone (Fig. 21.2b). It was introduced in the 1980s and is available in three sizes (40 mm, 50 mm, and 60 mm). The commonly used size for a term fetus is 50 mm. Soft cups should be considered for more straightforward occipitoanterior deliveries.

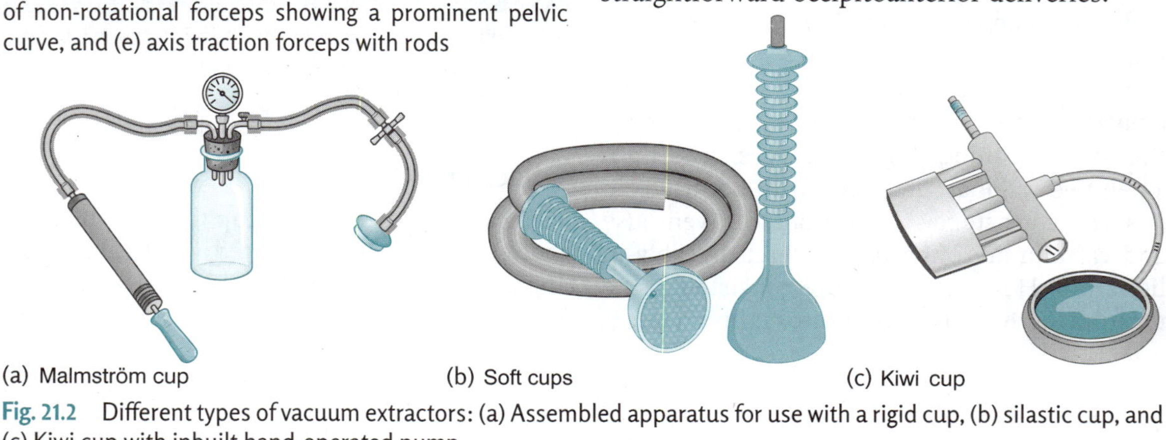

Fig. 21.2 Different types of vacuum extractors: (a) Assembled apparatus for use with a rigid cup, (b) silastic cup, and (c) Kiwi cup with inbuilt hand-operated pump

A recent systematic review of the Cochrane Database [3] compared soft and rigid vacuum extractor cups. The review concluded that failed delivery may be more likely with the soft vacuum cup because of more frequent detachments (pop-offs). However, soft cups have a lower rate of scalp trauma than rigid cups [2].

Kiwi handheld device

The Kiwi system is a disposable handheld device with a simple hand-operated pump that has gained popularity since its introduction in 2001 (Fig. 21.2c). The advantages of the Kiwi system are that it is associated with a significantly lower episiotomy rate, is easy to use and can be applied rapidly [4].

Random-allocation studies show that this device has a comparable safety profile but is less successful than conventional vacuum in achieving vaginal delivery [5,6]. Cup detachment occurs more often with the Kiwi cup [4].

> **Key Point**
>
> While a vaginal delivery is less likely to be achieved with a vacuum extractor than with forceps, the risk of third- and fourth-degree tears is lower with the vacuum extractor.

CHOOSING THE RIGHT INSTRUMENT

For most indications, the vacuum and forceps can be used interchangeably. The choice of the instrument depends on the clinical situation, personal preference, and operator skills [2].

Forceps and vacuum extraction are associated with different benefits and risks (see section on *Types of instruments*). Because of the lower risk of maternal trauma with vacuum, especially the soft cup, it is recommended as the first instrument of choice [2].

Obstetricians should be intimately familiar with the details and application of both devices. The forceps and metal cup are associated with a greater chance of successful delivery as compared to soft cups and the Kiwi device. The trade-off is a higher risk of maternal injury with forceps and a higher risk of fetal injury with the metal cup [7].

Vacuum extraction often needs more maternal effort to help achieve delivery when compared to forceps. This may need to be taken into consideration when making a choice where there is maternal exhaustion.

A comparison of instruments used for assisted birth is summarised in Table 21.1.

Table 21.1 Comparison of instruments used for assisted vaginal delivery (data extracted from the Cochrane Database [3] and the RCOG guidance on Assisted Vaginal Birth [2])

Type of instrument	Chance of successful delivery	Risk of failure to complete delivery with single instrument	Risk of maternal perineal trauma	Risk of neonatal cephalhematoma and retinal hemorrhage	Risk of neonatal scalp trauma
Forceps	More	Less	More	Less	Less
Rigid cups	More	More	Less	More	More
Soft cups	Less	More	Less	More	Less
Kiwi device	Less than other vacuum devices	More	Less	More	Less

CLASSIFICATION OF OPERATIVE VAGINAL DELIVERY

The classification and criteria for the various types of forceps delivery are presented in Table 21.2. Delivery is classified according to the following criteria:

- The station of the fetal head at application and
- The degree of rotation necessary for delivery.

This often dictates the type of device to use and the potential success of delivery. It must be noted that no indication is absolute and that competent clinical judgement is required in each case.

Key Point

The lower the fetal head and the lesser the rotation required, the lesser is the risk of injury to the woman and the fetus [8].

Table 21.2 Classification and criteria for the types of operative vaginal delivery (adapted from ACOG Practice Bulletin on Operative Vaginal Birth [8], and RCOG guidance on Assisted Vaginal Birth [2])

Classification of forceps	Criteria for applying forceps
Outlet forceps	• Fetal scalp visible at the introitus without separating the labia • Fetal skull has reached the pelvic floor • Sagittal suture is in the – Antero-posterior diameter or – Right or left occiput-anterior or occiput-posterior position (rotation does not exceed 45 degrees)
Low forceps	• Leading point of the skull (not caput) is at station +2 cm or more and not on the pelvic floor • Two subdivisions – Rotation of ≤45 degrees – Rotation >45 degrees
Midforceps	• Fetal head is 1/5 palpable per abdomen • Leading point of the skull is above station +2 cm but not above the ischial spines (engaged)

INDICATIONS FOR OPERATIVE VAGINAL DELIVERY

Operative vaginal delivery is performed when delivery needs to be expedited due to fetal compromise or maternal exhaustion or to shorten the second stage on account of maternal medical conditions.

The indications for instrumental delivery are often complex and interdependent, e.g., fetal malposition leading to prolonged labour and maternal exhaustion. The clinician will need to develop expert clinical judgement rather than take the following indications prescriptively. Broadly speaking, however, the indications for instrumental deliveries may be divided into maternal and fetal (Table 21.3).

Table 21.3 Indications for operative vaginal delivery (adapted from ACOG Practice Bulletin on *Operative Vaginal Birth* [8], and *Intrapartum care for healthy women and babies*, Clinical Guideline 190, NICE [9])

Indications	Clinical situation
Maternal	• Prolonged second stage • Maternal exhaustion • Epidural block with a diminished urge to push • Maternal medical conditions – Severe hypertensive disease – Cardiac disease – Myasthenia gravis – Proliferative retinopathy – Cerebral aneurysm
Fetal	• Suspected immediate or potential fetal compromise – Non-reassuring CTG trace – Thick (significant) meconium • Aftercoming head of breech (Piper forceps), if a clinician with expertise is available • Difficulty in delivering the head at cesarean
Combined	• Maternal and fetal indications for operative vaginal delivery frequently coexist

Maternal Indications

Prolonged second stage

A prolonged second stage is defined as an active second stage lasting more than 2 hours in a primigravida (3 hours with epidural) or more than 1 hour in a multipara (2 hours with epidural). It can lead to maternal and fetal compromise (see **Chapter 12**, *Abnormalities in the second stage of labour*). Hence, operative vaginal delivery is indicated in this situation unless delivery is imminent [2,10].

Maternal exhaustion

Maternal exhaustion is a common indication for assistance.

Maternal medical conditions

In women with medical conditions such as cardiac disease, cerebrovascular disease, myasthenia gravis, severe hypertensive disease, or spinal cord injury, it is beneficial to cut short the second stage of labour.

Fetal Indications

Malposition of the fetal head

This may result from non-rotation or partial rotation of the fetal head from the OP position. The initial step of management is augmentation with oxytocin after ruling out disproportion. Assistance is provided if spontaneous rotation does not occur within the timeframe mentioned above or if maternal or fetal compromise supervenes.

Suspected immediate or potential fetal compromise

Suspected fetal compromise in the form of non-reassuring CTG changes or thick (significant) meconium is an indication for instrumental delivery if the clinical situation allows it.

Breech delivery

The aftercoming head of breech can be delivered using long-shank forceps such as Piper forceps.

Cesarean delivery

Forceps (outlet) or vacuum (handheld) can be used at cesarean, especially if difficulty is anticipated in delivering the baby's head (see **Chapter 22**, *Cesarean section: Procedure and technique*).

CONTRAINDICATIONS TO OPERATIVE VAGINAL DELIVERY

Incompletely Dilated Cervix

Instrumental delivery should not be attempted before full dilatation. Doing so risks severe cervical lacerations. The only possible exceptions to this rule are the use of vacuum at 9 cm dilatation for the second of twins, with a cephalic presentation.

Unengaged Head

Forceps or vacuum should not be used when the head is palpable abdominally and is not engaged.

Non-vertex Deliveries

Operative vaginal delivery is contraindicated in non-vertex deliveries except for the aftercoming head of breech, where forceps (not vacuum) can be used by an experienced operator. There is no mechanism for the delivery of a fetus in the mentoposterior position; an instrumental delivery should not be attempted in this situation.

Increased Risk of Fetal Injury

Instrumental delivery should not be carried out when the procedure risks injury to the fetus as in cases of **pelvic disproportion, fetal demineralisation disease** (e.g., osteogenesis imperfecta), or **coagulopathy**. Suspected **fetal bleeding disorders** (e.g., hemophilia and alloimmune thrombocytopenia) are relative contraindications to operative vaginal delivery. Vacuum should be **avoided under 32 weeks** and should be used with caution between 32+0 and 36+0 weeks of gestation [2]. **The**

operator's unfamiliarity with the instrument precludes safe instrumental delivery.

The contraindications to operative vaginal delivery are summarised in Box 21.1.

Box 21.1 Contraindications to operative vaginal delivery

- Incompletely dilated cervix
- Unengaged head
- Fetal malpresentation (brow or face presentation)
- Unknown fetal position
- Suspected cephalopelvic disproportion/macrosomia
- Rotation >45° from occiput-anterior or occiput-posterior
- Fetal bleeding disorders, e.g., hemophilia and thrombocytopenia
- Fetal demineralising disease, e.g., osteogenesis imperfecta
- Fetal prematurity <32 weeks (for vacuum)

PREREQUISITES FOR OPERATIVE VAGINAL DELIVERY

Training

Obstetricians should be trained to carry out operative vaginal delivery as a prerequisite to commencing this highly skilled procedure. A senior obstetrician competent in performing midcavity deliveries should be present if a junior trainee is performing the delivery. See the section below on *Training in operative vaginal delivery.*

Informed Consent

Women should be informed about operative vaginal delivery as part of routine antenatal education, especially if they are primigravidas, in whom the chance of the need for forceps or vacuum birth is the highest. The intrapartum period can be a minefield as far as the legality of the given advice is concerned. This has prompted many experts to advocate the counselling of all pregnant women regarding operative vaginal delivery because as many as 10% of them may need it.

Before starting the procedure, it is crucial to get informed consent from the woman. The 2015 Montgomery Rules [11] strictly emphasise the clinician's role in informing women about the risks of the proposed procedure along with the risks of alternative procedures. The information provided to a woman in labour should be delivered **between contractions** when she can process and understand what is being said to her.

Verbal consent is the traditional route for labour room procedures, whilst written consent is a requirement for a trial of assisted vaginal birth in an operating theatre [12].

Key Points

- For labour room procedures, verbal consent should be obtained prior to operative vaginal birth, and the discussion should be documented in the notes.
- Written consent should be obtained for a trial of assisted vaginal birth in an operating theatre.

Examination of the Woman

On examination, the maternal abdomen should be palpated to confirm the engagement of the fetal head. A vaginal examination should be performed to assess the following:

- Full dilatation of the cervix
- Absence of membranes (operative delivery cannot be performed with intact membranes)
- Fetal position
- The presence or absence of caput or moulding
- The presence of thin or thick meconium-stained amniotic fluid
- Adequacy of the pelvis using the following landmarks:
  - The sacral hollow
  - The prominence of the ischial spines
  - The shape of the subpubic arch

The maternal bladder should be emptied. If a urinary catheter is in situ, it should be removed, or its bulb should be deflated.

Analgesia

Adequate analgesia should be ensured. This can be in the form of **regional** (epidural or spinal) or **local** anesthesia by perineal infiltration with a pudendal block.

Key Point

A neonatologist should be present for all instrumental deliveries to resuscitate the baby if needed and to examine the baby for birth injuries.

Antibiotics

Till recently, routine administration of prophylactic antibiotics was not recommended for operative vaginal delivery because of the potential adverse effects of unnecessarily exposing mothers and fetuses to antibiotics.

However, the RCOG recommends a single prophylactic dose of intravenous amoxicillin and clavulanic acid within 6 hours of assisted vaginal birth [2]. This is based on the ANODE trial [13], a recent multicentre randomised controlled trial from the UK. The latest systematic review of the Cochrane Database [14] has changed its recommendation in favour of a single dose of prophylactic antibiotic, as has the World Health Organization [15].

The ACOG does not feel this recommendation can be generalised to all women undergoing operative vaginal birth in the United States but recommends the judicious use of a single dose of antibiotic if a third- or fourth-degree tear occurs [8].

The antibiotic, dosage, and timing are as follows:

- A single dose of intravenous amoxicillin (1 g) and clavulanic acid (200 mg)
- Administered as soon as possible after birth and no more than 6 hours after birth

The feasibility of applying the results of a study from a high-income country to LMICs in terms of resources and cost has not been studied. See **Chapter 19,** *Antibiotic prophylaxis in labour and delivery,* for further details.

Intrapartum Ultrasound

Ultrasound assessment of the position of the fetal head prior to assisted vaginal birth is more reliable than clinical examination. It may be used to confirm the fetal head position if there is uncertainty following clinical examination [2] (see **Chapter 20,** *Role of ultrasound in the labour room*). Although ultrasound itself is not a prerequisite to operative vaginal delivery, it is important to note that knowing the correct fetal head position is essential.

Table 21.4 summarises the prerequisites for instrumental delivery.

APPLICATION AND TECHNIQUE FOR VACUUM-ASSISTED DELIVERY

Initial Steps

The woman is placed in the lithotomy position, and analgesia is ensured. Her bladder is emptied (by catheterisation if necessary) before the procedure. A vaginal examination is performed to determine the position and station of the fetal head.

Table 21.4 Prerequisites for operative vaginal delivery

Preparation of labouring woman	• Informed consent
	  – Verbal, if in the labour room
	  – Written, if trial in theatre
	• Availability of analgesia
	• Prophylactic antibiotic according to unit policy

Abdominal and vaginal examination	• Engaged head • Cervix fully dilated and membranes ruptured • Vertex presenting • Adequate pelvis • Presence or absence of caput/moulding • Correct diagnosis of fetal position – Confirm with ultrasound if there is doubt
Clinical requirements	• Empty bladder • Aseptic technique • Episiotomy, if there is a risk of perineal laceration
Staff and facility	• Experienced and trained staff • Facilities for cesarean delivery and neonatal resuscitation • Willingness to abandon procedure, if required

Determining the Flexion Point

Crucial to the success of vacuum delivery is the placement of the centre of the cup at the **flexion point**. This is a point on the sagittal suture 3 cm anterior to the posterior fontanelle (Fig. 21.3). Correct application facilitates flexion and synclitism of the fetal head and promotes delivery. Incorrect or paramedian applications are a common reason for failure and pop-offs.

Positioning the Cup

The labia are spread, and the soft cup is introduced by compressing and inserting it into the vagina while angling the device towards the occiput. If a rigid cup is used, the device is inserted sideways into the vagina while angling it posteriorly.

When contact is made with the fetal head, the centre of the cup is placed over the flexion point and symmetrically across the sagittal suture (Fig. 21.4a). The entire circumference of the cup must then be digitally inspected to ensure that no vaginal, cervical, or vulvar tissues are trapped between the cup and the fetal surface.

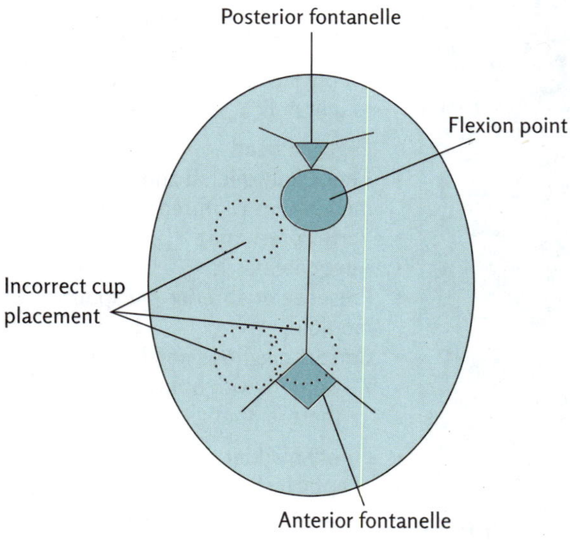

Fig. 21.3 Determination of the flexion point—the circle with the bold outline shows correct cup placement at the flexion point, which is over the sagittal suture, approximately 3 cm from the posterior fontanelle; the circles with the dotted outlines show incorrect cup placement, which may lead to failure and pop-offs

> **Key Point**
>
> Care must be taken not to cover either fontanelle with the ventouse cup.

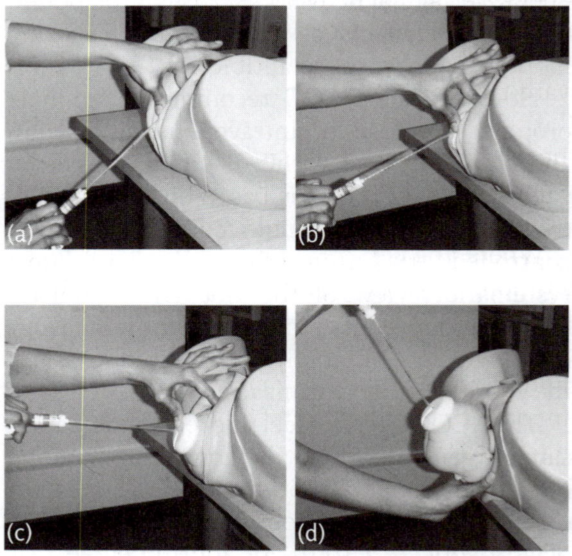

Fig. 21.4 Steps of a vacuum-assisted delivery: (a) Positioning the cup; (b) the thumb and index finger of one hand are kept on the edges of the cup to apply counterpressure while the other hand applies traction; (c) sustained downward traction applied along the pelvic curve; and (d) supporting the perineum while the head is delivered

Application of Suction

After the cup is applied, the vacuum is initially set at -0.2 Kg/cm^2, and a vaginal examination is carried out to confirm that the cup is free of the cervix. Once this is confirmed, the suction is turned up to the operating pressure of -0.6 to -0.8 Kg/cm^2 (-60 to -80 kPa/ -500 to -800 cm H_2O). An effective chignon (false caput) is formed in 2 minutes. It is not necessary to wait for longer than that before commencing traction.

Application of Traction

Once the chignon is formed, the operator uses her dominant hand to provide traction and her non-dominant hand to steady the cup with the index and middle fingers on the fetal scalp and the thumb on the cup. (Fig. 21.4b). Traction is applied perpendicular to the cup, changing direction as the head descends. Angular traction is avoided as it leads to pop-offs and 'cookie-cutter' injuries to the fetal scalp.

As the head descends, sustained downward traction is applied along the pelvic curve (Fig. 21.4c). Traction is applied gradually as the contraction builds and is maintained as long as the contraction lasts, in conjunction with the mother's expulsive efforts.

Where the fetal head is in the OT or OP position, autorotation occurs with traction. The upper limits of safety are not known but a traction force of 23 Kg is accepted as the maximum. Unless fetal compromise is suspected, it is important to deliver the fetal head slowly, allowing the perineum to stretch and to minimise tears. A modified Ritgen manoeuvre may also be used to minimise perineal trauma (Fig. 21.4d).

In the majority of cases, vacuum-assisted birth is completed with a maximum of **three pulls** to bring the fetal head onto the perineum. Three additional gentle pulls can be used to ease the head out of the perineum. Attempts at delivery should be halted when there is no descent of the fetal head with 2–3 pulls, and the clinical findings should be re-evaluated [2]. Vacuum delivery should also be stopped if there is suspicion of fetal injury.

Observational studies have shown that nearly all successful vacuum deliveries occur within 15 minutes of commencing the procedure. The risk of fetal injury increases with prolonged operative time [8]. Åberg et al. [16] investigated the impact of protracted vacuum extraction on the risk of neonatal intracranial hemorrhage in term infants and found that the safe limits for vacuum duration and the number of pulls are still unknown and that intracranial hemorrhage may occur even when performed in accordance with safety recommendations.

Thus, if fetal descent and delivery have not occurred within 20 minutes, the procedure should be abandoned, and the baby should be delivered by cesarean section.

> **Key Point**
>
> Traction should be applied in concert with uterine contractions and maternal expulsive efforts. The safe limits for vacuum duration and number of pulls are still unknown.

APPLICATION AND TECHNIQUE FOR FORCEPS DELIVERY

Initial Steps

After ensuring that aseptic precautions have been taken, the woman is placed in the lithotomy position. Her bladder is emptied and analgesia is ensured. A vaginal examination is performed, and using the posterior fontanelle and sagittal suture as guidelines, the position of the fetal head is accurately identified. This is particularly important in the presence of a caput.

Application of the Forceps Blades

The operator inspects the blades of the forceps to ensure that they belong to the same pair and that they lock easily. To facilitate the **identification of the right and left blades**, the forceps can be articulated and held in front of the perineum in the position in which the blades will be applied. This makes it easy to identify the left blade and the right (here, right and left refer to the woman's right and left).

After checking the fetal position, by convention, **the left blade is applied first**. The left blade is held in the operator's left hand and gently glided into the sacral hollow, with the operator's right hand guarding the maternal soft tissues. The blade is then moved to the left of the maternal pelvis to lie between the fetal head and pelvic wall. The **right blade** is then held in the operator's right hand and eased into place directly between the fetal head and the right maternal pelvic wall. The operator's left hand guards the maternal soft tissues.

Key Point

The blades of the forceps are applied with the pelvic curve directed anteriorly and the cephalic curve directed medially.

With proper application, the sagittal suture of the fetal skull lies in the midline of the blades, the blades are symmetrical, and the application and locking are smooth. Difficulty with locking signifies asymmetrical application on the fetal head and can cause fetal injuries. The operator then ensures there is no maternal tissue between the blades.

Traction

The forceps are held by the dominant hand supinated. The non-dominant hand deflects the traction downwards (Pajot's manoeuvre; Fig. 21.5a), following the J-shaped pelvic curve or the curve of Carus (Fig. 21.5b). As the head descends, traction is applied horizontally until the head crowns and the perineum bulges (Fig. 21.5c). As the fetal head is delivered, the handles are elevated almost to a vertical position (Fig. 21.5d). The delivery of the head should be slow, controlled and combined with the Ritgen manoeuvre. The operator or an assistant can guard the maternal perineum with a large swab to prevent excess trauma (Figs. 21.5b,d). Once the fetal head is delivered, the blades of the forceps are removed in the reverse order of application (first one in, last one out).

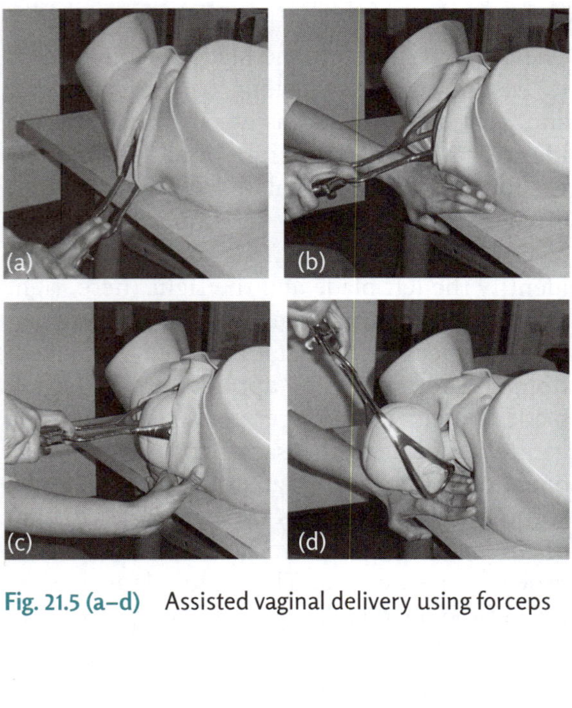

Fig. 21.5 (a–d) Assisted vaginal delivery using forceps

THE ROLE OF EPISIOTOMY IN OPERATIVE DELIVERY

The traditional teaching is to perform an episiotomy routinely with forceps delivery and selectively when vacuum is used. This is because forceps are thought to take up extra space around the fetal head and their rigid nature is thought to increase the risk of perineal tears. The risk of episiotomy is 50–60% with vacuum and ≥90% with forceps [12].

In a small retrospective series, a mediolateral episiotomy was found to be associated with fewer third- and fourth-degree perineal tears [17]. An observational study of 27,832 operative vaginal deliveries in the Netherlands found that mediolateral episiotomy protected against obstetric anal sphincter injuries (OASI) in both vacuum (9.4% compared to 1.4%) and forceps deliveries (22.7% compared to 2.6%) [18].

The American College of Obstetricians and Gynecologists [8] **does not recommend routine episiotomy** with operative vaginal birth because of the lack of data to support its use. Moreover, poor healing and prolonged discomfort have been reported with mediolateral episiotomy.

Key Point

Due to the absence of conclusive evidence, the decision to perform an episiotomy should be based on robust clinical judgement and decision-making in consultation with the woman [2].

ROTATIONAL INSTRUMENTAL DELIVERY

Rotational delivery can be achieved using either vacuum or rotational forceps like the Kielland forceps. The instrument used depends on the choice and expertise of the operator.

A rotational delivery is a clinically sound option in certain circumstances:

- Rotation of an occiput-posterior position to an occiput-anterior position in a forceps-assisted delivery prevents the more severe maternal perineal trauma that occurs with forceps-assisted delivery in the occiput-posterior position [19].
- Compared to rotational vacuum, Kielland forceps, in experienced hands, have been found to be effective and safe in preventing a cesarean section when malposition complicates the second stage of labour [20].

Key Point

Rotation, when needed, is performed between contractions.

Rotational delivery with the Kielland forceps should preferably be carried out by an appropriately trained and experienced operator as its use can be associated with additional risks [21,22]. Alternatively, rotational vacuum or manual rotation followed by traction forceps can be used to achieve delivery in cases of non-OA positions of the fetal head [23].

SEQUENTIAL USE OF INSTRUMENTS

In cases where the head is not delivered using either vacuum or forceps with adequate traction, another instrument may be applied to try to deliver the head. In other words, a vacuum device is followed by a forceps or vice versa. Both the RCOG and the ACOG advise against the routine sequential use of instruments since they are associated with increased rates of neonatal complications [2,8].

Key Point

If proper placement of forceps cannot be achieved or a vacuum device fails to achieve suction and no traction has been applied, switching to another device should not be considered a sequential attempt.

The sequential use of instruments leads to an increased risk of trauma to the fetus [24]. One needs to weigh the risks of an emergency cesarean section in the second stage following failed delivery using vacuum extraction against forceps application following a failed vacuum extraction. Second-stage cesarean sections are known to increase both maternal and perinatal morbidity and mortality [25]. It is good practice to involve a senior colleague if one is not able to achieve a delivery with the chosen instrument before switching to another device.

TRIAL VERSUS FAILED INSTRUMENTAL DELIVERY

Trial of Instrumental Delivery

The majority of instrumental vaginal deliveries are conducted in the delivery room as there is a high chance of successful delivery. In a small proportion, **a trial of instrumental vaginal delivery** is attempted because the operator anticipates **a chance of failure** [26,27]. A trial is usually conducted in the operating theatre with the intention of abandoning the procedure if fetal descent meets with resistance or if excessive force is required. This is so that facilities for cesarean section are immediately available should the need arise.

Key Point

Trial of instrumental delivery should be conducted by an experienced operator and in a facility where immediate recourse to cesarean section is possible. Most often, it is performed in the operating room.

Thus, most non-OA and midcavity instrumental deliveries, in which the chance of failure is high, should ideally be carried out in the operation theatre.

Failed Instrumental Delivery

This refers to failure to deliver the baby in the labour room in cases where **the possibility of failure was not considered**. A failed instrumental delivery could be due to a maternal body mass index >30 Kg/m^2, an estimated fetal weight >4000 g or a clinically big baby [25].

A failed instrumental delivery has the potential for causing panic for the woman and the staff looking after her. In most obstetric units, failed instrumental delivery is a risk-management trigger point, whereas a failed trial of instrumental delivery is considered acceptable.

MANAGEMENT AFTER OPERATIVE VAGINAL DELIVERY

Shoulder dystocia and uterine atony should be anticipated since they may occur after instrumental births. Prompt implementation of shoulder dystocia drill and the use of uterotonics will prevent catastrophic outcomes.

The woman should be reassessed for the risk factors of venous thromboembolism and be given thromboprophylaxis accordingly [2]. She should also be advised regarding good perineal care. Regular analgesics (such as non-steroidal anti-inflammatory drugs and paracetamol) should be considered in the absence of contraindications.

Most importantly, a post-operative review of the woman by the clinician who performed the procedure reflects good medical practice. A study of 5,332 women who delivered by different methods found that women value a post-procedure review to discuss concerns and potential implications for future births [28].

RISKS AND COMPLICATIONS OF OPERATIVE VAGINAL DELIVERY

Complications are common following instrumental delivery and can, on the rare occasion, be serious. However, the risk should be in the context of the alternative, which is a cesarean section in the second stage. There is no doubt that the skill of the operator in making a good situational judgement in the use of instruments is pivotal in achieving a safe delivery of the baby without compromising the safety of the woman.

The occurrence of any complications/incidents should be clearly reported and documented for ongoing risk management learning.

Fetal Complications

- **Forceps marks:** These are common and, in most cases, trivial. Rarely, excess pressure and incorrect application can cause serious injury to the fetal soft tissue or cranium.
- **Nerve injury**: Pressure from the blades can sometimes lead to **facial nerve palsy**. In most cases, spontaneous resolution occurs [29]. Fetal **cervical spine injuries** may occur rarely after rotational forceps delivery. Shoulder dystocia is more common in women who undergo instrumental delivery and can be associated with **injury to the brachial plexus** [6].
- **Cephalohematoma**: This is a collection of blood under the subperiosteal space and confined by the sutures of the skull. Cephalohematomas are of little clinical consequence and resolve spontaneously. They can sometimes be associated with **neonatal jaundice** because of the breakdown of the collected blood. A cephalohematoma is more likely to occur after the use of vacuum than with the use of forceps.
- **Ocular trauma**: **Retinal hemorrhage** is more common after vacuum application. It does not usually lead to long-term sequelae. **Eyelid** or **eye trauma** is an uncommon result of incorrect forceps application. Incorrect application of the vacuum to the face can **injure facial soft tissue.**
- **Intracranial hemorrhage**: Though this may occur even with a spontaneous delivery, the

risk increases with operative delivery. Rarely, it results from a bleeding tendency of the baby or poor application of the instrument.

- **Subgaleal/subaponeurotic hemorrhage**: This is a potentially serious injury with a mortality rate of 14–20%. It can occur after vacuum, forceps, or more uncommonly, normal birth. Prompt diagnosis and treatment are vital as delays may lead to cardiovascular collapse in the newborn [30]. The risk of hemorrhage is higher in preterm babies [2].

Table 21.5 summarises the fetal risks and complications of operative vaginal delivery.

Maternal Complications

- **Perineal or cervical tears and lacerations**: These are more common with the use of forceps as compared to vacuum, regardless of whether an episiotomy is used or not [31]. Rotational forceps can lead to **spiral tears** of the vagina. The operator should actively check for perineal and cervical tears by performing both a vaginal and a rectal examination, and carefully repair any injuries.
- **Urinary and fecal incontinence**: Damage to the pelvic floor (levator ani) or the anal sphincter during birth can lead to urinary and fecal incontinence. Operative vaginal delivery is associated with a significantly higher risk of anal incontinence and pelvic organ prolapse [33]. The incidence of such damage is increased by intervention with any instrument, rising from an approximate baseline incidence of 10–25% following vacuum to 40% following forceps. Correct identification and proper repair of anal sphincter injuries [32] along with pelvic floor physiotherapy can prevent long-term problems.
- **Psychological trauma:** Some women can become psychologically traumatised by an instrumental birth. If this is compounded by the need for neonatal resuscitation, the result is often a traumatic birth experience leading to postnatal depression and requests for cesarean birth in subsequent pregnancies. It is important to debrief the woman before discharge; in some complicated births, it is important to offer postnatal support and follow-up.

The maternal complications of operative vaginal delivery are summarised in Table 21.6.

Table 21.5 Fetal risks and complications of operative vaginal delivery (adapted from RCOG guidance on Assisted Vaginal Birth [2])

Fetal risk	Incidence
Cephalohematoma (predominantly with vacuum delivery)	1–12%
Facial or scalp lacerations	10%
Retinal hemorrhage (more common with vacuum than forceps, variable)	17–38%
Jaundice or hyperbilirubinemia	5–15%
Subgaleal hemorrhage (predominantly vacuum delivery)	0.3–0.6%
Intracranial hemorrhage: Vacuum and forceps	5 to 15 in 10,000
Cervical spine injury: Mainly with Kielland rotational forceps	Rare
Skull fracture: Mainly with forceps	Rare
Facial nerve palsy: Mainly with forceps	Rare
Fetal death	Very rare

Table 21.6 Maternal risks and complications of operative vaginal delivery (adapted from RCOG guidance on Assisted Vaginal Birth [2])

Maternal risk	Incidence
Episiotomy	Vacuum: 50–60% Forceps: 90%
Vulvovaginal tear	Vacuum: 10% Forceps: 20%
OASI	Vacuum: 1–4% Forceps: 8–12%
Urinary or bowel incontinence	Common at 6 weeks, improves over time
Postpartum hemorrhage	10–40%

OASI, obstetric anal sphincter injury

TRAINING IN OPERATIVE VAGINAL DELIVERY

Insufficient training, a reduction in working time and the fear of litigation have contributed to a reduction in the rates of instrumental deliveries and an explosion in the rates of cesarean section in recent times.

It is vital that in this present environment, operative vaginal delivery be carried out either by an expert or a well-supervised trainee. Lack of training is associated with adverse outcomes, which could otherwise be avoided with appropriate instructional guidance [34].

In addition to bedside training, courses like ALSO (Advanced Life Support in Obstetrics) and MOET (Management of Obstetric Emergencies and Trauma) use mannequins to teach the practical aspects of operative vaginal delivery. The training of obstetricians in the art of instrumental vaginal delivery is of crucial importance if the rates of emergency cesarean section in the second stage of labour are to be reduced. Practical procedures can be learnt using suitably designed mannequins under directed supervision, but only practice in a 'real' labour ward environment will enable these skills to mature.

RISK MANAGEMENT

Operative vaginal delivery carries risks if it is not performed with utmost care. Complaints and litigations are far too common following an operative birth gone wrong. Obstetrics has the greatest number of litigations in the UK [35]. Common allegations include inappropriate continuation of procedure, poor indication for intervention, improper choice of instrument, excessive use of force, lack of information, and poor supervision.

Attempts should be made to reduce the rates of instrumental deliveries by interventions like companionship in labour, enhanced mobility, avoidance of regional analgesia, maternal hydration, and prudent oxytocic use.

Good documentation is vital to any operative delivery and can prove to be invaluable to build up a defence in medicolegal cases.

CONCLUSION

The ability to perform an operative delivery is a critical skill for those who provide maternity care. However, the lack of proper training and fear of litigation have led to a decrease in these procedures and an increase in cesarean deliveries. The risks of a cesarean delivery in the second stage are high, and operative assisted delivery is a less invasive intervention. Forceps or vacuum are reasonable options when delivery has to be accomplished speedily for either a maternal or fetal indication. The risks and benefits of operative vaginal birth should be individualised for each woman. The obstetrician should assess whether an operative vaginal birth can be safely accomplished; if not, cesarean birth is the better option.

REFERENCES

1. Thomas FB. Operative vaginal delivery: A historical perspective. *Best Practice & Research Clinical Obset & Gynaecol.* 2019. 56:3-10.
2. Murphy DJ, Strachan BK, Bahl R. Royal College of Obstetricians and Gynaecologists. Assisted Vaginal Birth: Green-top Guideline No. 26. *BJOG.* 2020. 127(9):e70-e112.
3. Verma GL, Spalding JJ, Wilkinson MD, Hofmeyr GJ, Vannevel V, O'Mahony F. Instruments for assisted vaginal birth. *Cochrane Database Syst Rev.* 2021. Issue 9. Art. No.: CD005455.
4. Siggelkow W, Schwarz N, Beckmann MW, et al. Comparison of obstetric efficacy and safety of the Kiwi Omnicup with conventional vacuum extraction. *Geburtshilfe Frauenheilkd.* 2014. 74(2):146-151.
5. Attilakos G, Sibanda T, Winter C, et al. A randomised controlled trial of a new handheld vacuum extraction device. *Br J Obstet Gynaecol.* 2005. 112 (11):1510-5.
6. Groom KM, Jones BA, Miller N, Paterson-Brown S. A prospective randomised controlled trial of the Kiwi Omnicup versus conventional ventouse cups for vacuum-assisted vaginal delivery. *Br J Obstet Gynaecol.* 2006. 113(2):183-9.
7. O'Mahony F, Hofmeyr GJ, Menon V. Choice of instruments for assisted vaginal delivery. *Cochrane Database Syst Rev.* 2010.11:CD005455.9]

8. Operative vaginal birth. ACOG Practice Bulletin No. 219. American College of Obstetricians and Gynecologists. *Obstet Gynecol.* 2020;135:e149–59.
9. National Institute for Health and Care Excellence. Clinical Guideline 190. London: NICE. 2017.
10. ACOG-SMFM. American College of Obstetricians and Gynecologists, Society for Maternal-Fetal Medicine. Obstetric care consensus no. 1: Safe prevention of the primary cesarean delivery. *Obstet Gynecol.* 2014. 123:693.
11. Chan SW, Tulloch E, Cooper ES, Smith A, Wojcik W, Norman JE. Montgomery and informed consent: Where are we now? *BMJ.* 2017. 357: j2224.
12. Royal College of Obstetricians and Gynaecologists. Operative vaginal delivery. Consent Advice No. 11. *RCOG.* 2010. London.
13. Knight M, Chiocchia V, Partlett C, et al. Prophylactic antibiotics in the prevention of infection after operative vaginal delivery (ANODE): A multicentre randomised controlled trial. ANODE collaborative group [published erratum appears in *Lancet.* 2019.393:2394]. *Lancet.* 2019. 393:2395–403.
14. Liabsuetrakul T, Choobun T, Peeyananjarassri K, Islam QM. Antibiotic prophylaxis for operative vaginal delivery. *Cochrane Database Syst Rev.* 2020. Issue 3. Art. No.: CD004455.
15. World Health Organization. WHO recommendation on routine antibiotic prophylaxis for women undergoing operative vaginal birth. 2021. World Health Organization, Geneva. https://apps.who.int/iris/handle/10665/341862.
16. Åberg K, Norman M, Pettersson K, et al. Protracted vacuum extraction and neonatal intracranial hemorrhage among infants born at term: A nationwide case-control study. *Acta Obstet Gynecol Scand.* 2019. 98:523.
17. Bodner-Adler B, Bodner K, Kimberger O, et al. Management of the perineum during forceps delivery. Association of episiotomy with the frequency and severity of perineal trauma in women undergoing forceps delivery. *J Reprod Med.* 2003. 48(4):239-42.
18. de Leeuw JW, de Wit C, Kuijken JP, Bruinse HW. Mediolateral episiotomy reduces the risk for anal sphincter injury during operative vaginal delivery. *BJOG.* 2008. 115:104–8.
19. Bradley MS, Kaminski RJ, Streitman DC, et al. Effect of rotation on perineal lacerations in forceps-assisted vaginal deliveries. *Obstet Gynecol.* 2013. 122:132.
20. Tempest N, Hart A, Walkinshaw S, Hapangama DK. A re-evaluation of the role of rotational forceps: Retrospective comparison of maternal and perinatal outcomes following different methods of birth for malposition in the second stage of labour. *BJOG.* 2013. 120:1277.
21. Chiswick ML, James DK. Kielland's forceps: Association with neonatal morbidity and mortality. *BMJ.* 1979. 1:7–8.
22. Chow SL, Johnson CM, Anderson TD, Hughes JH. Rotational delivery with Kielland's forceps. *Med J Aust.* 1987. 146:616–9.
23. SOGC Clinical practice guideline No 148. Guidelines for operative vaginal birth. *J Obstet Gynaecol Can.* 2004. 26:747–53.
24. Edozien LC, Williams JL, Chatterjee IC, Hirsch PJ. Failed instrumental delivery: How safe is the use of a second instrument? *J Obstet Gynaecol.* 1999. 19(5):460-2.
25. Murphy DJ, Liebling RE, Verity L, et al. Early maternal and neonatal morbidity associated with operative delivery in second stage of labour: A cohort study. *Lancet.* 2001. 358:1203–7.
26. Lowe B. Fear of failure: A place for the trial of instrumental delivery. *Br J Obstet Gynaecol.* 1987. 94(1):60-6.
27. Majoko F, Gardener G. Trial of instrumental delivery in theatre versus immediate caesarean section for anticipated difficult assisted births. *Cochrane Database Syst Rev.* 2012. Issue 10. Art. no.:CD005545.
28. Rowlands IJ, Redshaw M. Mode of birth and women's psychological and physical wellbeing in the postnatal period. *BMC Pregnancy and Childbirth.* 2012. 12:138.
29. Duval M, Daniel SJ. Facial nerve palsy in neonates secondary to forceps use. *Arch Otolaryngol Head Neck Surg.* 2009. 135 (7):634-6.
30. Vacca A. Sub-aponeurotic haemorrhage: A rare but life-threatening neonatal complication associated with ventouse delivery. *Br J Obstet Gynaecol.* 2000. 107(3):433.
31. Christianson LM, Bovbjerg VE, McDavitt EC, Hullfish KL. Risk factors for perineal injury during delivery. *J Obstet Gynecol.* 2003. 189(1):255-60.
32. Sultan AH, Thakar R. Lower genital tract and anal sphincter trauma. *Best Pract Res Clin Obstet Gynaecol.* 2002. 16(1):99-115.
33. Blomquist JL, Muñoz A, Carroll M, Handa VL. Association of delivery mode with pelvic floor disorders after childbirth. *jama.* 2018. 320(23):2438–2447.
34. Hotton E, O'Brien S, Draycott TJ. Skills training for operative vaginal birth. *Best Practice & Research Clinical Obstetrics & Gynaecology.* 2019. 56: 11-22.
35. Lane J, Bhome R, Somani B. National trends and cost of litigation in UK National Health Service (NHS): A specialty-specific analysis from the past decade. *Scott Med J.* 2021. 66(4):168-174.

CHAPTER 22

Cesarean Section

Procedure and Technique

GITA ARJUN

INTRODUCTION

Cesarean section rates have increased over the past three decades. This is a global phenomenon that has concerned professional bodies, activists, women and the media (see **Chapter 23**, *Reducing cesarean rates*). Betrán and colleagues [1] analysed the latest available data (2010–2018) from 154 countries, covering 94.5% of the world's live births, and found that 21.1% of women (1 in 5) worldwide gave birth by cesarean.

Cesarean sections are life-saving procedures that are firmly entrenched in obstetric practice. Though advances in anesthetic services and improved surgical techniques have reduced the morbidity and mortality of this procedure, there is evidence that there are short- and long-term effects on the mother and infant (see **Chapter 23**).

Overuse of Cesarean Delivery

Overuse of cesarean, i.e., cesareans performed with no medical indication, has not shown benefits and may, in fact, cause harm and unnecessary wastage of resources. Maternal and perinatal deaths following cesarean sections are disproportionately high in LMICs—a quarter of all women who died in LMICs (72 studies, 27,651 deaths) had undergone a cesarean section [2].

In India, as in other LMICs, the rate of cesarean delivery increases with improved socio-economic status, higher education, lower birth order, higher age, and number of antenatal check-ups. In other words, delivering in a private facility increases the chances of having a cesarean.

Unmet Needs

The underuse of cesarean contributes to increased maternal and perinatal mortality and morbidity. Women in under-resourced areas do not receive the optimal rate of cesareans. It has been shown that a cesarean rate of <10% increases maternal and perinatal morbidity and mortality. Due to this, many LMICs face a double burden—the unmet requirement for cesarean coupled with unsafely performed cesarean delivery [1].

As the most common surgical procedure performed by an obstetrician, it is important to be up to date with evidence-based procedures and surgical techniques involved in a cesarean birth.

TYPES OF CESAREAN SECTION

- **Primary cesarean section:** When a cesarean section is performed for the first time on a pregnant woman, it is called a primary cesarean section. In India, approximately 70% of cesareans have been reported to be primary cesarean sections [3].
- **Repeat cesarean section:** When a woman has had one or more previous cesarean sections, it is known as a repeat cesarean. With the rising rate of primary cesareans, repeat cesareans are adding to the total cesarean section rate.
- **Lower segment cesarean section (LSCS):** In modern obstetrics, the uterine incision is made in the lower uterine segment.
- **Classical cesarean section:** In rare cases, a vertical incision is made in the upper uterine segment. This is called a classical cesarean

section. It is not routinely used in modern obstetrics because of the increased risk of uterine rupture in a subsequent pregnancy.

- **Cesarean hysterectomy:** This procedure is uncommon but may be life-saving. The most common indications are intractable hemorrhage due to uterine atony, placenta percreta or increta, and uterine rupture (see **Chapter 24**, *Peripartum hysterectomy*).

CLASSIFICATION OF CESAREAN SECTION (BASED ON INDICATION)

- **Emergency cesarean section:** A cesarean section performed on a labouring woman (intrapartum) is known as an **emergency** cesarean section.
- **Elective cesarean section:** A cesarean section performed on a woman before she is in labour is known as an **elective** cesarean section.
- **Cesarean on demand:** A cesarean performed on maternal request without a medical indication is called a cesarean on demand. In 2016, the World Health Organization issued a statement that cesareans should only be performed for a medical indication [4].

The American College of Obstetricians, in a Committee Opinion [5], recommends that in the absence of maternal or fetal indications for cesarean delivery, **vaginal delivery should be recommended as the safest and most appropriate option.** Given the high repeat cesarean delivery rate, women should be informed that the risks of placenta previa, placenta accreta spectrum, and peripartum hysterectomy increase with each subsequent cesarean delivery.

If a woman has severe anxiety about labour pain and vaginal birth, every effort should be made to understand her mental status and treat her with empathy [6]. She should be educated about pain relief in labour, especially epidural analgesia and the advantages of a birth companion. If, after offering counselling, the woman still wants a planned cesarean, then the following is recommended:

- Explain to the woman the short- and long-term effects of cesarean delivery on her and her baby
- Schedule the cesarean at or after 39 completed weeks of gestation

For Indian women, cesarean should be performed at or after 38 completed weeks of gestation (see the section on *Scheduling an elective cesarean section*).

If a woman and her family want to proceed with a cesarean based on cultural and social pressures (e.g., 'auspicious' time of birth, early delivery to meet social commitments such as a wedding in the family) and the obstetrician is not comfortable with performing a cesarean on demand, they can refer the woman to a colleague.

> **Key Point**
>
> An obstetrician is not under any ethical or professional obligation to perform a cesarean on demand, i.e., without a medical indication. It is acceptable to refer a woman early to another willing obstetrician in such cases [6,7].

EMERGENCY CESAREAN SECTION (INTRAPARTUM)

Indications for Emergency Cesarean Section

The majority of primary cesarean sections are performed as an emergency due to problems that arise in labour. The commonest indications for 85% of cesarean deliveries performed globally are:

- Failure to progress in labour
- Non-reassuring fetal status
- Breech presentation

Maternal indications

Dystocia or failure to progress **is the most common indication for an emergency cesarean delivery in a labouring woman** (see

Chapter 11, *Abnormalities in the latent phase and the first stage of labour* and **Chapter 12**, *Abnormalities in the second stage of labour*). Failure to progress in labour may occur due to the following:

- **Dysfunctional labour** resulting from abnormal uterine action, protraction, and arrest disorders may require a cesarean section if other treatment modalities fail.
- **Cephalopelvic disproportion (CPD)** is another reason for failure to progress in labour. It may occur due to an inadequate maternal pelvis. Although CPD can be suspected prior to labour, it is usually diagnosed during labour.
- **Failed induction**: When labour has been induced but does not progress to a vaginal delivery, it is termed failed induction. A cesarean section is indicated in this situation.

Fetal indications

- **Non-reassuring fetal status** (fetal distress) is the second most common indication for cesarean sections. Non-reassuring fetal status is diagnosed by:
  - The presence of abnormal fetal heart rate on auscultation (persistent tachycardia or bradycardia)
  - Abnormal fetal heart tracing on an electronic fetal monitor, which could be any of the following (see **Chapter 15**, *Identification and management of fetal distress*):
    - Absent baseline variability
    - Recurrent variable decelerations
    - Recurrent late decelerations
    - Bradycardia
- **Placental abruption** occurring during labour can be an acute indication for a cesarean section (see **Chapter 29**, *Antepartum hemorrhage*).
- **Fetal macrosomia** leading to CPD and prolonged labour is an indication for a cesarean section.
- **Second twin**—i.e., difficulty in the delivery of the second twin—may also necessitate a cesarean section.

Timing of Emergency (Intrapartum) Cesarean Section

Decision-to-surgery interval

Once a decision has been made to proceed with an emergency cesarean, it is recommended that the decision-to-surgery interval be 30 minutes or less. However, all indications are not the same. The time to delivery varies depending on the situation, which may be as follows:

- A life-threatening situation for the woman or the fetus
- Maternal or fetal compromise, but no immediate danger to either life
- Indication for delivery present, but no evidence of maternal or fetal compromise

The time to cesarean also depends on the infrastructure available at the facility and the availability of a theatre, staff, an anesthetist, and access to blood products.

ELECTIVE CESAREAN SECTION

Indications for Elective Cesarean Section

Maternal indications

An elective cesarean section can be performed for the following indications:

- **Previous cesarean section,** which is a leading indication; a previous **classical** cesarean section (though rare) is an absolute indication for an elective cesarean section
- **Placenta previa** partially or completely covering the internal os
- **Maternal HIV**—cesarean is performed to minimise transmission to the baby
- **Primary genital herpes** with visible lesions at the time of labour or rupture of membranes—to prevent congenital herpes in the infant

- An **elderly primigravida** who has conceived after extensive infertility treatment and may have associated complications such as gestational and pregestational diabetes, hypertension, and fetal growth restriction/ macrosomia
- **Soft tissue dystocia** resulting from uterine fibroids or ovarian tumours obstructing labour
- **Anomalies of the lower genital tract** such as vaginal septum, and scarring of the vagina or cervix
- **Previous vaginal surgery for pelvic organ prolapse**
- **Extensive vaginal lacerations** after a previous vaginal delivery may be an indication for an elective cesarean section
- **Cervical cancer** necessitates a cesarean section because a vaginal delivery can pose a risk of hemorrhage and dissemination of disease

Fetal indications

The following are the fetal indications for an elective cesarean section:

- **Fetal growth restriction** with oligohydramnios/abnormal Doppler findings—to prevent fetal compromise in labour
- **Twin pregnancy** with the first baby in a non-cephalic presentation
- **Malpresentations:**
  - Term singleton breech, if external cephalic version is contraindicated or has failed; however, each obstetric unit needs to work out its policy for allowing a vaginal delivery in selected cases of breech presentation (see **Chapter 27,** *Breech delivery [including external cephalic version]*)
  - Transverse lie
- **Suspected macrosomia** (estimated fetal weight >4000 g), especially in diabetic women
- **Fetal anomalies** such as severe hydrocephalus
- **A previous adverse perinatal event,** for example, stillbirth or a difficult vaginal delivery resulting in a severely asphyxiated infant

Scheduling an Elective/Planned Cesarean Section

An elective cesarean prior to the onset of labour, for a medical or obstetric indication, may need to be performed:

- Immediately, regardless of gestational age because of worsening maternal or fetal condition **or**
- At the best gestational age for the mother and fetus

If there is **no medical indication for the cesarean**, it is best scheduled at **38–39 completed weeks** to reduce the risk of respiratory distress syndrome (RDS).

ACOG [8] and NICE guidelines [6] have suggested scheduling surgery at 39 completed weeks for non-medically indicated cesareans. However, it is important to remember that Indian babies are born earlier and mature earlier in utero than Caucasian babies.

Median gestational age at birth among Indians

The median gestational age at delivery is <39 weeks in Indians. The WHO Multinational Longitudinal Study to establish growth charts for developing countries [9] found the median gestational age at birth was **38 weeks+4 d in India.**

A large study (122,000 women) conducted in a mixed-population hospital in London [10] reported the following findings:

- Normal gestational length is shorter among Indian, Pakistani, and Bangladeshi women.
- Meconium-stained amniotic fluid, which is a sign of fetal maturity, was significantly more frequent in preterm South Asian infants as compared to white European infants.

Key Point

Scheduling non-medically indicated cesareans at 38 completed weeks of gestation may be more suited for Indian women.

ENHANCED RECOVERY AFTER CESAREAN (ERAC)

Introduced a little more than a decade ago for colorectal surgery, enhanced recovery after surgery (ERAS) is an evidence-based concept that combines aspects of perioperative care to accelerate recovery. Now adapted to cesarean delivery (ERAC), it results in the following:

- A reduction in hospital stay, re-admissions, and postoperative complications
- Improved patient satisfaction

These core principles involve interventions that cover the **preoperative**, **intraoperative,** and **postoperative** periods. Recommendations focus on optimising the following [11]:

- Maternal recovery
- Maternal–infant bonding
- Perioperative outcomes after cesarean delivery

ERAC involves multidisciplinary team efforts, including those of an anesthetist, obstetrician, nursing staff, the hospital, and the woman undergoing surgery.

PREOPERATIVE PREPARATION

Recommendations for the preoperative steps included in ERAC are summarised in Table 22.1 [11].

SURGICAL CHECKLIST

As with any surgery, a woman undergoing a cesarean should have a safety checklist that is filled out by a nurse or physician before taking the woman to the operation theatre. The checklist is continued immediately before the start of surgery and is completed at the end of surgery. The WHO surgical checklist can be modified

Table 22.1 Recommendations for preoperative management to promote enhanced recovery after cesarean birth

Recommendations	Action	Advantages
Limiting the interval of preoperative fasting	• Solids up to 8 h preoperatively • Clear liquids (water) up to 2 h	• Reduces aspiration risk • Decreases hypovolemia, metabolic stress, and ketosis
Carbohydrate loading with non-particulate liquid	250 mL of clear apple juice (in a tetrapack) up to 2 h before cesarean delivery (non-diabetic women only)	Reduces preoperative thirst, hunger, and anxiety
Educating the woman about the process	• Instructions for preparing herself for the cesarean • Explanations of what to expect during cesarean delivery–provided at least 1 d before surgery	• Improves compliance with care pathways • Reduces anxiety and postoperative pain • Improves outcomes • Empowers the woman to participate in her own care
Lactation/breastfeeding preparation and education	Should be a part of prenatal classes, along with in-person lactation support in the hospital	Early breastfeeding improves newborn and maternal outcomes (see **Chapter 43**, *Routine care of the newborn*)
Optimisation of Hgb level following screening for anemia	Iron-deficiency anemia should be treated with supplemental oral or IV iron in addition to prenatal vitamins	Correcting anemia reduces the risk of low birth weight, preterm delivery, and perinatal mortality

for use for a cesarean section. The Society for Maternal–Fetal Medicine (SMFM) has designed a checklist for cesarean sections [12]. Fig. 22.1 is a sample safety checklist for cesarean sections.

The checklist is completed at the end of surgery by documenting the surgical (instrument and pad) count. A checklist ensures that important patient data is not overlooked and decreases mishaps occurring due to simple errors of omission.

ORAL INTAKE AND INTRAVENOUS ACCESS

The recommendations are as follows [11]:

- The uncomplicated pregnant woman undergoing elective cesarean delivery should not consume solids for 6 hours (light meal) or 8 hours (if it is high in fat content) prior to surgery. She may consume moderate amounts of clear liquids (water or clear juice) up to 2 hours before the induction of anesthesia (Table 22.1).
- A preoperative carbohydrate drink (250 mL of tetrapack clear apple juice) or a preoperative glucose infusion has been shown to reduce preoperative thirst, hunger, and anxiety as well as the degree of hyperglycemia that typically occurs after major surgery.
- Intravenous access should be established with an 18-gauge intravenous (IV) catheter. 5% dextrose in normal saline, 0.45% saline, or lactated Ringer's solution can be administered.

Key Point

If a labouring woman requires an emergency cesarean section, she may be given H_2-receptor antagonists (e.g., ranitidine 50 mg IV) and/or metoclopramide for preventing complications, in the rare case of anesthetic aspiration.

Sign in (before shifting to theatre)	Before start of procedure	Sign out (before shifting out of theatre)
Confirm the following: • Name and date of birth • Consent form signed • Recent lab results reviewed — Hemoglobin — Blood group and Rh type — Platelet count — Blood glucose (if diabetic) • Blood typed, cross-matched and reserved • Allergies documented on chart • Anesthetic team informed — Concerns about high BMI, difficult airway, or any others communicated • Neonatal team informed — Gestational age, EFW — Indication for cesarean • Personal items — Jewellery removed and handed to attendant — Glasses/contact lenses/dentures removed	**Confirm the following:** • Name and date of birth • Consent form signed • Procedure and indication **Review the following:** • Blood and blood products need and availability • Relevant medical history • Perform anesthesia safety check — Anesthetist aware of allergies and medical issues, if any **Before skin incision:** • IV line started • Prophylactic antibiotic dose administered • Pediatric/neonatal team in place • Presence of fetal heart tones documented • Surgical instrument and pad counts done • Skin prepped	• Lead surgical nurse announces pad and instrument count before closure of abdominal incision • Anesthetist and surgical teams confirm volume of blood loss — Rule out PPH • Urine output from catheter is checked — Urine clear — Intraoperative output noted • Pain management plan in place • Medication for prevention of nausea and vomiting • VTE prophylaxis • Mother and baby tagged

Fig. 22.1 A sample safety checklist for cesarean section (adapted from the SMFM Special Statement on surgical safety checklist)

HAIR REMOVAL AT SURGICAL SITE

- Women who are shaved are more likely to develop surgical site infection (SSI). Pubic hair need not be shaved routinely. Instead, hair that is likely to interfere with the operative area can be clipped on the day of the surgery.
- Shaving on the night before surgery increases the risk of wound infection, and therefore, should not be performed.

BATHING ON THE DAY OF SURGERY

In an elective surgery, bathing on the day of surgery has been shown to decrease surgical site infection. However, there is no clear evidence that an antiseptic solution like chlorhexidine is better than regular soap for cleaning [13].

PROPHYLACTIC ANTICOAGULATION

Anticoagulation to prevent venous thromboembolism (VTE) is not recommended for cesarean sections in low-risk pregnancies. It may be used in women at high risk for VTE. This includes women with previous VTE, high-risk thrombophilia (inherited or acquired), or a body mass index (BMI) >40 Kg/m^2.

Anticoagulation is initiated 6–12 hours postoperatively, after the risk of hemorrhage has decreased and is continued till ambulation. The following can be used:

- Unfractionated heparin 5000 units every 12 hours **or**
- Low-molecular-weight heparin (enoxaparin) 40 mg daily

INTRAOPERATIVE MANAGEMENT

Certain intraoperative steps can enhance the woman's recovery after surgery. The intraoperative recommendations for enhanced recovery after cesarean delivery (ERAC) are summarised in Table 22.2 [11].

PROPHYLACTIC ANTIBIOTICS

Cesarean delivery is the most important risk factor for postpartum maternal infection. Prophylactic antibiotics are strongly recommended as they reduce the risk of surgical site infection, endometritis, and postoperative urinary tract infection [14]. Antibiotics used for prophylaxis for cesarean delivery should be effective against gram-positive bacteria, gram-negative bacteria, and some anaerobic bacteria.

Choice of Antibiotic

For antibiotic prophylaxis for cesarean delivery, the World Health Organization recommends **a single dose of first-generation cephalosporin** or **penicillin** over other classes of antibiotics [15].

For further details about the choice of antibiotic, dosage, and timing, see **Chapter 19**, *Antibiotic prophylaxis in labour and delivery*.

ANESTHESIA FOR CESAREAN DELIVERY

Regional Anesthesia

- **Spinal anesthesia** is the most common type of anesthesia used for a cesarean delivery. It has the advantage of quick placement and rapid onset of anesthesia.
- **Epidural analgesia** is used when an epidural catheter is already in place for labour analgesia or when the cesarean section is not an emergency. Combined spinal–epidural is preferred by some anesthetists.

General Anesthesia

The indications for general anesthesia are as follows:

- Urgency of delivery of the baby
- Inadequate or failed regional anesthesia
- Coagulation disorders
- Spinal abnormalities (preventing spinal anesthesia)

See **Chapter 9**, *Labour analgesia*, for further details.

Table 22.2 Recommendations for intraoperative management to promote enhanced recovery after cesarean birth

Recommendations	Action	Advantages
Antibiotic prophylaxis	Administered before skin incision	Reduces the risk of surgical site infection, endometritis, and postoperative urinary tract infection
Optimal uterotonic administration	Administered as per protocols	Reduces the risk of uterine atony and PPH (see **Chapter 5**, *Management of the third stage of labour)*
Prophylaxis against postoperative nausea and vomiting	• Combination of at least 2 prophylactic IV antiemetics with different mechanisms of action • Examples: — Ondansetron 4 mg — Dexamethasone 4 mg (effective for PONV) — Metoclopramide 10 mg (effective for IONV) — Avoid or limit uterine exteriorisation	• Intraoperative and postoperative nausea and vomiting cause major distress to the woman • Actively avoiding nausea and vomiting is an important part of care
Multimodal analgesia	• Intrathecal morphine (50–150 mcg) or epidural morphine (1–3 mg) • Non-opioid analgesia, e.g., IV paracetamol started in the OT • Supplemental local anesthetic wound infiltration	• The emphasis is on regular, scheduled non-opioid analgesia commencing before the onset of pain and not on first pain request • The woman is kept as pain-free as possible
Optimisation of intravenous fluids	Limit IV fluids to <3 L intraoperatively for routine cases	Avoidance of fluid overload prevents the risk of hyponatremia due to oxytocin administration
Delayed cord clamping	Cord clamping delayed for 1–3 minutes	Reduces the risk of neonatal anemia

IONV, intraoperative nausea and vomiting; *IV*, intravenous; *OT*, operation theatre; *PPH*, postpartum hemorrhage; *PONV*, postoperative nausea and vomiting

TECHNIQUE OF CESAREAN DELIVERY

The steps of a cesarean section have been standardised over the years since it is the most common surgical procedure in obstetrics. The common steps are presented here, based on current evidence.

Vaginal Preparation with Antiseptic Agents

A recent systematic review and network meta-analysis [16] concluded that preoperative vaginal preparation with a swab soaked in an antiseptic solution significantly reduces the risk of post-cesarean infectious diseases (endometritis, postoperative fever, and wound infection). The recommended solution with the best results is 1% povidone-iodine, though the WHO [17] has also recommended a chlorhexidine solution. Only water-based solutions should be used and **not** alcohol-based ones.

> **Key Point**
>
> Vaginal preparation in a pregnant woman is an invasive procedure, and therefore, uncomfortable. The procedure should be explained to the woman beforehand and should be performed gently to avoid discomfort as much as possible. Vaginal preparation is a recent recommendation and should be adopted only if postoperative infectious morbidity in the institution has not been controlled with routine perioperative interventions. **Alcohol-based antiseptics should not be used.**

Bladder Drainage

An indwelling bladder catheter is placed and is usually removed 12–24 hours after surgery. An empty bladder helps in better visualisation of the lower uterine segment during surgery.

Skin Cleansing Techniques

A systematic review of the Cochrane Database [18] found insufficient evidence to recommend one agent over the other. Either 10% povidone–iodine solution or chlorhexidine (as soap or in an alcohol base) can be used to prep the skin.

Opening the Abdomen

Skin incision

The commonly used skin incisions for a cesarean delivery are as follows:

- Transverse incisions (Pfannenstiel, Joel–Cohen)
- Vertical (midline) incision

The type of incision is usually dictated by the clinical situation and the preferences of the operator.

> **Key Point**
>
> If a prominent scar or keloid from a previous cesarean is present, the incision may be made above or below it and the scar is excised after the cesarean section is completed.

Transverse skin incision

A low transverse skin incision is the preferred option for a cesarean delivery. It is associated with less postoperative pain, greater wound strength, less risk of incisional hernia, and better cosmetic results than the vertical midline incision [19]. The **Pfannenstiel** and the **Joel–Cohen** incisions are commonly used.

> **Key Point**
>
> The Joel–Cohen incision is associated with less fever, pain and analgesic requirements, less blood loss, and a shorter duration of surgery and hospital stay as compared to the Pfannenstiel incision [20].

Vertical skin incision

Though vertical incisions generally allow faster abdominal entry, are associated with less bleeding and nerve injury, and can be easily extended cephalad if more space is required for access, they do not improve neonatal outcomes. Vertical midline incisions are associated with a greater risk of postoperative wound dehiscence and the development of incisional hernia. The scar is also cosmetically less pleasing.

> **Key Point**
>
> A midline incision is the preferred vertical incision. Paramedian incisions are not recommended in modern obstetrics.

Length of skin incision: An incision measuring at least 15 cm in length (the length of a standard Allis clamp) is considered reasonable and avoids difficulty in delivering the fetus.

Subcutaneous tissue

The subcutaneous tissue is dissected sharply till the glistening fascia is seen.

Rectus fascia

One of two methods can be used with no difference between the two regarding post-operative pain:

- In the Pfannenstiel incision, the fascia is cut with a transverse incision and either side is raised as a flap.
- In the Joel–Cohen incision, the fascia is nicked in the midline and opened transversely with blunt finger dissection or by pushing laterally with slightly opened scissor tips. Care must be taken to avoid cutting the superficial and deep epigastric vessels.

Rectus muscles

- In the **Pfannenstiel technique**, the rectus muscles are separated in the midline with blunt finger dissection. Then, the rectus fascia is dissected from the muscle. This appears to be unnecessary and is less physiological.
- In the **Joel–Cohen technique**, the rectus muscles are separated by applying traction with the fingers.
- In the **Maylard muscle-cutting technique**, after incising the fascia transversely, the rectus muscles are undermined from the midline or the lateral edge with a finger. The muscles are then completely transected with sharp dissection or electrocautery, approximately 2 cm above the insertion into the pubic bone. This technique provides much greater exposure. Studies have shown that this is a safe option, and transecting the rectus muscle was not more deleterious than the Pfannenstiel incision. There was no difference in objectively measured abdominal wall strength [21,22].

Opening the peritoneum

The peritoneum is nicked open in the midline. The opening in the peritoneum is then widened sharply with fine scissors or widened bluntly using fingers. The CORONIS trial found no short- or long-term difference when the two techniques were compared [23].

Dextrorotation of the uterus

It is important to know that the uterus is often dextrorotated, with the left round ligament lying more anterior and closer to the midline than the right round ligament. Once the peritoneal cavity is accessed and the lower part of the uterus exposed, this dextrorotation can be quickly corrected by inserting a hand between the uterus and the right pelvic sidewall and lifting the uterus gently upwards and to the left.

Opening the Uterus (Hysterotomy)

Raising the bladder flap

The uterovesical fold of the peritoneum is grasped with toothed forceps, just above the upper margin of the bladder, and a small nick is made in the midline with fine scissors. The blades of the scissors are then inserted under the loose fold of the peritoneum and intermittently opened and closed to separate the peritoneum from the underlying tissue. This strip is then cut sharply to both sides, taking care to cut so that the incision forms a curve, with the lateral ends curving upwards.

The lower edge of the peritoneal flap is then grasped with toothed forceps or an artery clamp, and the bladder is separated gently by blunt dissection. In the presence of a previous cesarean scar, sharp dissection may be required to release the adherent bladder.

There is no strong evidence to either support or oppose the creation of a bladder flap. In women who are not in labour, the lower uterine segment may be better approached after creating a bladder flap. Similarly, creating a bladder flap may be helpful in women who have had a previous cesarean, and in whom the bladder is attached well above the lower uterine segment. Pushing the bladder out of harm's way may decrease the risk of inadvertent bladder injury.

> **Key Point**
>
> In women who have adhesions due to one or more previous cesarean deliveries, the location of the bladder is best delineated by palpating the bulb of the bladder catheter.

Uterine incision

A transverse uterine incision is made in the lower segment. Rarely, a vertical uterine incision is used. The low vertical incision has not found much favour in practice because of the possibility of extension upward into the uterine fundus or downwards into the bladder.

The type of uterine incision used is dictated by the fetal size, presentation, placental location, and the presence of large fibroids. The uterine incision must be large enough to allow the atraumatic delivery of the fetal head and trunk without tearing into or having to cut the uterine vessels at the lateral margins of the uterus.

A 'J' or **inverted 'T' extension** is often performed if a larger incision is required to deliver the infant, particularly in a breech or a transverse lie. The 'J' or 'T' incision may result in problems in future pregnancies because of the potential for uterine scar rupture. **If such an incision is made, it should be documented in the medical records for future reference.**

> **Key Point**
>
> It is important to be aware of the placental position while making the uterine incision, especially if an ultrasound scan has indicated a low-lying placenta or placenta previa. This helps in preventing entry into the placenta and averts significant hemorrhage.

Technique

A small incision is made in the midline with the scalpel, 1 cm below the upper margin of the peritoneal reflection. In women who have been in labour and have undergone significant cervical effacement and dilatation, it is prudent to place the incision relatively higher. This will not only prevent lateral extension into the uterine vessels but will also avoid opening into the vagina. If possible, the membranes should be left intact until the complete extension of the incision.

When entry into the uterine cavity is achieved, the hysterotomy incision can be extended using blunt side-to-side expansion with the surgeon's index fingers. Blunt expansion is fast and has a lower risk of inadvertent trauma to the fetus as compared to the use of scissors. It reduces lateral extension of the incision and decreases blood loss [24].

> **Key Points**
>
> The risk of nicking the baby's skin during hysterotomy is increased if:
> - The lower uterine segment is thinned out
> - The fetus is in breech presentation

Classical cesarean: A vertical incision that extends into the upper uterine segment/ fundus is termed a 'classical' incision and is rare in modern obstetrics because of the higher frequency of catastrophic uterine rupture in subsequent pregnancies. The only indication for a classical cesarean incision may be the need for a quick delivery in cases where the woman will be undergoing tubal ligation concomitantly.

Delivering the Fetus

After the uterine incision is made, the membranes (if still intact) are ruptured. Then, the obstetrician inserts a hand into the uterine cavity and quickly assesses the presentation (if not known earlier).

Cephalic presentation: When the fetus is in a cephalic presentation, the hand is used to scoop the head up and bring it to the level of the uterine incision. The head is then extracted through the uterine incision. To facilitate the delivery of the head through the uterine incision, the surgical assistant usually applies transabdominal fundal pressure.

Breech presentation: Delivery of the breech fetus may require the same manoeuvres used for vaginal breech delivery.

Transverse lie: The fetus is turned either to a vertex (cephalic version) or breech presentation (podalic version) and then delivered. Usually, podalic version followed by breech extraction is recommended (see section below on *Internal podalic version*). The shoulders are then delivered by gentle traction, and the rest of the body will readily follow (see **Chapter 35,** *Malpositions and malpresentations [other than breech]*, for further details).

The mouth and nostrils of the infant are immediately wiped gently. Once the infant's cord is clamped and cut, it is handed over to an appropriately trained clinician/nurse who will take over the care of the infant.

Special Situations

Instrumental delivery at cesarean

A systematic review of the Cochrane Database [25] found insufficient information from randomised trials to support or refute the routine or selective use of forceps or a vacuum device to facilitate infant birth at the time of difficult cesarean section.

Delivering the deeply impacted head

A deeply impacted fetal head may be encountered during a cesarean delivery following prolonged labour. The head is wedged deep in the pelvis and can be hard to disengage and deliver.

The fingers of one hand are insinuated between the fetal head and the cervix and vagina and wiggled gently. This releases the suction holding the fetal head in the pelvis. A sucking sound is heard as the air rushes into the space between the head and the pelvis, and then the head can be extracted.

However, with prolonged labour, the tissues may be edematous and friable. This could lead to the extension of the incision laterally into the broad ligament and uterine vessels. If this procedure fails, upward pressure applied by the assistant's hand in the vagina can push the head back through the vagina and out of the pelvis.

> **Key Point**
>
> The delivery of a deeply impacted head could also be facilitated by extending the uterine incision into an inverted 'T' shape.

Delivering the floating head

When the head is floating above the hysterotomy incision (a situation more likely in prelabour cesarean delivery), it is difficult to grasp it and bring it out through the hysterotomy. There are two options:

- **Internal podalic version:** Once both the feet of the fetus are identified, they are grasped by the obstetrician, and with gentle traction, guided out through the hysterotomy. External pressure on the uterus pushes the head towards the fundus, and the infant is delivered as a footling breech. A recent study [26] found internal podalic version to be a safe and rapid technique when compared to forceps or vacuum extraction in the presence of a floating head at cesarean.
- **Instrumental delivery:** Some obstetricians use forceps or a vacuum device to deliver the floating head.

Delivering the Placenta

Spontaneous delivery of the placenta is encouraged with gentle traction on the cord and the use of oxytocin to enhance uterine expulsive forces. A systematic review of the Cochrane Database [27] showed that manual extraction results in more postoperative endometritis, greater blood loss, and lower postpartum hematocrit.

Prophylaxis Against Postpartum Hemorrhage (PPH)

The uterus is massaged immediately after the delivery of the placenta to promote uterine contraction. The commonest uterotonic used is oxytocin. This is usually administered intravenously in a dose of 10–20 units in 500 mL of normal saline. The next three bottles of postoperative intravenous solutions should also contain the same dosage, and the fluid should be run at 125 mL/hour. Oxytocin has fewer side effects than ergot alkaloids, especially in hypertensive women.

CLOSURE OF HYSTEROTOMY

Exteriorisation of the Uterus

Closure of the uterine incision may be aided by the **exteriorisation** of the uterus. This involves the temporary removal of the uterus from the abdominal cavity to facilitate the repair of the uterine incision. It allows the direct massage of a non-contracted, flabby uterus. Exteriorisation is particularly valuable when exposure of the incision is difficult or there is a need for immediate hemostasis due to excessive bleeding. It also allows easy access to the tubes for tubal ligation.

A recent systematic review and meta-analysis comparing exteriorisation with in situ repair [28] showed an increased risk of intraoperative nausea and vomiting with exteriorisation.

Choice of Suture

The choice of suture is based on the operator's preference. In LMICs, the choice of suture is heavily influenced by the cost to the woman. Both chromic catgut and delayed absorbable synthetic suture, e.g., polyglactin 910 (Vicryl®) are used to close the uterine incision. The CORONIS trial [23] clearly showed that there were no differences in the short- and long-term outcomes of using chromic catgut and polyglactin 910. A recent meta-analysis [36] found that no specific type of suture material used for the closure of hysterotomy was superior in terms of maternal outcome.

Key Point

In the short- and long-term, chromic catgut, polyglactin 910, and barbed suture produced similar results [29].

Single-Layer Versus Double-Layer Closure

Traditionally, the uterine incision is closed by a **double-layer repair**. The first layer is closed with a continuous locking suture, which ensures hemostasis. This is followed by a continuous non-locking imbricating layer. A double (or even triple) layer closure may be necessary when the myometrium is thick, as may be the case with a classical cesarean, low vertical incision, or a 'T' extension.

Single-layer closure

The long-term risk of uterine rupture in a subsequent pregnancy following a single-layer closure has been a matter of debate. In the past, reports showed the risk of uterine rupture during subsequent vaginal deliveries with a single-layer closure to be increased two- to four-fold compared to deliveries with a double-layer closure. However, a recent meta-analysis [30] found that single- and double-layer closure of the uterine incision are associated with a similar incidence of cesarean scar defects as well as uterine dehiscence and rupture in a subsequent pregnancy. The CORONIS trial [23] also found no evidence of differences in maternal death or complications while comparing the long-term effects of single- and double-layer closure.

Key Point

With conflicting data, some of which are of poor quality, it is prudent to restrict single-layer closure to women undergoing tubal ligation.

Extension of the Incision

Extension of the incision to the vagina or upper segment or laterally involving the uterine vessels must be managed by careful suturing and ligation of uterine vessels.

Inspection of the Adnexae

It is good clinical practice to inspect the ovaries and tubes at the time of a cesarean section. This ensures that a cyst or mass is not missed. See the section below on *Incidental surgery during cesarean section.*

ABDOMINAL CLOSURE

Fascial Closure

This is probably the most important step in the closure of the abdomen. A properly done fascial closure is essential in preventing incisional hernia. It is important to place the sutures with the appropriate tension—**the aim is to reapproximate, not strangulate**.

Key Points

- The recommendation for fascial closure is a continuous non-locking technique, with the sutures placed 1 cm from the edge of the fascia and 1 cm apart [31].
- The suture material used for fascial closure can be a delayed absorbable material such as polydiaxonone or polyglactin 910 or a permanent suture like 1-0 nylon. In LMICs, nylon is a cost-effective permanent suture with a lower incidence of suture sinus formation than polypropylene.
- Prior to suturing the fascial edges, it is important to inspect the subfascial plane for bleeders and to achieve meticulous hemostasis.

Closure of the Subcutaneous Tissue

When the depth of the subcutaneous tissue is <2 cm, routine closure is not recommended. However, when the subcutaneous tissue is >2 cm in depth, closure with an interrupted delayed absorbable suture prevents the formation of seroma and subsequent wound breakdown [32].

Closure of the Skin

The options for skin closure are as follows:
- **Subcuticular sutures:** Better cosmesis and patient satisfaction can be achieved with subcuticular sutures using delayed-absorbable suture.
- **Mattress sutures**: The skin can be closed with vertical mattress sutures using fine nylon. This does not leave behind a cosmetic scar.
- **Adhesive paper strips**: These are the least painful and have excellent cosmetic results. The skin edges are cleaned with saline and dried. An adhesive skin prep like tincture benzoin can be used on the edges to help the strips stick better. The edges of the skin are held together with forceps, and the adhesive strips are applied by placing them on one edge and then pulling them gently across to the other skin edge.

Wound Dressing

A light protective gauze dressing is recommended. One or two narrow strips of adhesive tape can hold the dressing in place. Occlusive dressings or other advanced dressings including antimicrobial dressings do not decrease the risk of surgical site infection [33]. The dressing can be removed in 24–48 hours.

UNNECESSARY INTERVENTIONS DURING CESAREAN SECTION

Abdominal Irrigation

Other than suctioning out excessive amniotic fluid and blood which may have collected in the peritoneal cavity, there is no necessity for intra-abdominal irrigation, which has been shown to increase the risk of intraoperative and postoperative nausea [34].

Adhesion Barriers

Following cesarean section, the chances of intra-abdominal adhesions, with or without the use of adhesion barriers, are the same (11–70%). Evidence does not support their use.

Suturing of the Rectus Muscles

There is no necessity to reapproximate the rectus muscles if they are cut during surgery or electively (as in Maylard incision). When the fascial edges are approximated, the muscles will come together naturally. Suturing the rectus muscles has been shown to increase postoperative pain.

Closure of the Peritoneum

There is currently no evidence to justify the time taken to close the visceral or peritoneal peritoneum. There is no convincing data to show that closing the peritoneum decreases adhesion formation [35].

Irrigation of the Subcutaneous Tissue

Irrigation of the subcutaneous tissues at cesarean delivery is not recommended and has not been shown to reduce the incidence of surgical site infection [36].

Drains

Drains are not recommended in cesarean sections because the routine use of drains has **not** been shown to reduce the risk of seroma, hematoma, infection, or wound disruption [37], even in obese women.

Manual Cervical Dilatation

Postoperative manual cervical dilatation has no benefit, and there is no evidence to support it [38].

INCIDENTAL SURGERY DURING CESAREAN SECTION

The two common incidental findings at cesarean section are adnexal masses and fibroids.

Ovarian Mass

An ovarian cyst or mass identified incidentally at the time of cesarean section should be removed [39]. If malignancy is suspected and facilities for frozen section are available, then an oophorectomy is performed upon confirmation of malignancy. A staging laparotomy should be performed at a later date.

In LMICs, facilities for frozen section may not be readily available in all institutions. In such a case, the mass may be excised in toto. If it is proven to be malignant by histopathology, a staging laparotomy may be done at a later date.

Fibroids

The term uterus receives 17% of the cardiac output, and attempting a myomectomy at cesarean section can lead to significant hemorrhage. Myomectomy is generally contraindicated for this reason although excision of a pedunculated fibroid is acceptable (see **Chapter 36**, *Pregnancy and labour in women with fibroids*, for further details).

POSTOPERATIVE CARE

INTRAVENOUS FLUIDS

Intravenous fluids are continued for the first 24–48 hours after cesarean till the woman is able to tolerate and retain oral feeding. Typically, lactated Ringer solution or a similar crystalloid solution containing 5% dextrose is used. The usual volume administered is 500 mL every 4 hours. Urine output is recorded, and intake and output are charted.

PAIN RELIEF

Pain relief after cesarean requires a multimodal approach.

- **Paracetamol**: 1 g of paracetamol in a 100 mL vial is infused intravenously over 15 minutes as the surgery is coming to an end. This is repeated every 6–8 hours for the first 24 hours.
- **Opioid:** Tramadol is most commonly used in India for postoperative analgesia. It can be given intravenously or orally. It is associated with nausea.
- **NSAIDs:**
  - Diclofenac 100 mg rectal suppository can be used at the end of surgery and may be repeated every 8 hours for the first 24 hours
  - After 24 hours, oral ibuprofen 400 mg in combination with 500/650 mg of paracetamol will provide good pain relief
  - Ketorolac 10 mg may also be given orally after the first 24 hours
- **Transversus abdominis plane (TAP) block:** Using ultrasound guidance, a local anesthetic is injected into the neurovascular plane between the transversus abdominis (TA) and internal oblique (IO) muscles. TAP

block is now becoming part of the multimodal approach to postoperative pain relief.

FEEDING AFTER CESAREAN SECTION

Early oral intake after cesarean delivery (clear liquids or solids according to the mother's preference) can be resumed within 6 hours of surgery. This improves the return of gastrointestinal function without increasing the occurrence of gastrointestinal complications [40]. Early intake of oral fluids or food is associated with the following:

- Reduced time to first food intake
- Reduced time to return of bowel sounds
- Reduced postoperative hospital stay

FOLEY CATHETER

The urinary catheter may be removed after 12–24 hours. Routine urine culture after catheterisation is not recommended.

POSTOPERATIVE COMPLICATIONS AFTER CESAREAN SECTION

Postoperative complications following a cesarean section include wound infection, endometritis, and hemorrhage.

Long-term complications of a cesarean section include the following:

- Abnormal placentation in the subsequent pregnancy
- Scar dehiscence or rupture in the next pregnancy
- Ectopic pregnancy in the hysterotomy scar
- Subfertility
- Complications related to the uterine and abdominal scar include pain and numbness over the abdominal scar and scar endometriosis

Neonatal complications include transient tachypnea of the newborn or respiratory distress syndrome (due to unexpected prematurity).

CONCLUSION

A cesarean section can be a life-saving procedure for both the mother and baby. Every obstetrician should know and follow evidence-based guidelines for each step of the surgery. The Enhanced Recovery After Cesarean (ERAC) are guidelines for the perioperative care of women undergoing an elective or emergency cesarean delivery. These guidelines are focused on the pregnant woman and begin 30 to 60 minutes before the skin incision is made and end at hospital discharge. The aim is to reduce hospital stay, re-admissions, and postoperative complications along with improving patient satisfaction.

REFERENCES

1. Betrán AP, Ye J, Moller AB, Souza JP, Zhang J. Trends and projections of caesarean section rates: Global and regional estimates. *BMJ Glob Health*. 2021. 6(6):e005671.
2. Sobhy S, Arroyo-Manzano D, Murugesu N, et al. Maternal and perinatal mortality and complications associated with caesarean section in low-income and middle-income countries: A systematic review and meta-analysis. *Lancet*. 2019. 393:1973–82. 10.1016/S0140-6736(18)32386.
3. Mittal S, Pardeshi S, Mayadeo N, Mane J. Trends in cesarean delivery: Rate and indications. *J Obstet Gynaecol India*. 2014. 64(4):251-4. doi: 10.1007/s13224-013-0491-2. Epub 2014 Jan 3. PubMed PMID: 25136169; PubMed Central PMCID: PMC4126949.
4. Betrán AP, Torloni MR, Zhang JJ, Gülmezoglu AM. WHO Working Group on Caesarean Section. WHO Statement on Caesarean Section Rates. *BJOG*. 2016.123(5):667–670.
5. Cesarean delivery on maternal request. ACOG Committee Opinion No. 761. American College of Obstetricians and Gynecologists. *Obstet Gynecol*. 2019. Reaffirmed 2020. 133:e73–7.
6. NICE guideline (NG192). Cesarean birth. 2021. Updated 2023. www.nice.org.uk/guidance/ng192
7. Norwitz ER. Cesarean birth on patient request. Grobman W (Ed). *UpToDate*. 2023. Waltham, MA.
8. ACOG Committee Opinion No. 765. Avoidance of non-medically indicated early-term deliveries and associated neonatal morbidities. American College of Obstetricians and Gynecologists. *Obstet Gynecol*. 2019. 133:e156–63.

9. Kiserud T, Piaggio G, Carroli G, et al. The World Health Organization fetal growth charts: A multinational longitudinal study of ultrasound biometric measurements and estimated fetal weight. *PLoS Med.* 2017. 14: e1002220.
10. Patel RR, Steer P, Doyle P, et al. Does gestation vary by ethnic group? A London-based study of over 1,22,000 pregnancies with spontaneous onset of labour. *International Journal of Epidemiology.* Volume 33, Issue 1. 2004. 107–113.
11. Bollag L, Lim G, Sultan P, et al. Society for Obstetric Anesthesia and Perinatology: Consensus Statement and Recommendations for Enhanced Recovery After Cesarean. *Anesth Analg.* 2021.132(5):1362-1377.
12. Combs CA, Einerson BD, Toner, LE et al. Society for Maternal-Fetal Medicine Special Statement: Surgical safety checklists for cesarean delivery. *Am J Obstet Gynecol.* 2021.
13. Webster J, Osborne S. Preoperative bathing or showering with skin antiseptics to prevent surgical site infection. *Cochrane Database Syst Rev.* 2015. Issue 2. Art. No.: CD004985.
14. Smaill FM, Grivell R. Antibiotic prophylaxis versus no prophylaxis for preventing infection after cesarean section. *Cochrane Database Syst Rev.* 2014. Issue 10. Art. No.: CD007482.
15. WHO recommendation on prophylactic antibiotics for women undergoing caesarean section. 2021. WHO, Geneva.
16. Liu G, Liang J, Bai L, et al. Different methods of vaginal preparation before cesarean delivery to prevent postoperative infection: A systematic review and network meta-analysis. *Am J Obstet Gynecol.* 2023. 5:100990.
17. WHO recommendation on vaginal preparation with antiseptic agents for women undergoing caesarean section. 2021. WHO, Geneva.
18. Hadiati DR, Hakimi M, Nurdiati DS, et al. Skin preparation for preventing infection following caesarean section. *Cochrane Database Syst Rev.* 2018. Issue 10. Art. No.:CD007462.
19. Bickenbach KA, Karanicolas PJ, Ammori JB, et al. Up and down or side to side? A systematic review and meta-analysis examining the impact of incision on outcomes after abdominal surgery. *Am J Surg.* 2013. 206:400.
20. Mathai M, Hofmeyr GJ, Mathai NE. Abdominal surgical incisions for caesarean section. *Cochrane Database Syst Rev.* 2013. Issue 5. Art. No.:CD004453.
21. Ayers JW, Morley GW. Surgical incision for cesarean section. *Obstet Gynecol.* 1987. 70:706.
22. Giacalone PL, Daures JP, Vignal J, et al. Pfannenstiel versus Maylard incision for cesarean delivery: A randomized controlled trial. *Obstet Gynecol.* 2002. 99:745.
23. CORONIS collaborative group. Abalos E, Addo V, Brocklehurst P, et al. Caesarean section surgical techniques: 3-year follow-up of the CORONIS fractional, factorial, unmasked, randomised controlled trial. *Lancet.* 2016. 388:62.
24. Saad AF, Rahman M, Costantine MM, Saade GR. Blunt versus sharp uterine incision expansion during low transverse cesarean delivery: A meta-analysis. *Am J Obstet Gynecol.* 2014. 211:684.e1.
25. Waterfall H, Grivell RM, Dodd JM. Techniques for assisting difficult delivery at caesarean section. *Cochrane Database of Systematic Review.* 2016. Issue 1. Art. No.: CD004944.
26. Elshwaikh SL, Elsokary AA, Abuhamama AM. Internal podalic version for delivery of high floating head during cesarean section and neonatal outcome. *J Obstet Gynaecol Res.* 2019.
27. Anorlu RI, Maholwana B, Hofmeyr GJ. Methods of delivering the placenta at caesarean section. *Cochrane Database of Systematic Reviews.* 2008. Issue 3. Art. No.: CD004737.
28. Tan HS, Taylor CR, Sharawi N, et al. Uterine exteriorization versus in situ repair in cesarean delivery: A systematic review and meta-analysis. *Can J Anaesth.* 2022. 69:216.
29. Khanuja K, Burd J, Ozcan P, et al. Suture type for hysterotomy closure: A systematic review and meta-analysis of randomized controlled trials. *Am J Obstet Gynecol* MFM. 2022. 4:100726.
30. Di Spiezio Sardo A, Saccone G, McCurdy R, et al. Risk of Cesarean scar defect following single- vs double-layer uterine closure: Systematic review and meta-analysis of randomized controlled trials. *Ultrasound Obstet Gynecol.* 2017. 50:578.
31. Diener MK, Voss S, Jensen K, et al. Elective midline laparotomy closure: The INLINE systematic review and meta-analysis. *Ann Surg.* 2010. 251(5):843–56.
32. Chelmow D, Rodriguez EJ, Sabatini MM. Suture closure of subcutaneous fat and wound disruption after cesarean delivery: A meta-analysis. *Obstet Gynecol.* 2004. 103:974.
33. Wijetunge S, Hill R, Katie Morris R, Hodgetts Morton V. Advanced dressings for the prevention of surgical site infection in women post-caesarean section: A systematic review and meta-analysis. *Eur J Obstet Gynecol Reprod Biol.* 2021. 267:226.
34. Eke AC, Shukr GH, Chaalan TT, et al. Intra-abdominal saline irrigation at cesarean section: A systematic review and meta-analysis. *J Matern Fetal Neonatal Med.* 2016. 29:1588.
35. Berghella V. Cesarean birth: Surgical technique. Grobman W. (Ed). *UpToDate.* Waltham, MA. 2024.

36. Aslan Çetin B, Aydogan Mathyk B, Barut S, et al. The impact of subcutaneous irrigation on wound complications after cesarean sections: A prospective randomised study. *Eur J Obstet Gynecol Reprod Biol.* 2018. 227:67.
37. Gates S, Anderson ER. Wound drainage for caesarean section. *Cochrane Database Syst Rev.* 2013. Issue 12. Art. No.:CD004549.
38. Dahlke JD, Mendez-Figueroa H, Rouse DJ, et al. Evidence-based surgery for cesarean delivery: An updated systematic review. *Am J Obstet Gynecol.* 2013. 209:294.
39. Dede M, Yenen MC, Yilmaz A, et al. Treatment of incidental adnexal masses at cesarean section: A retrospective study. *Int J Gynecol Cancer.* 2007. 17:339.
40. Hsu YY, Hung HY, Chang SC, Chang YJ. Early oral intake and gastrointestinal function after cesarean delivery: A systematic review and meta-analysis. *Obstet Gynecol.* 2013. 121:1327.

CHAPTER 23

Reducing Cesarean Section Rates

GITA ARJUN

INTRODUCTION

Universal accessibility of cesarean section is crucial to the reduction of maternal and fetal mortality. A cesarean section is a life-saving procedure when it is performed for an appropriate and justifiable medical indication. However, this surgical intervention is also associated with short- and long-term effects on women and their children [1].

Cesarean section is well-recognised as a maternal healthcare indicator. Lack of facilities for cesarean can increase maternal and perinatal mortality. In 2016, the World Health Organization issued a statement [2] that when cesarean section rates rise towards 10–15% across a population, maternal and newborn deaths decrease. When the cesarean rate is less than 10%, it indicates that women and their babies are receiving less than optimum care.

Globally, the cesarean section rate has been growing at an alarming rate. Current rates of cesarean section, except in the least developed countries, are consistently higher than what is considered medically justifiable. This trend has received enormous attention from women, governmental agencies, public authorities, and the media.

Key Point

Available data predict that by 2030, 38 million women will give birth by cesarean annually, of which 33.5 million will be in LMICs [3].

A high rate of cesarean sections is a major public health concern and contributes to the healthcare cost burden of a country, particularly in emerging economies. Unfortunately, in the coming decade, South Asia (which includes India) and sub-Saharan Africa will face a complex situation where **both overuse and unmet needs are expected to coexist**. There is a call for global effective interventions to revert the trend, which will otherwise drain already scanty resources and result in avoidable morbidity and mortality.

Key Point

The latest available data show that almost 1 in 5 women in the world is now giving birth by cesarean [3]. Despite these high numbers, in low-resource areas, women and their babies are dying because of their inability to access facilities that offer safe cesarean births.

The obstetric community must take ownership of the problem and make sweeping changes to keep the cesarean section rate at a level that is beneficial to the woman and her child. Efforts must be made to reduce the number of unnecessary cesarean sections and, at the same time, make sure that women in need of a cesarean have access to it.

Key Point

Reducing the **primary** cesarean section rate should be the focus of all efforts.

SHORT- AND LONG-TERM HEALTH EFFECTS OF CESAREAN BIRTH

Maternal Risks

Short-term risks

As with any surgery, a cesarean can be associated with infection, hemorrhage, injury to other organs, and anesthetic risks. The risk of maternal mortality is higher after a cesarean than after vaginal birth.

Long-term risks

In a subsequent pregnancy, the presence of a uterine scar leads to an increased risk of the following complications:

- Uterine rupture (see **Chapter 18**, *Obstructed labour and uterine rupture*)
- Abnormal placentation (placenta previa and the placenta accreta spectrum; see **Chapter 29**, *Antepartum hemorrhage*)
- Cesarean scar pregnancy

Neonatal Risks

Short-term risks

Elective cesarean delivery is associated with neonatal respiratory morbidities (e.g., transient tachypnea of the newborn, respiratory distress syndrome), persistent pulmonary hypertension of the newborn, and admission to the neonatal intensive care unit (NICU).

Long-term risks

Emerging evidence shows that not passing through the vaginal canal prevents the baby from being exposed to maternal vaginal bacteria [1]. This could preclude proper colonisation of the fetal gut and lead to reduced neonatal intestinal gut microbiome diversity. This is now being linked to the following:

- Altered immune development
- Increased likelihood of allergy, atopy, and asthma in childhood

Babies who are delivered by cesarean section also have different hormonal, physical, and medical exposures (such as intrapartum antibiotics and uterotonic drugs), which can subtly alter neonatal physiology.

Long-term consequences may also include late childhood obesity.

> **Key Point**
>
> **Vaginal seeding** refers to the practice of applying a cotton swab with maternal vaginal fluids to the mouth, nose, or skin of an infant delivered by cesarean. This is done in an effort to transfer the maternal vaginal bacteria to the newborn. There is no evidence of the benefits of this practice and hence, it is **not recommended** [4]. A recent randomised clinical study found no effect of this intervention on gut microbiota, body mass index, and allergy risks [5].

OPTIMUM CESAREAN SECTION RATE

The optimum rate of cesarean deliveries has not been defined, though recommendations certainly exist. In 1985, the WHO released a statement that 'there is no justification for any region to have a cesarean section rate higher than 10–15%'. This was based on 'populations' and was not specific to the obstetric demographic that is served by the varied range of facilities around the world.

This 10–15% range has been misinterpreted, questioned, and criticised, which then led to the release of the 'WHO Statement on Cesarean Section Rates' [3]. In this statement, the WHO emphasised that cesarean should be undertaken when medically necessary, and rather than attempting to achieve a specific rate, efforts should focus on providing cesarean section to all women in need. However, the definition of a woman in need of a cesarean delivery can only be determined by the healthcare providers caring for the woman on a case-by-case basis and should be based on strong medical indications.

The greatest challenge in determining the optimal cesarean rate is the lack of a reliable and internationally accepted classification system to produce standardised data. The WHO has strongly recommended the Robson classification (see below) and expects that this will help healthcare facilities to:

- **Optimise the use of cesarean section** by identifying, analysing, and focusing interventions on specific groups of particular relevance for each healthcare facility
- **Assess the effectiveness** of strategies or interventions targeted at optimising the use of cesarean section

CESAREAN SECTION RATES IN INDIA

The National Family Health Survey (2019–2021) [6] charted several healthcare indicators, one of which is cesarean section rate.

The survey found a marked disparity between the cesarean rates at private and public facilities. In private facilities, 49.3% of urban women and 46% of rural women delivered by cesarean. On the other hand, the cesarean rate was 22.7% in urban and 11.9% in rural public facilities. In several states, public hospitals show cesarean rates well below 10%, leading to unacceptable and preventable maternal and perinatal mortality. The unfortunate fact is that private facilities in the same states have higher cesarean birth rates that are medically unjustified.

This inequity in healthcare delivery needs to be monitored. Guidelines need to be laid down by professional bodies to ensure that one segment is not receiving cesareans at a rate that is **too little too late,** while another segment is receiving **too many too early**.

FACTORS CONTRIBUTING TO INCREASED CESAREAN RATES

Maternal Perception

There is a widespread misconception that a cesarean is safer for the woman and her baby. This perception is sometimes fuelled by professionals and the media. Some women are terrified of the pain of labour, on account of which, they are unwilling to undergo a vaginal delivery. Exploring the cause behind this fear and addressing it coupled with empathetic counselling, offering support, and providing effective pain relief during labour can help to convince them to attempt labour. Some women and their partners may be concerned that vaginal delivery will lead to vaginal laxity, sexual dysfunction, and urinary/fecal incontinence.

Social Factors

Cesarean birth is considered to be a more 'modern' approach to delivery; hence, wealthier sections of society tend to opt for it. In many countries, one of the cultural pressures leading to scheduled cesareans arises from the belief that choosing an auspicious date and time for the baby's birth would somehow ensure a good future. Some families choose a cesarean for the convenience of a scheduled delivery that will allow the woman's husband and other family members to be present at the time of the delivery.

The Preference of Healthcare Professionals

Globally, there is evidence that some healthcare professionals opt for cesarean section due to the convenience of a scheduled delivery. In some healthcare settings, the lack of infrastructure and availability of medical personnel 24/7 drives an early decision for a cesarean section. The fear of medical litigation is becoming a driving force contributing to the increasing rate of cesareans. Women and their families have a much lower tolerance to any complications or outcomes that do not result in a 'perfect baby'. A neonatal complication is much better accepted by the mother and the family after a cesarean than with a vaginal delivery.

AUDITING TO REDUCE CESAREAN SECTION RATES

It is difficult to standardise the cesarean section rate across all obstetric units and populations—teaching hospitals, private hospitals, public hospitals, and hospitals catering to high-risk pregnancies. Auditing helps an obstetric unit understand where changes can be introduced to reduce cesarean rates.

To understand the cesarean rates in specific groups across different populations, the **Robson ten-group classification of cesarean sections** (Fig. 23.1) should be introduced into every unit providing maternity care. This allows for the auditing of cesareans across all type of hospitals and populations. This classification has proved useful in reducing cesarean rates in units that have implemented it [7].

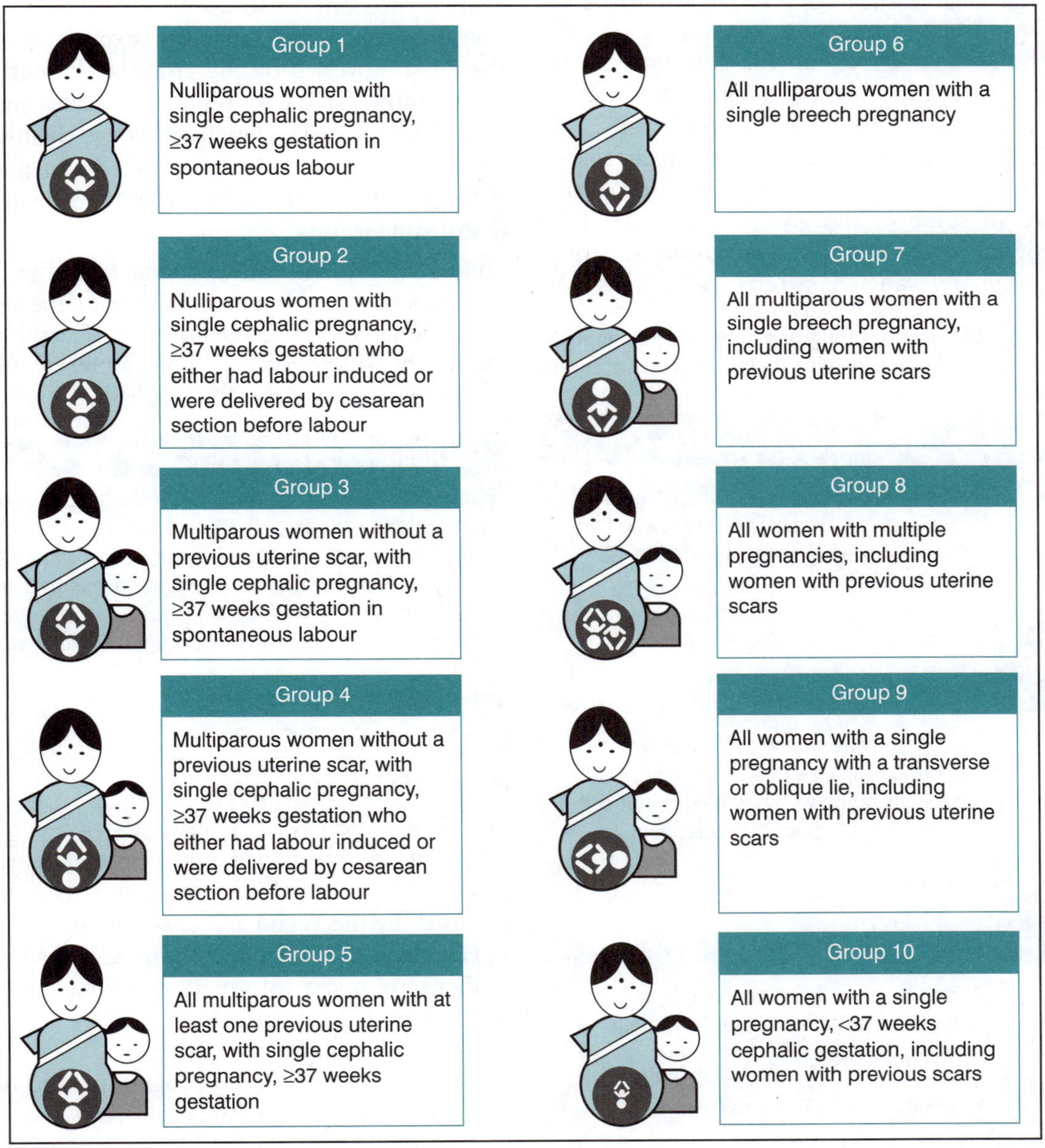

Fig. 23.1 The Robson ten-group classification of cesarean sections—adapted from the WHO Implementation Manual [8]

Key Point

Classifying an obstetric population using the Robson classification allows one to justify or decrease the cesarean rate for each individual group. For example, group 1 (nulliparous women with a single cephalic pregnancy, ≥37 weeks' gestation in spontaneous labour) should not have a cesarean rate exceeding 10%.

The Robson Ten-group Classification is easy to implement because of its simplicity, robustness, reproducibility, and flexibility [8]. To achieve better uniformity and homogeneity of the groups, certain subdivisions have been introduced in some of the groups (Table 23.1) by stratifying women within that group according to certain relevant characteristics. It does not, however, tell us what the actual indications were for the cesarean within a group.

Table 23.1 Subdivisions for groups 2, 4, and 5 to improve uniformity and homogeneity (helps in more accurate reporting and auditing)

Group	Obstetric population
2	Nulliparous women with a single cephalic pregnancy, ≥37 weeks' gestation who had labour induced or were delivered by CS before labour
2A	Labour induced
2B	Pre-labour cesarean
4	Multiparous women without a previous CS, with a single cephalic pregnancy, ≥37 weeks' gestation who had labour induced or were delivered by CS before labour
4A	Labour induced
4B	Pre-labour cesarean
5	All multiparous women with at least one previous CS, with a single cephalic pregnancy, ≥37 weeks' gestation
5.1	With one previous cesarean
5.2	With two or more previous cesareans

Classifying a Woman on Admission

Fig. 23.2 shows a simple flowchart that can help any healthcare worker classify the expectant woman into one of Robson's ten groups. The Robson groups are **mutually exclusive** (i.e., there is no overlap of one group with another) and **totally inclusive** (i.e., every category of labouring woman is covered in this classification).

Suggested Cesarean Rates for the Robson Groups

Table 23.2 presents the cesarean rates that are acceptable and to be aimed for, and at the same time, consistent with good outcomes of labour and childbirth. Groups 6 and 7 (breech presentation) have a cesarean rate of >90% globally.

Key Point

Groups 1, 2, and 5 contribute to 2/3rd of all cesareans performed. In units trying to reduce their cesarean rate, these are the groups on whom effort should be focused. Avoiding cesarean section in groups 1 and 2 will reduce the numbers in group 5 in subsequent years and, therefore, will bring down the overall rate.

STRATEGIES TO REDUCE CESAREAN SECTION RATES

Non-clinical Strategies

In 2018, the WHO released non-clinical interventions to reduce unnecessary cesarean sections [9]. Some of the important suggestions put forth by the WHO are listed below.

- **Educating women and their families** helps them to make informed decisions on the mode of delivery, utilising:
  - Childbirth classes
  - Relaxation training programmes to help a woman cope with labour pain
  - Counselling for those with anxiety and extreme fear of labour pain

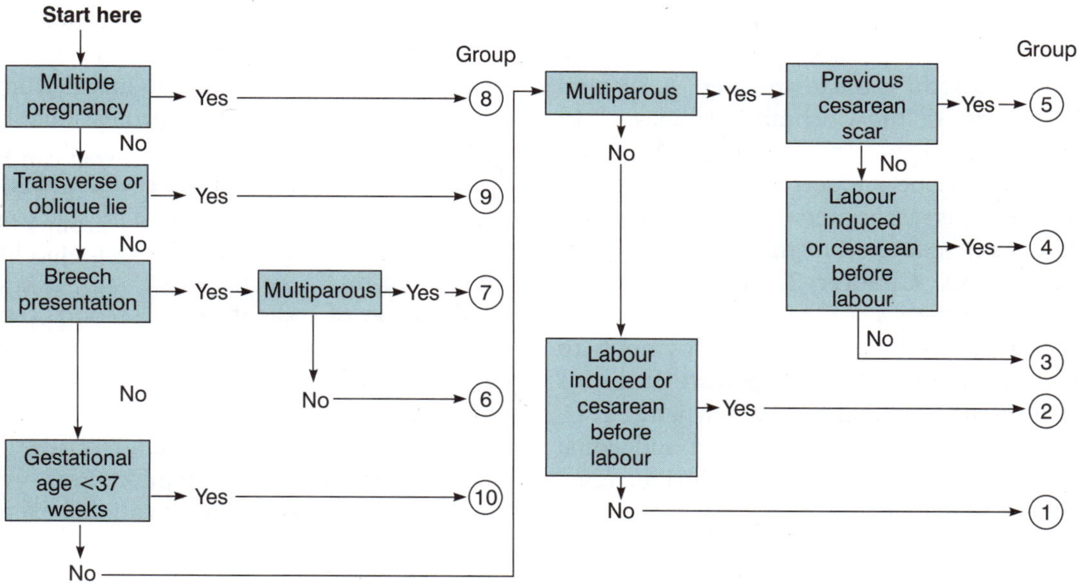

Fig. 23.2 A simple flowchart that can be used by any healthcare worker to place a woman in a Robson group (adapted from the WHO Robson Classification: Implementation Manual, 2017)

Table 23.2 Guidelines for acceptable cesarean section rates in different Robson groups

Group	Robson guideline for acceptable CS rate	Remarks
Group 1 (Nullipara, single cephalic, ≥37 weeks)	10% or less	This group should be the focus to reduce the overall CS rate
Group 2 (Nullipara, single cephalic, ≥37 weeks + induced labour **or** prelabour CS)	20–35%	If induction of labour is resulting in high CS rates, better selection of candidates for induction may bring down the rate
Group 3 (Multipara, single cephalic, ≥37 weeks, no CS scar)	No higher than 3.0%	A woman who has had a successful vaginal delivery with a previous pregnancy should be given every chance to have another vaginal delivery
Group 4 (Multipara, single cephalic, ≥37 weeks, no CS scar + induced labour **or** prelabour CS)	15%	A woman with a previous traumatic or prolonged labour may request a CS in the current pregnancy
Group 5 (Multipara, single cephalic, ≥37 weeks, with CS scar)	50–60%	The CS rate could be higher if the hospital does not allow VBAC
Group 8 (Multiple pregnancy, including women with previous CS scar)	60%	Rates will depend on the type of twin pregnancy; they are lowest when the first twin is in cephalic presentation

CS, cesarean section; *VBAC*, vaginal birth after cesarean

- **Continuous labour support** (with a companion of the woman's choosing) has been shown to reduce cesarean rates. A systematic review of the Cochrane Database [10] demonstrated that the presence of continuous one-on-one support during labour and delivery was associated with a statistically significant reduction in the rate of cesarean delivery (see **Chapter 3**, *Respectful obstetric care and the role of a birth companion*).
- **Changing fee-for-service employment to full-time employment in private facilities** changes the customer–hospital dynamic [11]. Working as a team rather than individual consultants takes the pressure off an individual and helps in making collaborative decisions that ultimately help the pregnant woman.

The initiative to reduce cesarean section rates, particularly in a private facility, requires a multi-pronged approach and requires the entire team to be invested in the cause. This is an achievable goal, as was demonstrated in a private hospital in New Delhi, India, where the cesarean rates were reduced from 52% to 18% between 2011 and 2016, and to 17–19% from 2016 to 2018. The greatest declines were for low-risk first-birth women (Robson groups 1 and 2), among whom, the rate declined from 48% to 12% [11].

In our own practice in a small private facility with a large high-risk obstetric population, we worked as a team practice, and our primary cesarean rate never exceeded 22%. In Robson group 1, our cesarean rate was consistently 9–11% with good perinatal outcomes.

Other strategies that can be used to reduce cesarean section rates are as follows:

- **Utilising clinical guidelines, audits of cesarean sections, and timely feedback** to health professionals about cesarean practices helps in reducing the cesarean rate. The Robson classification contributes greatly to this process.
- **Implementation** of evidence-based clinical practice guidelines is another important measure.
- **Policy** across the globe must be changed and should require audits of each and every facility delivering care to the pregnant woman. Individuals, hospitals, and professional bodies should work to create a culture where policy changes regarding cesarean delivery are incorporated voluntarily. The safe lowering of the primary cesarean rate should be encouraged.
- **Validation of indication**—a second opinion should be required for cesarean section indication at the point of care in settings with adequate resources. Team practice facilitates this since the expertise of a senior obstetrician is available for a second opinion. Peer review after the cesarean (as an educational exercise and not as a 'blame game') also contributes to a reduction in cesarean rates.
- **Introducing midwife-led obstetric units** has been shown to lower cesarean sections as compared to obstetrician-led units.
- **Financial strategies** in the form of incentives seem to be a strong driver for cesarean sections as shown by the much higher cesarean rates in private facilities. Equalising physician fees for vaginal births and cesarean sections might drive down the incidence of cesareans [12].

Clinical Strategies

A single strategy is unlikely to change practices; several clinical strategies, implemented together, are required to reduce cesarean rates.

- **Reducing surgical intervention in the first stage**—slow but progressive labour in the first stage of labour should not be an indication for cesarean delivery (see **Chapter 11**, *Abnormalities in the latent phase and the first stage of labour*).
- **Defining the active phase**—a cervical dilatation of 6 cm has been shown to be the beginning of the active phase for most women in labour. Thus, before 6 cm of dilatation is achieved, standards of active phase progress should not be applied (see **Chapter 11**).
- **Routine induction at 39 weeks of gestation for low-risk nulliparous women** has

been shown to decrease cesarean rates significantly [13]. Maternal and neonatal morbidity also decreased with this strategy. The need to manage deliveries and emergencies during the hours when staffing may be low is reduced. This is an important policy that can be implemented in obstetric facilities. In the presence of an unfavourable cervix, ripening should be achieved before formal induction.

- **Operative vaginal delivery** in the second stage of labour by experienced and well-trained physicians should be considered a safe, acceptable alternative to cesarean delivery. Training in operative vaginal delivery should be emphasised (see **Chapter 21,** *Operative vaginal delivery*).
- **Manual rotation of the fetal occiput** in the setting of fetal malposition in the second stage of labour is a reasonable intervention to consider before moving to operative vaginal delivery or cesarean delivery (see **Chapter 4,** *Management of the first and second stages of normal labour*). Assessing the fetal position in the second stage of labour, particularly when there is abnormal fetal descent, and then correcting malposition will reduce cesarean rates.
- **Early rather than delayed pushing** in women with epidural analgesia has been recommended by the ACOG [14]. The woman should be encouraged to commence pushing at full dilatation; pushing should not be delayed [15].
- **External cephalic version (ECV)**—fetal presentation should be assessed and documented beginning at 36 0/7 weeks of gestation to allow for ECV to be offered (see **Chapter 27,** *Breech delivery*).
- **Twin pregnancy**—perinatal outcomes for twin gestations in which the first twin is in cephalic presentation are not improved by cesarean delivery. Women with either cephalic–cephalic presenting twins or cephalic–non-cephalic presenting twins should be counselled for vaginal delivery [14].

CONCLUSION

Reducing cesarean rates requires commitment from healthcare providers, the healthcare system, and global policymakers. The rate can be safely reduced by complex interventions that initially require analysis of the birth data and which will lead to safe modifications of practice norms. Identification of barriers to change, both in the mindset of clinicians and the women they serve, is a major contributor to accomplishing this goal. Multidimensional strategies, based on audit using the Robson classification and implementation of safe guidelines, will improve clinical practice and effectively reduce the cesarean section rate.

REFERENCES

1. Sandall J, Tribe RM, Avery L, Mola G, Visser GH, Homer CS, et al. Short-term and long-term effects of caesarean section on the health of women and children. *Lancet.* 2018. 392(10155):1349–57.
2. Betrán AP, Torloni MR, Zhang JJ, Gülmezoglu AM. WHO Working Group on Caesarean Section. WHO Statement on Caesarean Section Rates. *BJOG.* 2016.123(5):667–670.
3. Betrán AP, Ye J, Moller AB, Souza JP, Zhang J. Trends and projections of caesarean section rates: Global and regional estimates. *BMJ Glob Health.* 2021. 6(6):e005671.
4. ACOG. Vaginal seeding. Committee Opinion No. 725. American College of Obstetricians and Gynecologists. *Obstet Gynecol.* 2017. 130:e274–8.
5. Liu Y, Li HT, Zhou SJ, et al. Effects of vaginal seeding on gut microbiota, body mass index, and allergy risks in infants born through cesarean delivery: A randomized clinical trial. *Am J Obstet Gynecol MFM.* 2023. 5:100793.
6. National Family Health Survey (NFHS-5) 2019–2021. Compendium of fact sheets. Ministry Of Health & Family Welfare, Government of India (available at https://main.mohfw.gov.in/sites/default/files/NFHS-5_Phase-II_0.pdf)
7. Tanaka K and Mahomed K. The Ten-Group Robson Classification: A Single Centre Approach Identifying Strategies to Optimise Caesarean Section Rates. *Obstetrics and Gynecology International.* 2017. Article ID 5648938.
8. WHO: Robson Classification: Implementation Manual. 2017. WHO, Geneva.
9. WHO recommendations: Non-clinical interventions to reduce unnecessary caesarean sections. 2018. WHO, Geneva.

10. Bohren MA, Hofmeyr GJ, Sakala C, et al. Continuous support for women during childbirth. *Cochrane Database of Systematic Reviews*. 2017. Issue 7. Art. No.: CD003766.
11. Bhartia A, Sen Gupta Dhar R, Bhartia S. Reducing caesarean section rate in an urban hospital serving women attending privately in India—a quality improvement initiative. *BMC Pregnancy Childbirth*. 2020. **20**, 556.
12. Opiyo N, Young C, Requejo JH, Erdman J, Bales S, Betrán AP. Reducing unnecessary caesarean sections: Scoping review of financial and regulatory interventions. *Reprod Health*. 2020. 31;17(1):133.
13. Grobman WA, Rice MM, Reddy UM, et al. Labor induction versus expectant management in low-risk nulliparous women. *N Engl J Med*. 2018. 379:513.
14. ACOG Committee Opinion No. 766. Approaches to limit intervention during labor and birth. *Obstet Gynecol*. 2019. 133:e164.
15. Cahill AG, Srinivas SK, Tita ATN, et al. Effect of immediate vs delayed pushing on rates of spontaneous vaginal delivery among nulliparous women receiving neuraxial analgesia: A randomized clinical trial. *JAMA*. 2018. 320:1444.

CHAPTER 24

Peripartum Hysterectomy

V P PAILY, G RAJI RAJ

INTRODUCTION

A **peripartum hysterectomy** is defined as the removal of the uterine body, either alone or with the cervix, at birth or in the immediate postpartum period. It is usually performed as a life-saving obstetric procedure in an emergency either following a vaginal delivery or cesarean section. The majority of cases are unplanned, but in some scenarios such as the placenta accreta spectrum (PAS), it may be a planned procedure.

Postpartum hemorrhage (PPH) is still the leading cause of maternal mortality worldwide [1]. The World Health Organization (WHO) considers peripartum hysterectomy a maternal near-miss event and uses it as a proxy for severe postpartum hemorrhage [2]. Since the majority of cases are unplanned, and performed on compromised women, surgery can be challenging.

Key Point

Peripartum hysterectomy is a devastating event since it results in the loss of fertility and is associated with significant maternal morbidity and mortality.

Obstetric hysterectomy in a broader sense can include the removal of a uterus that is pregnant but not associated with labour and delivery. If we follow this broad definition, additional conditions such as hysterectomy for septic abortion, a hydatidiform mole in situ, rupture of a scar pregnancy leading to broad ligament hematoma, or rupture of a poorly developed horn of the uterus in Mullerian anomalies have to be included. However, these constitute only a small percentage of obstetric hysterectomies.

The emphasis in this chapter will mainly be on peripartum hysterectomy for conditions such as placenta accreta spectrum (PAS), atonic PPH, uterine rupture, and sepsis.

HISTORY

Peripartum hysterectomy was first proposed by Joseph Cavallini in 1768. Cesarean hysterectomy was first performed by Horatio Storer in the United States in 1869, but the woman did not survive. Eduardo Porro of Milan performed the first successful cesarean hysterectomy in 1876; both the mother and baby survived the procedure. Porro's patient was a 25-year-old primipara with dwarfism. He used a constriction wire around the cervix to control bleeding.

INCIDENCE

The worldwide incidence of emergency peripartum hysterectomy is around 1 per 1000 deliveries [3,4]. A recent meta-analysis suggests that the incidence varies with settings, being highest in low- and middle-income countries (LMICs) (3 in 1000 births) and lowest in high-income countries (0.7 in 1000 births) [4]. In LMICs, uterine rupture was found to be the most common indication. However, the incidence in LMICs was based on data from only two hospitals, one in Tanzania and the other in Nepal. Studies from tertiary teaching hospitals in India showed an incidence ranging from 1.3 to 6.9/1000, with the placenta accreta spectrum as the leading cause, followed by atonic PPH, and uterine rupture [5,6].

Key Point

The incidence in India ranges from 1.3 to 6.9/1000, with PAS and atonic PPH being the leading causes.

Even in LMICs, the incidence of peripartum hysterectomy following atonic PPH is decreasing due to the availability of effective drugs and other methods to arrest bleeding quickly (e.g., uterine balloon tamponade, transvaginal uterine artery clamps [7], and SR suction cannula [8]). For more details, see **Chapter 13,** *Abnormalities in the third stage of labour: Postpartum hemorrhage and retained placenta.*

Variations in the incidence of peripartum hysterectomy across the world could be due to differences in standards of obstetric care, parity, cesarean section rates, availability of other methods to control bleeding, and the lack of availability of blood and blood products.

Studies have shown that the incidence of peripartum hysterectomy increases with the number of cesarean sections. Women who have had one cesarean section have double the risk as compared to women who have not had one, and women who have had two cesarean sections have 18 times the risk of peripartum hysterectomy [4].

RISK FACTORS FOR PERIPARTUM HYSTERECTOMY

Abnormal Placentation

With the rise in cesarean section rates, the incidence of placenta previa and the placenta accreta spectrum are on the rise, even in LMICs [5]. **In most high-income countries, the placenta accreta spectrum is now the leading cause of peripartum hysterectomy**. Early diagnosis of abnormal placentation is the key to preventing the morbidity and mortality from such cases and ultrasonography is the most commonly used tool to make the diagnosis.

Diagnosis of the placenta accreta spectrum

Although ultrasound evaluation is important, the absence of ultrasound findings does not preclude a diagnosis of PAS. In LMICs, access to ultrasonography may not be widespread, or ultrasonography expertise in identifying features of PAS may be limited. In such areas, clinical risk factors are equally important predictors.

See **Chapter 29,** *Antepartum hemorrhage,* for further details regarding the diagnosis of PAS by imaging.

Key Point

Placenta previa is present in more than 80% of cases of accretas and is perhaps the most important ultrasonographic association of PAS in the second and third trimesters [9].

Parity and Previous Cesarean Delivery

A previous cesarean delivery is the most significant risk factor for PAS. Silver et al. [10], in a prospective study, found that in the presence of placenta previa, the risk of PAS increases exponentially with an increasing number of cesarean deliveries—3% with the primary cesarean, 11% with the second cesarean, 40% with the third, 61% with the fourth, and 67% with the fifth and above.

The combination of placenta previa and a previous cesarean is an ominous risk factor for massive postpartum hemorrhage and peripartum hysterectomy. Ideally, a dedicated ultrasound should be performed in the third trimester (around 32–34 weeks) in every pregnancy with this combined risk factor to rule out the placenta accreta spectrum [11,12].

Key Point

One should carefully look for the ultrasound features of adherence in all women with low-lying placenta, especially if they have had a previous cesarean.

Higher Order Pregnancies

Compared to singletons, higher-order multiple gestations were found to have nearly a 24-fold increased risk of emergent peripartum hysterectomy [13].

Advanced Maternal Age

The incidence of hysterectomy has been reported to be 1% in mothers under 20 years and 13% in mothers who are 40 and above [14]. This may be related to increased parity with increasing age.

Other Risk Factors

Antepartum hemorrhage, preeclampsia, bleeding disorders, and pregnancy resulting from assisted reproductive techniques have been mentioned as risk factors for peripartum hysterectomy.

INDICATIONS FOR PERIPARTUM HYSTERECTOMY

The most common indication for peripartum hysterectomy is hemorrhage; the cause leading to hemorrhage varies in different settings. In low-income countries, it is uterine atony and uterine rupture. However, with increasing cesarean section rates, the placenta accreta spectrum is rapidly becoming a leading indication in LMICs too [5,6]. In high-income countries, peripartum hysterectomy is chiefly performed due to abnormal placentation. When all conservative methods to control postpartum hemorrhage fail, an immediate peripartum hysterectomy must be performed as a life-saving procedure. The indications for peripartum hysterectomy identified in a recent systematic review and meta-analysis [4] are presented in Table 24.1.

Globally, the placenta accreta spectrum is the most challenging of all the indications for obstetric hysterectomy and is rapidly becoming the most common indication as well. Hence, in this chapter, there will be an emphasis on hysterectomy for the placenta accreta spectrum.

TECHNIQUE FOR PERIPARTUM HYSTERECTOMY

The technique for peripartum hysterectomy will vary for different indications. In this chapter, techniques for the following indications will be discussed:

- Placenta accreta spectrum (PAS)
- PPH
- Uterine rupture
- Placental abruption

Table 24.1 Common indications for peripartum hysterectomy and their respective proportions (more than one indication can occur in the same woman [4])

Indications for peripartum hysterectomy	Proportion (%)
Placental pathology	38
Placenta accreta spectrum	23.9
Placenta previa	13.9
Combined or unspecified placental pathology	26.1
Uterine atony	27.0
Uterine rupture	21.2
Placental abruption	5.2

Hysterectomy for Placenta Accreta Spectrum

Hysterectomy for PAS should be performed in a tertiary–care centre, if possible. Without the presence of an experienced multidisciplinary care team, maternal morbidity and mortality are high. An experienced obstetrician should collaborate with a skilled pelvic surgeon. In addition, an obstetric anesthetist, urologist, general surgeon, and critical care physician should also be recruited into the team to safeguard the woman's health [15]. A neonatology team should be available to handle the preterm neonate.

The available infrastructure and the nursing team at the facility should be accustomed to managing significant postpartum hemorrhage. Reliable access to a blood bank capable of employing massive transfusion protocols is essential.

Challenges in peripartum hysterectomy for PAS

- The uterus is enlarged and the tissues are friable and edematous.
- The blood vessels are greatly dilated, which increases the risk of bleeding during surgery.
- **Neovascularisation**—a large number of new vessels develop from the surrounding organs, especially the bladder and vagina. These vessels are more prone to bleeding as they are thin-walled and do not have the muscular wall of arteries. For the same reason, electrocoagulation may not be an effective method of arresting bleeding from these vessels.
- Dense bladder adhesions from previous cesarean sections may make it difficult to separate the bladder from the uterus.
- The invasion of the placenta into the bladder–uterine interface, with the presence of large venous sinuses, can lead to torrential bleeding and also endanger bladder integrity.
- In the presence of low implantation of the placenta, the lower uterine segment may be grossly enlarged. In such cases, the placement of clamps laterally can **injure** or **kink the ureters**.

The management of a **diagnosed case of PAS** is different from the management of an **unanticipated case of PAS**. They will, therefore, be discussed separately. Ideally, the diagnosis of PAS should be made in the antenatal period, as this provides the obstetrician with an opportunity to plan the surgical procedure.

Management of a diagnosed case of PAS

Most guidelines on the surgical management of PAS depend on cohort studies, retrospective case series, and expert opinion as very few randomised clinical trials are available.

Timing of delivery

Elective surgery should be planned after taking the woman's condition and fetal maturity into consideration. In a woman who does not have any bleeding, it is suggested that the cesarean delivery/hysterectomy be scheduled between **34 0/7 and 35 6/7 weeks of gestation** [11,16]. This is because of the increased risk of bleeding after 36 weeks [15]. Approximately 50% of women with PAS will require an emergency delivery if they go beyond 36 weeks of gestation [11].

> **Key Point**
>
> Performing a cesarean delivery **before the onset of labour** followed immediately by a cesarean hysterectomy has been shown to improve maternal outcomes in PAS [17].

Surgical planning

- **Counselling:** The woman and her family should be counselled regarding the procedure and possible intraoperative and postoperative complications. They should be aware of the need for blood transfusion, prolonged catheterisation, mechanical ventilation, ICU stay, and prolonged hospitalisation.
- **Transfer to tertiary centre:** The centre should be capable of handling operative and postoperative complications.
- **Optimisation of hemoglobin levels:** Iron deficiency anemia should be tackled with oral replacement and/or intravenous infusions.
- **Ensuring availability of blood and blood products:** Blood grouping and cross-matching should be done, and **at least six units of packed red cells** and other blood products should be kept ready before the surgery. The blood bank should be warned about the possible need for **massive transfusion protocols**. If the facility for cell salvage is available, it should be used.
- **Intravenous lines**: Large-bore (16–18 gauge) IV cannulae should be used. At least two IV lines should be available.
- **Prophylactic antibiotics**: It is recommended that a single dose of antibiotic be administered within 60 minutes before making the skin incision [18]. See **Chapter 19**, *Antibiotic prophylaxis in labour and delivery,* for further details.

- **Ensuring adequate surgical instruments and supplies:** The availability of an adequate number of instruments should be ensured in addition to the usual laparotomy instruments (Fig. 24.1). The authors of this chapter keep 28 hysterectomy clamps, two transabdominal uterine artery clamps, two Green Armytage forceps, three Paily aorta clamps, a special Babcock forceps to lift up the aorta, Deaver retractors of different sizes, and a malleable retractor. Spare suction tips and needle holders are also kept ready, to avoid loss of time. Two suction units and electrosurgical instruments are kept available.
- **Anesthesia:** Epidural or combined spinal/epidural anesthesia may be used, but the facility to convert to general anesthesia should be immediately available [19]. It should be borne in mind that hypotension caused by regional anesthesia may complicate the clinical situation.
- **Antenatal corticosteroids**: This is indicated for fetal lung maturation in women with anticipated delivery before 36 0/7 weeks of gestation.

Technique of hysterectomy for PAS

- **Safeguarding the bladder and ureters**: In known cases of placenta percreta invading the bladder or parametrium, a cystoscopy with stenting/catheterisation of the ureters is recommended initially to help avoid inadvertent injury to the ureters. In such situations, the presence of a urologic surgeon is advisable. An indwelling Foley catheter is introduced into the urinary bladder. The catheter is inserted deep into the bladder so that the bulb can be moved around to identify the upper margins of the bladder during surgery.

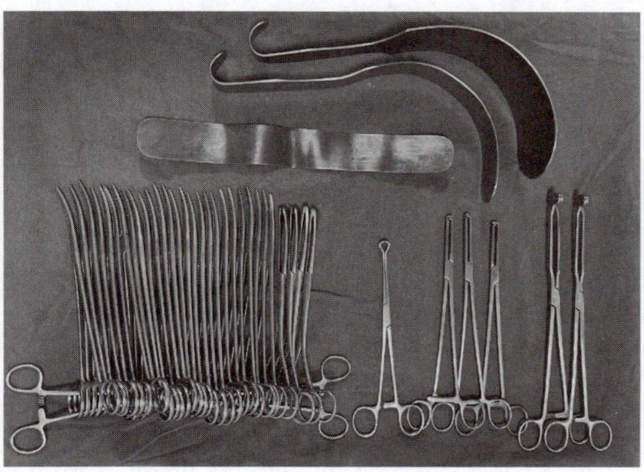

Fig. 24.1 Surgical instruments that should be kept available for peripartum hysterectomy (*Image courtesy*: Dr V P Paily, Rajagiri Hospital, Kerala)

- **Abdominal incision:** A vertical incision is preferred as it gives better exposure and access to the aorta and iliac vessels. A muscle-cutting transverse abdominal incision may also be used.
- **Uterine incision:** The uterine incision to deliver the fetus is placed at a site away from the placental location, at least two fingerbreadths above the placental edge. It is advisable to leave a myometrial margin between the placenta and the incision to avoid disruption of the placenta during the opening or closing of the uterus. The transverse or vertical incision may be placed in the upper segment or fundus. Prior knowledge of the location of the placenta helps in placing the uterine incision.
- **Delivery of the fetus:** The fetus is then delivered, the cord clamped and cut, and the neonate handed over to a neonatologist.
- **Managing the placenta:** Care is taken not to disturb the placenta. **No attempt should be made to separate the placenta** since doing so may result in massive hemorrhage.

Key Point

Prophylactic oxytocin is **not** routinely administered after the infant is delivered because it may result in increased bleeding from partial placental separation.

- **Control of bleeding:** Green Armytage clamps or the Paily uterine artery clamps are applied to the uterine wound margins to control bleeding. The uterus is exteriorised, and **the lower end of the aorta** or **both common iliac arteries are clamped with the**

Paily aorta clamp [20] to control bleeding. The aortic clamp may be kept on for 40–50 minutes (see section below on *Intraoperative bleeding*).

Even though the application of this clamp does not require a vascular surgeon's presence, it does require training and experience with this procedure. The clamp has to be specially ordered.

If the bleeding is profuse, the aorta clamp can be reapplied. In doing so, when the aorta clamp is released, it is not removed from the location. If excess bleeding is noted, re-clamping is easier. Such bleeding is most often noted on the bladder base and vaginal surface.

Procedure

Extensive vascularisation close to the placental site is the rule with PAS. Therefore, devascularisation of the uterine corpus in proximity to the placenta is of utmost importance.

Clamping is initiated at the cornual pedicles and is continued downwards until the uterine arteries are reached. Two clamps are applied laterally and one medially, and a cut is made in between. If there is no active bleeding from the uterine wound or from the premature separation of the placenta, the lateral pedicles are ligated in a stepwise fashion proceeding downwards until the uterine arteries are tied. On the other hand, if there is bleeding, the 'clamp, cut, and drop' technique is used until the uterine arteries are reached (the availability of an adequate number of clamps is essential, as mentioned above).

The parametrial structures below the level of uterine arteries are clamped after the bladder has been dissected free. Once the bladder has been separated low enough, palpation with fingers inserted anterior and posterior to the lower segment will help to identify whether the lower edge of the placenta has been reached. The cervix is then cross-clamped at that level and transected to remove the uterus. Inspection of the lower end of the uterus will confirm whether the placenta has been removed in its entirety.

Total or subtotal hysterectomy?

The decision regarding total or subtotal hysterectomy should be individualised depending on the clinical scenario. In obstetric hysterectomy, Wright et al. found that total hysterectomy is associated with more complications, though the same study showed a higher rate of reoperation and perioperative death with subtotal hysterectomy [21]. A recent retrospective study found subtotal hysterectomy to be safer and associated with less blood loss [22]. However, some authors found no difference in complication rates when the two were compared [23].

The authors of this chapter prefer subtotal hysterectomy (Fig. 24.2 and 24.3) unless the woman is already in labour with a dilated cervix, in which case, total hysterectomy is preferable. As a general principle, the cervix may have to be removed in cases with cervical injury or lower segment PPH, or when the placenta invades the cervical stroma.

The advantages of subtotal hysterectomy include a decrease in operative time and a reduction in total blood loss, which is of utmost importance in a hemodynamically unstable woman.

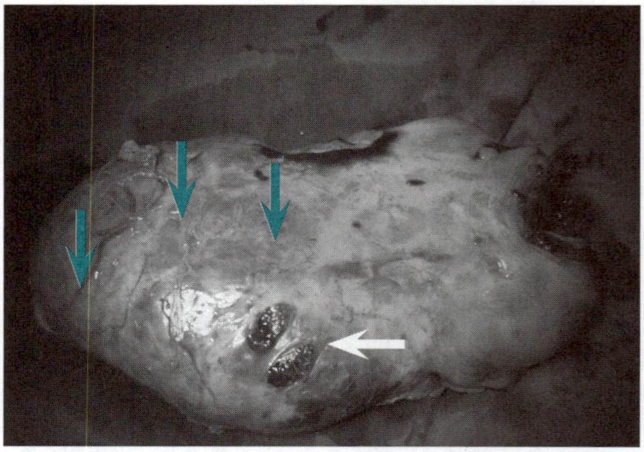

Fig. 24.2 Subtotal hysterectomy specimen with the placenta accreta spectrum. The ballooned-out lower segment—green arrows—shows areas where the placenta has penetrated through the uterine serosa—white arrow (*Image courtesy*: Dr V P Paily, Rajagiri Hospital, Kerala)

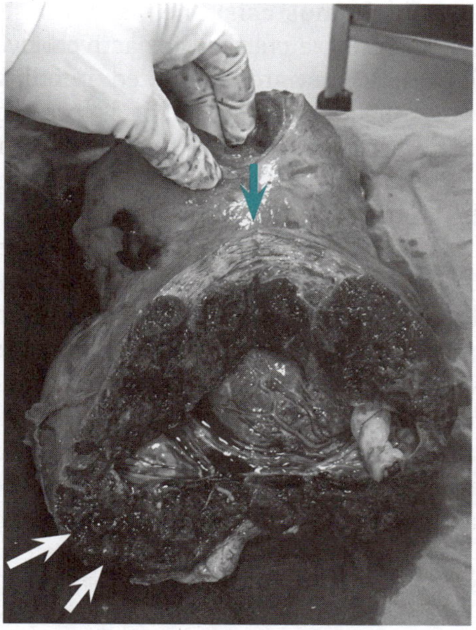

Fig. 24.3 Tangential section through the lower segment to demonstrate the different depths of invasion by the placenta. In some areas, the placenta has invaded through the myometrium and beyond the serosa—white arrows, whereas at about 12'o clock position, the myometrium is intact—green arrow (*Image courtesy*: Dr V P Paily, Rajagiri Hospital, Kerala)

Management of intraoperative bleeding

Application of the Paily aorta clamp [20], which is an atraumatic clamp, prevents intraoperative bleeding and provides a relatively dry field to operate in. Instead of the aorta, the common iliac arteries on both sides may also be clamped using the same instrument. With a transverse abdominal incision, clamping the common iliac arteries is technically easier.

Paily aorta clamp

The aorta clamp is a straight instrument resembling the Allis forceps but with blunt tips that overlap and prevent the vessel from slipping out of the clamp (Fig. 24.4a). The blades have a smooth surface. Even on full closure, there is a gap of 2 mm between the blades (Fig. 24.4b) to prevent crush injuries to the vessel wall and the vasa-vasorum of the aorta.

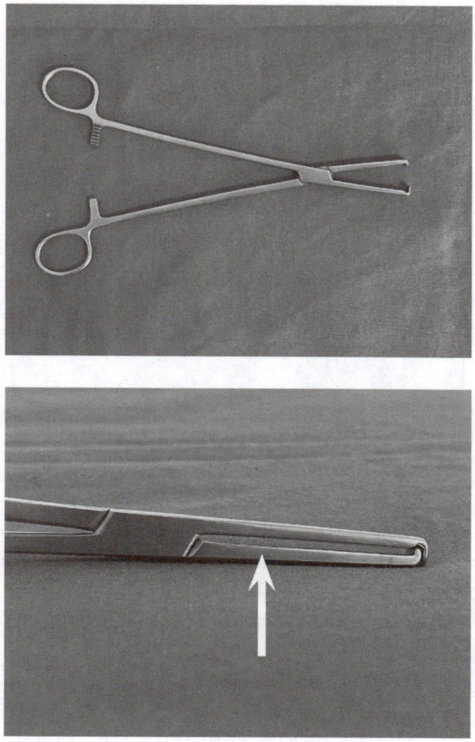

Fig. 24.4 (a) The Paily aorta clamp and (b) even after closing the clamp, there is a 2 mm gap between the blades (*Image courtesy*: Dr V P Paily, Rajagiri Hospital, Kerala)

Key Point

The application of the clamp does not require retroperitoneal dissection or vessel skeletonisation [20]. However, it should be used by experienced pelvic surgeons who are capable of complex surgery.

The operator lifts the aorta with a Babcock clamp just above the bifurcation of the aorta and applies the aorta clamp to include the full thickness of the aorta (Fig. 24.5). The pulsation of the common iliac arteries on both sides is checked to ensure that the clamp has effectively occluded the aorta. It is not all that uncommon to mistake the common iliac artery for the aorta and occlude only one common iliac artery while the other continues to supply the uterus.

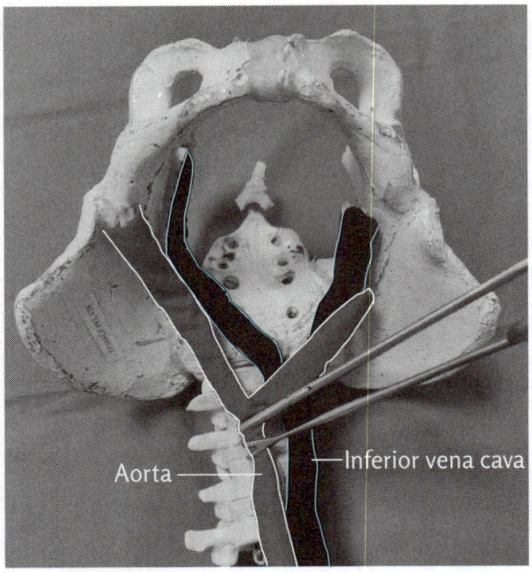

Fig. 24.5 Paily aorta clamp application: A Babcock clamp is used to lift the aorta and the Paily aorta clamp is applied on the aorta, just above the bifurcation into the iliac vessels. (*Image courtesy*: Dr V P Paily, Rajagiri Hospital, Kerala)

The concern commonly expressed about the use of the aorta clamp is the possibility of inadvertent injury to the inferior vena cava (IVC) and/or the lumbar vessels. To avoid injury to the IVC, the operator should ensure that neither the Babcock clamp nor the aorta clamp wanders towards the right, where the venous system lies. Lifting the thick-walled aorta with a Babcock helps in this regard. The lumbar arteries usually originate from the posterior aspect of the aorta (and not from the sides as shown in some textbooks) and lie at a higher level than where the clamps are applied.

A recent retrospective study of 33 women [20] with varying degrees of histopathology-confirmed PAS, in whom elective or emergency hysterectomy was performed in a tertiary-care setting in India showed a median-estimated intraoperative blood loss of 1000 ± 1500 mL. Only 21.2% of these women required transfusion of more than four units of PRBCs. The median time of application of the aorta was 55 +/–20 minutes. The application of the aorta clamp was not associated with any intraoperative or postoperative complication.

Confirming hemostasis: The bladder base and vaginal surface are checked for active bleeders, and if present, they are coagulated or tied. With extensive bladder dissection, it is prudent to routinely perform bilateral internal iliac artery ligation.

The aorta/common iliac artery clamps are now released, and the clamp time is recorded. The posterior surface of the bladder is inspected carefully for any bleeders after the aorta/common iliac artery clamps have been removed.

All bulky and vascular pedicles are double-ligated. An intraperitoneal tube drain is inserted into the pelvis and brought out through the anterior abdominal wall, lateral to the inferior epigastric artery.

Other options to control bleeding

Embolisation of the hypogastric arteries in cases of persistent or uncontrolled hemorrhage may be a useful option, if available. This is particularly useful when there is generalised bleeding, and a single point of bleeding is not identified. A systematic review of 108 studies worldwide found that only **3% of women globally had access to arterial embolisation to prevent hysterectomy** [24].

Pelvic pressure packing and **aortic compression** have been used as alternative methods in the presence of severe and intractable pelvic hemorrhage [11].

Aortic clamping by the conventional method of dissecting the lower end of the aorta free of surrounding tissues requires the expertise of a vascular surgeon.

Bladder separation and possible injuries

Separation of the adherent bladder from the lower segment of the uterus can be challenging. It may be adherent to a previous cesarean scar or to the percreta placenta. New vessels bridging the bladder and the uterus/placenta can bleed profusely. The following steps may help avert or reduce bleeding:

- The preoperative insertion of a ureteric stent or catheter helps in identifying the ureters while dissecting and clamping the pedicles.

- The upper border of the bladder can be identified by moving the Foley bulb inside the bladder. The uterovesical fold of the peritoneum over the protruded placenta should be avoided, and dissection should start about a centimetre or two above the bladder border.
- The surface of the placenta may be covered by a membranous coagulum. This should not be disturbed while separating the bladder. If the membrane gets torn, continuous bleeding will flood the surgical field. This can be temporarily controlled by applying and maintaining pressure with a sterile surgical pad.
- In the case of a previously diagnosed placenta percreta, it is prudent to have an experienced urologist as part of the surgical team. Injuries to the ureters or the bladder can be handled by the urologist, who may stent the ureters, especially before closing a trigonal tear.
- Postoperatively, continuous bladder drainage is advised after bladder injury—one week for a clean cut near the dome of the bladder and at least three weeks for tears on the trigone and for irregular tears. For long-term drainage, a silicone catheter is preferred over a latex catheter.

Some authors recommend deliberate incision of the bladder and resection of part of the bladder wall. However, the authors of this chapter, from their experience with the Paily aorta clamp, report relatively bloodless fields which allow for the dissection of the bladder from the uterine wall or the placenta. If the bladder wall is thinned out during dissection, that area is reinforced with a box stitch or purse string sutures.

Management of an unanticipated case of PAS

It is not rare to unexpectedly encounter PAS at the time of cesarean delivery. It may be suspected **before the uterine incision** or **after the delivery of the baby**, when difficulty is faced in delivering the placenta [11].

Before the uterine incision (best case scenario)

The appearance of the lower uterine segment upon opening the abdomen is characteristic of placenta previa with PAS (large vessels, placental bulging). In this situation, the following management would be appropriate:

- The surgery is not taken forward till the required surgical team is in place, the anesthetic team is prepared, and provisions for blood products are made.
- Once all these measures are in place, the baby is delivered, the uterine incision is closed, and a hysterectomy is performed.
- If the mobilisation of such a team is not possible, the woman should be stabilised and transferred to a tertiary centre. This is provided the maternal and fetal conditions are stable.

Inadvertent discovery of PAS immediately after the delivery of the baby

In this situation, after the uterus is opened and the fetus is delivered, difficulty is faced in delivering the placenta. In such cases, the following measures are recommended:

- The uterine incision is rapidly closed.
- All appropriate resources are mobilised, and a hysterectomy is performed.
- If the centre is not equipped to handle the surgery and the woman is stable after the delivery of the fetus, transfer to a tertiary centre should be considered.
- The abdomen should be packed, tranexamic acid infusion given, and transfusion with available blood products initiated to stabilise the woman before transfer.

Intraoperative and postoperative complications of peripartum hysterectomy for PAS

Emergency peripartum hysterectomy results in more complications than a planned one, as is to be expected. Transfusion, infection, urinary tract injury, and reoperation are more common with peripartum than with a non-obstetric hysterectomy.

The most common complication is **excessive blood loss** and **the need for blood transfusion**. In a worldwide study, the average blood loss was found to be 3.7 L [24]. The requirement for blood transfusion ranged from 46% [22] to 84% [25]. A recent meta-analysis of 20 studies evaluating red blood cell (RBC) use in nearly 1100 patients with the placenta accreta spectrum demonstrated the potential for uncontrollable hemorrhage in PAS [26]. It was found that an average of 5 units of RBCs were transfused per woman at delivery.

Maternal mortality has been reported as 5.2 per 100 hysterectomies (reported range 0–59.1). It is higher in resource-poor settings—11.9 as compared to 2.5 per 100 hysterectomies in resource-rich regions [25].

> **Key Point**
>
> It is recommended that at least 6 units of RBCs be kept available at delivery with PAS [26].

The triple P procedure

With the increasing incidence of PAS, there has been an effort to conserve the uterus in young women with PAS. Conservative surgery may be attempted in carefully selected women. The triple P procedure was introduced in the past decade as a conservative surgical approach [27]. It consists of the following steps:

- **P**erioperative localisation of the placental edge and delivery of the fetus above the upper border of the placenta
- **P**elvic devascularisation
- **P**lacental non-separation with myometrial excision

> **Key Point**
>
> Conservative surgery may be attempted in carefully selected women and should be performed by experienced surgeons who can manage massive bleeding if it occurs.

Hysterectomy for Postpartum Hemorrhage

Generally, uterine atony can be controlled by uterotonic medications alone or in combination with fertility-preserving procedures (e.g., uterine balloon tamponade, the B-Lynch and other uterine compression sutures, uterine artery/utero-ovarian artery ligation, and if available, arterial embolisation, as described in **Chapter 13**). However, if conservative procedures do not control atonic PPH, a hysterectomy may be the only option to prevent severe morbidity or death and should not be delayed in women with severe coagulopathy who require immediate control of uterine hemorrhage. **A subtotal hysterectomy is usually the best option in this situation. The hysterectomy is performed in the usual manner.** The abdomen is opened through a vertical midline incision, to improve the speed of the procedure.

The following special steps are recommended by the authors to control bleeding:

- The uterus is lifted and exteriorised.
- A transabdominal uterine artery clamp (the T clamp) may be applied on the sides of the isthmus over the uterine arteries without any dissection.
- Another pair of clamps may be used to occlude the anastomosing branch from the ovarian artery supplying the cornual region (Fig. 24.6 and 24.7). The T clamp has to be specially procured.

Hysterectomy for Uterine Rupture

In modern obstetrics, the classical presentation of obstructed labour leading to a ruptured uterus is not as common as dehiscence or rupture of a uterine scar (see **Chapter 18**, *Obstructed*

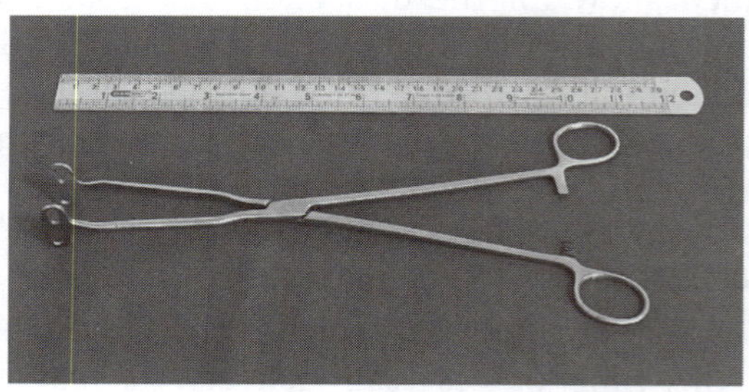

Fig. 24.6 A novel transabdominal uterine artery clamp (T clamp) (*Image courtesy*: Dr V P Paily, Rajagiri Hospital, Kerala)

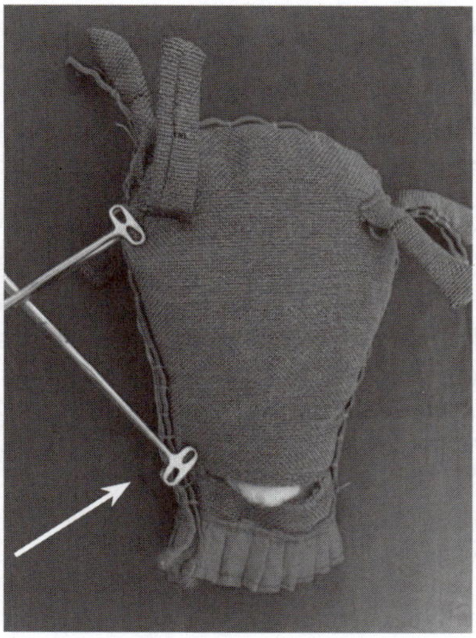

Fig. 24.7 A demonstration of how to use the T clamp: The T clamp has been applied to the cervical isthmus over the uterine arteries without the need for dissection (arrow), and another pair of clamps has been applied to occlude the anastomosing branch from the ovarian artery supplying the cornual region (*Image courtesy*: Dr V P Paily, Rajagiri Hospital, Kerala)

labour and uterine rupture). However, in LMICs, obstructed labour leading to uterine rupture may be complicated by the non-availability of surgical resources and may lead to maternal death.

For optimal access, a vertical midline incision should be used to enter the abdominal cavity. Injury to the uterine arteries and the bladder may be present and should be tackled carefully. Though a subtotal hysterectomy is usually performed, a total hysterectomy may be required if the rupture involves the cervix.

Hysterectomy for Placental Abruption

In the presence of massive abruption, a Couvelaire uterus is atonic and may lead to postpartum hemorrhage and coagulopathy (see **Chapter 29**, *Antepartum hemorrhage*). Atony in this situation is difficult to manage, and these women may require a hysterectomy.

Hysterectomy in the Presence of Disseminated Intravascular Coagulation (DIC)

In women with DIC, the postpartum uterus will provide a large surface area to bleed from. A rapid hysterectomy as described above for atonic PPH may be life-saving. The importance of a subtotal hysterectomy here is to be re-emphasised.

Postoperative Care

- **Monitoring:** The immediate postoperative period is very crucial in women who have undergone peripartum hysterectomy. They should be observed in an intensive care unit or a high-dependency unit.
- **Pain relief:** Epidural analgesia can be continued in the postoperative period for adequate pain relief. Other alternatives include opioid analgesics as patches or injections, paracetamol, and NSAIDs, as in any postoperative woman.
- **Antibiotics:** A hysterectomy is considered a clean-contaminated case and no postoperative antibiotics are indicated. Active infection should be treated appropriately [28]. Repeat intraoperative dosing should be considered when the duration of surgery is prolonged and when the blood loss is >1500 mL.
- **DVT prophylaxis:** Women undergoing peripartum hysterectomy are at high risk of developing venous thromboembolism. Low-dose heparin is initiated at least 6–12 hours postoperatively once the risk of hemorrhage has decreased, and is continued until the woman is fully ambulating [29].
- **Diet:** As with any other surgery, early feeding is recommended, and clear liquids may be started 6–8 hours postoperatively [29]. The intake can be increased depending on how the woman tolerates food and fluids. Signs of paralytic ileus should be recognised early and treated with intravenous fluids, restriction of oral intake, and in severe cases, insertion of a nasogastric tube.

- **Ambulation:** Early ambulation is essential and decreases the risk of venous thromboembolism.
- **Bladder:** Bladder injuries are common, especially in the case of hysterectomy for PAS. The Foley catheter can be removed after 24 hours but with bladder injury and repair, extended catheterisation may be required. If a ureteric catheter or stent had been placed, it may be removed after surgery, or retained if there had been a ureteric injury.
- **Wound care:** The wound dressing may be removed after 24 hours. Sutures are usually removed on the 7th–10th postoperative day.

CONCLUSION

Even though peripartum hysterectomy is a major life-saving procedure, it is associated with significant morbidity and mortality. Rising trends of cesarean section rates continue to increase the incidence of the placenta accreta spectrum. Early diagnosis of these cases by dedicated ultrasonography in women at risk for PAS will help plan surgery in a more optimal setting. In case of uncontrolled bleeding following delivery, delay in taking a decision increases the risk of maternal mortality.

REFERENCES

1. Say L, Chou D, Gemmill A, et al. Global Causes of Maternal Death: A WHO Systematic Analysis. *Lancet Global Health*. 2014. 2(6): e323-e333.
2. World Health Organization. Evaluating the quality of care for severe pregnancy complications: The WHO near-miss approach for maternal health. 2011.World Health Organization, Geneva. https://apps.who.int/iris/handle/10665/44692.
3. Govindappagari S, Wright JD, Ananth CV, Huang Y, D'Alton ME, Friedman AM. Risk of peripartum hysterectomy and center hysterectomy and delivery volume. *Obstet Gynecol*. 2016 128(6):1215-1224.
4. Kallianidis AF, Rijntjes D, Brobbel C, Dekkers OM, Bloemenkamp KWM, van den Akker T. Incidence, indications, risk factors, and outcomes of emergency peripartum hysterectomy worldwide: A systematic review and meta-analysis. *Obstet Gynecol*. 2023.1;141(1):35-48.
5. Sharma B, Sikka P, Jain V, et al. Peripartum hysterectomy in a tertiary care hospital: Epidemiology and outcomes. *J Anaesthesiol Clin Pharmacol*. 2017. 33(3):324-328.
6. Chaudhary V, Singh M, Nain S, et al. Incidence, management and outcomes in women undergoing peripartum hysterectomy in a tertiary care centre in India. *Cureus*. 2021. 29;13(3):e14171.
7. Paily VP, Raj G R, Sidhik A, Sudhamma A, Neelankavil JJ, Usha MG, George R, Cheriyan S, Ramakrishnan S, John TE, Vishnu D, Pradeep M. Arresting post-partum hemorrhage using the novel transvaginal uterine artery clamp. *Eur J Obstet Gynecol Reprod Biol*. 2022. 272:6-15.
8. Hemmanur SR, Samyukthallla S. Prophylactic SR PPH suction cannula application for high-risk women for atonic PPH. *IOSR Journal of Dental and Medical Sci*. 2019. 18(4):23-27.
9. Dwyer BK, Belogolovkin V, Tran L, et al. Prenatal diagnosis of placenta accreta: Sonography or magnetic resonance imaging? *J Ultrasound Med*. 2008. 27(9):1275-81.
10. Silver RM, Landon MB, Rouse DJ, et al. Maternal morbidity associated with multiple repeat cesarean deliveries. *Obstet Gynecol*. 2006. 107:1226.
11. ACOG. Placenta accreta spectrum. Obstetric Care Consensus No. 7. American College of Obstetricians and Gynecologists. *Obstet Gynecol*. 2018. 132:e259–75.
12. Why Mothers Die: Kerala 2010–2020 observations and recommendations. VP Paily, K Ambujam, Betsy Thomas, V Rajasekharan Nair, Prameela Menon, Megha Jayaprakash, Deepthy M, Afshana Sidhik (Eds). *Kerala Federation of Obstetrics and Gynaecology*. 2021. Page 107.
13. Francois K, Ortiz J, Harris C, Foley MR, Elliott JP. Is peripartum hysterectomy more common in multiple gestations? *Obstetrics and Gynecology*. 2005. 105(6):1369-1372.
14. Huque S, Roberts I, Fawole B, et al. Risk factors for peripartum hysterectomy among women with postpartum haemorrhage: analysis of data from the WOMAN trial. *BMC Pregnancy Childbirth*. 2018. 18(1):186.
15. Shamshirsaz AA, Fox KA, Salmanian B, et al. Maternal morbidity in patients with morbidly adherent placenta treated with and without a standardized multidisciplinary approach. *Am J Obstet Gynecol*. 2015. 212:218.e1 – 9.
16. Society for Maternal-Fetal Medicine (SMFM) Consult Series #44: Management of bleeding in the late preterm period. *Am J Obstet Gynecol*. 2018. 218(1):B2-B8.
17. Silver RM, Barbour KD. Placenta accreta spectrum: accreta, increta, and percreta. *Obstet Gynecol Clin North Am*. 2015. 42:381–402.
18. ACOG. Use of prophylactic antibiotics in labor and delivery. Practice Bulletin No. 120. American College of Obstetricians and Gynecologists. *Obstet Gynecol*. 117:1472–83.

19. Markley JC, Farber MK, Perlman NC, Carusi DA. Neuraxial anesthesia during cesarean delivery for placenta previa with suspected morbidly adherent placenta: A retrospective analysis. *Anesth Analg*. 2018. 127:930.
20. Paily VP, Sidhik A, Girijadevi RR, Sudhamma A, Neelankavil JJ, Menon UG, George R, Ramakrishnan S, Cheriyan S, John TE, Pradeep M. Managing placenta accreta spectrum in low-resource settings using a novel dissection-free aorta clamp: Operative technique. *Int J Gynaecol Obstet*. 2022. 158(2):469-475.
21. Wright JD, Devine P, Shah M, et al. Morbidity and mortality of peripartum hysterectomy. *Obstet Gynecol*. 2010. 115(6):1187.
22. Bulbul M, Karacor T, Peker N, et al. The effect of surgical procedure on surgical outcomes in patients undergoing emergency peripartum hysterectomy: A retrospective multicenter study. *J Matern Fetal Neonatal Med*. 2022. 35:5768.
23. Imudia AN, Hobson DT, Awonuga AO, Diamond MP, Bahado-Singh RO. Determinants and complications of emergent cesarean hysterectomy: supracervical vs total hysterectomy. *Am J Obstet Gynecol*. 2010. 203(3):221.e1-5.
24. van den Akker T, Brobbel C, Dekkers OM, Bloemenkamp KWM. Prevalence, indications, risk indicators, and outcomes of emergency peripartum hysterectomy worldwide: A systematic review and meta-analysis. *Obstet Gynecol*. 2016. 128(6):1281-1294.
25. Shellhaas CS, Gilbert S, Landon MB, et al. Eunice Kennedy Shriver National Institutes of Health and Human Development (NICHD) Maternal–Fetal Medicine Units Network (MFMU). The frequency and complication rates of hysterectomy accompanying cesarean delivery. *Obstet Gynecol*. 2009. 114(2 Pt 1):224-229.
26. Miller SE, Leonard SA, Meza PK, et al. Red blood cell transfusion in patients with placenta accreta spectrum: A systematic review and meta-analysis. *Obstet Gynecol*. 2023. 141(1):49. Epub 2022 Nov 30.
27. Piñas-Carrillo A, Chandraharan E. Conservative surgical approach: The triple P procedure. *Best Pract Res Clin Obstet Gynaecol*. 2021; 72:67.
28. Carusi DA. Cesarean birth: Peripartum hysterectomy for management of hemorrhage. Lockwood CJ (Ed). *UpToDate*. 2023, Waltham, MA.
29. Berghella V. Cesarean birth: Preoperative planning and patient preparation. Grobman W (Ed), *UpToDate*. 2023. Waltham, MA.

CHAPTER 25

Prevention and Management of Perineal Trauma Occurring in Childbirth

STERGIOS K DOUMOUCHTSIS, MARIA PATRICIA ROMAN

INTRODUCTION

Childbirth-related perineal tears are common during vaginal delivery, with varying degrees of severity. Perineal trauma affects millions of women worldwide with an incidence of over 91% in nulliparous women and over 70% in multiparous women [1]. Anal sphincter injury is clinically diagnosed in 1–11% of vaginal births [2]. In low- and middle-income countries (LMICs), the prevalence of severe perineal tears is higher. The reported incidence appears to have increased globally in recent years, probably because of improved training in the diagnosis of anal sphincter injuries [2,3,4].

Perineal trauma may result in short- and long-term effects on the daily activities of the mother and her overall health. These effects may have a negative impact on psychological well-being, sexual function, and quality of life.

Short-term consequences include the following[5]:

- Pain
- Difficulty in physical activities such as walking and sitting
- Impaired sexual function

Long-term effects include the following [5]:

- Urinary and fecal incontinence
- Pelvic organ prolapse
- Sexual dysfunction

DEFINITIONS

Obstetric perineal injury is defined as an injury to the perineum occurring at the time of vaginal childbirth [3]. This is usually classified using the Royal College of Obstetricians and Gynaecologists (RCOG) criteria. The RCOG classification defines perineal or vaginal injuries caused by spontaneous tearing or episiotomy as follows (Fig. 25.1):

- **First-degree**—cutaneous trauma to the vaginal epithelium or perineal skin only
- **Second-degree**—injury to the perineal muscles but not the anal sphincter
- **Third-degree**—injury to the perineum involving the anal sphincter complex
  - Tears involving the external anal sphincter (EAS) can be:
    - Partial EAS tears
    - Complete EAS tears
  - Tears involving the anal sphincter complex are further divided into three categories:
    - 3a—less than 50% of the external anal sphincter thickness torn
    - 3b—50% or more of the external anal sphincter thickness torn
    - 3c—internal anal sphincter torn
- **Fourth degree**—injury to the perineum involving the anal sphincter complex (external and internal anal sphincter) and anal epithelium

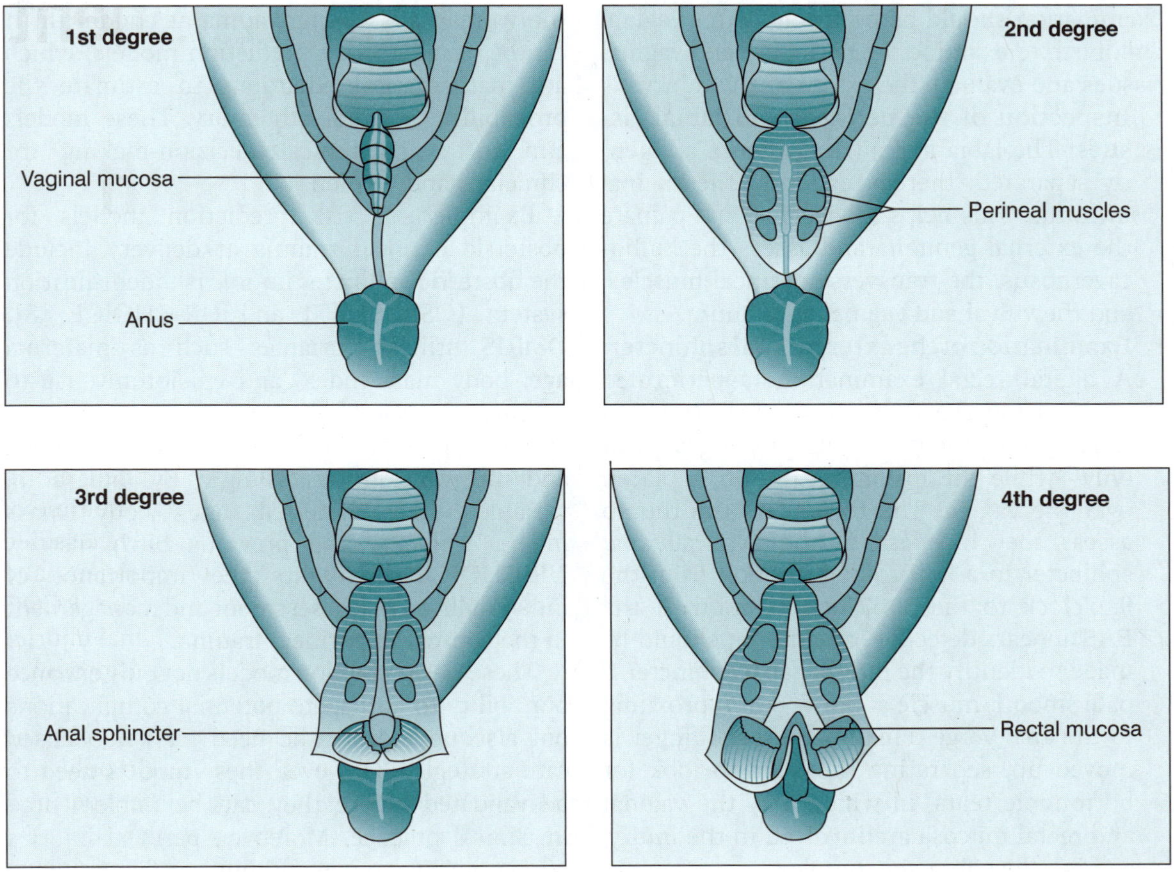

Fig. 25.1 Classification of obstetric perineal injury

Obstetric rectovaginal perforation (also known as 'buttonhole' tears) involves trauma (injury) to the anal mucosa and the vaginal epithelium without any involvement of the anal sphincters.

A **cloacal defect** refers to a confluence of the anus and vagina with no perineum to divide the vagina and anus, leaving one large opening.

New terminology has been introduced to describe **fistulas** occurring after childbirth [6]:

- An **obstetric fistula** (OF) is a de novo fistula that occurs due to prolonged obstructed labour causing ischemia and pressure necrosis of the soft pelvic tissues caught between the impacted fetal presenting part and the bony maternal pelvis, which results in an abnormal communication between the urinary/colorectal tract and the vagina or perineal area.
- An **iatrogenic childbirth-related postpartum fistula** (ICRF) occurs due to inadvertent injury to the urinary/colorectal tract during operative delivery (cesarean section/cesarean hysterectomy or instrumental delivery including episiotomy).

DIAGNOSIS OF PERINEAL INJURY AFTER CHILDBIRTH

Clinical Examination

The diagnosis of perineal tears is established by clinical examination. Vaginal and perineal examination should be performed after vaginal childbirth to examine the perineum and vaginal tissues and evaluate the extent of any injury.

- **Inspection of the perineal and labial tissues**: The labia majora and minora are gently separated, thereby exposing the vaginal introitus. This helps to visualise and palpate the external genitalia and assess the bulbocavernosus, the transverse perineal muscles, and the vulval and vaginal epithelium.
- **Examination of the external anal sphincter:** A digital rectal examination is performed by inserting the index finger into the anal canal—up to the distal interphalangeal joint only—while the ipsilateral thumb is placed over the vagina. The finger and the thumb assess the thickness of the external anal sphincter in a 'pill-rolling' motion from the 9 o'clock to the 3 o'clock position. If the EAS appears defective, an attempt should be made to identify the internal anal sphincter, a pale smooth muscle about 6–8 mm proximal to the anal verge. Finally, the rectal finger is moved up, separating the labia to look for buttonhole tears, in which only the vaginal and rectal mucosa are involved in the injury, sparing the sphincter complex.
- **Speculum examination:** A speculum examination allows the inspection of the deeper tissues and the fornices. Cervical tears can be diagnosed or ruled out by using sponge-holding forceps and gently grasping the cervix to systematically inspect for tears.
- **Palpation of the levator muscles**: This is undertaken to detect an avulsion injury or muscle defect.

Key Point

A rectal examination needs to be performed after every vaginal delivery to identify perineal tears.

PREDICTION OF PERINEAL INJURY

Prediction of obstetric perineal trauma is a process of prospectively evaluating the risk of the woman sustaining trauma at childbirth. It can be based on risk prediction models, which are mathematical equations to estimate the probability of childbirth injury. These models aim to assist clinical decision-making for clinicians and women.

Examples of risk prediction models for obstetric perineal trauma at delivery include the obstetric sphincter injury risk identification system (OSIRIS) [7] and UR-CHOICE [8]. OSIRIS utilises variables such as maternal age, body mass index, and episiotomy use to estimate the risk of obstetric sphincter injuries, aiding clinicians in tailoring their approach and interventions accordingly. By integrating variables like maternal age, body mass index, ethnicity, and previous birth history, UR-CHOICE highlights the importance of individualised risk assessment and management in the context of perineal trauma.

These risk prediction models not only enhance our ability to anticipate potential complications but also underscore the need for personalised care strategies. However, these models need to be validated before they can be implemented in clinical practice. Moreover, perineal injuries often occur in women without risk factors.

Antenatal Predictors

Several risk factors for perineal tears during vaginal delivery have been identified and include maternal, fetal, and obstetric factors [9].

Ethnicity

Asian women are considered to be at an increased risk of severe perineal trauma [10]. However, a systematic review by Wheeler et al. [11] concludes that this increased risk is limited to Asian women living in Western countries and has not been noted for Asian women living in Asia.

The higher prevalence of severe perineal tears among Asian women living in Western countries has been attributed to a shorter perineum or higher birth weights, possibly related to dietary factors. Another potentially contributing factor could be the limitations of language and communication between women and midwives during labour and delivery [11].

Parity

Nulliparity is a non-disputable risk factor for obstetric anal sphincter injuries (OASI). Reduced tissue elasticity seems to play a role. Anal sphincter injuries were associated with nulliparity [12]. Smith et al. showed that 6.6% of nulliparous and 2.7% of multiparous women sustained OASI after vaginal delivery [1]. The incidence of intact perineum was 9.6% and 31.2% in nulliparous and multiparous women respectively [1].

A retrospective cohort study of 20,674 deliveries also concluded that anal sphincter trauma occurred in 16% of women with first vaginal deliveries and 18% with vaginal birth after cesarean section (VBAC) [5].

Maternal age

Hornemann et al. [13], in a retrospective study of 2,967 women, found advanced maternal age to be the second most important risk factor for severe perineal trauma.

Obesity

Obesity (body mass index [BMI] >30 Kg/m^2) is not a risk factor for perineal injury during childbirth and does not lead to obstetric anal sphincter injuries [14]. However, obesity is associated with pelvic floor disorders in the long term [15].

Birth weight

A birth weight >4 Kg is associated with higher rates of perineal trauma, especially obstetric anal sphincter injuries. Shoulder dystocia and the manoeuvres to manage it are also risk factors for perineal injuries and OASI [16].

Intrapartum Predictors

Intrapartum risk factors include instrumental delivery, especially forceps, and a prolonged second stage [17]. In addition, a midline episiotomy and persistent occipitoposterior position have been associated with the highest risk of severe perineal trauma [18].

Instrumental delivery

Instrumental delivery of any kind is an independent risk factor for severe perineal trauma (see **Chapter 21**, *Operative vaginal delivery*). The use of forceps has been associated with higher risks compared to vacuum use. Forceps delivery markedly increases the risk of third- and fourth-degree tears and may also cause pelvic neuropathy. Unlike a long-held belief that rotational forceps causes more perineal trauma, Gauthaman et al. [19] found that the incidence of third and fourth-degree tears following rotational Kielland's forceps delivery is comparable to that associated with other non-rotational forceps deliveries.

Duration of the second stage of labour

A prolonged second stage of labour carries increased risks of both maternal and perinatal complications in nulliparous as well as multiparous women. A prolonged second stage increases the rates of OASI and is associated with neuromuscular injury [20].

Episiotomy

Episiotomy is the commonest procedure performed in obstetrics (see **Chapter 7**, *Episiotomy: What does the evidence say?*). Routine episiotomy offers little to the prevention of obstetric trauma. Choosing not to perform routine episiotomy for every 4.4 women could prevent one instance of perineal trauma that necessitates suturing [21]. A case control study of over 28,000 births in India [20] reported an increased risk of OASI with episiotomy.

While a mediolateral episiotomy does not protect the anal sphincter, a median episiotomy certainly increases the risk of anal sphincter injuries. Midline episiotomy is associated with an approximately threefold increase in the risk of OASI [22].

> **Key Point**
>
> Liberal episiotomy does not reduce the incidence of pain or dyspareunia. On the other hand, routine episiotomy results in an increased risk of OASI.

Malpresentation and malposition

Persistent occipitoposterior position leads to a larger presenting diameter and consequently, a difficult delivery; this increases the risk of perineal trauma. Face and brow presentations also increase the risk of trauma. Breech deliveries do not appear to increase the risk of severe perineal trauma.

Epidural analgesia

The reports are conflicting regarding the occurrence of OASI in women who receive epidural analgesia. Epidural analgesia is associated with increased rates of prolonged second stage, leading to operative deliveries and episiotomies, which may increase the risk of OASI. Gundabattula and colleagues [23], in a study of 28,000 births in India found epidural analgesia to be a contributing factor. Similarly, Eshkoli and colleagues found epidural analgesia to be an independent risk factor for OASI in their population [24]. However, Putri and associates [25] found a reduction in anal sphincter injuries with the use of epidural analgesia.

PREVENTION OF PERINEAL INJURY

Several interventions have been proposed to prevent perineal injuries during vaginal delivery.

Primary Prevention

Measures for primary prevention of perineal injuries at delivery aim to prevent the occurrence of perineal trauma or postpartum pelvic floor dysfunction by modifying risk factors.

Prepregnancy and antepartum measures

Prepregnancy measures include lifestyle modifications such as controlling diabetes mellitus and optimising the body mass index. Other options include screening for gestational diabetes mellitus, ultrasound assessment for fetal macrosomia, perineal massage, pelvic floor muscle training, induction of labour for suspected macrosomia, and elective cesarean delivery.

Elective cesarean delivery has been advocated as the only true strategy for the primary prevention of perineal trauma.

Intrapartum measures

Several intrapartum interventions have been recommended for the prevention of perineal injury during a vaginal delivery.

- **Perineal massage**, antenatally [26] or during the second stage of labour [27], is a technique involving the insertion of one or two fingers into the vagina to massage the posterior vaginal wall in a U-shaped movement. The aim is to stretch the perineum and the surrounding structures. Moderate-quality evidence suggests that perineal massage may reduce third- and fourth-degree tears, but the evidence is inconsistent [26]. The most recent NICE guidance on intrapartum care [28] recommends offering a perineal massage with a water-soluble lubricant if it is acceptable to the woman.
- **Warm compresses** are towels or pads soaked in comfortably warm water and applied to the perineum at the commencement of perineal stretching in the second stage [28,29].
- **Manual perineal support (protection)** at birth is a bimanual technique that requires support of the posterior fourchette with one hand and cupping of the fetal head with the other to prevent the head from coming out with uncontrolled force as it progresses at crowning. The NICE guidance [28] advises that either the **'hands on'** (guarding the perineum with the hand and flexing the baby's head) or the **'hands poised'** (with hands off the perineum and baby's head but kept close in readiness) technique can be used to facilitate spontaneous birth. However, a recent study from the UK [30] showed that **perineal support resulted in a 23% reduction of OASI and a 71% reduction of major OASI.**

- **Avoiding episiotomy** can contribute to preserving perineal integrity and reducing unnecessary trauma. When an episiotomy is deemed necessary, the recommended technique involves a mediolateral approach originating at the vaginal fourchette and generally directed towards the right side. Ensuring the correct angle in relation to the vertical axis, ideally ranging from 45 to 60 degrees, is essential for optimising outcomes [31].
    - **Vaginal births after previous third- or fourth-degree trauma:** It is advised not to routinely offer episiotomies. This tailored approach considers individual medical history and aims to minimise additional trauma, aligning with the overarching goal of optimising maternal well-being. Lastly, the guidelines stress the importance of clinical judgment. Performing an episiotomy is recommended when there is a clinical need, such as during instrumental births or in situations of suspected fetal compromise.
- **Perineal hyaluronidase injection** in the second stage aims to relax the connective tissue around the skin or subcutaneous muscles and render them less vulnerable to mechanical stress or extension during the passage of the fetus through the vaginal canal. However, a systematic review found little evidence to recommend its use [32].
- **Maternal position** during delivery may be associated with the risk of perineal trauma, though the data is unclear. A population-based study of 113,000 spontaneous births found that the dorsolithotomy position and squatting were associated with an increased risk of anal sphincter injuries [33].

MANAGEMENT OF OBSTETRIC PERINEAL INJURY

Conservative Treatment

Conservative management of perineal tears involves non-surgical methods such as pain management, wound care, and pelvic floor exercises, and aims to promote healing and reduce pain after childbirth.

- **Pain management:** Pain relief is an important aspect of the conservative management of perineal tears. Non-steroidal anti-inflammatory drugs (NSAIDs) and local anesthetic agents such as lidocaine are used to manage pain after childbirth and to numb the area during wound care procedures [34]. Cold packs may be used over the menstrual pad for pain relief. After 24 hours, warm water soaks can be started.
- **Wound care**: Proper wound care is crucial for the healing of perineal tears. This includes regular cleaning of the area with warm water and mild soap. This may be followed by the application of a topical antiseptic or antibiotic ointment in the presence of infection. Sitz baths can also be used to soothe the area and promote healing [3].
- **Non-surgical treatment of vaginal/perineal tears**: Non-surgical management allows spontaneous healing of surgical trauma, and includes topical hygiene measures (avoiding irritant soaps, detergents, and douches) and expectant management.
    - *Vulval hygiene* involves regular washing of the vulval and perineal area and wearing cotton underwear. Shampoo, perfumed creams, or soap may cause vulval irritation and should be avoided.
    - *Anal hygiene* involves keeping the perianal area clean, especially in cases of fecal seepage and incontinence. Using water to wash after a bowel movement and patting the area dry afterwards, the use of soft toilet paper or moist wipes, avoidance of alcohol wipes, and wiping from the front to the back are recommended.

Surgical Management of Perineal Tears

In cases of perineal tears of the second degree or more or when there are other complications such as bleeding from the tear, surgical intervention may be warranted.

The surgical repair of vaginal and perineal trauma involves suturing for anatomical restoration of the perineum.

Assessment of the extent of bleeding and the injury to the perineum, vagina, and anorectum by inspection, and digital vaginal and rectal examination requires good exposure, with the woman ideally in the lithotomy position. Adequate lighting and effective analgesia are also important. A woman's informed consent should be obtained prior to suturing.

Second-degree tears

Suturing for a second-degree laceration is done using the same technique as that used for an episiotomy (see **Chapter 7**, *Episiotomy: What does the evidence say?*). The first suture is applied above the apex of the vaginal component of the tear to ensure hemostasis. For the vaginal part of the wound, a continuous, non-locking technique is commonly applied, as it is associated with less pain and dyspareunia compared to interrupted sutures.

The perineal muscles are apposed and sutured with the same continuous suture, aiming to approximate and align the muscles. Then, the skin can be closed without tension. When there is a deep perineal muscle tear, two layers of continuous sutures may be required. The perineal skin is apposed and closed with continuous subcuticular suturing.

Following repair, the vaginal and rectal examination is repeated to ensure that the repair is complete, that there are no sutures placed through the rectum inadvertently, and that there is no other trauma [34].

Third- and fourth-degree tears

The repair of anal sphincter injuries should be undertaken by a clinician who is competent and experienced, and who preferably has had formal training in the repair of severe perineal injury. A third- or fourth-degree tear may also be repaired by a junior consultant under adequate supervision. Ideally, these injuries should be promptly repaired after childbirth. Nevertheless, delaying the repair by a few hours, for instance, due to the unavailability of a trained practitioner, does not appear to impact functional outcomes.

The repair should take place in an operating theatre environment under regional or general anesthesia for a more complete examination and easier identification of the anatomy.

A **rectovaginal perforation (buttonhole tear)** should be repaired using two layers of interrupted polyglactin sutures.

Repair of anal mucosa (fourth-degree tear)

In the case of a fourth-degree tear, trauma to the anal epithelium should be repaired with continuous non-locking or interrupted 3-0 polyglactin sutures [3]. Interrupted sutures will leave more foreign material behind because of the increased number of knots.

Repair of the anal sphincter

The repair of the torn anal sphincter and restoring its anatomy are an important part of the repair of the perineum.

Internal anal sphincter: The internal anal sphincter should be properly identified and repaired as a separate layer. It appears as a thickened, pale pink, shiny tissue just above the anal mucosa and is often referred to as the perirectal fascia. Reapproximation of this layer is important for the strength and integrity of the repair and for achieving anal continence.

Any trauma to the internal anal sphincter should be repaired separately with interrupted horizontal mattress sutures using 3-0 polydioxanone (PDS) or 2-0 polyglactin [3]. Others recommend continuous suturing.

External anal sphincter: The ruptured edges of the external anal sphincter are grasped with Allis tissue forceps (Fig. 25.2) and sutured. The cut ends of the external sphincter tend to retract and, therefore, it may be necessary to push the Allis clamp deep into the surrounding connective tissue to locate the sphincter.

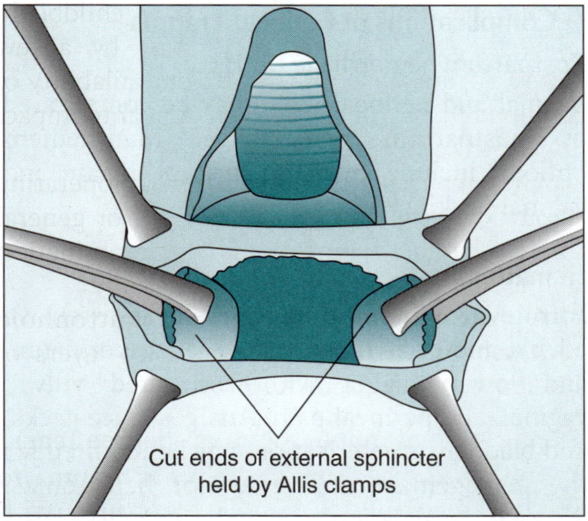

Fig. 25.2 The cut ends of the external anal sphincter are held with Allis clamps

An **incomplete** external or internal sphincter injury could be repaired with an end-to-end technique, while a **complete** external sphincter injury can be repaired by an end-to-end (Fig. 25.3) or overlapping technique [35] (Fig. 25.4) using 3-0 polydioxanone (PDS) or 2-0 polyglactin.

The **end-to-end technique** involves apposition of the injured ends of the sphincter by applying interrupted horizontal mattress sutures.

The **overlapping technique** involves using vertical mattress sutures to overlap one edge of the injured sphincter over the other. When overlapping suturing is applied, one or both sphincter ends may need to be dissected from the surrounding tissue and mobilised to allow sufficient length for the overlap. There is no difference between the two techniques in terms

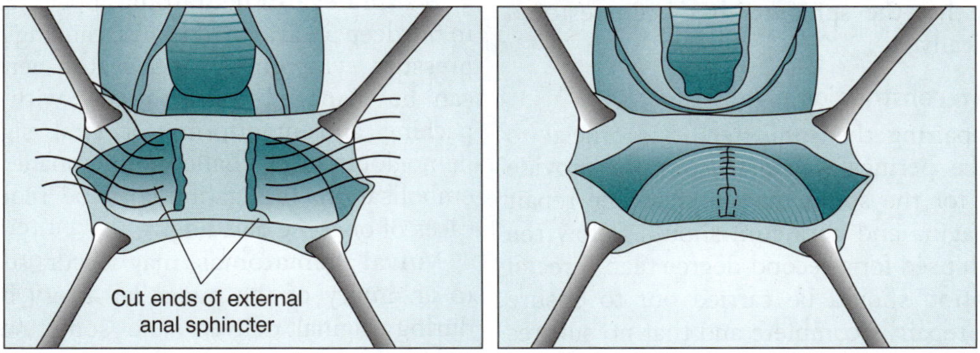

Fig. 25.3 The end-to-end technique for repairing the external anal sphincter: (a) The cut ends are apposed and (b) sutured with interrupted horizontal mattress sutures

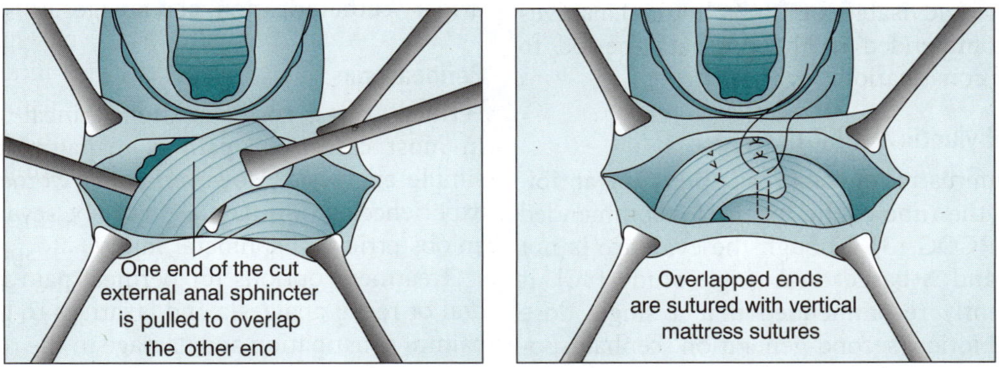

Fig. 25.4 The overlapping technique for the repair of the external anal sphincter: (a) One end of the cut external anal sphincter is pulled over the other end to overlap it and (b) the overlapped ends are sutured with vertical mattress sutures

of perineal pain, dyspareunia, fecal incontinence, or flatal incontinence, although there is some evidence of a lower incidence of fecal urgency and lower anal incontinence symptom scores in the overlap group [4].

> **Key Point**
>
> The overlap technique can only be used for a complete tear of the external sphincter. There is no difference between the end-to-end and overlapping techniques in terms of perineal pain, dyspareunia, fecal incontinence, or flatal incontinence.

At the end of the repair, the skin next to the anus should be stroked with a blunt instrument. If the sphincter has been properly approximated, the anus will pucker in its entirety. This will confirm that the sphincter has been restored anatomically.

Perineal reconstruction

After repairing the sphincter, it is crucial to undertake perineal reconstruction to provide support for the sphincter muscles. The repair of the vagina and perineum should follow the approach used for a second-degree tear. A rectal examination should be carried out to ensure that the repair is complete and that no sutures have been placed inadvertently through the rectal mucosa. The anus should easily admit one finger following the procedure. An indwelling catheter is advisable for 12–24 hours. Laxatives are recommended in the postnatal period to prevent constipation.

Prophylactic Antibiotics

The administration of broad-spectrum antibiotics at the time of the repair is recommended by the RCOG [3]. Though the evidence is not strong and is based on a single study [36], it is currently recommended that a single dose of antibiotic (second-generation cephalosporin, e.g., cefuroxime or cefoxitin) at the time of repair is reasonable [37].

Complications of Perineal Trauma

Postpartum hemorrhage (PPH)

Vaginal and perineal tears may be complicated by postpartum hemorrhage. Management options include primary surgical repair and vaginal packing.

Hematomas

Infralevator hematomas present as extensive edema and ecchymosis of the labia, perineum, and lower vagina with associated vulval, vaginal, and perineal pain. Analgesia, ice packs, and bladder catheterisation may be required for the management of infralevator hematomas. Surgical evacuation is indicated in large hematomas, to arrest hemorrhage and prevent tissue ischemia and necrosis.

A **supralevator hematoma** appears as a mass in the deep paravaginal tissues, causing pain and pressure symptoms. Supralevator hematomas can be managed conservatively with vaginal packing and monitoring of vital signs and hemoglobin levels. Balloon tamponade, arterial embolisation, or ligation may be required in cases of ongoing bleeding.

Vulval hematomas may occur secondary to an injury of the pudendal artery branches during vaginal delivery and sometimes after an episiotomy. Large hematomas require evacuation and ligation of the bleeding vessels in the theatre, followed by antibiotic cover, urinary catheterisation, and analgesia.

Perineal pain

Perineal pain is common after perineal trauma. In most cases, the pain is manageable with simple analgesia. However, some women may experience chronic pain. Pain can be severe after an obstetric anal sphincter injury.

Treatment options for perineal pain include oral or rectal analgesia and laxatives to prevent painful constipation and damage to the repaired sphincter muscles. Chronic pain, refractory to conservative measures, may be treated with local perineal injections with hydrocortisone, marcaine, or hyaluronidase.

Dyspareunia

Perineal trauma is associated with an increased risk of dyspareunia. Dyspareunia secondary to scarring following suturing can be initially treated with massage, dilators, and topical estrogens. Significant scarring and constriction of the vagina or introitus may require surgical revision. Surgical approaches include Fenton's procedure, Z-plasty, incision of constriction ring, or skin grafts. Perineal scar revision involves the surgical excision of the perineal scar and the creation of a new scar. Fenton's procedure is a surgical technique aimed at increasing the genital hiatus and widening the introitus by excising scar tissue and/or an area of constriction at the entrance of the vagina.

Perineal wound infection and breakdown

One in ten women with a perineal tear that required suturing may experience perineal wound infection with perineal pain, wound dehiscence, or vaginal discharge. Most perineal infections resolve with antibiotics and good perineal hygiene. Broad-spectrum antibiotics are recommended.

In cases of wound dehiscence, conservative management—allowing healing by secondary intention—is often adequate. Secondary repair can be considered in select cases with re-suturing of the perineal wound dehiscence within the first two weeks following childbirth.

Follow-up

Women with OASI require a clinic review postnatally by a professional with expertise in perineal trauma. Endoanal ultrasound and anal manometry should be available. The diagnosis of sphincter defects by ultrasound can be predictive of the development of fecal incontinence in later life.

Mild symptoms of fecal urgency and incontinence can be managed by dietary regimes, constipating agents, and physiotherapy with biofeedback. Women with more severe incontinence should be assessed by a colorectal surgeon. The mode of delivery in a future pregnancy should also be discussed.

CONCLUSION

Childbirth should be a happy event in the life of a woman. It may become physically and emotionally traumatising if there is major perineal trauma. The long-term consequences of OASI increase the risk of chronic pain, sexual dysfunction, and difficulty or inability to control the bladder, stools, or flatus. If an OASI is diagnosed and repaired immediately following childbirth, it gives women the best chance at better short- and long-term outcomes.

REFERENCES

1. Smith LA, Price N, Simonite V, Burns EE. Incidence of and risk factors for perineal trauma: A prospective observational study. *BMC pregnancy and childbirth*. 2013.13(1):1-9.
2. Dudding TC, Vaizey CJ, Kamm MA. Obstetric anal sphincter injury: Incidence, risk factors, and management. *Annals of surgery*. 2008. 247(2):224-37.
3. Fernando R, Sultan A, Freeman R, Williams A, Adams E. The management of third-and fourth-degree perineal tears (Green-top Guideline No. 29). London: Royal College of Obstetricians and Gynaecologists. 2015. 19.
4. Fernando RJ, Sultan AH, Kettle C, Thakar R. Methods of repair for obstetric anal sphincter injury. *Cochrane Database of Systematic Reviews*. 2013. (12).
5. Macarthur AJ, Macarthur C. Incidence, severity, and determinants of perineal pain after vaginal delivery: A prospective cohort study. *American journal of obstetrics and gynecology*. 2004. 191(4):1199-204.
6. Goh J, Romanzi L, Elneil S, Haylen B, Chen G, Ghoniem G, et al. An International Continence Society (ICS) report on the terminology for female pelvic floor fistulas. *Neurourol Urodyn*. 2020. 39(8):2040-71.
7. Webb SS, Hemming K, Khalfaoui MY, Henriksen TB, Kindberg S, Stensgaard S, et al. An obstetric sphincter injury risk identification system (OSIRIS): Is this a clinically useful tool? *International urogynecology journal*. 2017. 28:367-74.
8. Jelovsek JE, Chagin K, Gyhagen M, Hagen S, Wilson D, Kattan MW, et al. Predicting risk of pelvic floor disorders 12 and 20 years after delivery. *American journal of obstetrics and gynecology*. 2018. 218(2):222. e1-e19.

9. Meister MR, Cahill AG, Conner SN, Woolfolk CL, Lowder JL. Predicting obstetric anal sphincter injuries in a modern obstetric population. *American journal of obstetrics and gynecology*. 2016. 215(3):310. e1-. e7.
10. Pergialiotis V, Vlachos D, Protopapas A, Pappa K, Vlachos G. Risk factors for severe perineal lacerations during childbirth. *International Journal of Gynecology & Obstetrics*. 2014. 125(1):6-14.
11. Wheeler J, Davis D, Fry M, Brodie P, Homer CS. Is Asian ethnicity an independent risk factor for severe perineal trauma in childbirth? A systematic review of the literature. *Women Birth*. 2012. 25. 107–113
12. Zetterström J, Lopez A, Anzen B, Norman M, Holmström B, Mellgren A. Anal sphincter tears at vaginal delivery: risk factors and clinical outcome of primary repair. *Obstetrics & Gynecology*. 1999. 94(1):21-8.
13. Hornemann A, Kamischke A, Luedders DW, Beyer DA, Diedrich K, Bohlmann MK. Advanced age is a risk factor for higher grade perineal lacerations during delivery in nulliparous women. *Archives of gynecology and obstetrics*. 2010. 281:59-64.
14. Durnea CM, Jaffery AE, Gauthaman N, Doumouchtsis SK. Effect of body mass index on the incidence of perineal trauma. *International Journal of Gynecology & Obstetrics*. 2018. 141(2):166-70.
15. Dolan LM, Hilton P. Obstetric risk factors and pelvic floor dysfunction 20 years after first delivery. *International urogynecology journal*. 2010. 21:535-44.
16. Gauthaman N, Walters S, Tribe I-A, Goldsmith L, Doumouchtsis SK. Shoulder dystocia and associated manoeuvres as risk factors for perineal trauma. *International urogynecology journal*. 2016. 27:571-7.
17. Caudwell–Hall J, Kamisan Atan I, Martin A, Guzman Rojas R, Langer S, Shek K, et al. Intrapartum predictors of maternal levator ani injury. *Acta obstetricia et gynecologica Scandinavica*. 2017. 96(4):426-31.
18. Pergialiotis V, Bellos I, Fanaki M, et al. Risk factors for severe perineal trauma during childbirth: An updated meta-analysis. *Eur J Obstet Gynecol Reprod Biol*. 2020. 247:94.
19. Gauthaman N, Henry D, Ster IC, Khunda A, Doumochtsis SK. Kielland's forceps: Does it increase the risk of anal sphincter injuries? An observational study. *International urogynecology journal*. 2015. 26:1525-32.
20. Gundabattula SR, Surampudi K. Risk factors for obstetric anal sphincter injuries (OASI) at a tertiary centre in south India. *Int Urogynecol J*. 2018. 29:391.
21. Eason E, Labrecque M, Wells G, Feldman P. Preventing perineal trauma during childbirth: A systematic review. *Obstetrics & Gynecology*. 2000.95(3):464-71.
22. Ramm O, Woo VG, Hung YY, et al. Risk factors for the development of obstetric anal sphincter injuries in modern obstetric practice. *Obstet Gynecol*. 2018. 131:290.
23. Gundabattula SR, Surampudi K. Risk factors for obstetric anal sphincter injuries (OASI) at a tertiary centre in south India. *Int Urogynecol J*. 2018. 29:391. Cited in *UptoDate*.
24. Eshkoli T, Baumfeld Y, Yohay Z, Binyamin Y, Speigel E, Dym L, Weintraub AY. Is epidural analgesia an independent risk factor for OASIS? A population-based cohort study. *Arch Gynecol Obstet*. 2023 Jul 16.
25. Putri I, Simons K, Nettle J, Woodward A. Obstetric anal sphincter injuries (OASIS) in multiparous women with the use of epidural anaesthesia: A retrospective cohort study. *Aust N Z J Obstet Gynaecol*. 2021. 61: 30-34.
26. Beckmann MM, Stock OM. Antenatal perineal massage for reducing perineal trauma. *Cochrane Database Syst Rev*. 2013. CD005123.
27. Aasheim V, Nilsen ABV, Reinar LM, Lukasse M. Perineal techniques during the second stage of labour for reducing perineal trauma. *Cochrane Database Syst Rev*. 2017. 6:CD006672.
28. NICE guideline. NG 235. Intrapartum care. Published: 29 September 2023.www.nice.org.uk/guidance/ng235.
29. Magoga G, Saccone G, Al-Kouatly HB, et al. Warm perineal compresses during the second stage of labor for reducing perineal trauma: A meta-analysis. *European Journal of Obstetrics & Gynecology and Reproductive Biology*. 2019. 240:93-8.
30. Naidu M, Sultan AH, Thakar R. *Int Urogynecol J*. 2017. 28: 381.
31. Royal College of Obstetricians and Gynaecologists. Green-top guideline No. 26: Operative vaginal delivery. 2011. https://www.rcog.org.uk/globalassets/documents/guidelines/gtg26.pdf
32. Zhou F, Wang XD, Li J, Huang GQ, Gao BX. Hyaluronidase for reducing perineal trauma. *Cochrane Database of Systematic Reviews*. 2014(2).
33. Elvander C, Ahlberg M, Thies-Lagergren L, et al. Birth position and obstetric anal sphincter injury: A population-based study of 113,000 spontaneous births. *BMC Pregnancy Childbirth*. 2015. 15, 252.
34. Andrews V, Sultan AH, Thakar R, Jones PW. Occult anal sphincter injuries—myth or reality? *BJOG*. 2006.113(2):195-200.
35. Sultan AH, Monga AK, Kumar D, Stanton SL Primary repair of obstetric anal sphincter rupture using the overlap technique. *Br J Obstet Gynaecol*. 1999. 106(4): 318-23.
36. Duggal N, Mercado C, Daniels K, et al. Antibiotic prophylaxis for prevention of postpartum perineal wound complications: A randomized controlled trial. *Obstet Gynecol*. 2008. 111:1268.
37. ACOG Practice Bulletin No. 195: Prevention of Infection After Gynecologic Procedures. *Obstet Gynecol*. 2018. 131:e172. Reaffirmed 2022.

CHAPTER 26

Vaginal Birth After Cesarean Delivery

PRANATHI REDDY

INTRODUCTION

Pregnant women who have had a previous cesarean section can deliver in one of the following ways:

- Trial of labour after previous cesarean delivery (TOLAC) ending in vaginal birth after cesarean (VBAC)
- Trial of labour after previous cesarean delivery ending in emergency cesarean section
- Planned or elective repeat cesarean delivery (ERCD)

There is widespread public and professional debate about the increasing proportion of births by cesarean section, the definition of an acceptable cesarean delivery rate, and what rate achieves optimal maternal and infant outcomes [1,2] (see **Chapter 23,** *Reducing cesarean rates*). The overall cesarean delivery rate in India in 2019–2021 was 21.5%. In private health facilities, the rate was 47.4% (with some states reaching 65.34 %) and in public health facilities, it was 14.3% [1].

The increase in cesarean birth worldwide is attributed to multiple factors and interactions, both clinical and non-clinical. Increasing rates of primary cesarean section have led to an increase in the proportion of the obstetric population with a history of a uterine scar.

Large cohort studies in the 80s and 90s established that the majority of women with a previous cesarean section may have a VBAC with reported figures of success between 70% and 80% [3]. However, new evidence has emerged to indicate that a successful VBAC may not be as safe as they were thought to be [4,5,6]. There are infrequent but significant and serious risks which have led to decreasing rates of VBAC.

In 2010, the National Institutes of Health convened a consensus conference to examine the safety and outcomes of TOLAC and VBAC as well as factors associated with their decreasing rates. They concluded that planned VBAC is a clinically safe choice for the majority of women with a single previous lower-segment cesarean delivery and called on organisations to facilitate access to TOLAC while recognising concerns over liability [7].

ADVANTAGES OF ACHIEVING VBAC

Women who achieve a successful VBAC avoid major abdominal surgery, and consequently are at lower risk of hemorrhage and infection, and have a shorter recovery time compared to women who have an elective repeat cesarean delivery [8].

Additionally, for those considering having more children in the future, VBAC may avoid potential maternal consequences of multiple cesarean deliveries such as hysterectomy, bowel or bladder injury, transfusion, infection, and abnormal placentation such as placenta previa and placenta accreta [9,10].

Key Point

Attempting a vaginal birth after a single previous lower-segment cesarean delivery is a safe and appropriate choice that should be offered to select women who fulfil the criteria for the possibility of a successful VBAC [7,8].

RISKS OF TOLAC

Trial of labour after a previous cesarean is not without risks. However, the success rate is likely to be high with careful selection of candidates who can undergo TOLAC.

Uterine Rupture

One of the major determinants of severe adverse outcomes associated with TOLAC is the occurrence of uterine rupture (Table 26.1). Its incidence is generally estimated to be in the region of 0.5–1.0%. The overall risk of symptomatic uterine rupture at term has been reported to be 74/10,000 with TOLAC, whereas, in women undergoing elective repeat cesarean delivery (ERCD), the risk of this outcome is zero [5].

The reported incidence of uterine rupture varies, in part, because some studies have grouped true, catastrophic uterine rupture with asymptomatic scar dehiscence. Additionally, early case series did not stratify rupture rates by the type of prior cesarean incision (i.e., low transverse vs. classical) [11]. When uterine rupture occurs, there is a significant risk of bladder injury, transfusion, and infection [8]; approximately 25% may end in peripartum hysterectomy (see **Chapter 18**, *Obstructed labour and uterine rupture* and **Chapter 24**, *Peripartum hysterectomy*). Maternal death from uterine rupture in TOLAC occurs in 4/100,000 cases in the developed world; this estimate is based on information from case reports [12,13]. This risk is higher in low-resource areas.

Table 26.1 Composite maternal risks from elective repeat cesarean section and trial of labour after previous cesarean delivery at term [7,8,14]

Maternal risks	TOLAC (%)	ERCD (%) (After one cesarean)
Infectious morbidity	4.6	3.2
Surgical injury	0.37–1.3	0.30–0.60
Blood transfusion	0.66	0.46
Hysterectomy	0.14	0.16
Uterine rupture	0.71	0.02
Maternal death	0.0019	0.0096

ERCD, elective repeat cesarean delivery

Failed TOLAC

The major determinant of morbidity associated with a decision for TOLAC is whether the attempt is successful. The incidence of composite morbidity among women who had a VBAC is reported to be 2.4%, whereas, among women in whom TOLAC failed and led to an emergency cesarean delivery, it was found to be 14.1% [14].

Fetal and Neonatal Risks

TOLAC carries the additional risk of birth-related perinatal death in 2–3/10,000 cases when compared with ERCD [15]. The absolute risk of such birth-related perinatal loss is comparable to women having their first birth. TOLAC also carries a risk of the infant developing hypoxic–ischemic encephalopathy (HIE) in 8/10,000 cases [5]. The effect on the long-term outcomes of an infant with HIE are unknown (Table 26.2).

Table 26.2 Composite neonatal morbidity from trial of labour after previous cesarean delivery (TOLAC) and elective repeat cesarean delivery in term infants [5,15]

Neonatal risks	TOLAC (%)	ERCD (%)
Antepartum stillbirth	0.10	0.21
Intrapartum stillbirth	0.01–0.04	0–0.004
HIE	0–0.89	0–0.32
Perinatal mortality	0.13	0.05
Neonatal mortality	0.11	0.06
NICU admission	0.8–26.2	1.5–17.6
Respiratory morbidity	5.4	2.5
Transient tachypnea	3.6	4.2

HIE, hypoxic–ischemic encephalopathy; *NICU*, neonatal intensive care unit

SELECTING WOMEN FOR TOLAC

The ideal candidate for a planned TOLAC is a woman in whom the risks (as low as possible) are balanced out by the chances of success (as high as possible) in a manner that is acceptable to the woman and her healthcare provider. The balance of risks and benefits appropriate for one woman may seem unacceptable for another [8].

Ideal Candidates for a TOLAC

TOLAC is appropriate for, and may be offered to, the majority of women with a singleton pregnancy with a cephalic presentation at 37+0 weeks or beyond who have had a single previous lower-segment cesarean delivery with or without a history of previous vaginal birth [16].

Contraindications to TOLAC

There is limited evidence on whether maternal or neonatal outcomes are significantly influenced by the number of prior cesarean births or the type of the prior uterine scar. Nonetheless, due to the higher absolute risks of uterine rupture or other complications, planned TOLAC is contraindicated in women with the following [16,17,18]:

- Previous uterine rupture or dehiscence, since the risk of recurrent rupture is unknown
- Previous classical, T, or J incisions at cesarean birth (the incidence of uterine rupture is 200–900/10,000)
- A uterine incision that has involved the whole thickness of the myometrium, as in a previous myomectomy
- Three or more previous cesarean deliveries (there is no reliable estimate of the risk of rupture)
- A major degree of placenta previa (and some cases of minor placenta previa), which is a contraindication to vaginal delivery, including VBAC
- Refusal of the woman to attempt TOLAC

> **Key Point**
>
> Women with a prior history of a classical, T, or J incision at cesarean birth should not undergo TOLAC and should be advised to give birth by ERCD [16].

Role of Prediction Models

Neither elective repeat cesarean delivery nor TOLAC is without maternal and neonatal risks [11]. However, it is abundantly clear that a successful VBAC has the fewest complications, whereas a failed TOLAC leading to an emergency cesarean section has the greatest risk of adverse outcomes [16].

These findings underline the importance of developing methods to predict the likelihood of success of a VBAC in relation to maternal characteristics. Several investigators have attempted to create scoring systems to assist in the prediction of a successful VBAC.

A model that was developed specifically for women undergoing TOLAC at term with one prior low-transverse cesarean delivery incision, a singleton pregnancy, and cephalic fetal presentation showed reasonable accuracy [19], but most others have had limited success [20,21].

Rather than the use of scoring systems, the RCOG guidelines recommend the implementation of a TOLAC versus an ERCD checklist or clinical care pathway to facilitate the best practice in antenatal counselling, shared decision-making, and documentation [16].

FACTORS THAT INCREASE THE SUCCESS OF VBAC

The following factors have been shown to increase the rate of success of a VBAC:

- **A previous vaginal birth**, particularly a previous successful VBAC, is the single best predictor for a successful VBAC and is associated with an approximately 87–90% success rate for a planned VBAC [20,21].

Though the risk of rupture rises with each successive labour, a prior vaginal delivery also increases the chances of a successful VBAC.

- **Spontaneous onset** of labour and a **gestational age <40 weeks** at the onset of labour further contribute to a greater chance of having a successful VBAC.
- An **interpregnancy interval** of at least 24 months between the date of the last cesarean birth and the due date for the current pregnancy improves the rate of success [17].

Key Point

A previous vaginal birth, particularly a previous VBAC, is the single best predictor for successful VBAC [21,22].

FACTORS THAT LEAD TO UNSUCCESSFUL VBAC

The following factors reduce the chances of a successful VBAC [8,22,23]:

- Induced labour
- No previous vaginal birth
- Body mass index >30 Kg/m^2
- Recurrent indication for initial cesarean delivery (labour dystocia)
- Gestation beyond 41 weeks
- Maternal diabetes
- Estimated fetal weight >4000 g
- Previous preterm cesarean birth
- Cervical dilatation at admission <4 cm
- Short inter-pregnancy interval (<2 years from the previous cesarean birth)
- Advanced maternal age
- Short stature

Where relevant to the woman's circumstances, this information should be shared during the antenatal counselling process to enable the woman to make the best-informed choice. Women with a previous cesarean delivery are not always able to decide on the mode of delivery in their current pregnancy and are unhappy about taking responsibility for this decision. They expect appropriate guidance from their healthcare provider depending on their clinical situation [24].

ANTENATAL MANAGEMENT IN A WOMAN WITH A PREVIOUS CESAREAN SECTION

Counselling regarding the mode of delivery should ideally start at the time of the sentinel cesarean. Women should be offered information regarding the need for the first cesarean and the implications it may have for future pregnancies and deliveries.

Risk Assessment for TOLAC

At the first antenatal visit, women who have had a previous cesarean section or have a uterine scar should be identified. They should be assessed by a senior consultant. Factors to note at the booking visit include the following:

- Number and type of previous uterine scar/s
- Indication/s for prior cesarean
- Are the notes available?
- Were there any puerperal complications?
- Gestation at the time of the prior cesarean
- Anticipated family size is important, keeping in mind the long-term risks from repeat cesarean sections
- Has the woman had a successful vaginal delivery and was this before or after the uterine scar?
- Is the inter-conception interval >2 years?
- Are there other associated medical problems?

The role of antenatal ultrasonography in predicting the risk of uterine rupture in TOLAC

In an attempt to predict whether a previous cesarean scar would rupture during TOLAC, ultrasound imaging has been used to assess the uterine scar in pregnancy. However, a systematic review that included 21 studies [25] found that it was **not useful in clinical practice**. No myometrial thickness threshold value was entirely accurate in predicting whether a hysterotomy scar would rupture during labour or remain intact.

A thinned uterine scar has a very low positive predictive value [26] for rupture. There have been reports of uterine rupture in labour even with normal lower uterine segment thickness [27].

> **Key Point**
>
> Routine measurement of the lower uterine segment thickness in women with a prior cesarean is not recommended [28].

Antenatal Counselling

- **Booking visit:** The counselling of the women about choices regarding the mode of delivery should begin at the booking visit. Many of the factors related to the chance of successful VBAC or the risk of uterine rupture are known early in pregnancy. The potential risks and benefits of both TOLAC and elective repeat cesarean delivery should be discussed [8,16].

> **Key Point**
>
> Women with a prior history of one uncomplicated lower-segment transverse cesarean section in an otherwise uncomplicated pregnancy at term with no contraindication to vaginal birth should be able to discuss the option of TOLAC and the alternative of an elective repeat cesarean delivery (ERCD).

Educating the woman and her family

- **The risks and benefits of both options should be discussed with women:** The chances of a successful planned VBAC in a carefully selected candidate are 72–76%. [5,7]. Women should also be informed that this assessment would be an ongoing process and that the ultimate decision would depend on the course of the current pregnancy [8,16].
- **Decision regarding family size:** Women should be counselled regarding intended family size and the risk of additional cesarean deliveries with clear explanations that future reproductive plans may be uncertain or may change [8].
- **Antenatal transfer of care:** A woman's wishes in the matter must be respected. When conflicts arise between her and the obstetrician or another obstetric care provider, facility policy, or both, careful explanation and, if appropriate, transfer of care to facilities supporting TOLAC should be offered. A woman should not be forced to have an elective repeat cesarean because the facility does not support TOLAC.
- **Birth plan:** The woman and her obstetrician should agree upon the final decision for the mode of birth before the expected/planned delivery date (ideally before 36 weeks of gestation) [3]. A clear birth plan should be documented, which states the boundaries of safe practice to which they have agreed, and the circumstances under which the woman would request a repeat cesarean delivery. Equally, the possible scenarios where a section would be medically necessary or advised should also be discussed and documented.

  In women who choose ERCD, it is important to remember that up to 10% of them are likely to go into labour before 39+0 weeks. It is good practice to discuss and document a plan for delivery if labour starts before the scheduled date [16].
- **General measures:** Placenta previa/accreta should be excluded with ultrasonography. Identifying and treating anemia early on is important in these women.
- **Instructions and advice:** If the decision is in favour of TOLAC, the woman should be advised on the following:
  - To present to the facility early in labour or if there is spontaneous rupture of membranes.
  - The decision made in the clinic is not binding and she has the autonomy to change her mind.
- **Documentation:** The antenatal counselling of women with a prior cesarean birth should be documented in the notes. Providing the

woman with an information leaflet during the consultation can be useful [24].

INTRAPARTUM MANAGEMENT

Prerequisites for Units Offering TOLAC

Women who have had a previous cesarean should be offered care during labour in a unit where the following are available:

- Immediate access to facilities required for cesarean delivery (within 30 minutes or less of the indication arising)
- Facilities for continuous electronic fetal heart rate monitoring
- Experienced obstetrician/s capable of monitoring labour and performing an emergency cesarean delivery
- Anesthetists and neonatologists available on-site around the clock
- On-site blood transfusion services

At least 20–30% of all women attempting VBAC are likely to need repeat emergency cesarean section, and in a significant proportion of these cases, this may be very urgent due to an immediate threat to the life of the mother or baby, or both. Hospitals that do not have on-site theatre staff and anesthetic staff around the clock should have provisions for calling in staff at very short notice to enable a theatre to be opened quickly.

Close Monitoring of Labour

Effective and close monitoring of labour is essential for early identification of impending uterine rupture. A modified partograph may be used to facilitate the documentation of the progress of labour. The WHO's Labour Care Guide starts recording only at 5 cm dilatation so may miss signs of uterine rupture, the majority of which occur at 4–5 cm dilatation.

Maternal tachycardia can be an early indication of scar dehiscence. Monitoring the intensity, duration and frequency of uterine contractions is best accomplished manually.

Key Point

The routine use of intrauterine pressure catheters in the early detection of uterine scar rupture is not recommended.

The duration of labour should be closely monitored. Available data suggest that labour progress is similar in women with or without a previous cesarean delivery. However, clinicians tend to have a lower threshold for diagnosing failure to progress in women undergoing TOLAC than they do in women with an unscarred uterus. Prolongation of labour is an important sign of dystocia and imminent rupture or dehiscence [31].

Key Point

In cases of prolonged first or second stage of labour, it is prudent to have a lower threshold for resorting to repeat cesarean delivery than in women with an intact uterus.

Most uterine ruptures (>90%) occur during labour (the peak incidence being at 4–5 cm cervical dilatation), with around 18% occurring in the second stage of labour and 8% being identified after vaginal delivery [32].

Continuous Electronic Fetal Monitoring

Continuous electronic fetal monitoring is recommended following the onset of uterine contractions for the duration of TOLAC. An abnormal cardiotocograph (CTG) trace is the most consistent finding in uterine rupture and is present in 55–87% of these cases [29]. Over half of these cases present with a combination of an abnormal CTG and abdominal pain [29,30]. The relative and absolute risks of severe adverse events in the absence of continuous electronic fetal monitoring are unknown.

Analgesia

Epidural analgesia for labour may be used as part of TOLAC, and the availability of adequate pain relief may encourage more women to choose TOLAC. Epidural appears to have no effect on the rates of failed TOLAC or operative vaginal delivery [33].

In addition, effective regional analgesia does not mask signs and symptoms of uterine rupture, particularly since the most common sign of rupture is fetal heart abnormalities.

However, a case–control study showed frequent epidural dosing to be an independent risk factor for impending uterine rupture in TOLAC. The increasing pain and analgesia requirement that is likely to precede uterine rupture may explain the association between uterine rupture and increasing epidural dosing in TOLAC that progresses to uterine rupture [34].

Early Diagnosis of Uterine Scar Rupture

Early diagnosis of uterine scar rupture followed by expeditious laparotomy and resuscitation is essential to reduce associated morbidity and mortality in the mother and infant (see **Chapter 18**).

There is no single pathognomic clinical feature that is indicative of uterine rupture but the presence of any of the following should raise a concern about the possibility of this event [16,35]:

- Abnormal CTG tracing
- Severe abdominal pain, especially if persisting between contractions
- Chest pain or shoulder tip pain, with sudden onset of shortness of breath
- Acute onset scar tenderness
- Abnormal vaginal bleeding or hematuria
- Cessation of previously efficient uterine activity
- Maternal tachycardia, hypotension, or shock
- Loss of station of the presenting part

The diagnosis is ultimately confirmed at emergency cesarean section or postpartum laparotomy.

> **Key Point**
>
> The hospital should have a plan for managing uterine rupture, and clinical drills may be useful in preparing for these emergencies.

DELIVERY

- **Spontaneous vaginal delivery:** The same techniques used for the delivery of the fetus and the placenta in any other vaginal birth are used for VBAC (see **Chapter 4**, *Management of the first and second stages of normal labour*).
- **Operative vaginal birth:** The indications, contraindications, prerequisites, and procedure for operative vaginal birth are the same as in women without a previous cesarean birth (see **Chapter 21**, *Operative vaginal delivery*).

Induction and Augmentation of Labour

Induction and augmentation are not contraindicated in women with a previous cesarean delivery. However, induction and augmentation during TOLAC are associated with a 2- to 3-fold increased risk of uterine rupture and around a 1.5-fold increased risk of cesarean delivery compared to spontaneous labour [36].

The risk of uterine rupture is increased in the following:

- Women with a previous cesarean delivery who have not previously given birth vaginally
- Women with an unfavourable cervix
- Women undergoing induction with prostaglandins (especially misoprostol)

> **Key Point**
>
> A mechanical method of induction such as an **intracervical Foley catheter** is preferable to other methods of induction in a scarred uterus as it is less likely to be associated with uterine hyperstimulation. The use of **misoprostol is contraindicated.**

The points to be kept in mind for augmentation during TOLAC include the following:

- Although augmentation is not contraindicated, it should be preceded by careful assessment by an experienced obstetrician and appropriate maternal counselling.
- Oxytocin augmentation should be titrated to not exceed the maximum rate of contractions

of 4 in 10 minutes. The ideal contraction frequency would be 3-4 in 10 minutes.

- Careful serial cervical assessments, preferably by the same person, are necessary to confirm adequate progress, thereby allowing augmentation to continue.
- The decisions regarding intervals for serial vaginal examination and the selected parameters of progress that would necessitate discontinuing TOLAC should be made by a senior obstetrician.

Uterine Exploration After VBAC

Manual uterine exploration after VBAC and subsequent repair of asymptomatic scar dehiscence has not been shown to improve outcomes. Excessive vaginal bleeding or signs of hypovolemia may indicate uterine rupture and should prompt a complete evaluation of the genital tract [8].

TOLAC IN SPECIAL CIRCUMSTANCES

Preterm Labour

Women who are preterm and considering the options for birth after a previous cesarean should be informed that planned preterm VBAC has similar success rates to planned term VBAC but with a lower risk of uterine rupture. Therefore, in a carefully selected population, planned VBAC may be offered as an option to women undergoing preterm birth with a history of prior cesarean birth.

More Than One Previous Cesarean Delivery

Though a meta-analysis showed no significant difference in the rates of successful VBAC in women with two previous cesarean births and those with a single previous cesarean birth, there was a higher risk of uterine rupture in the former group [37].

Planned VBAC may be supported in women with two previous low-transverse cesarean deliveries, provided that the woman has been fully informed by a senior obstetrician of the increased risks. However, labour should be conducted in a tertiary centre with suitable facilities and recourse to immediate surgical delivery.

Multiple Gestation

Women with one previous cesarean delivery with a low transverse incision who are otherwise appropriate candidates for twin vaginal delivery may be considered candidates for TOLAC. In two analyses of large populations, women with twin gestations had a similar chance of achieving VBAC as women with singleton gestations, and the multiple gestation did not lead to any greater risk of uterine rupture or maternal/perinatal morbidity [38].

ELECTIVE REPEAT CESAREAN DELIVERY (ERCD)

Women considering ERCD should be counselled that delivery after 39+0 completed weeks has the least risk of respiratory morbidity and a lower risk of transient tachypnea of the newborn (see **Chapter 22**, *Cesarean section: Procedure and technique,* for details).

All women undergoing ERCD should receive a dose of prophylactic antibiotic in accordance with existing guidelines for cesarean delivery.

CONCLUSION

After careful assessment to rule out any contraindications, a woman with one previous transverse lower segment cesarean section may be offered a trial of labour (TOL) with appropriate discussion of maternal and perinatal risks and benefits.

To ensure safe labour after a prior cesarean section, a woman should deliver in a well-equipped tertiary facility with round-the-clock availability of obstetric, anesthetic, pediatric, and theatre staff.

REFERENCES

1. National Family Health Survey, NHFS 5, 2019–21, Ministry of Health & Family Welfare, GOI.
2. Goetzinger KR, Macones GA. Operative vaginal delivery: Current trends in obstetrics. *Women's Health.* 2008. 4:281–90.

3. Flamm BL, Newman LA, Thomas SJ, et al. Vaginal birth after cesarean delivery: Results of a 5-year multicenter collaborative study. *Obstet Gynecol*. 1990. 76:750–4.
4. Flamm BL. Once a cesarean, always a controversy. *Obstet Gynecol*. 1997. 90:312–5.
5. Landon MB, Hauth JC, Leveno KJ, Spong CY, Leindecker S, Varner MW, et al. National Institute of Child Health and Human Development Maternal–Fetal Medicine Units Network. Maternal and perinatal outcomes associated with a trial of labor after prior cesarean delivery. *N Engl J Med*. 2004. 351:2581–9.
6. Smith GC, Pell JP, Cameron AD, Dobbie R. Risk of perinatal death associated with labor after previous cesarean delivery in uncomplicated term pregnancies. *JAMA*. 2002. 287:2684–90.
7. National Institutes of Health Consensus Development conference statement: Vaginal birth after cesarean: New insights March 8–10, 2010. *Obstet Gynecol*. 2010. 115: 1279–95.
8. ACOG. Vaginal birth after cesarean delivery. ACOG Practice Bulletin No. 205. American College of Obstetricians and Gynecologists. *Obstet Gynecol*. 2019. 133:e110–27.
9. Silver RM, Landon MB, Rouse DJ, Leveno KJ, Spong CY, Thom EA, et al. Maternal morbidity associated with multiple repeat cesarean deliveries. National Institute of Child Health and Human Development Maternal–Fetal Medicine Units Network. *Obstet Gynecol*. 2006. 107:1226–32. (Level II).
10. Nisenblat V, Barak S, Griness OB, Degani S, Ohel G, Gonen R. Maternal complications associated with multiple cesarean deliveries. *Obstet Gynecol*. 2006. 108:21–6.
11. Leung AS, Leung EK, Paul RH. Uterine rupture after previous cesarean delivery: Maternal and fetal consequences. *Am J Obstet Gynecol*. 1993. 169: 945–50.
12. Wen SW, Rusen ID, Walker M, et al. Comparison of maternal mortality and morbidity between trial of labor and elective cesarean section among women with previous cesarean delivery. *Am J Obstet Gynecol*. 2004. 191:1263–9.
13. Farmer RM, Kirschbaum T, Potter D, et al. Uterine rupture during trial of labor after previous cesarean section. *Am J Obstet Gynecol*. 1991. 165:996–1001.
14. Guise JM, Eden K, Emeis C, Denman MA, Marshall N, Fu R, et al. Vaginal Birth After Cesarean: New Insights. Evidence Reports/Technology Assessments, No. 191. Rockville, Maryland, USA: Agency for Healthcare Research and Quality. 2010.
15. Smith GC, Pell JP, Dobbie R. Caesarean section and risk of unexplained stillbirth in subsequent pregnancy. *Lancet*. 2003. 362:1779–84.
16. RCOG Green-Top Guideline Number 45: Birth after Previous Cesarean Birth. 2015.
17. Landon MB, Leindecker S, Spong CY, Hauth JC, Bloom S, Varner MW, et al. The MFMU Cesarean Registry: Factors affecting the success of trial of labor after previous cesarean delivery. *Am J Obstet Gynecol*. 2005. 193:1016–23.
18. Guise JM, Hashima J, Osterweil P. Evidence–based vaginal birth after cesarean section. *Best Prac Res Clin Obstet Gynaecol*. 2005. 19:117–30.
19. Grobman WA, Lai Y, Landon MB, et al. Development of a nomogram for prediction of vaginal birth after cesarean delivery. National Institute of Child Health and Human Development (NICHD) Maternal–Fetal Medicine Units Network (MFMU). *Obstet Gynecol*. 2007. 109:806–12.
20. Macones GA, Hausman N, Edelstein R, Stamilio DM, Marder SJ. Predicting outcomes of trials of labor in women attempting vaginal birth after cesarean delivery: A comparison of multivariate methods with neural networks. *Am J Obstet Gynecol*. 2001. 184:409–13.
21. Srinivas SK, Stamilio DM, Stevens EJ, Odibo AO, Peipert JF, Macones GA. Predicting failure of a vaginal birth attempt after cesarean delivery. *Obstet Gynecol*. 2007. 109:800–5.
22. Gyamfi C, Juhasz G, Gyamfi P, Stone JL. Increased success of trial of labor after previous vaginal birth after cesarean. *Obstet Gynecol*. 2004. 104:715–19.
23. Goodall PT, Ahn JT, Chapa JB, Hibbard JU. Obesity as a risk factor for failed trial of labor in patients with previous cesarean delivery. *Am J Obstet Gynecol*. 2005. 192:1423–6.
24. Moffat MA, Bell JS, Porter MA, Lawton S, Hundley V, Danielian P, et al. Decision making about mode of delivery among pregnant women who have previously had a caesarean section: A qualitative study. *BJOG*. 2007. 114:86–93.
25. Kok N, Wiersma IC, Opmeer BC, et al. Sonographic measurement of lower uterine segment thickness to predict uterine rupture during a trial of labor in women with previous Cesarean section: a meta-analysis. *Ultrasound Obstet Gynecol*. 2013. 42:132.
26. Rozenberg P, Goffinet F, Phillippe HJ, Nisand I. Ultrasonographic measurement of lower uterine segment to assess risk of defects of scarred uterus. *Lancet*. 1996. 347:281.
27. Cheung VY. Sonographic measurement of the lower uterine segment thickness: is it truly predictive of uterine rupture? *J Obstet Gynaecol Can*. 2008. 30:148.
28. Landon MB, Frey H. TD. Uterine rupture: After previous cesarean delivery. Berghella V (Ed), *UpToDate*. 2020. Waltham, MA.
29. Fitzpatrick KE, Kurinczuk JJ, Alfirevic Z, Spark P, Brocklehurst P, Knight M. Uterine rupture by intended mode of delivery in the UK: a national case-control study. *PLoS Med*. 2012. 9:e1001184.

30. Craver Pryor E, Mertz HL, Beaver BW, et al. Intrapartum predictors of uterine rupture. *Am J Perinatol.* 2007. 24:317–21.
31. Grantz KL, Gonzalez-Quintero V, Troendle J, Reddy UM, Hinkle SN, Kominiarek MA, et al. Labor patterns in women attempting vaginal birth after cesarean with normal neonatal outcomes. *Am J Obstet Gynecol.* 2015. 213:226.e1–6.
32. Zwart JJ, Richters JM, Ory F, et al. Uterine rupture in The Netherlands: A nationwide population-based cohort study. *BJOG.* 2009. 116:1069–78.
33. Sakala EP, Kaye S, Murray RD, Munson LJ. Epidural analgesia: Effect on the likelihood of a successful trial of labor after cesarean section. *J Reprod Med.* 1990. 35:886–90.
34. Cahill AG, Odibo AO, Allsworth JE, Macones GA. Frequent epidural dosing as a marker for impending uterine rupture in patients who attempt vaginal birth after cesarean delivery. *Am J Obstet Gynecol.* 2010. 202:355.e1–5.
35. Turner MJ. Uterine rupture. *Best Prac Res Clin Obstet Gynaecol.* 2002; 16:69–79.
36. Grobman WA, Gilbert S, Landon MB, Spong CY, Leveno KJ, Rouse DJ, et al. Outcomes of induction of labor after one prior cesarean. *Obstet Gynecol.* 2007. 109:262–9.
37. Tahseen S, Griffiths M. Vaginal birth after two caesarean sections (VBAC-2): A systematic review with meta-analysis of success rate and adverse outcomes of VBAC-2 versus VBAC-1 and repeat (third) caesarean sections. *BJOG.* 2010. 117:5.
38. Varner MW, Thom E, Spong CY, Landon MB, Leveno KJ, Rouse DJ, et al. Trial of labor after one previous cesarean delivery for multifetal gestation. National Institute of Child Health and Human Development (NICHD) Maternal-Fetal Medicine Units Network (MFMU). *Obstet Gynecol.* 2007. 110:814–9.

CHAPTER 27

Breech Delivery

LAKSHMI SESHADRI

INTRODUCTION

The delivery of a singleton fetus presenting as breech is a challenge to the obstetrician. The mode of delivery is widely debated and remains controversial. The incidence of breech presentation varies with gestational age. At term, it is 3–4%; at 32 weeks, it is 7%; and at 28 weeks, it is 25% [1].

TYPES OF BREECH PRESENTATION

Breech presentation is of three types (Fig. 27.1):

- **Frank breech** is one in which both the hips are flexed and both knees are extended. This is the most common type. The breech fits snugly in the lower uterine segment and has the best prognosis for vaginal delivery.
- **Complete breech** is one in which the hips and knees are both flexed. The irregular breech does not fit well in the lower segment. Therefore, cord prolapse is more common and the chances of vaginal delivery are lower.
- **Incomplete breech** is one in which one or both the hips are extended, and the knee or foot presents below the breech. This is also referred to as **footling presentation**. Cord prolapse and head entrapment are common in this type of breech.

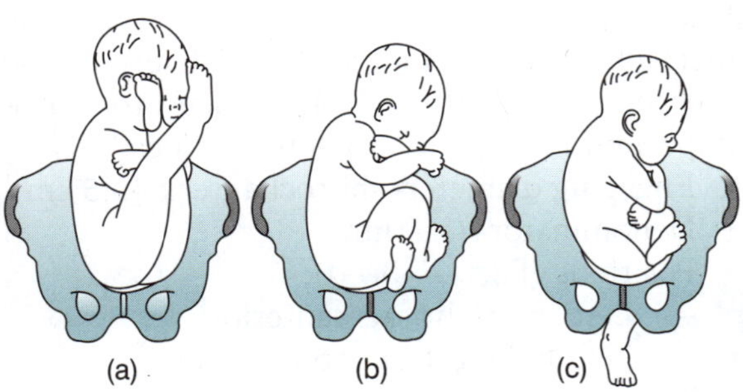

Fig. 27.1 Types of breech presentation: (a) Frank breech, (b) complete breech, (c) incomplete or footling breech

ETIOLOGY OF BREECH PRESENTATION

Prematurity, advanced maternal age, amniotic fluid abnormalities, placenta previa, low birth weight, and fetal anomalies are the common causes of breech presentation [2,3,4]. The causes of breech presentation are listed in Table 27.1.

Table 27.1 Causes of breech presentation

Maternal	Fetal

• Advanced maternal age
• Uterine anomalies
• Placenta previa
• Grand multiparity/ nulliparity
• Polyhydramnios
• Previous cesarean delivery
	• Prematurity
	• Low birth weight
	• Multifetal pregnancy
	• Pregnancy after assisted reproductive techniques
	• Congenital anomalies of the fetus
	  – Hydrocephalus
	  – Anencephaly
	• Chromosomal abnormalities

Key Point

Prematurity, placenta previa, and congenital anomalies of the fetus should be excluded when the fetus presents as breech.

DIAGNOSIS OF BREECH

The diagnosis of breech presentation is made by clinical examination and confirmed by ultrasonography.

Clinical Examination

Abdominal examination reveals the hard, ballotable head at the uterine fundus and the soft, broad breech at the pelvic inlet (Fig. 27.2).

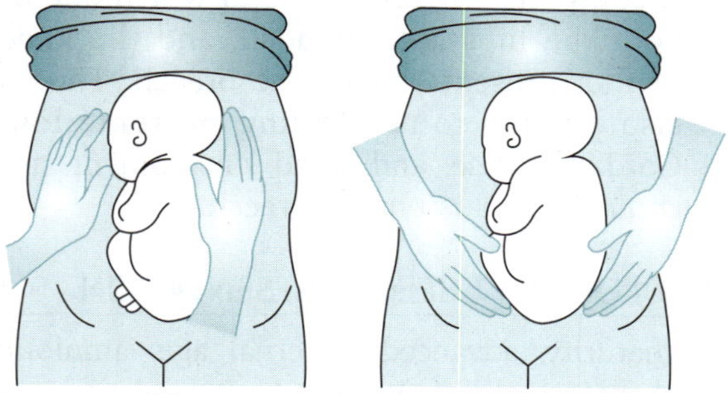

Fig. 27.2 Abdominal examination: (a) Ballotable head is felt at the fundus and (b) breech is felt at the lower pole of the uterus

On vaginal examination, the fetal sacrum, ischial tuberosities, anus, external genitalia, and the feet or knee are felt.

A frank breech may be mistaken for a face presentation. In a frank breech presentation, the anus and ischial tuberosities lie in a straight line, whereas in a face presentation, the mouth and malar prominences are in a triangular configuration.

In complete breech and footling presentations, one foot or both feet may be felt.

Ultrasonography

Ultrasonography is mandatory if breech presentation persists after 34 weeks. Apart from confirming the diagnosis, ultrasonography provides the following important information, which plays a major role in decision-making regarding the mode of delivery:

- Type of breech
- Location of the placenta
- Fetal anomalies
- Uterine anomalies
- Volume of amniotic fluid
- Estimated weight of the fetus
- Flexion/extension of the fetal head

Key Point

Ultrasonography is an essential tool in the diagnosis of breech presentation and also helps in making a decision regarding the mode of delivery.

COMPLICATIONS OF BREECH PRESENTATION

Complications of breech presentation and delivery may be due to inherent problems in the fetus [5,6] or may result from complications of vaginal breech delivery as listed in Box 27.1.

Box 27.1 Complications associated with breech presentation

- Inherent problems in the fetus in breech presentation
  - Congenital and chromosomal abnormalities
  - Prematurity
  - Neuromuscular disorders
- Complications of vaginal breech delivery
  - Cord accidents
  - Birth asphyxia
  - Birth trauma
- Entrapment of the aftercoming head

MECHANISM OF LABOUR IN BREECH DELIVERY

When the fetus presents as breech, the mechanism of labour includes delivery of the breech, shoulders, and head, in that order. The important information to note includes:

- Engaging diameter—bitrochanteric (9.5 cm)
- Denominator—sacrum
- Positions (Figs. 27.3a–d):
  - — Left and right sacroanterior
  - — Left and right sacroposterior

The **cardinal movements** for breech delivery are as follows:

- The right sacroanterior is the most common position. Here, the bitrochanteric diameter

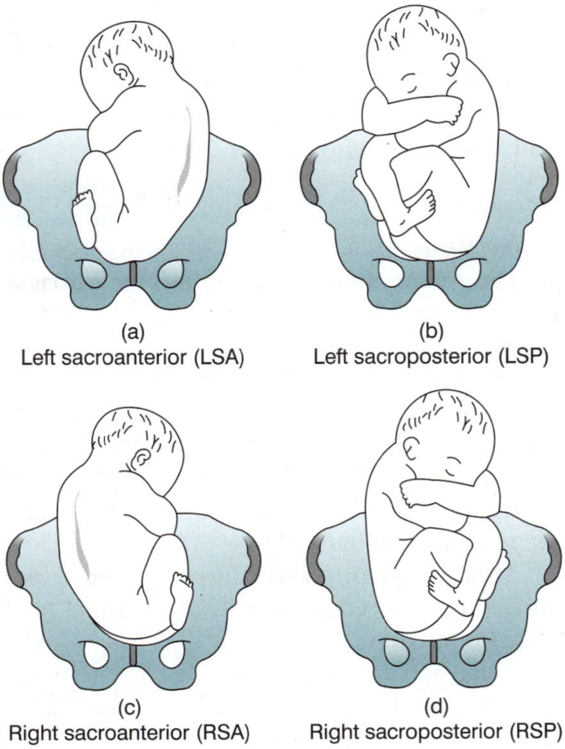

Fig. 27.3 Fetal positions in breech presentation: (a) Left sacroanterior (LSA), (b) left sacroposterior (LSP), (c) right sacroanterior (RSA), (d) right sacroposterior (RSP)

engages in the right oblique diameter (Fig. 27.4a).

- The fetus descends with compaction, with the limbs and trunk coming closer. The anterior buttock rotates by 45 degrees and hitches under the pubic symphysis (Fig. 27.4b).
- By a process of lateral flexion, the posterior buttock is born first, followed by the anterior buttock (Fig. 27.4c).
- The rest of the trunk is delivered until the bisacromial diameter of the shoulder comes to lie in the right oblique diameter of the pelvis (Fig. 27.4d).
- The anterior shoulder rotates through 45 degrees and hitches under the pubic symphysis.
- The posterior shoulder is born first, followed by the anterior shoulder (Fig. 27.4e).

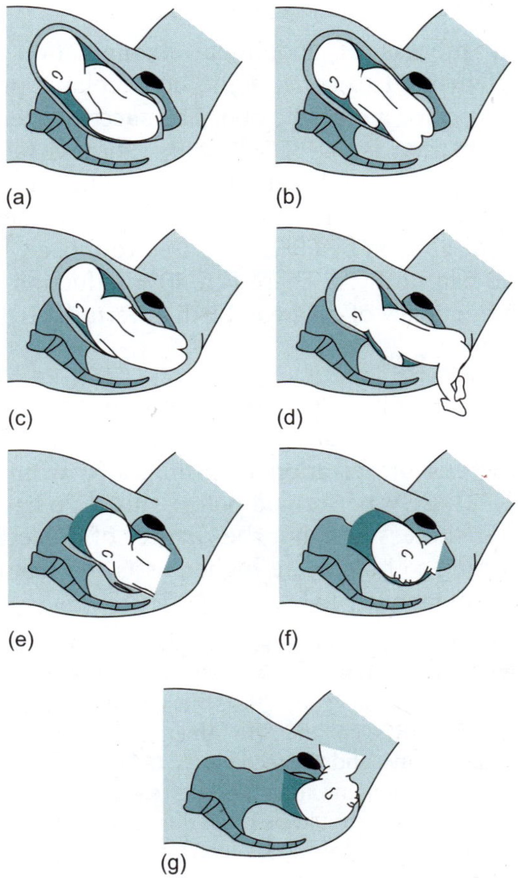

Fig. 27.4 Mechanism of labour in breech presentation

- The suboccipitofrontal diameter engages in the left oblique diameter of the pelvis. The occiput rotates through 45 degrees and hitches under the pubic symphysis (Fig. 27.4f) and the head is born by flexion. (Fig. 27.4g).

MANAGEMENT OF BREECH PRESENTATION

In all women, fetal presentation may keep changing till 34 weeks of gestation. If breech presentation persists after 34 weeks, converting the presentation to cephalic by **external cephalic version** increases the chances of vaginal delivery and reduces the risk of cesarean section [7].

External Cephalic Version (ECV)

This process of abdominal manipulation is implemented to convert the non-cephalic presentation to a cephalic one. The success rate of this method is 50–60% [7,8,9]. Success rates are higher in a multipara than in a nullipara [7]. External version reduces non-cephalic presentations at term by 60% compared to those who have had no ECV. There is a 40% reduction in the frequency of cesarean birth at term [7,10].

Timing of ECV

External cephalic version is recommended at 37 weeks of gestation in multigravidas and at 36 weeks of gestation in primigravid women [11,12]. ECV performed before this time has a better success rate, but the chances of the fetus reverting to breech are higher, as is the risk of preterm labour. [13].

> **Key Point**
>
> The Royal College of Obstetricians and Gynaecologists (RCOG) and the American College of Obstetricians and Gynecologists (ACOG) recommend that women with a breech presentation at or after 36 weeks should be offered external cephalic version after appropriate counselling regarding the risks and benefits unless there is an absolute contraindication.

Success of ECV

The factors that reduce the success rate of ECV are nulliparity, extended breech, decreased amniotic fluid volume, obesity, and an anterior placenta.

Risks associated with ECV

There are few risks associated with ECV. They may include transient fetal heart rate abnormalities, rupture of membranes, placental abruption, cord prolapse, or fetomaternal transfusion and can occur in 6% of women [7,14].

Contraindications to ECV

The contraindications to ECV include multifetal pregnancy, hypertensive disorders, placenta previa, uterine anomalies, ruptured membranes, and oligohydramnios. A previous cesarean delivery or myomectomy, fetal macrosomia, and fetal growth restriction are relative contraindications.

Procedure

Preparation

Pre-procedure counselling regarding the risks and benefits is mandatory. The procedure should be explained to the woman and her informed consent should be obtained.

Ultrasonography should be performed to assess the type of breech, location of the placenta, and quantity of amniotic fluid. It is also used during the procedure to monitor fetal heart rate and to guide manipulation.

Cardiotocography is usually performed before starting the procedure to ensure a normal fetal heart rate pattern.

Analgesia is not used. Tocolysis is useful for relaxing the uterus [7]. Either of the following tocolytic agents are used:

- **Terbutaline** 0.25 mg is administered subcutaneously 15–30 minutes prior to ECV.
- **Nifedipine** 10 mg orally may be given 30 minutes before the procedure and has been shown to be an effective tocolytic for the procedure [15].

It is advisable to apply either talc powder or ultrasound jelly over the maternal abdomen to reduce friction over the skin as the version is attempted.

Steps of ECV

The breech is disengaged, and the fetal head is manipulated towards the pelvis. A 'forward roll' is easier and generally preferred, but a backward flip may be used in some cases (Fig. 27.5). Which method is used is dictated by the position of the fetal spine and the location of the placenta.

The fetal heart rate is monitored frequently throughout the procedure. Cardiotocography is repeated after the procedure to look for fetal heart changes, especially bradycardia.

External version may be repeated, even in early labour, if the presentation reverts to breech.

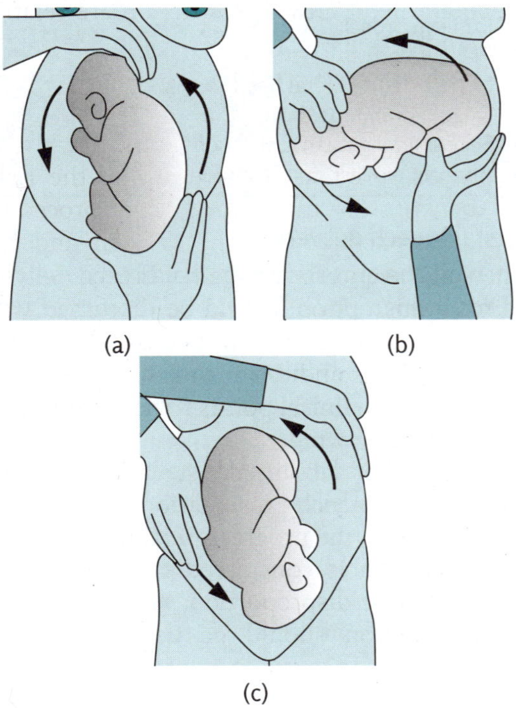

Fig. 27.5 External cephalic version: (a) The breech is disengaged from the pelvis, (b) the head is turned in the forward direction ('forward roll'), (c) the version is complete, with the fetal head in the lower pole

> **Key Point**
>
> Anti-D immunoglobulin must be administered after the procedure if the mother is Rh-negative [7].

MODE OF DELIVERY OF TERM SINGLETON BREECH

The mode of delivery of a term singleton breech has been controversial. There have been several observational and randomised trials comparing vaginal delivery and cesarean birth. The Term Breech Trial, a large randomised controlled trial, showed significantly higher perinatal mortality and morbidity in the planned vaginal delivery group [16]. The findings of a study by the World Health Organization (WHO) and other studies were similar [17,18,19]. A systematic review of the Cochrane Database in 2015 endorsed the same findings [20].

However, the PREMODA study from France and Belgium [21] and an earlier study from France [22] showed no difference in the perinatal outcomes of planned vaginal delivery and planned cesarean birth. The follow-up of infants delivered vaginally at 18 months [23] and 2 years [20] also revealed no neurodevelopmental delay.

A recent meta-analysis comparing four national evidence-based guidelines including the PREMODA trial demonstrated that **perinatal mortality and morbidity are slightly higher with vaginal delivery, but that the absolute risk is low** [24]. Further, the skill and experience of the obstetrician in vaginal breech delivery should also be taken into account. Hence, the mode of delivery in breech presentation is a challenge. Elective vaginal breech delivery should be undertaken only after due consideration of the benefits and risks, under hospital-specific protocols and guidelines, and following a detailed discussion with the mother.

> **Key Point**
>
> The decision regarding cesarean section or vaginal breech delivery should be individualised, based on the centre, the obstetrician's experience, and the woman's preference.

Elective Cesarean Delivery in Breech Presentation

If a cesarean section has been decided upon, it should be a planned one, performed prior to the onset of labour, at or after 39 weeks of gestation. It is important to remember that delivery of the fetus by breech at the time of cesarean section involves all the manoeuvres of vaginal breech delivery.

Planned Vaginal Delivery for Breech Presentation

Vaginal delivery can be undertaken for a primigravida after appropriate counselling and for a multigravida with a previous vaginal delivery provided that the criteria discussed below are met.

Criteria for vaginal breech delivery

Guidelines have been published by professional bodies for the selection of candidates for vaginal breech delivery [25,26]. All guidelines emphasise the following criteria for vaginal breech delivery:

- Informed consent
- Availability of:
  - Obstetrician skilled at vaginal breech delivery
  - Intrapartum fetal monitoring
  - Facilities for immediate cesarean delivery
  - Pediatrician/neonatologist at the time of delivery

Contraindications to vaginal breech delivery

It is mandatory that there should be no contraindications to vaginal breech delivery. A fetal weight of 3.8–4 Kg is considered the upper limit by the American College of Obstetricians and Gynecologists [26]. However, since Indian women are smaller, a fetal weight of 3.5 Kg may be considered the upper limit.

The vaginal delivery of the preterm breech is associated with a poorer outcome [27,28]. The preterm fetal head is larger than the abdomen; therefore, the body tends to slip through a partially dilated cervix, leading to head entrapment, asphyxia, and fetal death. Hence, cesarean birth is recommended for preterm breech <34 weeks. For late preterm fetuses, the route of delivery must be individualised.

The contraindications to vaginal breech delivery are listed in Box 27.2.

Box 27.2 Contraindications to vaginal breech delivery

- Estimated fetal weight >4 Kg
- Incomplete (footling) breech
- Preterm breech
- Placenta previa
- Hyperextended fetal head
- Oligohydramnios
- Severe fetal growth restriction
- Abnormal pelvic configuration

Vaginal breech delivery

When all the criteria for vaginal breech delivery are met, this option should be discussed with the woman, and her informed consent should be obtained. Contraindications must be excluded. The important clinical points to be remembered include the following:

- Induction of labour is usually not recommended in breech presentation [29]
- Any delay in the progress of labour in breech presentation is considered to be indicative of fetopelvic disproportion. Hence, oxytocin augmentation should be used with great caution
- Membranes should not be ruptured early
- Electronic fetal monitoring is recommended

When the woman is admitted to the labour suite with spontaneous labour pains, preparations should be made for the conduct of assisted breech delivery. A skilled senior obstetrician, an assistant, and a neonatologist must be available. Epidural analgesia may be used if available. Uterine contractions and the progress of labour should be monitored. A partograph should be maintained. Alternative birthing positions may be considered over the supine position.

Procedure of assisted breech delivery

When the cervix is fully dilated and the mother has pushing pains, she is placed in the lithotomy position, and brought to the edge of the delivery table. An episiotomy is performed when the fetal anus is visible at the introitus between contractions. **The fetus should be allowed to deliver spontaneously till the umbilicus.** The feet may be hooked out if required.

If the legs are extended, a hand should be passed along the fetal thigh to the popliteal fossa, and gentle pressure should be applied to flex the leg (**Pinard manoeuvre**). The foot can then be grasped and pulled down.

The umbilical cord is moved to one side to avoid compression while the rest of the baby is born.

The fetus is wrapped in a towel to avoid cutaneous stimulation and is held in a **femoropelvic grip** by placing the thumbs on the sacrum and the index fingers on the iliac crests (Fig. 27.6). The back of the fetus should face the obstetrician throughout the procedure.

When the inferior angle of the scapula is visible, the anterior arm may be helped out by bringing it down over the chest, simultaneously rotating the fetus a little toward the opposite side.

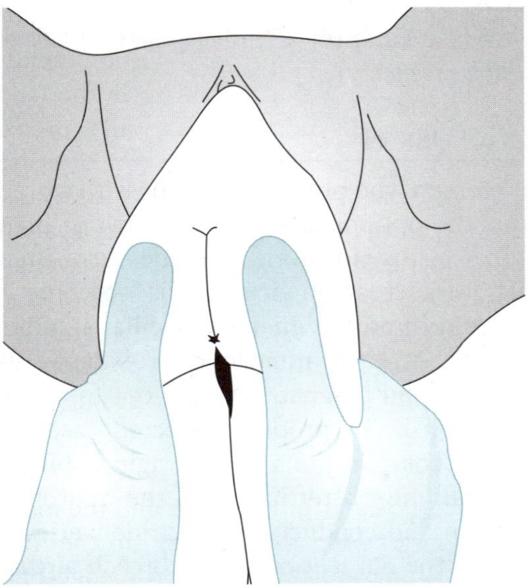

Fig. 27.6 The fetus is held in the femoropelvic grip

If the arms are extended, the fetus should be rotated through 90 degrees and then in the opposite direction through 180 degrees to bring the posterior arm to lie under the pubic symphysis (**Loveset manoeuvre**). This allows the baby to be delivered easily.

If the forearms are behind the occiput (**nuchal arms**), the fetus should be rotated in the direction in which the fetal fingers point.

The **aftercoming head** is delivered by one of the two commonly used manoeuvres described below, or with forceps (see **Chapter 26**, *Operative vaginal delivery*).

Burns–Marshall technique: After the shoulders are delivered, the baby is allowed to hang by its own weight until its hairline becomes visible (Fig. 27.7a).

- Flexion of the head is facilitated by suprapubic pressure applied by the assistant.
- The baby is held with the obstetrician's thumb and ring finger on either side of the feet and the index or middle finger between the heels and swung in an arc over the mother's abdomen (Fig. 27.7b).
- The head is delivered with the assistant providing perineal support.

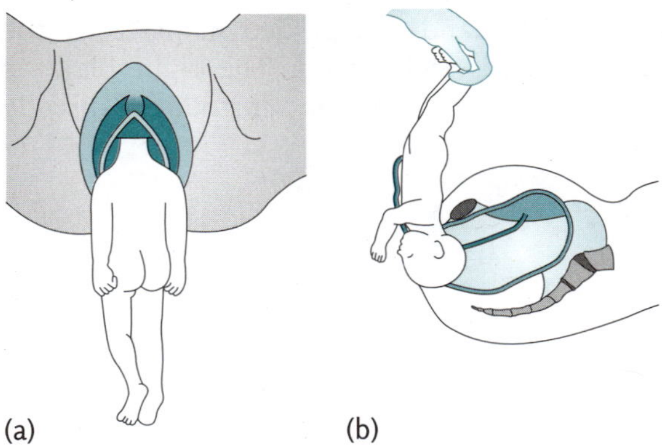

Fig. 27.7 Delivery of the head by the Burns–Marshall technique: (a) The body is allowed to hang by its weight till the hairline is visible and (b) the baby is swung in an arc over the mother's abdomen

Mauriceau–Smellie–Veit technique: After the shoulders are delivered, the baby is held astride the obstetrician's left forearm. The index finger of the right hand is placed on one shoulder and the middle and ring fingers on the other shoulder.

The index and middle fingers of the obstetrician's left hand are placed on each maxilla (Fig. 27.8). Gentle downward traction is applied with the right hand till the nape of the neck is visible. The assistant applies suprapubic pressure. There is no pressure exerted by the left hand which is placed on the maxilla. One should avoid placing a finger in the baby's mouth.

The fetus is lifted toward the mother's abdomen and the mouth, nose, and forehead are delivered in that order.

Delivery by forceps: Forceps delivery may be used as the method of choice. Piper's forceps have the advantage of a good perineal curve for the delivery of the aftercoming head. However, any low forceps can be used.

Once the nape of the neck is visible, the baby is wrapped in a sterile towel and lifted up by the assistant. The blades of the forceps are applied from below. The left blade is held in the left hand and guided in place by the obstetrician's right hand. The right blade is held in the right hand and introduced directly (Fig. 27.9).

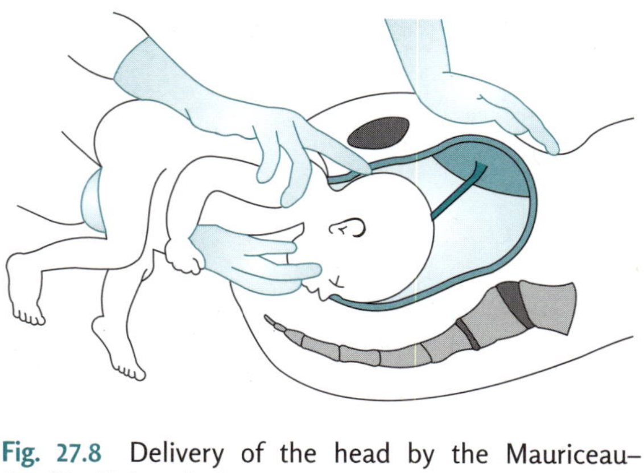

Fig. 27.8 Delivery of the head by the Mauriceau–Smellie–Veit technique

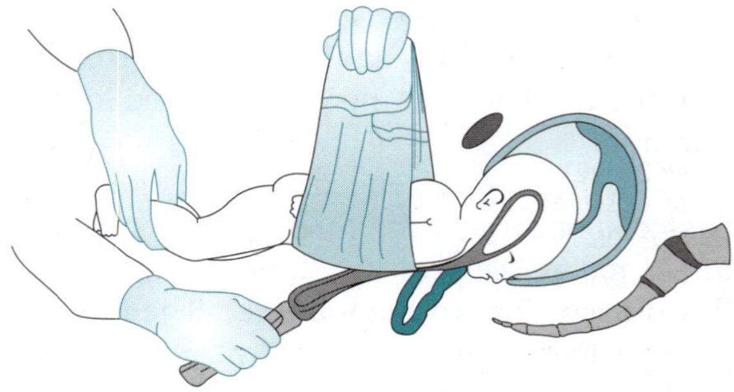

Fig. 27.9 Delivery of the aftercoming head by forceps

Key Point

In assisted breech delivery, there should be no intervention till the fetus is delivered up to the umbilicus. The preferred method of delivery of the aftercoming head is by forceps.

Breech extraction

This refers to the complete extraction of the breech without allowing spontaneous delivery till the umbilicus. Breech extraction is usually performed following internal podalic version and is used in the delivery of the second of twins (see **Chapter 17**, *Management of labour in multiple pregnancy*).

CONCLUSION

For women who present in labour with a breech fetus, the options are cesarean birth or breech vaginal birth. However, after the Term Breech Trial [15], cesarean delivery has become the preferred approach in most facilities offering obstetric care. A minority of obstetric care providers and pregnant women opt for vaginal breech birth. In properly selected cases, the risk of complications with vaginal birth is low. Training obstetricians in the appropriate selection and conduct of breech deliveries can increase the number of vaginal breech births.

REFERENCES

1. Hickok DE, Gordon DC, Milberg JA, et al. The frequency of breech presentation by gestational age at birth: A

large population-based study. *Am J Obstet Gynecol.* 1992. 166:851.

2. H Cammu, N Dony, G Martens, R Colman. Common determinants of breech presentation at birth in singletons: A population-based study. *European Journal of Obstetrics & Gynecology Reproductive Biology.* 2014. 177: 106.
3. Noli SA, Baini I, Parazzini F, et al. Preterm birth, low gestational age, low birthweight, parity, and other determinants of breech presentation: Results from a large retrospective population-based study. *Biomed Res Int.* 2019. 9581439.
4. Toijonen AE, Heinonen ST, Gissler MVM, Macharey G. A comparison of risk factors for breech presentation in preterm and term labor: A nationwide, population-based case-control study. *Arch Gynecol Obstet.* 2020. 301:393.
5. Macharey G, Gissler M, Toijonen A, et al. Congenital anomalies in breech presentation: A nationwide record linkage study. *Congenit Anom* (Kyoto). 2021. 61:112.
6. Mostello D, Chang JJ, Bai F, et al. Breech presentation at delivery: A marker for congenital anomaly? *J Perinatol.* 2014. 34:11.
7. Hofmeyer GJ, Kulier R, West HM. External cephalic version for breech presentation at term. *Cochrane Database Syst Rev.* 2015. Issue 4. Art. No.:CD000083.
8. Grootscholten K, Kok M, Oei SG, et al. External cephalic version-related risks: A meta-analysis. *Obstet Gynecol* 2008. 112:1143.
9. Melo P, Georgiou EX, Hedditch A, et al. External cephalic version at term: A cohort study of 18 years' experience. *BJOG.* 2019. 126(4):493.
10. Devold Pay AS, Johansen K, Staff AC, et al. Effects of external cephalic version for breech presentation at or near term in high-resource settings: A systematic review of randomized and non-randomized studies. *Eur J Midwifery.* 2020. 4:44.
11. External Cephalic Version. ACOG Practice Bulletin, Number 221. *Obstet Gynecol.* 2020. 135:e203.
12. Impey LWM, Murphy DJ, Griffiths M, Penna LK on behalf of the Royal College of Obstetricians and Gynaecologists. External Cephalic Version and Reducing the Incidence of Term Breech Presentation. *BJOG2017*; 124: e178–e192.
13. Hutton EK, Hofmeyr GJ, Dowswell T. External cephalic version for breech presentation before term. *Cochrane Database Syst Rev.* 2015. Issue 7. Art. No.:CD000084.
14. Collins S, Ellaway P, Harrington D, et al. The complications of external cephalic version: Results from 805 consecutive attempts. *BJOG.* 2007. 114:636.
15. Hannah ME, Hannah WJ, Hewson SA, et al. Planned caesarean section versus planned vaginal birth for breech presentation at term: A randomised multicentre trial. Term Breech Trial Collaborative Group. *Lancet.* 2000. 356:1375.
16. Lumbiganon P, Laopaiboon M, Gülmezoglu AM, et al. Method of delivery and pregnancy outcomes in Asia: The WHO global survey on maternal and perinatal health 2007–08. *Lancet.* 2010. 375(9713):490.
17. Berhan Y, Haileamlak A. The risks of planned vaginal breech delivery versus planned caesarean section for term breech birth: A meta-analysis including observational studies. *BJOG.* 2016. 123(1):49.
18. Lyons J, Pressey T, Bartholomew S, Liu S, Liston RM, Joseph KS. The Canadian Perinatal Surveillance System (Public Health Agency of Canada). Delivery of breech presentation at term gestation in Canada, 2003–2011. *Obstet Gynecol.* 2015. 125:1153.
19. Hofmeyr GJ, Hannah M, Lawrie TA. Planned caesarean section for term breech delivery. *Cochrane Database Syst Rev.* 2015. Issue 7. Art. No.:CD000166.
20. Goffinet F, Carayol M, Foidart JM, et al. Is planned vaginal delivery for breech presentation at term still an option? Results of an observational prospective survey in France and Belgium. *Am J Obstet Gynecol.* 2006. 194:1002.
21. Michel S, Drain A, Closset E, et al. Evaluation of a decision protocol for type of delivery of infants in breech presentation at term. *Eur J Obstet Gynecol Reprod Biol.* 2011. 158(2):194.
22. Martel-Santiago CR, Arencibia-Díaz RD, Romero-Requejo A, et al. Delivery in breech presentation: Perinatal outcome and neurodevelopmental evaluation at 18 months of life. *Eur J Obstet Gynecol Reprod Biol.* 2020. 255:147.
23. Wängberg Nordborg J, Svanberg T, Strandell A, Carlsson Y. Term breech presentation-Intended cesarean section versus intended vaginal delivery. A systematic review and meta-analysis. *Acta Obstet Gynecol Scand.* 2022. 101:564.
24. Tsakiridis I, Mamopoulos A, Athanasiadis A, Dagklis T. Management of breech presentation: A comparison of four national evidence-based guidelines. *Am J Perinatol.* 2020. 37(11):1102.
25. ACOG Committee Opinion No. 745: Mode of Term Singleton Breech Delivery. *Obstet Gynecol* 2018. 132:e60.
26. Reddy UM, Zhang J, Sun L, et al. Neonatal mortality by attempted route of delivery in early preterm birth. *Am J Obstet Gynecol.* 2012. 207(2):117.
27. Bergenhenegouwen L, Vlemmix F, Ensing S, et al. Preterm breech presentation: A comparison of intended vaginal and intended cesarean delivery. *Obstet Gynecol.* 2015. 126(6):1223.
28. Sun W, Liu F, Liu S, et al. Comparison of outcomes between induction of labor and spontaneous labor for term breech: A systemic review and meta-analysis. *Eur J Obstet Gynecol Reprod Biol.* 2018. 222:155.

CHAPTER 28

Shoulder Dystocia
Prevention and Management

B S SUSHEELA RANI

INTRODUCTION

Shoulder dystocia is a dreaded emergency during vaginal delivery which adversely affects fetal and maternal outcomes. It occurs when one or both shoulders become impacted in the maternal pelvis. Quite often described as the 'obstetrician's nightmare', it can happen when least expected and can challenge the most experienced obstetricians.

Shoulder dystocia is also one of the most common obstetric situations leading to litigation.

Definition

Shoulder dystocia is defined as a condition where after the delivery of the head, the shoulders fail to be delivered by the usual gentle traction and require additional obstetric manoeuvres.

An objective definition of shoulder dystocia as proposed by Spong and colleagues [1] is "prolonged head-to-body delivery time (e.g., more than 60 seconds) or the need for ancillary obstetric manoeuvres".

Incidence

Shoulder dystocia occurs in 0.2–3% of deliveries [2]. There is a wide variation in the incidence since it may not be reported uniformly.

MECHANISM OF LABOUR IN SHOULDER DYSTOCIA

At the beginning of normal labour, the shoulders are above the anteroposterior diameter of the pelvic inlet. As labour progresses, they enter the pelvic inlet through the oblique diameter or the larger transverse diameter. The posterior shoulder descends ahead of the anterior shoulder. By the time the head is delivered, the shoulders have entered the pelvis, the shoulders rotating to the anteroposterior diameter of the pelvic outlet. The delivery of the shoulders quickly follows the delivery of the head, and the baby is born.

When there is shoulder dystocia, the shoulders are unable to enter the pelvic inlet even after the head is born. Generally, the posterior shoulder enters the sacral hollow, and the anterior shoulder remains just above the pubic symphysis. Occasionally, the posterior shoulder is lodged behind the maternal sacral promontory. Rarely, both shoulders remain at the pelvic inlet and with the head delivered, all that remains in the pelvic cavity is the fetal neck.

Key Point

When there is shoulder dystocia, one or both shoulders are unable to enter the pelvic inlet even after the head is born.

RISK FACTORS FOR SHOULDER DYSTOCIA

Though there are a number of factors associated with the risk of shoulder dystocia, they are not sensitive enough to predict shoulder dystocia by themselves [3]. 50% of cases of shoulder dystocia can occur in women with no risk factors. Based on the known risk factors, several scoring systems have been developed to predict shoulder dystocia, though none have proven useful clinically. The risk factors for shoulder dystocia can be categorised as follows (Table 28.1):

- Preconceptional
- Antepartum
- Intrapartum

Table 28.1 **Risk factors for shoulder dystocia**

Preconceptional factors	Antepartum factors	Intrapartum factors
• History of shoulder dystocia or baby with brachial plexus injury • Maternal diabetes • Maternal obesity • Increased maternal age • Multiparity	• Macrosomia • Gestational diabetes • Excessive weight gain • Postdated pregnancy • Male baby	• Prolonged labour • Precipitate labour • Instrumental delivery

Key Point

It is important to remember that 50% of cases of shoulder dystocia occur in women with no risk factors.

Preconceptional Factors

A woman with a history of shoulder dystocia has a 10–15% risk of facing shoulder dystocia in the next pregnancy. Increased BMI, diabetes, obesity, and advanced maternal age are some of the maternal risk factors. Many of these risk factors are interrelated and contribute to increasing the risk when they occur together.

Antepartum Factors

Macrosomia

Macrosomia is defined as a fetus that is large for gestational age (>90th per centile). Western countries define macrosomia as an infant weighing >4000–4500 g at any gestational age [4]. However, this is not applicable to Indian babies. The data from the World Health Organization's Global Survey on Maternal and Perinatal Health showed that only 0.5% of babies in India are born weighing >4000 g as compared to 5–20% in high-income countries (HICs) [5]. Even within the country, the definition of macrosomia may differ between the urban and the rural populations and between different socio-economic classes.

In India, if the definition of macrosomia being >90th percentile is applied, a fetus weighing >3250 g at term would be considered to have macrosomia. Even if the cut-off were the 95th percentile, a fetus weighing >3500 g would be considered macrosomic [5].

In a study by Acker et al. [6], the incidence of shoulder dystocia in non-diabetic gravidas delivering an infant weighing 4000–4499 g and 4500+ g vaginally was 10.0 and 22.6% respectively. **For the same weights, the incidence doubled when the mother was diabetic** (Table 28.2). See the section below on *Maternal diabetes*.

Key Point

In India, a fetus weighing >3250–3500 g at term is considered to have macrosomia by definition [5] and may be at risk of shoulder dystocia.

Table 28.2 **Fetal weights in non-diabetic and diabetic pregnant women and the corresponding incidence of shoulder dystocia [2]**

Estimated fetal weight	Rate of shoulder dystocia (%)	
	Non-diabetic pregnant women	Diabetic pregnant women
<4000 g	1.1	3.7
4000–4499 g	10	23.1
>5000 g	22.6	50

Excessive gestational weight gain and post-dated pregnancies are associated with macrosomia and therefore contribute to shoulder dystocia. A higher birth weight in male babies could similarly contribute to shoulder dystocia.

Estimation of fetal weight

The estimation of fetal weight can be done clinically and by ultrasound. However, the sensitivity of the clinical and ultrasonographic prediction of macrosomia (defined as a birth weight >4000 g) is 68% and 58% respectively.

Predictability of birth weight by ultrasound is poorer at higher birth weights (see **Chapter 34**, *Management of labour with fetal macrosomia*). 70–90% of macrosomic infants are delivered vaginally without any shoulder dystocia. On the other hand, 40–60% of cases of shoulder dystocia occur in infants who weigh <4000 g.

> **Key Point**
>
> The sensitivity of clinical and ultrasonographic prediction of macrosomia (defined as birth weight >4000 g) is 68% and 58% respectively. The predictability by ultrasound is poorer at higher birth weights.

Maternal diabetes

The body composition and weight distribution of infants born to diabetic mothers differ from the norm even in the absence of macrosomia. Such infants have larger shoulder and extremity circumferences, a decreased head-to-shoulder ratio, significantly higher body fat, and thicker upper extremity skinfolds compared to non-diabetic control infants of similar birth weight and birth length. These differences in body composition can make the descent of the shoulders into the pelvis difficult and contribute to shoulder dystocia [7].

Intrapartum Risk Factors

Instrumental vaginal delivery

The risk of shoulder dystocia is significantly higher in operative vaginal delivery when the intervention is associated with macrosomia, a prolonged second stage of labour, and mid-pelvic delivery [3]. In such a situation, the incidence of shoulder dystocia can be as high as 21% [8].

Abnormal progress of labour

A large multicentre study found that a prolonged second stage was not associated with a statistically significant increase in the risk of shoulder dystocia among both nulliparous and multiparous women [9].

DIAGNOSIS OF SHOULDER DYSTOCIA

Shoulder dystocia is typically diagnosed when, once the head is delivered, the face and chin are delivered with difficulty, the chin has to be hooked over the perineum, or the perineum has to be pushed back to allow the chin to be delivered. In some cases, the head attempts to recede into the vulva, the face turns blue, the baby's cheeks bulge out—resembling a turtle pulling its head back into its shell ('turtle sign'), and despite good bearing down efforts by the mother and gentle traction on the fetal head, there is no further progress.

COMPLICATIONS OF SHOULDER DYSTOCIA

The incidence of complications associated with shoulder dystocia increases with the number of manoeuvres required to deliver the baby. The delivery of the posterior shoulder is most successful in delivering the infant and should be resorted to early to avoid multiple manoeuvres [10].

Neonatal Complications

In a large series of 132,098 women who delivered a term cephalic liveborn fetus vaginally, 2018 had shoulder dystocia and 101 (5.2%) of these incurred a neonatal injury [10].

Brachial plexus injury

The most common complication of shoulder dystocia is unilateral brachial plexus injury (BPI) [3,11]. Downward lateral traction (i.e., bending the neck away from the anterior shoulder and toward the posterior shoulder) causes more stretching of the brachial plexus than downward axial traction (i.e., applying force parallel to the fetal spine). BPI is seen in 2–16% of deliveries with shoulder dystocia.

It is important to remember that brachial plexus injury may occur even in the absence of shoulder dystocia or identifiable risk factors [12]. It has been documented even without excessive traction being applied in the following clinical situations:

- In the posterior arm of infants whose anterior shoulder was impacted behind the symphysis pubis
- In vertex-presenting fetuses delivered by cesarean section where there was absolutely no difficulty in delivering the fetus
- Without any apparent relationship to the type or number of manoeuvres used to disimpact the fetal shoulder
- In association with other peripheral nerve injuries

Key Point

Though brachial plexus injury is the commonest neonatal complication of shoulder dystocia, its presence alone is not evidence that shoulder dystocia has occurred [3]. Cases of severe brachial plexus palsy have been documented in the absence of shoulder dystocia and without identifiable risk factors [12].

Erb palsy

50% of the cases of BPI result in **Erb palsy** (C5 and C6 injury) [13]. This leads to weakness of the deltoid, infraspinatus, and biceps muscles. The upper arm is abducted and internally rotated and the forearm is extended. **Erb palsy plus** (C5, C6, and C7 injury) accounts for 35% of cases of BPI [13] and manifests as the adduction and internal rotation of the arm, extension and pronation of the forearm, and flexion of the wrists and fingers resulting in the typical 'policeman's tip' posture.

Most infants with BPI recover in the first three months after birth and a few recover within one year. 10% of BPI cases result in permanent neurological injury. Surgical intervention may be required in a few.

Fractures

Fracture of the **humerus** is more commonly seen in cases of manual removal of the posterior arm. **Clavicular fracture** is less common and when it does occur, heals well without any major intervention.

Hypoxic–ischemic encephalopathy (HIE)

Shoulder dystocia may lead to hypoxic–ischemic encephalopathy and death. Compression of the umbilical cord leading to hypoxia is the proposed mechanism.

Neonatal hypovolemia and cardiac asystole

Rare cases of cardiac asystole at birth have been reported that occur even though the fetus may have had a reassuring tracing just before birth. Mercer and colleagues [14] hypothesised that severe hypovolemia due to umbilical cord compression, which occurs in shoulder dystocia, results in asystole at birth. Cord compression transfers blood to the placenta via the firm-walled arteries but prevents blood from returning to the infant via the soft-walled umbilical vein, resulting in the loss of blood into the placenta. When immediate cord clamping is done to resuscitate the neonate, it further limits the newborn's access to this blood after birth. In a neonate so resuscitated, the loss of this large a blood volume may initiate an inflammatory response that can enhance neuropathologic processes including seizures, hypoxic–ischemic encephalopathy, and death. Leaving the cord intact (allowing for the return of the umbilical cord circulation) for several minutes after birth may allow most of the sequestered blood to return to the infant [14]. Umbilical cord milking may return enough of the blood volume to restart the heart. When a fetus is more depressed than anticipated or is born with pallor and an absent heart rate after delivery in cases of shoulder dystocia, **the obstetrician should delay cord ligature, and neonatologists should consider volume resuscitation.**

Maternal Complications

- **Postpartum hemorrhage** is seen in 11% of cases of shoulder dystocia [3]. PPH can be a result of uterine atony resulting from prolonged labour, overdistension of the uterus, or trauma following instrumental delivery. It is not related to the manoeuvres used to resolve dystocia.

- **Cervical and vaginal lacerations** and **third- and fourth-degree tears** are often due to manipulations to resolve shoulder dystocia.
- **Rupture of the uterus** can occur due to manoeuvres to resolve shoulder dystocia.
- **Bladder atony** can result due to pressure on the bladder by the anterior shoulder against the maternal pubic symphysis.
- **Separation of the symphyseal joint** and damage to the lateral femoral cutaneous nerve can occur as a result of overaggressive hyperflexion of the maternal legs during attempts to resolve the shoulder dystocia.

Neonatal and maternal complications of shoulder dystocia are summarised in Table 28.3.

Table 28.3 Neonatal and maternal complications of shoulder dystocia

Neonatal	Maternal
Brachial plexus injury	Postpartum hemorrhage
Fractures	Cervical/vaginal lacerations
Asphyxia	Bladder injury
Hypoxic–ischemic encephalopathy	Perineal damage
Neonatal hypovolemia, hypoxia	Uterine rupture
Death	Psychological impact and postpartum depression

TIME AVAILABLE TO RESOLVE SHOULDER DYSTOCIA

Wood et al. [15] studied the progress of acidemia in a neonate during normal birth and reported that the pH of umbilical artery blood diminishes at the rate of 0.04 pH units per minute. Based on this, it was believed that a delay beyond 7 minutes could result in dangerous acidemia in the neonate. The data Wood et al. referred to concerned normal births without any difficulty, and the results cannot be extrapolated to cases with shoulder dystocia where other factors come into play such as the following [16]:

- Traction of the neck with consequent vagal stimulation
- Compression of the abdomen and chest with the consequent transfer of blood from the body to the placenta

A previously well-oxygenated term fetus will tolerate up to 5 minutes of a head-to-body delivery interval before the risk of asphyxial injury increases [17]. However, the deterioration of the fetal condition can be rapid and hence, shoulder dystocia should be resolved as quickly as possible.

MANAGEMENT OF SHOULDER DYSTOCIA

General Guidelines

Though shoulder dystocia might be anticipated in some cases, most often, it comes as a surprise to the labour room team.

- Once a diagnosis is made, the situation needs to be quickly explained to the woman and her birth companion and their cooperation is solicited.
- The pre-arranged protocol should be activated, and more senior/trained staff should be brought into the labour room. Help should be sought from a colleague or a senior obstetrician, an anesthetist, and a neonatologist/pediatrician.
- The woman should be brought to the edge of the labour table.
- An episiotomy is not essential but may be performed to allow better access to the fetus if internal manoeuvres are to be performed.
- If the cord is wound around the neck, it **should not** be clamped and cut. Doing so can cause or aggravate hypovolemia in the fetus (see the section below on *Procedures to be avoided in shoulder dystocia*).
- One member of the labour room staff should be assigned to keep track and call out the time and document the manoeuvre/s employed.

Manoeuvres to Resolve Shoulder Dystocia

McRoberts manoeuvre

The woman is placed in the McRoberts position (legs hyperflexed; Fig. 28.1a–c). This position causes the rotation of the symphysis pubis superiorly by a distance of 8 cm. The angle of inclination is reduced from 26 to 10 degrees, and although the manoeuvre does not actually change the dimensions of the pelvis, it may free the impacted shoulder. Around 40% of cases of shoulder dystocia are resolved by the McRoberts manoeuvre alone. Using a computer simulation model, Gonik et al. [18] studied the effect on the stretching of the brachial plexus by the maternal bearing down forces and traction on the fetal neck applied by the clinician. They found that McRoberts positioning reduces the stretching significantly.

Key Point

Around 40% cases of shoulder dystocia are resolved by the McRoberts manoeuvre alone. This position also significantly reduces the stretching of the brachial plexus caused by maternal bearing down forces and the traction on the fetal neck applied by the clinician.

McRoberts manoeuvre with suprapubic pressure (Rubin I manoeuvre)

While the obstetrician performs gentle downward traction on the fetal head, another member of the team applies pressure suprapubically (**not** fundally) over the anterior shoulder (Fig. 28.2). Pressure is applied over the fetal back in order to adduct the shoulder, with the heel of the assistant's hand (cardiopulmonary resuscitation fashion) moving in a downward and lateral motion on the posterior aspect of the impacted shoulder. Initially, the pressure can be continuous, but if delivery is not accomplished, a rocking motion is recommended to dislodge the shoulder from behind the pubic symphysis.

If McRoberts manoeuvre combined with suprapubic pressure is not successful in resolving shoulder dystocia, any/all of the following manoeuvres are performed.

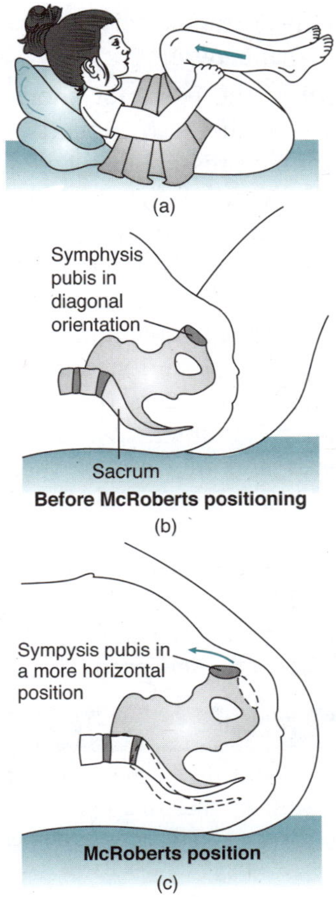

Fig. 28.1 McRoberts manoeuvre: (a) The woman hyperflexes her legs, causing the diagonally-oriented pubic sympyhsis (b) to become more horizontal, along with flattening of the sacrum, (c) allowing the anterior shoulder to deliver

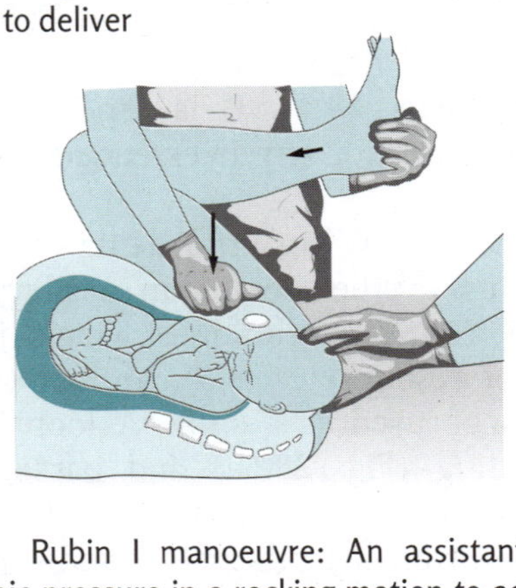

Fig. 28.2 Rubin I manoeuvre: An assistant applies suprapubic pressure in a rocking motion to adduct the fetal shoulder

Delivery of the posterior arm (Jacquemier manoeuvre)

The delivery of the posterior shoulder should be the next step if the McRoberts manoeuvre with suprapubic pressure has failed to deliver the baby. Delivery of the posterior shoulder is associated with the highest rate of delivery when compared to other manoeuvres [10]. The need for additional manoeuvres is associated with higher rates of neonatal injury.

Extracting the posterior arm reduces the diameter of the shoulders that needs to pass through the pelvic inlet. When the posterior arm is flexed and in front of the chest, the Jacquemier manoeuvre is useful (Fig. 28.3). Here, the operator's hand is introduced into the posterior vagina, passed along the humerus, and the elbow is identified and flexed (Fig. 28.3a). Then, the forearm is grasped (Fig. 28.3b), swept across the chest and delivered (Fig. 28.3c).

> **Key Point**
>
> For the delivery of the posterior arm, if the fetal abdomen faces the maternal right, the operator's left hand is used, and if the fetal abdomen faces the maternal left, the right hand is used.

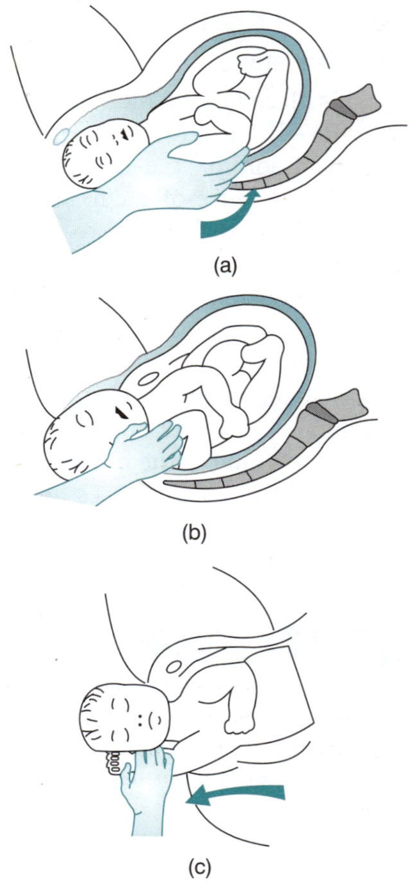

Fig. 28.3 Delivery of the posterior arm using the Jacquemier manoeuvre: (a) The operator's hand is passed along the humerus and the elbow identified, (b) the elbow is flexed, and the forearm is grasped; (c) the forearm is swept across the chest and delivered

Posterior axillary traction (Menticoglou manoeuvre)

This technique involves applying traction on the posterior axilla by hooking the middle fingers of both hands under it [19] while an assistant holds the fetal head and flexes it upward and anteriorly (Fig. 28.4). It is especially useful when the posterior arm is extended and above the pelvic brim.

Traction on the posterior axilla can also be applied using the **posterior axillary sling traction** (PAST) technique, which involves the use of a sling (Fig. 28.5). An infant feeding tube can be used as a sling. A loop is made in the sling (Fig. 28.5a) and passed under the posterior axilla (Fig. 28.5b). The sling is brought out on the other side, and traction is applied (Fig. 28.5c). The sling can also be used to apply lateral traction towards the fetal back

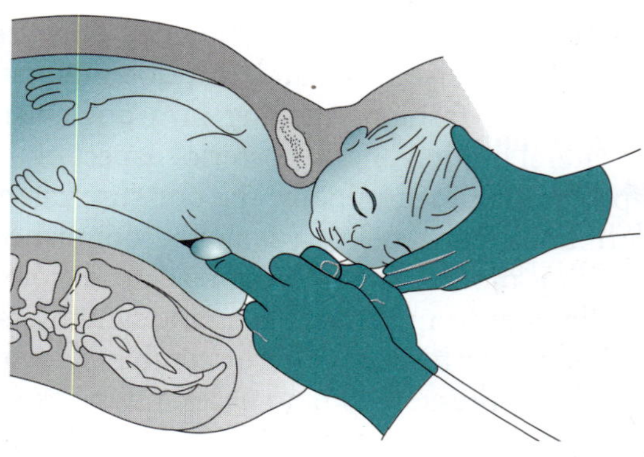

Fig. 28.4 Menticoglou manoeuvre

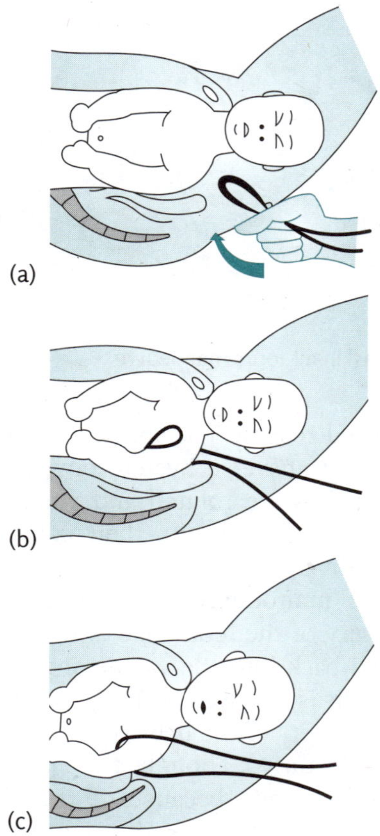

Fig. 28.5 Posterior axillary sling traction with a catheter or infant feeding tube used as a sling: (a) A loop is made in the sling, (b) the loop is passed under the posterior axilla, and (c) the sling is brought out on the other side and traction is applied

while an assistant applies suprapubic pressure, thereby assisting the shoulders to rotate to the oblique diameter of the inlet.

Secondary manoeuvres

Rubin II manoeuvre

The operator's hand is inserted into the vagina anteriorly and used to apply digital pressure to the posterior aspect of the anterior shoulder, pushing it towards the fetal chest (Fig. 28.6). This should bring the impacted anterior shoulder from the anteroposterior diameter of the pelvic inlet into the larger oblique diameter, allowing the anterior shoulder to slip into the pelvis.

Woods screw manoeuvre

If the Rubin II manoeuvre is unsuccessful, the other hand is inserted in the vagina posteriorly and used to apply digital pressure to the anterior aspect of the posterior shoulder to push it away from the chest (Fig. 28.7). This, combined with the pressure on the anterior shoulder, will bring the bisacromial diameter from the anteroposterior diameter of the pelvic inlet to the larger oblique diameter so that the anterior shoulder can move into the pelvis.

Reverse Woods screw manoeuvre

In this manoeuvre, the direction of the pressure is reversed. The anterior shoulder is pushed away from the chest and the posterior shoulder is pushed towards the chest in a clockwise direction (Fig. 28.8). The objective is to push

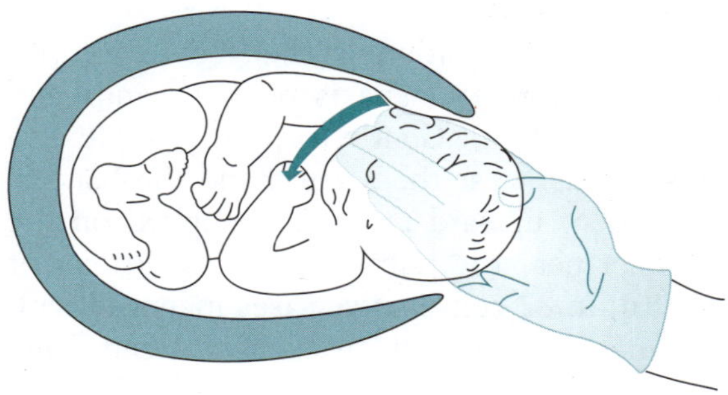

Fig. 28.6 Rubin II manoeuvre

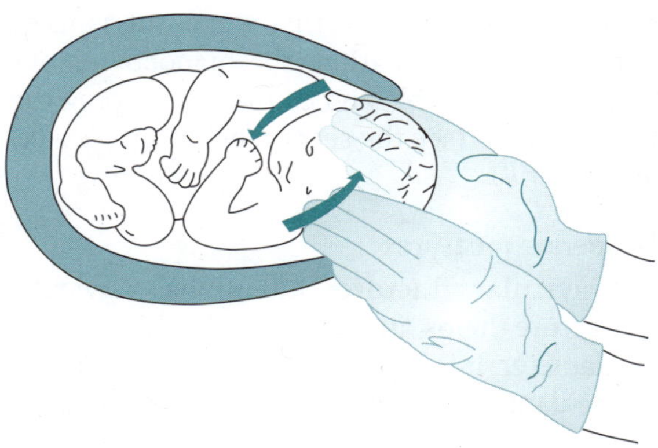

Fig. 28.7 Combined Rubin II and Woods manoeuvre

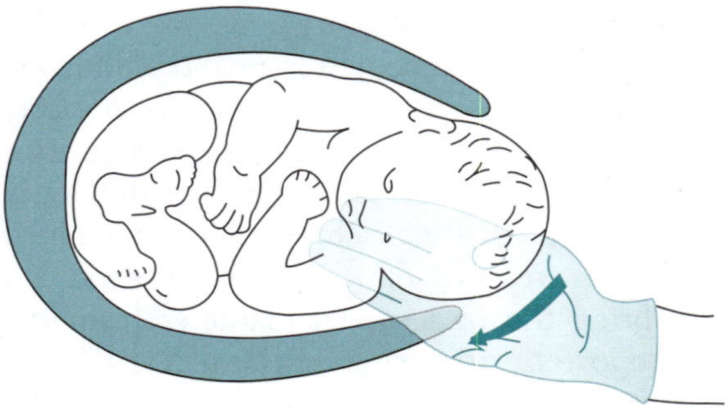

Fig. 28.8 Reverse Woods screw manoeuvre

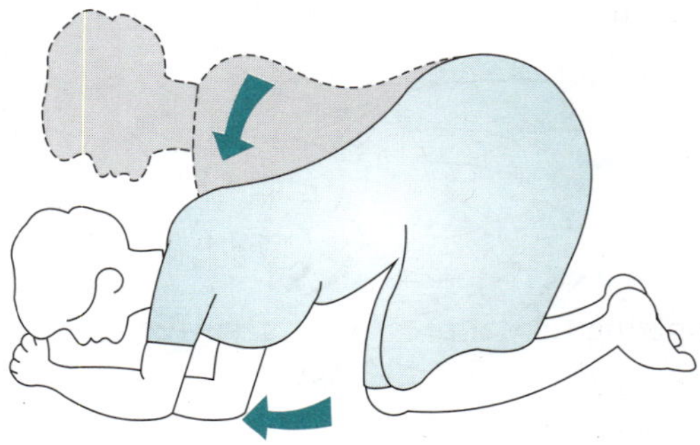

Fig. 28.9 Gaskin all-fours manoeuvre

the shoulders so that the bisacromial diameter moves from the anteroposterior diameter of the pelvic inlet to the other oblique diameter of the inlet.

Other manoeuvres

Gaskin manoeuvre

The woman's position is changed to the all-fours position, i.e., she is on her hands and knees (Fig. 28.9). Gentle traction is applied to the shoulder near the sacrum and the hand is released or upward traction is applied on the shoulder near the pubic symphysis. Bruner et al. [20], in 82 consecutive cases managed with this manoeuvre, found it to be a rapid, safe, and effective technique for resolving shoulder dystocia.

It is imperative for an obstetrician to be adept at performing all the manoeuvres. Periodic drills should be organised so that when one is faced with a real-life situation, the manoeuvres one is most comfortable and confident of doing can be performed (see the section below on *Shoulder dystocia drill*).

Desperate measures

- **Clavicular fracture:** Intentional clavicular fracture helps in reducing the bisacromial diameter. It is technically difficult and carries the danger of injury to major vessels and the fetal lungs.
- **Abdominal rescue**: The abdomen is opened and a low transverse hysterotomy is done. The shoulders are rotated and pushed into the pelvis. An assistant then conducts a vaginal delivery.
- **Zavanelli manoeuvre**: The mechanism of the delivery of the fetal head is reversed—it is pushed back into the vagina and into the uterus. This is followed by a cesarean section and the delivery of the baby.
- **Symphysiotomy**: Though this procedure is not often done because of the lack of expertise and resources, it may save the lives of both the mother and baby in LMICs. A review of literature suggests that, in terms of maternal risk, a symphysiotomy compares favourably with a cesarean birth [21].

Technique

A Foley catheter is inserted into the bladder. The mons pubis over the symphysial joint is infiltrated with a local anesthetic. A finger is placed in the anterior vaginal wall and used to gently push the urethra to the side and guard the fetal head. A sharp incision is made on the mons, through the skin, subcutaneous tissue, and cartilage. This separation provides an additional 3 cm for the shoulders to pass through. Although the ensuing pain keeps the mother bound to the bed for the next three weeks, both the mother and baby generally do well. Abduction at the hip joint should be avoided for the next 7–10 days.

Procedures to be Avoided in Shoulder Dystocia

Fundal pressure

Applying fundal pressure can further aggravate the impaction of the shoulder at the symphysis pubis. It is associated with a high rate of brachial plexus injury, uterine rupture, and hemorrhage from the potential detachment of the fundal placenta.

Clamping or cutting of the nuchal cord before delivering the shoulders

Cutting a tight nuchal cord prior to the birth of the shoulders may increase the infant's risk of asphyxia, cerebral palsy, and even death in the presence of severe shoulder dystocia. It is advisable to maintain an intact cord as far as possible. Once the shoulders are delivered, it is best to slip the cord over the head or down around the shoulders and slide the baby through the cord.

Episiotomy

Since the primary problem in shoulder dystocia is a bony impaction, **an episiotomy by itself will not release the impaction.** However, if internal rotation manoeuvres are required, an episiotomy does provide additional room for the physician's hand.

POSTPARTUM DOCUMENTATION

Shoulder dystocia is among the four most common causes of litigation in obstetrics.

Documentation in the Immediate Postpartum Period

This is an extremely important step. Complete and accurate information regarding any difficulty in delivery, the manoeuvres used, and the condition of the neonate and the mother at the end of the procedure should be recorded. The following facts should be documented [22]:

- Time of delivery of the head
- Time at which shoulder dystocia was first noted
- Who was called for help
- Which shoulder was anterior
- Manoeuvres performed and their order
- The force used, described in comparative terms such as average, maximal, etc.
- Time of delivery of the baby
- Condition of the baby
- Condition of the mother

Discussion and Debriefing with the Woman and Family

It is important to speak to the woman and her family about the delivery and outcome. This is particularly essential when there has been a difficult resolution of shoulder dystocia and there is a high possibility of neonatal complications.

Medicolegal Aspects of Shoulder Dystocia

When there is a permanent brachial plexus injury following shoulder dystocia, the obstetrician is often held responsible for either not foreseeing it or for mishandling it. However, brachial plexus injury can occur even without excessive pressure being applied [23]. See the section above on *Brachial plexus injury*.

SUBSEQUENT PREGNANCY

Shoulder dystocia can recur in about 12–15% of cases. Maternal obesity, excessive weight gain during pregnancy, a prolonged second stage of labour, and an estimated fetal weight >4000 g contribute to the recurrence. The mode of delivery, cesarean or vaginal, is best decided jointly by the woman and her caregivers after considering the risk factors in the current pregnancy.

PREVENTION OF SHOULDER DYSTOCIA

It is not possible to prevent shoulder dystocia because it is not possible to predict it accurately in the first place [24].

Prophylactic cesarean section is not recommended. In non-diabetic women with macrosomia diagnosed by ultrasonography, 3695 elective cesarean deliveries would be required to prevent one permanent injury. Similarly, in diabetic women with an ultrasonographic diagnosis of macrosomia, 443 cesareans would have to be performed to prevent one permanent injury [25].

Elective induction of labour in women suspected to have macrosomic babies has **not been shown to decrease the incidence of shoulder dystocia** [3].

Identifying a fetus with disproportionate trunk or shoulder girdle growth by ultrasonography has a positive predictive value of only 5.7% and is not useful [26].

Shoulder Dystocia Drill

All obstetric units should diligently practice a shoulder dystocia drill. The specific protocols for the management of shoulder dystocia should be written down and emphasised. The proper protocol would be in the following order—McRoberts manoeuvre, suprapubic pressure, delivery of the posterior arm, and internal rotation manoeuvres.

Studies have demonstrated that simulated drills improved both the management and documentation of shoulder dystocia [27].

CONCLUSION

Shoulder dystocia is one of the most frightening emergencies in the delivery room. Although risk factors exist, most cases occur with no warning. Along with an immediate call for help from senior staff, calm and effective management of this emergency are required. Recognition of shoulder dystocia and stepwise institution of manoeuvres such as the McRoberts manoeuvre, suprapubic pressure, removal of the posterior arm or internal rotation, help relieve the impacted shoulder and allow for spontaneous delivery of the infant. All manoeuvres aid in completing one of three actions: enlarging the maternal pelvis through cephalad rotation of the symphysis and flattening of the sacrum, collapsing the fetal shoulder width, or altering the orientation of the longitudinal axis of the fetus to the plane of the obstruction. Shoulder dystocia drills should be routinely instituted in every obstetric unit. The obstetrician must ensure that the neonatal team is available for immediate resuscitation. Careful and complete documentation along with debriefing the couple are extremely important.

REFERENCES

1. Spong CY, Beall M, Rodrigues D, Ross MG. An objective definition of shoulder dystocia: Prolonged head-to-body delivery intervals and/or the use of ancillary obstetric maneuvers. *Obstet Gynecol*. 1995. 86(3):433–436.
2. Gherman RB, Chauhan S, Ouzounian JG, Lerner H, Gonik B, Goodwin TM. Shoulder dystocia: The unpreventable obstetric emergency with empiric management guidelines. *Am J Obstet Gynecol*. 2006. 195;657–72.
3. Shoulder dystocia. Practice Bulletin No. 178. American College of Obstetricians and Gynecologists. *Obstet Gynecol*. 2017 (reaffirmed 2020). 129:e123–33.
4. Macrosomia. ACOG Practice Bulletin No. 216. American College of Obstetricians and Gynecologists. *Obstet Gynecol*. 2020 (reaffirmed 2023). 135:e18–35.
5. Koyanagi A, Zhang J, Dagvadorj A, et al. Macrosomia in 23 developing countries: An analysis of a multicountry, facility-based, cross-sectional survey. *Lancet*. 2013. 381:476.
6. Acker DB, Sachs BP, Friedman EA. Risk factors for shoulder dystocia. *Obstet Gynecol*. 1985. 66(6):762-8. PMID: 4069477.
7. McFarland MB, Trylovich CG, Langer O. Anthropometric differences in macrosomic infants of diabetic and nondiabetic mothers. *J Matern Fetal Med*. 1998. 7(6):292-5. doi: 10.1002/(SICI)1520-6661(199811/12)7:6<292::AID-MFM7>3.0.CO;2-A. PMID: 9848695.
8. Benedetti TJ, Gabbe SG. Shoulder dystocia. A complication of fetal macrosomia and prolonged second stage of labor with midpelvic delivery. *Obstet Gynecol*. 1978. 52(5):526-9. PMID: 724169.
9. Laughon SK, Berghella V, Reddy UM, Sundaram R, Lu Z, Hoffman MK. Neonatal and maternal outcomes with prolonged second stage of labor. *Obstet Gynecol*. 2014. 124:57–67.
10. Hoffman MK, Bailit JL, Branch DW, et al. A comparison of obstetric maneuvers for the acute management of shoulder dystocia. *Obstet Gynecol*. 2011. 117:1272.

11. MacKenzie IZ, Shah M, Lean K, Dutton S, Newdick H, Tucker DE. Management of shoulder dystocia: Trends in incidence and maternal and neonatal morbidity. *Obstet Gynecol*. 2007. 110(5):1059-68.
12. Torki M, Barton L, Miller DA, Ouzounian JG. Severe brachial plexus palsy in women without shoulder dystocia. *Obstet Gynecol*. 2012. 120:539–41.
13. Selcen D. Neonatal brachial plexus palsy. Patterson MC (Ed). *UpToDate*. 2023. Waltham, MA.
14. Mercer J, Erickson-Owens D, Rabe H, Andersson O. Cardiac asystole at birth re-visited: Effects of acute hypovolemic shock. *Children* (Basel). 2023. 15;10(2).
15. Wood C, Ng KH, Hounslow D, Benning H. The influence of differences of birth times upon fetal condition in normal deliveries. *J Obstet Gynaecol Br Common*. 1973. 80: 289-294.
16. Beer E, Folghera MG. Time for resolving shoulder dystocia. *Am J Obstet Gynecol*. 1998. 179(5):1376-7.
17. Leung TY, Stuart O, Sahota DS, et al. Head-to-body delivery interval and risk of fetal acidosis and hypoxic ischaemic encephalopathy in shoulder dystocia: A retrospective review. *BJOG*. 2011. 118:474.
18. Gonik B, Zhang N, Grimm MJ. Prediction of brachial plexus stretching during shoulder dystocia using a computer simulation model. *Am J Obstet Gynecol*. 2003. 189(4):1168-72. doi: 10.1067/s0002-9378(03)00578-7. PMID: 14586372.
19. Menticoglou S. Shoulder dystocia: Incidence, mechanisms, and management strategies. *Int J Womens Health*. 2018. 9;10:723-732. doi: 10.2147/IJWH.S175088. PMID: 30519118; PMCID: PMC6233701.
20. Bruner JP, Drummond SB, Meenan AL, Gaskin IM. All-fours maneuver for reducing shoulder dystocia during labor. *J Reprod Med*. 1998. 43(5):439-43.
21. Björklund K. Minimally invasive surgery for obstructed labour: A review of symphysiotomy during the twentieth century (including 5000 cases). *BJOG*. 2002. 109(3):236-48.
22. Acker DB. A shoulder dystocia intervention form. *Obstet Gynecol*. 1991;78(1):150–1.
23. Steer PJ. Shoulder Dystocia and Erb's palsy: Is the accoucheur always guilty of negligence? *BJOG: Int J Obstet Gy*. 2014. 121: 43-43.
24. Hill MG, Cohen WR. Shoulder dystocia: Prediction and management. *Womens Health* (Lond). 2016. 12(2):251-61.
25. Rouse DJ, Owen J. Prophylactic cesarean delivery for fetal macrosomia diagnosed by means of ultrasonography—A Faustian bargain? *Am J Obstet Gynecol*. 1999. 181:332–8.
26. Gerber S, Goldsmith S, Sharkey J, Grobman W. Ultrasonographic prediction of shoulder dystocia risk. *Am J Obstet Gynecol*. 2008. S76.
27. Dahlberg J, Nelson M, Dahlgren MA, Blomberg M. Ten years of simulation-based shoulder dystocia training: Impact on obstetric outcome, clinical management, staff confidence, and the pedagogical practice—a time series study. *BMC Pregnancy Childbirth*. 2018. 18(1):361.

CHAPTER 29

Antepartum Hemorrhage

NISHITA MEHTA, AMARNATH BHIDE

INTRODUCTION

Antepartum hemorrhage (APH) is defined as bleeding from or into the genital tract, occurring from 24+0 weeks of pregnancy and before the birth of the baby [1]. Some guidelines define it as bleeding occurring after 20 weeks of gestation [2]. It remains a major cause of perinatal mortality and maternal morbidity even in high-income countries (HICs) [1]. In approximately half of all women presenting with APH, a diagnosis of **placental abruption** or **placenta previa** will be made; no firm diagnosis will be made in the other half even after investigations.

DEFINITION OF SEVERITY

Although there is a lack of uniformity regarding the definitions of the severity of APH, it is recognised that the amount of blood lost is generally more than what is estimated. Thus, clinical signs of shock and fetal compromise are important indicators of the severity of blood loss. The classification of APH based on volume of bleeding is presented in Table 29.1 [1]. When bleeding occurs on more than one occasion, it is called **recurrent APH**.

Table 29.1 Classification of antepartum hemorrhage based on volume of blood loss [1]

Type of APH	Blood loss
Minor hemorrhage	Blood loss of <50 mL, which has settled
Major hemorrhage	Blood loss of 50–1000 mL with no signs of clinical shock
Massive hemorrhage	Blood loss >1000 mL and/or signs of clinical shock

Key Point

In cases presenting with APH, thorough clinical evaluation including a detailed history and physical examination is key to making an initial clinical diagnosis, starting supportive treatment, and guiding further investigations and management. Once the woman is stabilised, imaging tests are useful to support or revise the initial diagnosis.

CAUSES OF ANTEPARTUM HEMORRHAGE

The causes of antepartum hemorrhage are as follows:

- Placental abruption
- Placenta previa
- APH of indeterminate origin
- Uterine rupture (in women with previous uterine surgery)
- Heavy show
- Vasa previa
- Bleeding from the lower genital tract

PLACENTAL ABRUPTION

DEFINITION

Placental abruption is the premature separation of a normally situated placenta from the uterine wall, resulting in hemorrhage before the delivery of the fetus. Abruption is a significant cause of both maternal and neonatal morbidity and mortality, particularly when it occurs preterm.

INCIDENCE

Large epidemiological studies performed recently report an incidence of placental abruption ranging from 2–10 per 1000 singleton births and up to 12.2 per 1000 twin births [3,4].

It is estimated that abruption is implicated in 10% of preterm births. Perinatal mortality rates range from 3–12% in births complicated by abruption (versus 0.6% in births without abruption) [5]. The risk of abruption recurring in a subsequent pregnancy is increased as much as 10-fold [6].

PATHOPHYSIOLOGY OF ABRUPTION

The precise cause of abruption is unknown. Abruption arises from hemorrhage into the decidua basalis of the placenta, which results in the formation of a hematoma and an increase in hydrostatic pressure, leading to the separation of the adjacent placenta. The resultant hematoma may be small and self-limiting or may continue to dissect through the decidual layer.

However, the bleeding may be **in whole** or **in part concealed** if the hematoma does not reach the margin of the placenta and cervix for the blood loss to be revealed. Therefore, the correlation between the amount of revealed hemorrhage and the degree of actual blood loss is poor. The bleeding may infiltrate the myometrium, turning the uterus deep purple, resulting in the **Couvelaire uterus**.

> **Key Point**
>
> The bleeding may not reach the edge of the placenta and may be concealed. The correlation between the amount of revealed hemorrhage and the degree of actual blood loss is poor.

RISK FACTORS

The most predictive risk factor for placental abruption is **abruption in a previous pregnancy**. The risk is estimated to be up to 5% in women who have had one, and up to 25% in women who have had two previous pregnancies complicated by abruption. Other conditions associated with abruption include the following [7,8]:

- Preeclampsia
- Fetal growth restriction
- Non-vertex presentations
- Sudden uterine decompression as may occur in
  - Membrane rupture with polyhydramnios
  - Delivery of the first twin
- Chorioamnionitis
- Advanced maternal age
- Multiparity
- Pregnancy following assisted reproductive techniques
- Intrauterine infection
- Abdominal trauma (accidental or resulting from domestic violence)
- Maternal thrombophilias (especially heterozygous factor V Leiden and heterozygous prothrombin 20210A gene mutation)
- First-trimester bleeding, especially when recurrent or associated with a significant intrauterine hematoma on ultrasound scan
- Potentially preventable risk factors include maternal use of recreational drugs such as cocaine and amphetamine, and smoking

> **Key Point**
>
> Abruption in a previous pregnancy is the most predictive risk factor. The risk is estimated to be up to 5% in women who have had one and up to 25% in women who have had two previous pregnancies complicated by abruption.

First- and Second-Trimester Maternal Serum Biomarkers as Predictors of Placental Abruption

Unexplained elevation of maternal serum alpha-fetoprotein (MSAFP) levels in the second trimester or low pregnancy associated plasma protein-A (PAPP-A) in the first trimester is associated with pregnancy complications such as growth restriction and placental abruption [9]. However, the clinical usefulness of this test is limited due to low sensitivity and a high false-positive rate.

Hypertension and Abruption

The existence of a causal relationship between hypertension and abruption is controversial.

In hypertension, the muscular arterioles fail to transform to low-resistance, dilated vessels as in normal pregnancy and there is a lack of trophoblastic invasion of the uterine vessels; these factors are thought to result in decreased placental blood flow and abnormal endothelial responses to vasoactive substances. These abnormal placental vessels may predispose to ischemia and rupture of the involved vessels, thus causing placental abruption.

CLINICAL PRESENTATION

The diagnosis of placental abruption is clinical, based on characteristic signs and symptoms. This is then confirmed by the evaluation of the placenta after delivery.

Classical Presentation

Placental abruption classically presents with the following signs and symptoms:

- Vaginal bleeding
- Abdominal pain—the pain is continuous, i.e., persisting between contractions
- Uterine contractions and tenderness

However, it is important to remember that not all signs may be present simultaneously.

- **Revealed abruption:** Blood trickles from between the membranes and escapes through the vagina and cervix. This occurs in 65–80% of cases [10].
- **Concealed abruption:** Blood collects behind the placenta with no evidence of vaginal bleeding. This occurs in 10–20% of cases. In such cases, the diagnosis of placental abruption may not be obvious, and it may be misdiagnosed as idiopathic preterm labour. Thus, it is important to have a strong index of suspicion.

Clinical Examination

The uterus may be irritable with an increased baseline tone. A typical labour pattern with rapid progress is also possible.

Maternal signs and symptoms

In severe cases, the woman may show signs and symptoms of **hypovolemia.** Severe cases of hypovolemic shock may lead to acute kidney injury, adult respiratory distress syndrome, multiorgan failure and rarely, maternal death. The clinical signs of blood loss are often more pronounced than the amount of visible vaginal bleeding, especially in a concealed abruption.

There is a serious risk of **disseminated intravascular coagulopathy (DIC)** in the woman due to the consumption of clotting factors.

In severe abruption, blood may extravasate into the myometrium, turning the uterus deep purple **(Couvelaire uterus)**. Due to the accumulation of blood between the muscle fibres, atonic **postpartum hemorrhage** may result. The atony may not respond to standard management, and a hysterectomy may be required to control the bleeding.

In a recent abruption, the diagnosis may be confirmed postpartum on gross examination of the placenta, which will reveal a clot and/or depression in the maternal surface, known as a **delle**.

Fetal signs

Abruption is commonly associated with fetal compromise due to fetal hypoxia. There may be evidence of fetal distress, i.e., an abnormal cardiotocograph (CTG) trace. In severe cases, fetal cardiac activity may be absent.

The majority of cases of fetal morbidity are thought to be caused by hypoxia and prematurity. Low birth weight, fetal growth restriction, neonatal anemia, and hyperbilirubinemia are significantly more common in cases of placental abruption [11].

The incidence of **stillbirth** is related to the size of the abruption and the uterine irritability that causes tachysystole and sustained uterine contractions.

Key Point

The separation of the placental surface exceeding 50% of the placenta causes a marked elevation in the stillbirth rate.

Role of Ultrasonography

Ultrasound imaging is an insensitive and unreliable tool for detecting or excluding placental abruption, as **negative sonographic findings are common with clinically significant abruption**. The value of ultrasound is to exclude low-lying placenta or placenta previa.

Key Point

The diagnosis of placental abruption is clinical, based on characteristic signs and symptoms. Ultrasound has a limited role in the diagnosis.

MANAGEMENT OF PLACENTAL ABRUPTION

Once placental abruption is suspected, action should be swift and decisive because the prognosis for the pregnant woman and fetus is worsened by delay. Treatment consists of initial resuscitation and stabilisation of the woman, as in all cases of antepartum hemorrhage, and the recognition and management of complications. Maternal resuscitation and treatment of hypovolemic shock are a subject of a review in their own right, and out of the scope of this chapter. See the section on *Resuscitation and the role of transfusion therapy* in **Chapter 13**, *Abnormalities in the third stage of labour: Postpartum hemorrhage and retained placenta*.

Key Point

Once placental abruption has been suspected, action should be swift and decisive because the prognosis for the pregnant woman and her fetus is worsened by delay.

Classification by Degree of Severity

For the purpose of management, Sher and Statland [12] classified placental abruption into three degrees of severity. These are as follows:

- **Mild (Grade 1):** The abruption is not recognised clinically before delivery and is usually diagnosed by the presence of a retroplacental clot. This is a retrospective diagnosis.
- **Moderate (Grade 2):** This is an intermediate grade in which the classical clinical signs of abruption are present but the **fetus is still alive**. The frequency of fetal heart rate abnormalities is high.
- **Severe (Grade 3):** The **fetus is dead** and **coagulopathy** may be present. The volume of blood loss is appreciable in this condition. If a woman presents with Grade 3 abruption, the following arrangements should be made immediately
  - — Cross-match at least 4 units of blood
  - — Start blood transfusion early, with appropriate replacement of platelets and clotting factors since abruption large enough to lead to fetal demise is associated with significant blood loss and DIC

Management Options

There are three practical options for management:

- Expectant management
- Immediate cesarean section
- Rupture of membranes, with the aim of vaginal delivery

The management of abruption is individualised based on the following:

- Extent of the abruption
- Maternal and fetal reaction to this insult
- Gestational age of the fetus

Stable maternal condition and reassuring fetal status

Expectant management

Gestational age <34 weeks

In this situation, expectant management is a reasonable option [13.14]. In mild placental abruption, the bleeding may stop and the symptoms gradually resolve with satisfactory findings on fetal monitoring. Conservative management with the aim of delivering a more mature fetus is the main goal, especially before 34+0 weeks of gestation with no evidence of ongoing major blood loss or onset of labour.

The woman can often be discharged after a few days and managed as an outpatient. Multiple studies have shown that expectant management, with or without tocolytics, is safe and effective in a select population of women with preterm placental abruption provided that the fetal heart rate tracing is normal. In practice, this is likely to be diagnosed as:

- APH of uncertain origin or
- Threatened preterm labour

Only postpartum placental pathological examination may show evidence of long-standing abruption and associated placental changes.

These women should be monitored regularly because there is a risk of recurrent bleeding associated with the development of placental ischemia, resulting in oligohydramnios (**termed chronic abruption-oligohydramnios sequence**) [15], fetal growth restriction, and/or preeclampsia. **Antenatal corticosteroids** are recommended.

The use of **tocolytics** is controversial. In one observational study, tocolysis allowed a median delay of delivery of several days without increasing neonatal or maternal morbidity, including the need for transfusion or delivery by cesarean section [16]. However, in the absence of randomised controlled trials, the benefit of tocolysis remains uncertain.

Gestational age 34–36 weeks

For women between 34 and 36 weeks of gestation, management should be individualised.

Gestational age >36 weeks

Delivery should be strongly considered in women presenting with mild abruption beyond 36 weeks due to the relatively low neonatal morbidity of the near term newborn.

Unstable maternal condition and/or non-reassuring fetal status

The management of moderate or severe placental abruption includes the following:

- Resuscitation
- Delivery of the fetus
- Investigation for and correction of any coagulation defect that arises

Trial of labour and vaginal delivery

A trial of labour and vaginal delivery are recommended whenever tolerated by the maternal–fetal pair. This requires management in the labour ward with intensive monitoring of both the woman and the fetus. Labour is usually rapid, and progress should be monitored with continuous fetal heart rate monitoring. Delivery should be expedited in the form of an **emergency cesarean section** if fetal distress is evident.

Management of Complications

Moderate to severe abruption should be regarded as an emergency, requiring multidisciplinary input from the obstetrician, anesthetist, hematologist, and neonatologist. A **fulminant maternal DIC** can ensue within hours of a complete abruption. Immediate delivery should be arranged as it is the only way to halt the DIC. Replacement of blood and its components should begin before surgery.

Abruption also places the woman at a high risk of **severe postpartum hemorrhage** due to the combination of uterine atony and coagulation failure. Invasive monitoring with arterial lines and central venous access may be necessary, and these women are best treated in the high-dependency unit. Urine output should be closely monitored, as acute kidney injury is a potential complication.

> **Key Point**
>
> Major abruption should be regarded as an emergency, requiring multidisciplinary inputs from the obstetrician, anesthetist, and hematologist. **Fulminant maternal DIC** should be managed by immediate delivery along with replacement of clotting factors, as it is the only means with which to halt the DIC.

RECURRENCE OF ABRUPTION

The probability of a recurrence of abruption increases in future pregnancies following a history of placental abruption. There are no reliable predictors of the timing in a pregnancy at which this may happen, and there are no known interventions proven to reduce recurrence.

A meta-analysis of randomised trials [17] concluded that prophylactic low-dose aspirin (at a daily dose of ≥100 mg) may decrease the risk of abruption if initiated at ≤16 weeks of gestation rather than >16 weeks.

The practice of elective delivery is reasonable after fetal maturity is reached in the subsequent pregnancy.

PLACENTA PREVIA

DEFINITION

The insertion of the placenta partially or entirely in the lower uterine segment with the placental tissue extending up to or over the internal os is known as placenta previa. At the time of delivery, the position of the placenta precedes the baby.

CLASSIFICATION

The American Institute of Ultrasound in Medicine (AIUM), in a multidisciplinary meeting, recommended the following definitions based on transabdominal sonography (TAS) or transvaginal sonography (TVS) in pregnancies >16 weeks of gestation [18]:

- **Placenta previa**: The placenta lies directly over the internal os.
- **Low-lying placenta**: The leading placental edge is within 20 mm of the internal os.

They recommended discontinuing the use of the terms **'partial'** and **'marginal' previa**. The description of the location of the edge of the placenta should be documented in the report. **When the placental edge is ≥20 mm from the internal os at the 36 weeks follow-up scan, it should be reported as normal.** As this new classification better defines the risks of perinatal complications and improves the obstetric management of placenta previa, it has been adopted by professional bodies internationally, including the RCOG and ACOG.

Key Point

As per current definitions, **placenta previa** is the term used when the placenta lies directly over the internal os; the term **low-lying placenta** is used when the leading placental edge is within 20 mm of the internal os.

EPIDEMIOLOGY

The prevalence of placenta previa depends on the gestational age. It may be as high as 2–5% at 18–20 weeks' gestation [19] but is 4–5 per 1000 pregnancies at term.

Placenta previa and the placenta accreta spectrum (PAS) are clinically significant causes of APH because not only are they associated with high maternal and neonatal morbidity and mortality, but unlike abruption, their incidence has increased and will continue to do so. The following are important contributors to the increasing rates of placenta previa and PAS:

- Rising rates of cesarean deliveries
- Use of assisted reproductive technology (ART)
- Rising maternal age

The highest complication rates for both mother and newborn are observed when these conditions are only diagnosed at delivery, stressing further on the importance of accurate early diagnosis and planned management (see **Chapter 24**, *Peripartum hysterectomy*).

ETIOLOGY AND ASSOCIATED FACTORS

Placenta previa is caused by the implantation of the blastocyst low in the uterine cavity. Factors associated with the development of placenta previa include the following:

- Previous cesarean delivery is the most common factor, and the risk rises as the number of prior cesarean sections increases
- Previous history of placental previa
- Increasing maternal parity and advancing maternal age
- Increasing placental size (e.g., multiple pregnancy)

- Endometrial damage (e.g., previous dilatation and curettage)
- Uterine scarring from previous myomectomy or endometritis
- Placental pathology such as marginal cord insertions and succenturiate lobes
- Artificial reproductive techniques
- Maternal smoking

CLINICAL PRESENTATION AND DIAGNOSIS

Placenta previa may present as one of the following clinical scenarios:

- An incidental finding in the mid-trimester ultrasound scan
- Vaginal bleeding after 20 weeks of gestation

Follow-up of Low-Lying Placenta/Previa in the Mid-Trimester Ultrasound Scan

In women who have a routine scan between 18+6 and 22 weeks, the placenta may be low-lying in some, necessitating a repeat scan later in pregnancy.

A transvaginal or transperineal scan can be done, which will help to delineate the distance from the internal os more accurately and reduce the number of women for whom follow-up will be needed.

- **Low-lying placenta (edge <20 mm from the internal os) or previa (covering the os):**
  - The RCOG [20] recommends a repeat TVS at 32 weeks of gestation to diagnose persistent low-lying placenta and/or placenta previa.
  - If low-lying placenta or placenta previa persist at 32 weeks, an additional TVS is recommended at around 36 weeks of gestation to help guide the plan for delivery.
- **Cervical length measurement**: A short cervical length (≤30 mm) on TVS at sonographic diagnosis of placenta previa predicts the risk of emergency cesarean delivery at <34 weeks due to massive hemorrhage in women with complete placenta previa [21].

Key Point

25% of placentas are found to be low lying on ultrasound examination in the early second trimester. 90% of these resolve at the 32 weeks' scan and 50% of those remaining resolve by the 36 weeks' scan. This is due to **placental migration.** Placenta previa at term will not be encountered unless the placental edge is at least reaching the internal cervical os at mid-pregnancy [22].

MANAGEMENT

Most cases presenting with APH would already be known to have a low-lying placenta. Some of these women will present with antepartum bleeding. Initial hemorrhages, referred to as 'warning hemorrhages', are often small and tend to stop spontaneously. When a woman with placenta previa presents with vaginal bleeding, a comprehensive clinical assessment should be carried out.

Detailed Clinical Examination

This must include an abdominal and speculum examination to assess the tone of the uterus, cervical dilatation, and any local causes of bleeding. When there is no prior knowledge about the placental position, this detailed clinical assessment assumes even more importance.

Key Point

Digital vaginal examination should be **avoided** in suspected placenta previa as it can further aggravate the bleeding. Transvaginal ultrasound, however, is safe.

General Measures

Initial multidisciplinary management, common to all women with antepartum hemorrhage, includes inserting two wide-bore IV cannulae, sending urgent blood investigations including a complete blood count, urea, creatinine, and electrolytes, clotting factors, and a group and cross-match, and initial stabilisation and resuscitation of the woman. With any new episode of antepartum hemorrhage, anti-D should be administered to Rh-negative women.

Further Management

Further management of placenta previa depends upon the following:

- Clinical presentation
- Gestational age
- Severity of bleeding
- Degree of previa

Diagnosis at the mid-trimester scan

In asymptomatic women (no episodes of painless bleeding after 20 weeks of gestation) with a low-lying placenta, the mode of delivery should be based on the clinical background and the woman's preferences and supplemented by ultrasound findings, including the distance between the placental edge and the fetal head position relative to the leading edge of the placenta on TVS.

Low-lying placenta

The success rates of vaginal delivery when **the placental edge is between 10 and 20 mm away from the cervical os** vary widely, and are reported to be 56 and 93% respectively. There is still a risk of significant bleeding. Thus, although an attempt at vaginal delivery may be considered, it would not be unreasonable to plan a cesarean section for women with low-lying placentas at the 36 weeks' scan. It is also important to remember that the risk of postpartum hemorrhage remains high in this group [22].

Placenta previa

Cesarean section is the recommended mode of delivery for persistent placenta previa. The delivery timing should be individualised according to antenatal symptoms and, for women presenting with uncomplicated placenta previa, **delivery should be considered between 36+0 and 38+0 weeks of gestation**. The timing of surgery may be deferred to 38 weeks, if possible, in order to reduce neonatal morbidity.

Recurrent bleeding

The management of women with recurrent bleeding should be individualised based on the woman's needs, social circumstances, and current clinical picture, e.g., the distance between her home and the hospital and availability of transportation, previous bleeding episodes, the absence of active current bleeding, stable hematology laboratory results, and acceptance of receiving donor blood or blood products.

Any home-based care requires close proximity to the hospital, the constant presence of a companion, and full informed consent from the woman. She should be advised to contact the hospital early in the event of abdominal pain or vaginal bleeding.

Late preterm delivery (34+0 to 36+6 weeks of gestation) should be considered for women with a history of vaginal bleeding, especially if it is recurrent or associated with other risk factors for preterm delivery.

Prior to the delivery, a discussion about the delivery plan, risks of severe hemorrhage, the need for blood transfusion, and the possibility of surgical intervention, including peripartum hysterectomy, should take place. Delivery should be arranged in a maternity unit with on-site blood transfusion services and access to critical care.

Key Point

Women with placenta previa who have previously bled may be admitted and managed as inpatients from 34 weeks of gestation.

Antenatal corticosteroids

A single course of antenatal corticosteroid therapy should be considered for women at higher risk of preterm birth. Tocolysis may be considered for women presenting with symptomatic placenta previa or a low-lying placenta for 48 hours to facilitate the administration of antenatal corticosteroids, as long as immediate delivery is not indicated due to maternal or fetal concerns. The maternal hemoglobin level should be optimised antenatally.

Acute hemorrhage

Emergent delivery may be needed for severe, intractable, or recurrent bleeding. Fetal morbidity is associated with iatrogenic prematurity.

Important points to remember during surgery are as follows:

- Preoperative and/or intraoperative ultrasonography should be used to precisely determine placental location and fetal position to help plan the uterine incision and delivery.
- The most experienced surgeon available should be operating, especially if the woman has a previous uterine scar, an anterior placenta, or is suspected to have placenta accreta [20].
- If the placenta is traversed during the uterine incision, in order to avoid excessive fetal blood loss, the umbilical cord should be immediately clamped after delivery.
- Control of hemorrhage should be proactive. Intrauterine tamponade, compression sutures, and surgical hemostatic techniques should be undertaken. A hysterectomy should be performed, sooner rather than later, if bleeding persists despite conservative medical and surgical interventions.
- Four units of cross-matched blood and other blood products should be kept ready.
- Delivery of women with placenta previa **should not** be planned in units where blood transfusion facilities are unavailable. Rapid infusion, fluid warming devices, and cell salvage should be used if available.

VASA PREVIA

Vasa previa has been defined as a fetal vessel running in the free placental membranes within 2 cm of the cervix. As it is not protected by placental tissue or Wharton's jelly of the umbilical cord, a vasa previa is likely to rupture in active labour or when an amniotomy is performed to induce or augment labour. Though rare, its consequences are catastrophic if not prenatally diagnosed.

INCIDENCE AND RISK FACTORS

Vasa previa has an incidence of between 1 in 1200 and 1 in 5000 pregnancies [23,24]. Risk factors for vasa previa include placenta previa, bilobed placenta, succenturiate placental lobes, conception by assisted reproductive technology, and velamentous cord insertion.

> **Key Point**
>
> A strong risk factor for vasa previa is a low-lying placenta, which resolves in later pregnancy. The diagnosis should also be kept in mind in IVF pregnancies with a low-lying placenta.

DIAGNOSIS

In the hands of an experienced sonographer, antenatal diagnosis by a combination of both transabdominal and transvaginal ultrasound with colour Doppler imaging has a high diagnostic accuracy with a low false-positive rate. Echogenic parallel or circular lines near the cervix representing the umbilical cord, seen by grey-scale ultrasound, should raise the suspicion of vasa previa.

Oyelese et al. [25] demonstrated the importance of prenatal diagnosis. In the group where prenatal diagnosis of vasa previa had been made, 97% of infants survived, as opposed to only 44% in cases where the diagnosis was not made before birth.

PRESENTATION

Undiagnosed vasa previa classically presents with vaginal bleeding following the spontaneous rupture of membranes, or amniotomy, with subsequent severe fetal heart rate decelerations or bradycardia.

The diagnosis of this condition before these events is difficult, but the experienced observer may be able to feel vessels below the presenting part on digital examination. A speculum examination may also reveal the vessels on inspection.

MANAGEMENT

Rupture of Vasa Previa Undiagnosed Antenatally

If the gestational age is viable, immediate cesarean delivery and neonatal resuscitation—including the use of blood transfusion, if indicated—are essential in the management of ruptured vasa previa diagnosed during labour. Neonatologists should be alerted to expect a severely hypovolemic fetus. After delivery, placental pathological examination should be performed to confirm the diagnosis of ruptured vasa previa (fetal vessels running unsupported in fetal membranes), especially in cases of acute fetal compromise or stillbirth.

Key Point

Prenatal diagnosis of vasa previa has a major impact on improving fetal survival. The perinatal mortality in cases undetected prior to delivery is high (56%), but it can be reduced to 3% with prenatal diagnosis [26].

Vasa Previa Diagnosed Antenatally

In cases diagnosed antenatally, prophylactic hospitalisation from 30–32 weeks of gestation may be considered, especially in women with multiple pregnancy, a history of antepartum hemorrhage, a previous preterm birth, and threatened premature labour [27]. Hospitalisation may be considered for logistic reasons if a quick transfer to the maternity unit is difficult. The woman should be instructed to carry her notes with her and warn the caregivers of the diagnosis so that precious time is not lost in an emergency.

A plan should be in place for **elective delivery by cesarean section at 34–36 weeks** after the administration of steroids for fetal pulmonary maturity. In women with vasa previa who develop premature rupture of membranes and/or go into labour at viable gestational ages, a cesarean section should be performed without delay [24].

PLACENTA ACCRETA SPECTRUM (PAS)

Although the placenta accreta spectrum is very rare (4/100,000) in women with a normally situated placenta, data from Southern California [28] showed an incidence of 9.3% among women with placenta previa. In a recent systematic review [29] that included 7001 cases of PAS, the overall pooled prevalence was 0.17% (the range being 0.01–1.1%). Although the incidence of PAS is rising, the maternal mortality associated with it has declined over the years. This can be attributed to early diagnosis and good multidisciplinary management.

Based on the depth of villous tissue invasion, PAS is classified as follows:

- **Placenta accreta**: The villi adhere superficially to the myometrium without an interposing decidua.
- **Placenta increta**: The villi penetrate deeply into the uterine myometrium, reaching the serosa.
- **Placenta percreta**: The villi perforate through the entire uterine wall and may invade the surrounding pelvic organs, such as the bladder.

RISK FACTORS

The most important risk factors for PAS are the following:

- A history of accreta in a previous pregnancy
- Placenta previa after a prior cesarean delivery—the risk rises as the number of prior cesarean sections increases, being 3%, 11%, 40%, 61%, and 67% for one, two, three, four, and five or more cesarean deliveries, respectively [30]

Other risk factors include the presence of a cesarean scar pregnancy, a history of uterine surgery (e.g., myomectomy entering the uterine cavity), some hysteroscopic surgeries, dilatation and curettage, endometrial ablation, maternal age >35 years, multiparity, a history of pelvic irradiation, manual removal of the placenta, postpartum endometritis, infertility and/or infertility procedures.

DIAGNOSIS

Ultrasound Imaging

All women with a previous cesarean section or other risk factors and an anterior low-lying placenta or placenta previa at the routine mid-trimester scan should be specifically screened for the placenta accreta spectrum. Ultrasound imaging is highly accurate in diagnosing PAS when performed by an experienced operator, with a sensitivity of 90–97% and a specificity of 96–97% [31,32].

Ultrasound findings suggestive of placenta accreta spectrum include the following:

- Presence of multiple vascular lacunae within the placenta (Swiss-cheese appearance) with turbulent blood flow (Figs. 29.1 and 29.2)
- The loss of a normal hypoechoic retroplacental zone and increased vascularity of the placental bed with large feeder vessels entering the lacunae (the best predictive accuracy)
- Abnormalities of the uterine serosa–bladder interface have the best specificity of 99.8% [32] (Fig. 29.3)
- Colour Doppler abnormalities (Fig. 29.4)

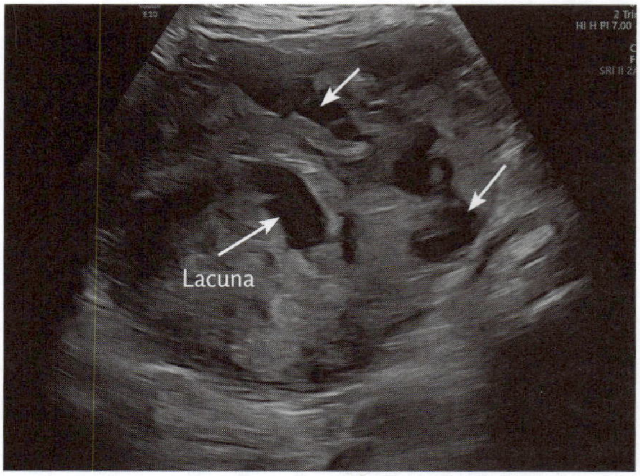

Fig. 29.1 Ultrasound image of the placenta showing lacunae (arrows) in the body of the placenta (*Image courtesy:* Dr Amarnath Bhide, St. George's Hospital, London, UK)

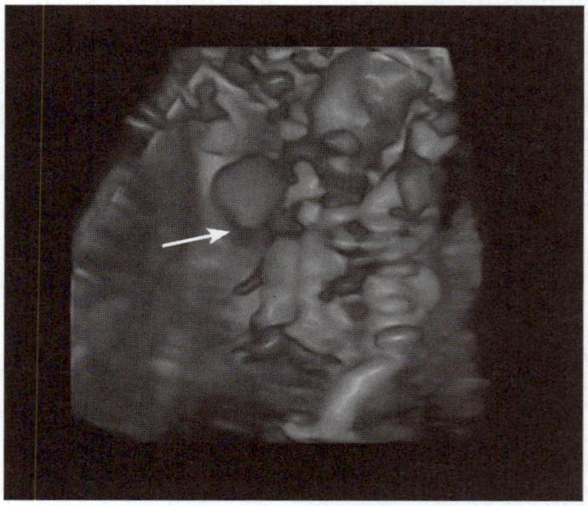

Fig. 29.2 Ultrasound image of the placenta showing turbulent blood flow (arrow) in the lacunae on Doppler flow study (*Image courtesy:* Dr Amarnath Bhide, St. George's Hospital, London, UK)

> **Key Point**
>
> Placenta previa is present in more than 80% of cases of accretas, and is perhaps the most important ultrasonographic association of PAS in the second and third trimesters.

Magnetic Resonance Imaging (MRI)

MRI can also be used in the diagnosis of PAS. It has a similar diagnostic value to ultrasound imaging and may be used to complement ultrasound imaging to assess the depth of invasion and lateral extension of myometrial invasion, especially with posterior placentation and/or in women with ultrasound signs suggesting parametrial invasion [33]. However, MRI is not easily accessible in LMICs.

MANAGEMENT

Once PAS is diagnosed, management should ideally be at a tertiary centre by a multidisciplinary team with expertise in complex pelvic surgery,

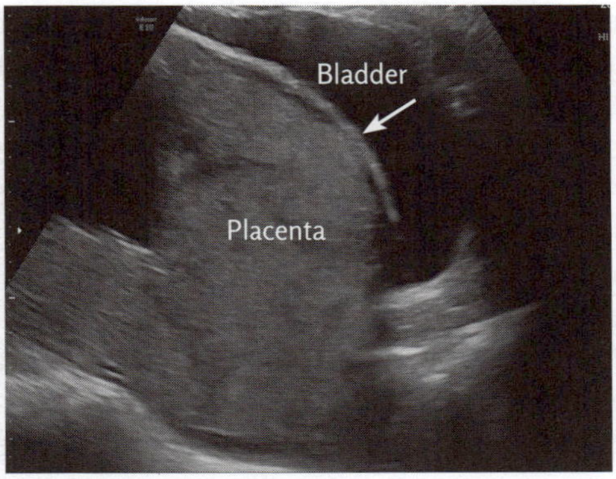

Fig. 29.3 Ultrasound image of the placenta showing a discontinuity in the uterine wall (arrow) between the placenta and the bladder (*Image courtesy:* Dr Amarnath Bhide, St. George's Hospital, London, UK)

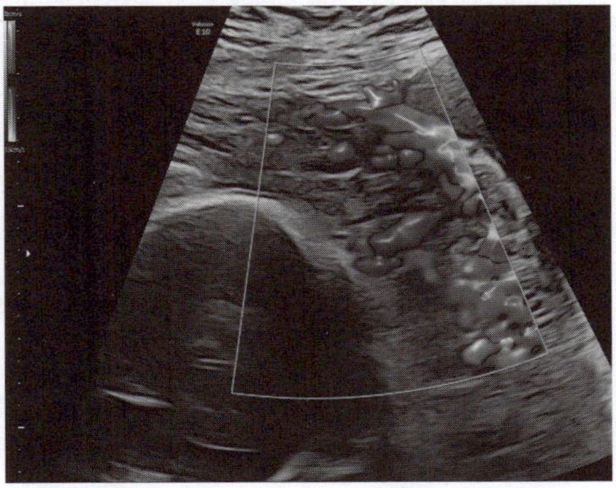

Fig. 29.4 Ultrasound colour Doppler findings in placenta accreta showing vascular channels at the interface between the placenta and the bladder (*Image courtesy:* Becky Liu, St. George's Hospital, London, UK)

with immediate access to blood products, an adult intensive care unit and NICU. The maternal risks from placenta accreta include massive hemorrhage, injury to the urinary tract or the pelvic viscera, vascular injuries, hysterectomy, infection, and even maternal death. Neonatal morbidity is chiefly associated with prematurity. See **Chapter 24,** *Peripartum hysterectomy* for detailed management of PAS.

Methotrexate administration, in order to accelerate the process of absorption of the adherent placenta that has been left in situ, is **not recommended**, as it has significant adverse effects and its benefit has not been proven. Following a decision of leaving the placenta in situ, the woman should be closely monitored for delayed hemorrhage, as some women may require a secondary hysterectomy.

> **Key Point**
>
> Methotrexate is **not** recommended to accelerate the process of absorption of the adherent placenta which had been left in situ. It is associated with significant adverse effects and its benefit has not been proven.

BLEEDING OF INDETERMINATE ORIGIN

This is the most common cause of APH, and is seen in around 2–5% of pregnancies [34]. It may be a case of placenta previa that has not been diagnosed on ultrasound imaging, especially in cases of accessory lobes or abnormally-shaped placentas, or milder forms of abruption that do not present with typical clinical signs and symptoms.

In a small proportion of cases, where placenta previa and placental abruption have been excluded, a cause may still be found. They include the following:

- Cervicitis or vaginitis
- Trauma
- Vulval varicosities
- Genital tract tumours
- Cervical polyps or fibroids
- Hematuria
- Genital infections

Many of these conditions are evident on the initial speculum examination. 'Heavy show' is a diagnosis of exclusion and should be considered in women with bleeding in latent or established labour. Approximately 15–20% of women with unexplained APH will go into spontaneous labour within two weeks of the initial bleed [35]. Antepartum bleeding of indeterminate origin has been reported to increase the risk of preterm birth two- to three-fold [36].

MANAGEMENT

- Thorough clinical assessment including details about present symptoms, review of past obstetric and medical history, a speculum examination, and ultrasound, if deemed appropriate, are key to planning further management.
- Older reports including blood results and ultrasound should be reviewed to look for risk factors for the various etiologies of APH.
- Investigations should include blood grouping and cross-match, and clotting screen. Anti-D prophylaxis and Kleihauer test should be performed when indicated, as well as a cardiotocograph for fetal assessment.

In the majority of cases, the bleeding is mild and settles spontaneously. Further management will either be expectant, or delivery will be expedited, based on the clinical situation.

Expectant Management

If a policy of expectant management is adopted, fetal well-being should be monitored. If the gestational age is below 34–36 weeks, antenatal steroids should be administered in view of the risk of preterm delivery.

Delivery

Labour should be managed as high-risk, with continuous fetal monitoring, access to blood products, maternal and neonatal HDU/ ICU, and active management of the third stage.

If the pregnancy is beyond 37 weeks' gestation and the bleeding is recurrent, or is associated with fetal growth restriction, delivery is the management of choice.

CONCLUSION

Antepartum hemorrhage is one of the main causes of obstetric hemorrhage. The cause of APH remains undetermined in about half of the cases. The diagnosis of placental abruption is clinical, whereas that of placenta previa is based on ultrasound imaging. Cesarean section for placenta previa should involve a senior and experienced obstetrician and an experienced anesthetic team. The possibility of placenta accreta should be kept in mind in cases of placenta previa. Vasa previa though rare, is a cause of acute fetal compromise and can be diagnosed antenatally by experienced operators.

If episodes of bleeding are recurrent and significant, there may be a need for **immediate delivery** even if the gestation is below 37 weeks.

REFERENCES

1. *Antepartum Haemorrhage*. Green-top Guideline No. 63. Royal College of Obstetricians and Gynaecologists. 2011.
2. Gyamfi-Bannerman C. Society for Maternal-Fetal Medicine (SMFM) Consult Series #44: Management of bleeding in the late preterm period. *Am J Obstet Gynecol*. 2018. 218:B2.
3. Lueth A, Blue N, Silver RM, Allshouse A, Hoffman M, Grobman WA, et al. Prospective evaluation of placental abruption in nulliparous women. *J Matern Fetal Neonatal Med*. 2022. 35(25):8603-10.
4. Maeland KS, Morken NH, Schytt E, Aasheim V, Nilsen RM. Placental abruption in immigrant women in Norway: A population-based study. *Acta Obstet Gynecol Scand*. 2021. 100(4):658-65.
5. Tikkanen M, Luukkaala T, Gissler M, Ritvanen A, Ylikorkala O, Paavonen J, et al. Decreasing perinatal mortality in placental abruption. *Acta Obstet Gynecol Scand*. 2013. 92(3):298-305.
6. Ruiter L, Ravelli AC, de Graaf IM, Mol BW, Pajkrt E. Incidence and recurrence rate of placental abruption: A longitudinal linked national cohort study in the Netherlands. *Am J Obstet Gynecol*. 2015. 213(4):573 e1-8.
7. Ananth CV, Oyelese Y, Yeo L, Pradhan A, Vintzileos AM. Placental abruption in the United States, 1979 through 2001: Temporal trends and potential determinants. *Am J Obstet Gynecol*. 2005. 192(1):191-8.
8. Tikkanen M. Placental abruption: Epidemiology, risk factors and consequences. *Acta Obstet Gynecol Scand*. 2011. 90(2):140-9.
9. Ananth CV, Wapner RJ, Ananth S, et al. First-trimester and second-trimester maternal serum biomarkers as predictors of placental abruption. *Obstet Gynecol*. 2017. 129:465.
10. Oyelese Y, Ananth CV. Placental abruption. *Obstet Gynecol*. 2006. 108(4):1005-16.
11. Ananth CV, Berkowitz GS, Savitz DA, Lapinski RH. Placental abruption and adverse perinatal outcomes. *JAMA*. 1999. 3;282(17):1646-51.

12. Sher G, Statland BE. Abruptio placentae with coagulopathy: A rational basis for management. *Clin Obstet Gynecol*. 1985. 28(1):15-23.
13. Combs CA, Nyberg DA, Mack LA, Smith JR, Benedetti TJ. Expectant management after sonographic diagnosis of placental abruption. *Am J Perinatol*. 1992. 9(3):170-4.
14. Bond AL, Edersheim TG, Curry L, Druzin ML, Hutson JM. Expectant management of abruptio placentae before 35 weeks gestation. *Am J Perinatol*. 1989. 6(2):121-3.
15. Elliott JP, Gilpin B, Strong TH Jr., Finberg HJ. Chronic abruption-oligohydramnios sequence. *J Reprod Med*. 1998. 43(5):418-22.
16. Towers CV, Pircon RA, Heppard M. Is tocolysis safe in the management of third-trimester bleeding? *Am J Obstet Gynecol*. 1999. 180(6 Pt 1):1572-8.
17. Roberge S, Bujold E, Nicolaides KH. Meta-analysis on the effect of aspirin use for prevention of preeclampsia on placental abruption and antepartum hemorrhage. *Am J Obstet Gynecol*. 2018. 218(5):483-9.
18. Reddy UM, Abuhamad AZ, Levine D, Saade GR, Fetal imaging workshop invited participants. fetal imaging: Executive summary of a joint Eunice Kennedy Shriver National Institute of Child Health and Human Development, Society for Maternal-Fetal Medicine, American Institute of Ultrasound in Medicine, American College of Obstetricians and Gynecologists, American College of Radiology, Society for Pediatric Radiology, and Society of Radiologists in Ultrasound Fetal Imaging Workshop. *J Ultrasound Med*. 2014. 33(5):745-57.
19. Taipale P, Hiilesmaa V, Ylostalo P. Transvaginal ultrasonography at 18–23 weeks in predicting placenta previa at delivery. *Ultrasound Obstet Gynecol*. 1998. 12(6):422-5.
20. Jauniaux E, Alfirevic Z, Bhide AG, Belfort MA, Burton GJ, Collins SL, et al. Placenta praevia and placenta accreta: Diagnosis and management: Green-top Guideline No. 27a. *BJOG*. 2019. 126(1):e1-e48.
21. Ghi T, Contro E, Martina T, Piva M, Morandi R, Orsini LF, et al. Cervical length and risk of antepartum bleeding in women with complete placenta previa. *Ultrasound Obstet Gynecol*. 2009. 33(2):209-12.
22. Bhide A, Thilaganathan B. Recent advances in the management of placenta previa. *Curr Opin Obstet Gynecol*. 2004. 16(6):447-51.
23. Silver RM. Abnormal placentation: Placenta previa, vasa previa, and placenta accreta. *Obstetrics and gynecology*. 2015. 126(3):654-68.
24. Society of Maternal-Fetal (SMFM) Publications Committee. Sinkey RG, Odibo AO, Dashe JS. #37: Diagnosis and management of vasa previa. *Am J Obstet Gynecol*. 2015. 213(5):615-9.
25. Oyelese Y, Smulian JC. Placenta previa, placenta accreta, and vasa previa. *Obstetrics and gynecology*. 2006.107(4):927-41.
26. Oyelese Y, Catanzarite V, Prefumo F, Lashley S, Schachter M, Tovbin Y, et al. Vasa previa: The impact of prenatal diagnosis on outcomes. *Obstet Gynecol*. 2004. 103(5 Pt 1):937-
27. Jauniaux E, Alfirevic Z, Bhide AG, Burton GJ, Collins SL, Silver R, et al. Vasa praevia: Diagnosis and management: Green-top Guideline No. 27b. *BJOG*. 2019. 126(1):e49-e61.
28. Miller DA, Chollet JA, Goodwin TM. Clinical risk factors for placenta previa-placenta accreta. *American Journal of Obstetrics and Gynecology*. 1997. 177(1):210-4.
29. Jauniaux E, Bunce C, Gronbeck L, Langhoff-Roos J. Prevalence and main outcomes of placenta accreta spectrum: A systematic review and meta-analysis. *Am J Obstet Gynecol*. 2019. 221(3):208-18.
30. Silver RM, Landon MB, Rouse DJ, Leveno KJ, Spong CY, Thom EA, et al. Maternal morbidity associated with multiple repeat cesarean deliveries. *Obstet Gynecol*. 2006. 107(6):1226-32.
31. D'Antonio F, Iacovella C, Bhide A. Prenatal identification of invasive placentation using ultrasound: Systematic review and meta-analysis. *Ultrasound in Obstetrics & Gynecology*. 2013. 42(5):509-17.
32. Jauniaux E, Bhide A. Prenatal ultrasound diagnosis and outcome of placenta previa accreta after cesarean delivery: A systematic review and meta-analysis. *Am J Obstet Gynecol*. 2017. 217(1):27-36.
33. D'Antonio F, Iacovella C, Palacios-Jaraquemada J, Bruno CH, Manzoli L, Bhide A. Prenatal identification of invasive placentation using magnetic resonance imaging: Systematic review and meta-analysis. *Ultrasound in Obstetrics & Gynecology*. 2014.44(1):8-16.
34. McCormack RA, Doherty DA, Magann EF, Hutchinson M, Newnham JP. Antepartum bleeding of unknown origin in the second half of pregnancy and pregnancy outcomes. *BJOG*. 2008. 115(11):1451-7.
35. Yeung SW, Tam WH, Cheung RY. The risk of preterm delivery prior to 34 weeks in women presenting with antepartum haemorrhage of unknown origin. *Aust N Z J Obstet Gynaecol*. 2012. 52(2):167-72.
36. Bhandari S, Raja EA, Shetty A, Bhattacharya S. Maternal and perinatal consequences of antepartum haemorrhage of unknown origin. *BJOG*. 2014. 121(1):44-50; discussion-2.

CHAPTER 30

Preterm Labour and Preterm Prelabour Rupture of Membranes

SAREENA GILVAZ, DEEPTHI D NAIR

INTRODUCTION

Delivery occurring before 37 completed weeks of gestation is considered preterm birth. Approximately 70–80% of preterm births (PTB) are spontaneous and follow **preterm labour** (PTL) or **preterm prelabour rupture of membranes** (PPROM). The remaining 20–30% of PTB are iatrogenic and result from clinician interventions for maternal or fetal conditions that complicate pregnancy.

Every year, an estimated 15 million babies are born early, and the data show a rising trend. Preterm birth and its associated complications cause approximately 1 million deaths per year [1], making prematurity one of the leading causes of neonatal death. India is a major contributor to the global preterm birth numbers; estimates suggest that India contributes 23–24% to the global average [2].

The timing of birth is important, as the risks of neonatal death, severe morbidity, prolonged hospital admissions, and long-term sequelae increase as the gestational age decreases. Despite improvements in neonatal care, infants born prematurely have a high rate of mortality; those who survive may have neurodevelopmental and medical disabilities [3,4].

Fetal Viability

Fetal viability is the ability of a human fetus to survive outside the uterus. Viability is generally considered to be between 20 and 24 weeks' gestational age (depending on the country) and is influenced by factors such as birth weight, gestational age, and the availability of advanced medical care.

PRETERM LABOUR

DEFINITION OF PRETERM LABOUR

Preterm labour is defined as the presence of uterine contractions of sufficient frequency and intensity to result in progressive effacement and dilatation of the cervix after the period of viability and before 37 completed weeks of gestation. Preterm delivery can be classified based on gestational age [5] or birth weight.

Based on Gestational Age

- **Moderate to late preterm**: Between 32 and 36+6 weeks of gestation
- **Very preterm**: Between 28 and 31+6 completed weeks of gestation
- **Extreme preterm**: Before 28 completed weeks of gestation

Based on Birth Weight

- **Low birth weight**: <2500 g
- **Very low birth weight**: <1500 g
- **Extremely low birth weight**: <1000 g

INCIDENCE OF PRETERM LABOUR

The average preterm birth rate is 10.6% worldwide, ranging from 8.7% to 13.4% across regions [2]. The preterm birth rate also varies significantly across countries, with the United States and Greece among HICs to have rates exceeding 10% [5]. In 2020, India had the highest number of preterm births (3.02 million), accounting for over 23% of all preterm births worldwide, though it ranked fourth in preterm birth rate after Bangladesh, Malawi, and Pakistan [5].

> **Key Point**
>
> The rising trend of preterm birth may be due to increasing assisted reproductive techniques, multiple pregnancy, and earlier termination for associated comorbidities in pregnancy due to the availability of better neonatal facilities.

RISK FACTORS FOR PRETERM BIRTH

Previous History of Preterm Labour

One of the strongest risk factors contributing to preterm birth is a prior history of spontaneous preterm labour before 34 weeks [6]. The recurrent preterm delivery risk for a woman whose first delivery was preterm is three times higher than a woman with a prior term delivery.

Demographic, Social, and Behavioural Factors

The following factors are associated with a higher incidence of preterm labour and birth:

- Extremes of maternal age (<17 and >35 years)
- Maternal educational status (the incidence is higher in lesser-educated women)
- Low socio-economic status and malnourishment (including anemia)
- Lack of prenatal care
- Low prepregnancy BMI, obesity, inadequate maternal weight gain
- Smoking, tobacco use, substance abuse
- Excessive physical activity
- Psychological factors like depression, anxiety, and stress

Pregnancy-Related Factors

Threatened miscarriage (vaginal bleeding) in early pregnancy and previous spontaneous miscarriages are associated with an increased risk of preterm birth. Several obstetric complications such as placenta previa, placenta accreta spectrum, PPROM, oligohydramnios or polyhydramnios, hypertensive disorders, poorly controlled gestational diabetes, and intrahepatic cholestasis of pregnancy may require an indicated PTB to safeguard the mother and/or the fetus.

Uterine Overdistension

Multiple pregnancy and polyhydramnios are factors that can result in the overdistension of the uterus. This predisposes to preterm labour by affecting the placental–fetal–endocrine cascade that initiates uterine activation and premature cervical ripening.

Congenital Malformations

Fetal birth defects increase the risk of preterm labour.

Genetic Factors

In a genome-wide association study, variants of certain gene loci were associated with PTB [7].

Cervical Factors

- **A short cervix,** as measured by transvaginal ultrasonography (<25 mm at 16–24 weeks of gestation), has been associated with an increased risk of preterm birth [8]. Clinically, the shorter the cervix, the greater the risk of preterm birth. However, a short cervix on ultrasound examination is most predictive of preterm birth in women with a history of preterm birth.
- Dysfunction of the cervical epithelium or extracellular stroma causes an ascending infection and, thereby, preterm labour.
- The mechanical competence of the cervix may be affected by prior surgeries on the cervix, including a D&E, ablative and

excisional procedures like conization, or loop electrosurgical excision (LEEP). These can lead to preterm labour.

Key Point

A short cervix on ultrasound examination is most predictive of preterm birth in women with a history of preterm birth.

Uterine Abnormalities

Developmental abnormalities such as unicornuate, bicornuate, or septate uterus, and fibroids distorting the cavity, have been shown to cause preterm labour.

Infections

Inflammatory responses drive the pathogenesis of infection-induced preterm labour (PTL). Intra-amniotic infections with intact membranes account for about 25–40% of PTB. The following infections are associated with preterm labour and birth:

- **Urinary tract infections**, especially pyelonephritis, have been studied as a cause of preterm birth.
  - **Asymptomatic bacteriuria** in the first and early second trimesters may lead to cystitis and pyelonephritis later in pregnancy. To avoid this, routine screening for asymptomatic bacteria at 12–16 weeks has been recommended in Western guidelines. However, this may not be performed routinely in LMICs due to resource constraints.
- **Periodontitis** (inflammation of the gums) is a chronic anaerobic infection that affects many pregnant women and may be a causative factor of PTB if not treated.
- **Malaria** is associated with PTB and low-birth-weight babies.
- **Genital tract infections** caused by *Mycoplasma hominis* or *Ureaplasma urealyticum*, bacterial vaginosis, and group B streptococcal infections have been associated with preterm labour.

Pregnancies Following Assisted Reproduction (ART)

Pregnancies conceived by assisted reproduction are at a higher risk of spontaneous PTB. The risk of preterm birth in singleton pregnancies resulting from IVF-ET is twice that of naturally conceived pregnancies [9]. Both female-factor infertility and the transfer of fresh embryos are independently associated with preterm birth and low birth weight for both singletons and twins after ART [10].

PATHOGENESIS OF PRETERM BIRTH

- Inflammation is the key to the pathogenesis of preterm labour [11]. It leads to intracellular signalling and the release of pro-inflammatory cytokines and chemokines, which activate toll-like receptors (TLR), leading to uterine contractility and cervical ripening, and thus promotes preterm labour and birth.
- Progesterone (P4) withdrawal initiates the onset of parturition at term and in preterm labour. Inflammation triggers P4 withdrawal.
- The normal maternal immune tolerance to the fetus helps to maintain pregnancy. When immune tolerance is lost due to a hostile immunogenic environment, it leads to preterm birth.
- Fetal stress as caused by uteroplacental insufficiency, or, less commonly, maternal stress, can induce the premature activation of the fetal hypothalamic–pituitary–adrenal (HPA) axis, resulting in a cascade of hormonal changes leading to PTB.

PREDICTION OF PRETERM LABOUR

The prediction of preterm labour is difficult, especially in women with no prior history of preterm birth. The risk of PTB must be assessed by obtaining a detailed history, which includes the following:

- Prior preterm birth and the gestational age at which it occurred

- Documented uterine abnormalities or surgeries performed on the cervix
- Other risk factors as mentioned above

The clinical examination should include the following:

- General physical examination
- BMI
- Gentle speculum and vaginal examination to check for any discharge, dilatation, and effacement of the cervix

Measurement of Cervical Length

The risk of spontaneous PTB increases as cervical length decreases. The shortening of the cervix precedes preterm labour by several weeks. **Routine cervical length measurement in a low-risk woman is controversial** and is recommended only in the following cases:

- Women with risk factors for PTB
- Women with a short cervix identified in the mid-trimester scan

Cervical length assessment (Fig. 30.1) is best achieved with transvaginal sonography (TVS) as per standard recommendations [12,13]. Measurement with TVS is not affected by maternal obesity, cervix position, or shadowing from the fetal presenting part. Transabdominal sonography is unreliable for calculating cervical length.

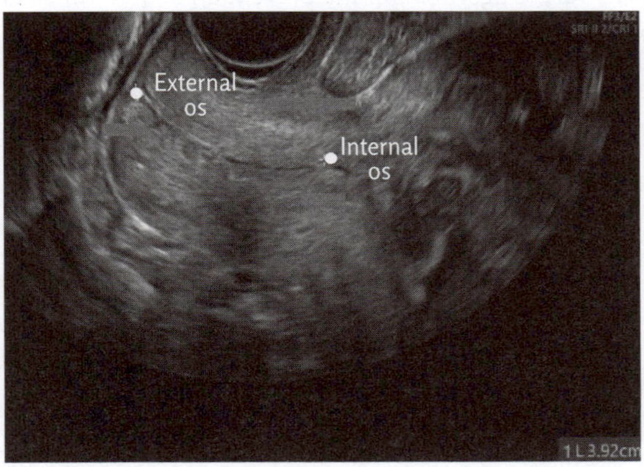

Fig. 30.1 Normal cervical length measurement—from internal os to external os (*Image courtesy*: Seethapathy Clinic and Hospital, Chennai)

Initiation of screening

The screening for cervical length is done between 16 weeks and up to 24 weeks. The measurement is taken transvaginally, avoiding excessive probe pressure on the cervix. Three measurements are taken, from the internal os to the external os, and the shortest is considered.

- Serial measurements are taken from 16–24 weeks. A shortening of cervical length of >10% within a 3-week period has been found to be associated with an increased risk of preterm birth [12].
- In asymptomatic twin pregnancies, cervical length measurement is a poor predictor of PTB <32 weeks' gestation.

Fetal Fibronectin fFN

Fetal fibronectin is a glycoprotein produced by amniocytes and cytotrophoblasts. It binds the chorionic membranes to maternal decidua. When labour contractions disrupt the decidual–chorionic interface, fFN is released. The presence of fFN in cervicovaginal secretions is a marker of true preterm labour. It is normally found in cervicovaginal fluids before 22 weeks of gestation but at very low levels.

Levels ≥50 ng/mL at or after 22 weeks have been associated with an increased risk of spontaneous preterm birth within 7–14 days, especially if associated with contractions and sonographic evidence of cervical shortening [14]. However, a systematic review of the Cochrane Database [15] did not find enough evidence to conclude whether or not the fFN test should be used in the management of women showing signs of preterm labour.

Key Point

Studies have shown that clinicians do not base their clinical management protocols on fFN results and that outcomes are not improved by knowing the fFN status [15]. Moreover, this test is not easily available in LMICs such as India and is expensive.

Other Biomarkers

Though more than 30 biomarkers have been described, a systematic review found that none of the biomarkers evaluated met the criteria to be considered clinically useful for predicting spontaneous preterm birth [16].

PREVENTION OF PRETERM LABOUR

As the mortality and morbidity associated with preterm birth are high, strategies have been described to prevent preterm labour and birth. These include the following:

- Progesterone supplementation
- Cervical cerclage
- Infection prevention strategies

Progesterone Supplementation

Over the past two decades, progesterone supplementation became part of international guidelines for the prevention of preterm labour. A recent meta-analysis and a few studies have raised doubts about the efficacy of the routine use of progesterone in women with a past history of preterm birth especially **if they do not have a short cervix on screening** [17,18,19,20]. There is a clear reduction of PTB and hence respiratory distress and composite neonatal morbidity with the use of progesterone in women with both singleton [21] and twin [22] pregnancies **with a short cervix.** The absolute risk reduction is greater for women with a short cervix [17,23,24].

The rationale for progesterone supplementation is that endogenous progesterone is responsible for uterine quiescence before labour begins. Exogenous progesterone supplementation may enhance this action. However, this hypothesis has been questioned. Circulating levels of endogenous progesterone in the third trimester are already very high, and exogenous progesterone administration does not increase these levels. It is unclear why exogenous supplementation should have biological effects [24].

Vaginal Progesterone

- **Asymptomatic women without a previous history of preterm labour**: Vaginal progesterone is recommended for these women [17,23] and is effective in a woman with:
  — A singleton pregnancy
  — Mid-trimester short cervix of ≤25 mm

  The daily dosage recommended varies between 100 and 200 mg in various studies. It is used till 36 completed weeks of gestation (Fig. 30.2).

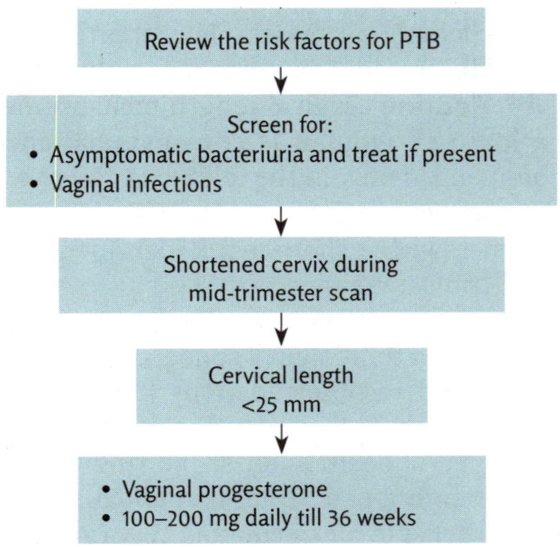

Fig. 30.2 Algorithm for the prevention of preterm birth (PTB) in a singleton pregnancy with no history of prior spontaneous preterm labour (screening for cervical length is not a routine recommendation in women at low risk for PTB)

- **Women with a previous history of PTB without a short cervix:** The use of vaginal progesterone in this situation is controversial. Currently, ACOG does not recommend vaginal progesterone for women with a prior history of preterm birth who have no cervical shortening [17]. However, other studies [23,25] consider vaginal progesterone to be the best preventive measure against preterm birth for asymptomatic women with a singleton pregnancy who are at high risk for PTB.

Key Points

- Currently, the ACOG does not recommend vaginal progesterone for women with a prior history of preterm birth who have no cervical shortening.
- There is very limited evidence for the use of oral progesterone for the prevention of PTB.

- **Women with twin pregnancy with a short cervix:** The efficacy of vaginal progesterone in twin pregnancy with a shortened cervix remains unclear [26]. While a few studies have shown some benefit, the numbers are small and need to be validated with larger studies.
- The algorithm for the prevention of preterm labour in a singleton pregnancy with a history of prior spontaneous preterm labour is presented in Fig. 30.3.

17-Alpha-hydroxyprogesterone Caproate (17-OHPC)

The recent PROLONG study (2020), which was a randomised placebo-controlled multicentre international trial, analysed the efficacy of 17-OHPC in over 1700 women with a singleton gestation and a past history of preterm birth. The study concluded that the intervention **did not significantly reduce preterm birth <35 weeks or fetal/early infant death** [20]. If used, it may be considered in women with a shortened cervix in the 18–22 weeks scan [23].

In April of 2023, the US Food and Drug Administration (FDA) withdrew approval for the use of 17-OHPC for the prevention of recurrent spontaneous PTB [27].

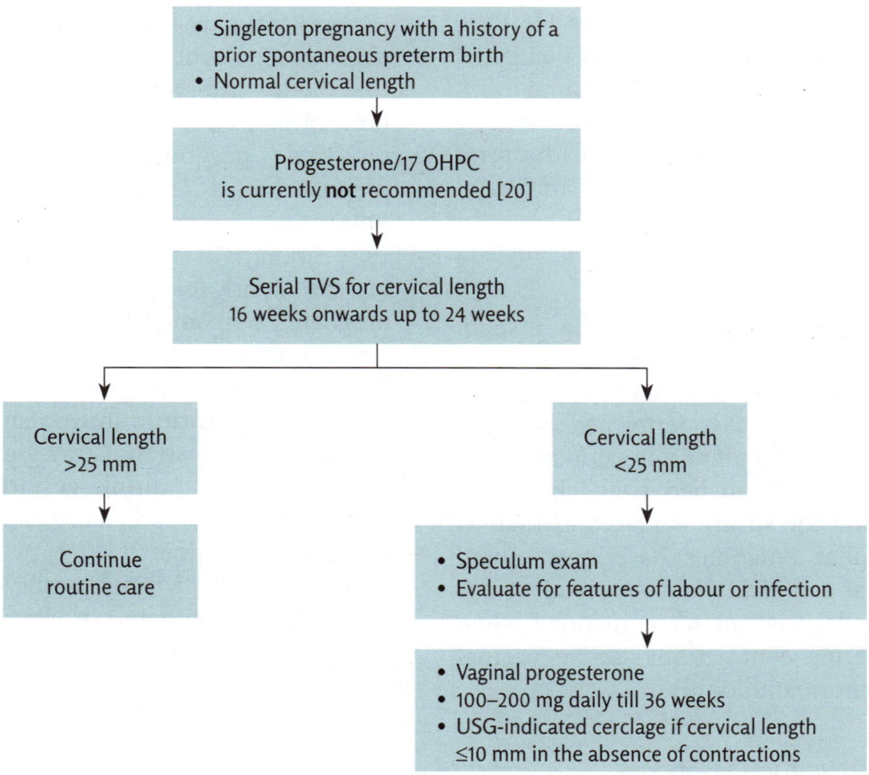

Fig. 30.3 Algorithm for the prevention of preterm labour in a singleton pregnancy with a history of prior spontaneous preterm labour

17-OHPC, 17-hydroxyprogesterone caproate; *TVS*, transvaginal sonography; *USG*, ultrasonography

Key Point

Recent studies have questioned the efficacy of 17-OHPC in preventing PTB. The USFDA no longer approves its use for the prevention of PTB.

Cervical Cerclage

History-indicated cerclage

Cervical cerclage is indicated in women with a history suggestive of preterm birth due to cervical insufficiency (multiple second-trimester pregnancy losses/PTBs associated with painless cervical dilatation).

USG-indicated cerclage

In those without a prior preterm birth, cerclage for a sonographically detected short cervix alone offers no advantage. In women with a singleton pregnancy with no other risk factors for PTB, cerclage is not recommended for an incidental finding of a short cervix on ultrasound [28]. Cerclage may be considered in those with a singleton pregnancy and who have had a prior preterm birth, cervical length <10 mm, and gestational age <24 weeks [26].

Rescue cerclage

This procedure is performed in the case of dilated/shortened cervix. The membranes may be exposed and may be seen through the external os. It is usually performed between 16 and 27+6 weeks under regional anesthesia. The membranes are pushed back above the internal os, and the suture is placed as high as possible. Similar outcomes have been noted with Shirodkar and McDonald's method.

Rescue cerclage is not recommended when there are uterine contractions, active vaginal bleeding, or chorioamnionitis.

Infection Prevention Strategies

Infection prevention strategies include periodontal care and diagnosing and treating asymptomatic bacteriuria and bacterial vaginosis.

Potentially Effective Interventions for the Prevention of PTB

- **Managing maternal medical disorders**: Identification and optimisation of chronic medical disorders before and during pregnancy can improve maternal health and, in turn, the outcome of pregnancy.
- **Aspirin for women at high risk of preeclampsia:** In women at high risk of developing preeclampsia, a daily dose of low-dose aspirin (80–150 mg) starting at 12–16 weeks of gestation can reduce the chances of preeclampsia and thus, iatrogenic PTB.
- **Substance abuse:** Avoidance of tobacco, cigarette smoking, alcohol, and substance abuse helps reduce the risk for PTB.
- **Diet and weight:** Pregnant women with adequate nutrition and a normal body mass index (BMI) have better pregnancy outcomes than women who do not, thus suggesting that dietary interventions may have a role in preventing PTB in selected populations.
- **Optimal pregnancy spacing:** Spacing pregnancies at least 18 months apart is important as short interpregnancy intervals (<6 months) are associated with an increased risk of PTB and other adverse pregnancy outcomes. However, an interval of ≥60 months also increases the risk of PTB.
- **Reducing the iatrogenic occurrence of multifetal gestation:** In women undergoing assisted reproduction, strategies to reduce the chance of a multiple gestation, particularly higher-order pregnancies (triplets and above), are of value.
  - This is done by single embryo transfer in women undergoing in vitro fertilisation (IVF).
  - Ovulation induction is performed with the use of either clomiphene citrate or aromatase inhibitors rather than gonadotropins.
  - In women with an excessive number of mature follicles, conversion to IVF or cycle cancellation is to be considered.

— If a high-order multiple gestation occurs, multifetal pregnancy reduction can improve neonatal outcomes and prevent preterm births.

- **Consider effects of cervical/uterine surgery on future pregnancies:** Procedural termination may be associated with higher rates of subsequent PTB than medical abortion. The use of cervical ripening agents rather than forceful dilatation before procedural evacuation may help reduce the risk of cervical injury.
- **Surgical correction of congenital uterine abnormalities**: Surgical correction of a uterine septum may reduce the risk for recurrent miscarriage or early PTB/miscarriage.

Ineffective and Unproven Interventions

- **Progesterone supplementation for women with a prior preterm birth**: Vaginal progesterone appears to be useful only in women with a short cervix. Cerclage is also another option in these women. Neither hydroxyprogesterone caproate nor vaginal progesterone reduce the risk of recurrent PTB in this population. These women should be followed sonographically to identify those with a short cervix between 16 and 24 weeks.
- **Monitoring uterine contraction frequency**: Although an increase in uterine activity is a prerequisite for labour, randomised trials have shown that measuring the frequency of uterine contractions by self-palpation/detection of the signs of labour or by using an ambulatory home uterine activity monitor is not beneficial in the management of PTB. Home uterine activity monitoring is not recommended as a strategy for predicting and preventing PTB.
- **Prophylactic tocolytics**: Prophylactic tocolytic therapy for the prevention of PTB in high-risk asymptomatic pregnant women is not effective in randomised trials.
- **Low-dose aspirin**: Low-dose aspirin should not be used in an attempt to prevent spontaneous PTB but should be considered for women with risk factors for preeclampsia to prevent this disorder and its consequences, including indicated PTB.
- **Pessary:** There is no evidence to support the use of pessaries in prolonging gestation or preventing preterm birth.
- **Bed rest**: Bed rest may improve uteroplacental blood flow and can lead to a slight increase in birth weight. However, there is **no evidence** that it decreases the incidence of PTB even in women with a short cervix.
- **Dietary modification**: Vitamin and protein supplements have not been found to reduce the rate of PTB. However, there may be potential benefits of micronutrient supplementation in specific subpopulations of pregnant women, such as those who are undernourished or infected with HIV.
- **Social support and stress reduction:** Although social support during pregnancy has resulted in improvements in short-term psychosocial outcomes, it has not significantly reduced the rate of PTB.

There are limited data on other interventions for reducing stress in pregnant women (e.g., meditation, massage, yoga, breathing exercises, music therapy, aroma therapy).

DIAGNOSIS OF PRETERM LABOUR

One of the most common reasons for hospital admission in pregnancy is suspected preterm labour.

Signs and Symptoms of Preterm Labour

Women may experience these prodromal signs and symptoms:

- Pelvic pressure
- Intermittent menstrual-like cramps
- Watery vaginal discharge
- Lower back pain

Regular contractions before 37 weeks that are associated with cervical changes are indicative of preterm labour [26]. Contractions with a frequency of at least 2 every 10 minutes or 6 per hour are significant. Cervical dilatation

≥3 cm, cervical length <10 mm, and 'show' or rupture of membranes confirm labour.

MANAGEMENT OF PRETERM LABOUR

Those with suspected preterm labour must be hospitalised, and interventions that have been shown to improve perinatal outcome should be implemented.

Tocolysis

Tocolysis is likely to be beneficial in uncomplicated preterm labour and may help in the short-term prolongation of pregnancy, thereby providing time for the corticosteroid to act and for in utero transfer to be achieved. However, tocolysis is not recommended prior to 24 weeks of gestation.

Nifedipine is the first drug of choice for tocolysis [29]. If a woman is already on magnesium sulphate for fetal neuroprotection, beta-adrenergic receptor agonists and calcium-channel blockers should be used with caution for tocolysis in combination with it because of the possibility of respiratory depression [30]. Terbutaline is associated with significant maternal side effects and is not recommended except under strict in-patient monitoring and for short durations.

The drugs available for tocolysis are listed in Table 30.1.

Table 30.1 Commonly used tocolytics for women with preterm labour and intact membranes

Drug	Class of drug	Route and dose	Maternal side effects
Nifedipine	Calcium channel blocker	• Loading dose of 30 mg orally • Followed by 20 mg 8th hourly for 48 hours • A maximum dose of 180 mg/day	Hypotension, tachycardia, headache
Terbutaline	β-adrenergic receptor agonist	For short-term inpatient use • 0.25 mg SC every 20 to 30 minutes up to 4 doses till tocolysis is achieved • Followed by 0.25 mg SC every 4 hours for 24–48 hours	Tachycardia, hypotension, palpitations, tremors, shortness of breath, chest discomfort
Magnesium sulphate*	Calcium antagonist	• 4–6 g IV load over 20 minutes • Followed by a continuous infusion of 2 g/hour	Respiratory and cardiac depression, cardiac arrhythmias, hypocalcemia
Indomethacin**	Cyclo-oxygenase inhibitor	• 50 mg loading dose orally • Followed by 25 mg orally every 4–6 hours for 48 hours	Nausea, vomiting, gastric reflux, platelet dysfunction
Nitroglycerine	Nitric oxide donor	• Nitroderm patch 10 mg • Oral vs transdermal vs IV showed no proven benefit	Significant maternal hypotension and headache
Atosiban	Oxytocin receptor antagonist	• Initial bolus dose 6.75 mg over 1 minute • Followed by an infusion of 18 mg/hour for 3 hours, then 6 mg/hr for up to 45 hours	Hypersensitivity to the drug

* Urine output and renal function should be monitored carefully while administering magnesium sulphate.

** Indomethacin should be avoided in women with bronchial asthma or gastrointestinal ulcerative disease. It may also cause fetal renal dysfunction, oligohydramnios, and premature closure of the ductus venosus. It should not be used after 32 weeks' gestation.

Contraindications

- Intrauterine fetal demise and lethal fetal anomalies
- Non-reassuring fetal status
- Preeclampsia with severe features or eclampsia
- Antepartum hemorrhage in a hemodynamically unstable woman
- Chorioamnionitis
- Medical contraindications to the tocolytic drug

Maintenance therapy

Maintenance therapy with tocolytics has been proven to be ineffective. Tocolysis is currently not recommended for more than 48 hours.

Corticosteroids

A single course of corticosteroids is recommended for pregnant women between 24+7 weeks and 33+6 weeks of gestation who are at risk of preterm delivery within 7 days, including those with ruptured membranes and multiple pregnancies in both singleton and multiple pregnancy.

Drugs and dosage

- Inj. betamethasone 12 mg IM 24 hours apart, 2 doses
- Inj. dexamethasone 6 mg IM 12 hrs apart, 4 doses

Studies have shown no difference between the outcomes of the two drugs, though betamethasone is less expensive and requires fewer doses. Though they do not reduce the incidence of cerebral palsy, steroids help in reducing the risk of the following:

- Perinatal death
- Respiratory distress
- Necrotising enterocolitis
- Intraventricular hemorrhage

A single **rescue course** of antenatal corticosteroids should be considered in women who are <34 weeks of gestation, who are at a risk of preterm delivery within the next 7 days, and to whom a prior course of antenatal corticosteroids was administered more than 14 days previously [30].

Magnesium Sulphate for Fetal Neuroprotection

When a woman is at high risk of giving birth before 32 weeks, the administration of magnesium sulphate reduces the risk of cerebral palsy [31]. It is of proven benefit when offered to women between 24 and 32 weeks of gestation.

Magnesium sulphate should be administered when early preterm birth is planned or expected in the next 24 hours. **However, it should be stopped if the woman has not delivered within 24 hours**. The dose can be repeated if labour does not progress, and the woman returns again with preterm labour.

Mechanism of action

Magnesium sulphate acts by blocking the N-methyl-D-aspartate (NMDA) receptors in the oligodendrocytes, thereby leading to vasodilatation and protection against white matter injury and hypoxia-induced ischemic injury. This reduces the risk of cerebral palsy.

Dosage

The recommended dosage is as follows:

- 4 g IV bolus over 15 minutes
- Followed by an infusion of 1 g/hour till the birth of the baby or for 24 hours, whichever is the earliest

The administration of magnesium sulphate for more than 5 days has been shown to be associated with skeletal adverse effects like fetal osteopenia, hypocalcemia, and hypermagnesemia in neonates.

Antibiotics in Preterm Labour

Preterm delivery is often associated with evidence of chorioamnionitis, and the earlier the gestational age at delivery, the greater the risk. However, the ORACLE-II trial [32] showed conclusively that **antibiotics should not be**

routinely prescribed for women in spontaneous preterm labour with intact membranes in the absence of evidence of clinical infection.

Management After Resolution of Acute Preterm Labour

- Women whose symptoms subside after treatment may be sent home with instructions to return if the pain recurs. Bed rest is not recommended. The woman may be advised to avoid sexual activity and strenuous work.
- Routine fetal fibronectin testing and home uterine activity monitoring devices have not proven useful in high-resource settings [30]. There is no role for long-term tocolytics or prophylactic antibiotics.

Management if the Woman Proceeds to Active Labour

- If the woman continues to have contractions despite all measures, the delivery should preferably be carried out in a tertiary-care centre with adequate facilities for monitoring the mother and a neonatal intensive care unit (NICU) for the care of the newborn.
- Continuous fetal monitoring is recommended.
- Fetuses in cephalic presentation can be delivered vaginally. A routine episiotomy is not required.
- Cesarean delivery is reserved for non-cephalic presentations and fetal growth restriction.
- When operative vaginal delivery is decided upon, vacuum is best avoided in a preterm baby <34 weeks due to the risk of intracranial hemorrhage and subdural hematoma.
- Delayed cord clamping is recommended (see **Chapter 5**, *Routine care of the third stage of labour*). This facilitates cardiopulmonary transition by expanding intravascular volume and reduces iron and hemopoietic stem cell loss.
- The neonatal team must be alerted and must be available to receive the preterm baby.

NEONATAL COMPLICATIONS OF PRETERM LABOUR

Complications of the preterm infant (gestational age <37 weeks) are divided into short-term complications that occur in the neonatal period and long-term sequelae in babies who survive and are discharged from the NICU.

Short-term Complications

- Hypothermia
- Hypoglycemia
- Respiratory distress syndrome
- Cardiovascular abnormalities
- Intraventricular hemorrhage
- Necrotising enterocolitis
- Risk of infection
- Retinopathy of prematurity due to increased oxygen use

Long-term Sequelae

- Neurodevelopmental disabilities such as cerebral palsy
- Failure to thrive
- Infant mortality

PRETERM PRELABOUR RUPTURE OF MEMBRANES (PPROM)

DEFINITION OF PROM AND PPROM

The rupture of membranes before the onset of labour but after 37 weeks of gestation is termed **prelabour rupture of membranes (PROM)**. Membrane rupture before 37 weeks is referred to as **preterm prelabour rupture of membranes (PPROM)**. The management of preterm and term PROM is influenced greatly by the gestational age. The presence of complicating factors such as infection, placental abruption, preterm labour, or non-reassuring fetal status will dictate further interventions.

INCIDENCE OF PROM AND PPROM

PROM complicates approximately 8% of all pregnancies [33]. PPROM occurs in up to 3% of pregnancies, of which 2% occur in pregnancies between 27 and 37 weeks; it is associated with approximately 30% of preterm births.

PATHOPHYSIOLOGY OF PPROM

The mechanism of spontaneous membrane rupture is poorly understood [34]. Extracellular collagen is the most important factor in maintaining the tensile strength of fetal membranes. When pregnancy progresses, the membranes thin out, and rupture occurs when the internal forces exceed the tensile strength of the chorioamnion. Matrix metalloproteins (MMPs) are associated with collagen degradation and tissue remodelling and are seen in higher levels in PPROM.

The inflammatory response to subclinical or overt infection as well as mechanical stress and bleeding have been implicated in PPROM. Bacterial infections release endotoxins and TNF-α, which releases fetal fibronectin and, in turn, activates MMPs and prostaglandins.

Key Point

In bacterial infections, fetal fibronectin is released, which activates MMPs and prostaglandins. Thus, membrane rupture is often accompanied by cervical ripening and uterine contractions.

RISK FACTORS FOR PPROM

Though many factors predispose to PPROM, no obvious identifiable risk factor may be found in many women. The following risk factors have been implicated:

- A **history of PPROM** in a previous pregnancy is a strong risk factor for recurrence
- **Infections** caused by *Chlamydia trachomatis*, *Trichomonas vaginalis*, group B β-hemolytic streptococci
- **Uterine factors** related to overdistension of the uterus, such as multiple pregnancy and polyhydramnios
- **Molecular changes** related to oxidative stress, and premature cell maturity, leading to thinning and breaking of the amniochorion
- **Demographic factors and lifestyle factors** similar to those explained in the risk factors for preterm labour
- **Connective tissue disorders**, e.g., Ehlers-Danlos syndrome
- **Invasive procedures** such as amniocentesis and fetal blood sampling

CLINICAL FEATURES OF PPROM

The symptoms of a woman presenting with PROM or PPROM may include the following:

- Sudden gush of clear or pale-yellow fluid from the vagina
- Intermittent or constant trickling of small amounts of fluid
- Sensation of wetness within the vagina; some women may mistake it for an involuntary passage of urine

DIAGNOSIS OF PROM AND PPROM

A speculum examination may reveal fluid gushing from the cervical os that may increase with the application of abdominal pressure. It may also reveal a pool of fluid in the vagina.

Key Point

A digital examination should be avoided in suspected cases of PPROM as it may increase the risk of intrauterine infection.

Diagnostic Tests

- **Nitrazine test**: The nitrazine paper strip changes colour from yellow to blue on exposure to the alkaline pH of the amniotic fluid, which is 7.3–7.8. The vaginal pH is usually

3.8–4.5. False positive tests may be seen in the presence of blood or semen, antiseptics, or bacterial vaginosis.

- **Fern test**: This is a bedside test in which fluid from the posterior vaginal fornix is swabbed onto a glass slide and allowed to dry for at least 10 minutes and then examined under a microscope. The characteristic ferning pattern of amniotic fluid will be observed.
- **Extended pad test**: If the diagnosis of ROM has still not been established, the woman is asked to wear a sanitary pad and walk around. On checking after two hours, if the pad is wet, ROM may be confirmed.
- **Commercial tests**: If, on speculum examination, no amniotic fluid is observed, clinicians should consider performing an insulin-like growth factor-binding protein-1 (IGFBP-1) or placental alpha macroglobulin-1 (PAMG-1) test on the vaginal fluid to guide further management. **These test kits are not commonly available in India and other LMICs.**
- **Ultrasound:** ROM can be confirmed by an ultrasound which may show marked oligohydramnios or anhydramnios.

COMPLICATIONS OF PPROM

Complications include both maternal and fetal complications.

Maternal Complications

- Chorioamnionitis is caused by ascending infection and occurs in 15–25% of women with PPROM. It leads to increased maternal and neonatal morbidity and mortality. Clinical features of chorioamnionitis include the following:
  - Fever (temperature >39°C or an additional clinical sign when the temperature is between 38–38.9°C)
  - Foul-smelling vaginal discharge
  - Uterine tenderness
  - Blood investigations showing leukocytosis and increased C-reactive protein (CRP)
  - Fetal tachycardia
- **Puerperal endometritis** may occur following PPROM. The risk is more with cesarean than it is with vaginal delivery.
- **Maternal sepsis** could be a sequel to chorioamnionitis or endometritis.
- **Placental abruption** may occur in 2–5% of women with PPROM [35]. The risk is 7- to 10-fold in women who have intrauterine infections or oligohydramnios.

Fetal and Neonatal Complications

Fetal infectious morbidity is high in the presence of chorioamnionitis and may present as pneumonia or sepsis. Prolonged NICU admissions and increased mortality and morbidity can result. Cord prolapse and cord compression may occur. The consequences of preterm birth may result in short-term and long-term sequelae (see section above on *Neonatal complications of preterm birth*).

MANAGEMENT OF PPROM

Initial Evaluation

All women who present with PPROM should be evaluated for the following:

- Gestational age
- Fetal presentation
- Fetal well-being

A confirmed case of PPROM should ideally be hospitalised. The majority of women will go into labour within a week of PPROM [34]. The two modes of management available are:

- **Immediate delivery** (by induction of labour or by cesarean delivery)
- **Expectant management**

Immediate Delivery

There does not seem to be much benefit to prolonging the pregnancy if prelabour ROM has occurred at ≥37+0 weeks. Immediate delivery is recommended and preferred by women.

Pregnancies between 34+0 to 36+6 weeks may be managed either by immediate delivery or with expectant management based on the resources available for neonatal care, the risk of infection, and the woman's choice. The advantages of immediate delivery include a decreased risk of chorioamnionitis and infection-related neonatal admission and a lower cost of treatment.

Prompt delivery of women with PPROM irrespective of gestational age is indicated in the presence of the following:

- Active labour
- Non-reassuring fetal status
- Signs and symptoms of chorioamnionitis
- Placental abruption
- A high risk of cord prolapse

Expectant Management

Expectant management is the preferred choice when the gestational age is between 24 and 34 weeks in the absence of a non-reassuring fetal status, chorioamnionitis, or placental abruption [31]. Expectant management is usually undertaken to carry the pregnancy up to 34 weeks, and if possible, 37 weeks [33,36]. A policy of expectant management with careful monitoring is associated with better outcomes for the mother and fetus [37]. Hospitalisation is recommended for at least 5–7 days for women who have a viable fetus. If necessary, this might be extended until the time of delivery.

Key Point

Expectant management is the preferred choice when the gestational age is between 24 and 34 weeks in the absence of a non-reassuring fetal status, chorioamnionitis, or placental abruption.

In low-resource areas, expectant management before 24 weeks may increase the risk of maternal infection without the possibility of salvaging the fetus. Prolonged oligohydramnios may also be associated with fetal lung hypoplasia, limb contractures, and facial compression. This should be explained to the couple in clear and sensitive language.

Prophylactic antibiotic therapy

The use of prophylactic antibiotics to prolong pregnancy has been proven to be beneficial. Various antibiotic regimens have been described. The maternity unit should adopt one to be used in all cases of PPROM. In addition to prolonging pregnancy, antibiotics also reduce the risk of maternal and neonatal infection and reduce neonatal morbidity associated with prematurity.

Recommended drugs and dosage

It is not clear which antibiotic regimen should be used. Any of the following regimens may be used, with similar results:

- Erythromycin 250 mg orally 4 times a day for 10 days [38,39] **or**
- IV ampicillin (2 g every 6 hours) and IV erythromycin (250 mg every 6 hours) for 48 hours followed by oral amoxicillin (250 mg every 8 hours) and erythromycin base (333 mg every 8 hours) [33] **or**
- Azithromycin 1 g orally on admission PLUS IV ampicillin (2 g every 6 hours for 48 hours) followed by oral amoxicillin (500 mg 3 times daily) for another 5 days

Key Point

Amoxicillin/clavulanic acid is contraindicated because of the increased risk of necrotising enterocolitis in neonates exposed to this antibiotic.

Tocolysis

There is insufficient evidence to conclude on the benefits or possible harms of tocolysis in women with PPROM [29]. Nifedipine can be considered in women with ruptured membranes to allow time to administer a course of steroids, as long as there are no contraindications such as intrauterine infection.

Corticosteroids for lung maturation

Antenatal corticosteroids are recommended in the latest WHO guidelines for preterm birth if the PPROM occurs between 24 and 34 weeks, delivery is expected within 7 days, there are no signs of infection, and facilities are available to manage a premature neonate [40].

Monitoring for signs of infection

If expectant management has been chosen, it is important to be alert for signs of infection. In the absence of fever, uterine tenderness or leukocytosis are not sensitive signs. Fetal tachycardia may occur after chorioamnionitis has set in.

The management of pregnancies with PPROM with a reassuring fetal status is summarised in Table 30.2.

Table 30.2 Management of PPROM according to gestational age [33,38,39,40]

Gestational age	Management of pregnancies with reassuring fetal status
34+0 to 36+6 weeks	• Expectant management or plan delivery (induction or cesarean as appropriate) • Single course of corticosteroid may be considered up to 36+6 weeks if not given previously (delivery need not be delayed for steroids)
24–33+6 weeks	• Explain prognosis to the couple • Expectant management • Antibiotics to prolong the pregnancy • Single course of corticosteroid • Magnesium sulphate for neuroprotection if <32 weeks
<24 weeks (previable)	• Explain poor fetal prognosis to couple and weigh it against maternal infectious morbidity • Depending on couple's decision, expectant management or induction of labour • Steroids and tocolysis not recommended before viability

CONCLUSION

The incidence of preterm birth and PPROM is increasing globally. However, it is seen more often in countries with low resources. The significance of preterm birth lies in the consequences of prematurity for the infant and the impact of these on the infant's survival and subsequent development. Neonatal mortality rates due to prematurity may vary among different geographical regions as well as among racial and ethnic groups. Preterm birth is a challenge for both the obstetrician and the neonatologist in LMICs like India. Screening for risk factors and appropriate initiation of preventive strategies including progesterone and cerclage can help prevent preterm births. Good facilities and adequate care with individualised treatment are the key to the management of preterm labour and PPROM.

REFERENCES

1. Perin J, Mulick A, Yeung D, Villavicencio F, Lopez G, Strong KL, et al. Global, regional, and national causes of under-5 mortality in 2000–19: An updated systematic analysis with implications for the Sustainable Development Goals. *Lancet Child Adolesc Health.* 2022. 6(2):106-15. doi:10.1016/S2352-4642(21)00311–4.
2. Chawanpaiboon S, Vogel JP, Moller A-B, Lumbiganon P, Petzold M, Hogan D, et al. Global, regional, and national estimates of levels of preterm birth in 2014: A systematic review and modelling analysis. *The Lancet Global Health.* 2019. 7(1): e37–e46. pmid:30389451.
3. Ramenghi LA. Late preterm babies and the risk of neurological damage. *Acta Biomed.* 2015. 86 (suppl 1): 36–40.
4. Mwaniki MK, Atieno M, Lawn JE, Newton CR. Long-term neurodevelopmental outcomes after intrauterine and neonatal insults: A systematic review. *Lancet.* 2012. 379: 445–52. https://www.who.int/news-room/fact-sheets/detail/preterm-birth. Accessed February 2023.
5. World Health Organization. Born too soon: Decade of action on preterm birth. WHO, Geneva. 2023.
6. Laughon SK, Albert PS, Leishear K, Mendola P. The NICHD Consecutive Pregnancies Study: Recurrent preterm delivery by subtype. *Am J Obstet Gynecol.* 2014. 210(2):131.e1-8.
7. Zhang G, Feenstra B, Bacelis J, et al. Genetic associations with gestational duration and spontaneous preterm birth. *N Engl J Med.* 2017. 377(12):1156–1167.

8. Berghella V. Short cervix before 24 weeks: Screening and management in singleton pregnancies. Simpson LL (Ed). *UpToDate*. 2023. Waltham, MA.
9. McGovern PG, Llorens AJ, Skurnick JH, et al. Increased risk of preterm birth in singleton pregnancies resulting from in vitro fertilization-embryo transfer or gamete intrafallopian transfer: A meta-analysis. *Fertil Steril*. 2004. 82:1514.
10. Wang YA, Sullivan EA, Black D, et al. Preterm birth and low birth weight after assisted reproductive technology-related pregnancy in Australia between 1996 and 2000. *Fertil Steril*. 2005. 83:1650.
11. Romero R, Espinoza J, Goncalves LF, et al. Inflammation in preterm and term labour and delivery. *Semin Fetal Neonatal Med*. 2006. 11(5):317–326. doi: 10.1016/j.siny.2006.05.001.
12. Berghella V, Bega G, Tolosa JE, Berghella M. Ultrasound assessment of the cervix. *Clin. Obstet. Gynecol*. 2003. 46:947–962. doi: 10.1097/00003081-200312000-00026.
13. Berghella V, Palacio M, Ness A, Alfirevic Z, Nicolaides KH, Saccone G. Cervical length screening for prevention of preterm birth in singleton pregnancy with threatened preterm labor: Systematic review and meta-analysis of randomized controlled trials using individual patient-level data. *Ultrasound Obstet Gynecol*. 2017. 49:322–329. doi: 10.1002/uog.17388.
14. Hezelgrave NL, Abbott DS, Radford SK, et al. Quantitative fetal fibronectin at 18 weeks of gestation to predict preterm birth in asymptomatic high-risk women. *Obstet Gynecol*. 2016. 127:255.
15. Berghella V, Saccone G. Fetal fibronectin testing for reducing the risk of preterm birth. *Cochrane Database Syst Rev*. 2019. 7(7):CD006843.
16. Conde-Agudelo A, Papageorghiou AT, Kennedy SH, Villar J. Novel biomarkers for the prediction of the spontaneous preterm birth phenotype: a systematic review and meta-analysis. BJOG 2011; 118:1042.
17. ACOG Practice Advisory. Updated clinical guidance for the use of progesterone supplementation for the prevention of recurrent preterm birth. 2023. https://www.acog.org/en/clinical/clinical-guidance/practice-advisory/articles/2023/04/updated-guidance-use-of-progesterone-supplementation-for-prevention-of-recurrent-preterm-birth?utm_source=higher-logic&utm_medium=email&utm_content=apr-07&utm_campaign=acog2023-rounds. (Accessed August 2023)
18. Conde-Agudelo A, Romero R. Vaginal progesterone does not prevent recurrent preterm birth in women with a singleton gestation, a history of spontaneous preterm birth, and a midtrimester cervical length >25 mm. *Am J Obstet Gynecol*. 2022. 227:923-6.
19. Nelson DB, Lafferty A, Venkatraman C, McDonald JG, Eckert KM, McIntire DD, et al. Association of vaginal progesterone treatment with prevention of recurrent preterm birth. *JAMA Netw Open*. 2022. 5:e2237600.
20. Blackwell SC, Gyamfi-Bannerman C, Biggio JR Jr, et al. 17-OHPC to Prevent Recurrent Preterm Birth in Singleton Gestations (PROLONG Study): A multicenter, international, randomized double-blind trial. *Am J Perinatol*. 2020. 37:127.
21. Romero R, Conde-Agudelo A, Da Fonseca E, et al. Vaginal progesterone for preventing preterm birth and adverse perinatal outcomes in singleton gestations with a short cervix: A meta-analysis of individual patient data. *Am J Obstet Gynecol*. 2018. 218, 161–180.
22. Romero R, Conde-Agudelo A, Rehal A, et al.Vaginal progesterone for the prevention of preterm birth and adverse perinatal outcomes in twin gestations with a short cervix: an updated individual patient data meta-analysis. *Ultrasound Obstet Gynecol*. 2022. 59(2):263.
23. Evaluating Progestogens for Preventing Preterm birth International Collaborative (EPPPIC): Meta-analysis of individual participant data from randomised controlled trials. 2021. *Lancet*. 397(10280), 1183-1194.
24. Norwitz ER. Progesterone supplementation to reduce the risk of spontaneous preterm labor and birth. Lockwood CJ (Ed). *UpToDate*. *2023*. Waltham, MA.
25. Care A, Nevitt SJ, Medley N, et al. Interventions to prevent spontaneous preterm birth in women with singleton pregnancy who are at high risk: Systematic review and network meta-analysis. *BMJ*. 2022. 376:e064547.
26. Prediction and prevention of spontaneous preterm birth. ACOG Practice Bulletin No. 234. American College of Obstetricians and Gynecologists. *Obstet Gynecol*. 2021;138:e65–90.
27. https://www.fda.gov/drugs/postmarket-drug-safety-information-patients-and-providers/makena-hydroxyprogesterone-caproate-injection-information (Accessed August 2023).
28. Shennan AH, Story L. the Royal College of Obstetricians and Gynaecologists. Cervical Cerclage. *BJOG*. 2022.129:1178–1210.
29. World Health Organization, WHO recommendation on tocolytic therapy for improving preterm birth outcomes. WHO, Geneva. 2022.
30. Management of preterm labor. Practice Bulletin No. 171. American College of Obstetricians and Gynecologists. *Obstet Gynecol*. 2016 (Reaffirmed 2022). 128:e155–64.
31. Doyle LW, Crowther CA, Middleton P, et al. Magnesium sulphate for women at risk of preterm birth for neuroprotection of the fetus. *Cochrane Database of Systematic Reviews*. 2009. Issue 1. Art. No.: CD004661.

32. Kenyon SL, Taylor DJ, Tarnow-Mordi W. ORACLE Collaborative Group. Broad-spectrum antibiotics for spontaneous preterm labour: The ORACLE II randomised trial. ORACLE Collaborative Group. *Lancet.* 200131;357(9261):989-94.
33. Prelabor rupture of membranes. ACOG Practice Bulletin No. 217. American College of Obstetricians and Gynecologists. *Obstet Gynecol.* 2020. 135:e80–97.
34. Duff P. Preterm prelabor rupture of membranes: Clinical manifestations and diagnosis. Lockwood CJ (Ed). *UpToDate.* 2023. Waltham, MA.
35. Ananth CV, Oyelese Y, Srinivas N, Yeo L, Vintzileos AM. Preterm premature rupture of membranes, intrauterine infection, and oligohydramnios: Risk factors for placental abruption. *Obstet Gynecol.* 2004. 104:71–7.
36. Thomson AJ. On behalf of the Royal College of Obstetricians and Gynaecologists. Care of women presenting with suspected preterm prelabour rupture of membranes from 24+0 weeks of gestation. *BJOG.* 2019. 126:e152–166
37. Bond DM, Middleton P, Levett KM, et al. 2017. Planned early birth versus expectant management for women with preterm prelabour rupture of membranes prior to 37 weeks' gestation for improving pregnancy outcome. *Cochrane Database Syst Rev.* Issue 3. Art. no.:CD0047.
38. Kenyon S L, Taylor D J, Tarnow–Mordi W. ORACLE Collaborative group. Broad–spectrum antibiotics for spontaneous preterm labour: The ORACLE I randomized trial. *Lancet.* 2001. 357979–988.
39. World Health Organization. WHO recommendations on interventions to improve preterm birth outcomes. WHO, Geneva. 2015.
40. World Health Organization. WHO recommendations on antenatal corticosteroids for improving preterm birth outcomes. WHO. Geneva. 2022a.

CHAPTER 31

Late Term and Postterm Pregnancy

NOZER SHERIAR

INTRODUCTION

For mammals, **gestation** is the period in which a fetus develops, beginning with fertilisation and ending at birth. The duration of this period varies between species. For humans, the period of gestation is 266 days or 38 weeks.

Gestational age is the term commonly used to describe the length of the pregnancy and is measured in weeks, from the first day of the woman's last menstrual cycle to the current date. The gestational age of a human term pregnancy is **280 days** or 40 weeks.

Postterm pregnancy is defined as a pregnancy that extends to 42 weeks and beyond [1]. While the reported frequency of postterm pregnancy is up to 12%, the actual incidence is probably less, because inaccurate dating is the most frequent cause of diagnosing a postterm pregnancy [2].

The timely onset of labour at and around term is an important determinant of a favourable perinatal outcome. While it has long been known that there is a small absolute increase in perinatal mortality in postterm pregnancies, the ideal gestational age to achieve delivery is still debated.

CLASSIFICATION OF PREGNANCIES AT AND AROUND TERM

Singleton pregnancies usually have a gestational period that lasts an average of 40 weeks. A pregnancy is said to be full term when it reaches 39 and 40 weeks. The upper limit of a full-term pregnancy is marked by the **estimated date of delivery (EDD)** which is **280 days** or **40 completed weeks** from the first day of the woman's last menstrual period (LMP), when the woman's menstrual cycles are regular and at or around 28 days in length. Besides the LMP date, the regularity and length of cycles must be taken into account when estimating gestational age [3].

The terms used for pregnancy subgroups, as listed below, are all defined relative to the full term pregnancy [2]:

- **Full term** 39+1 to 40+6 weeks' gestation
- **Early term** 37+1 to 38+6 weeks' gestation
- **Late term** 41+1 to 41+6 weeks' gestation
- **Postterm** Over 42 weeks' gestation (over 294 days from the LMP and 14 days from the EDD)

Key Point

Although the LMP has been traditionally used to calculate the EDD, there are many inaccuracies while using this method, particularly in women who have irregular cycles, those who have recently been on hormonal birth control, and those who have had bleeding in the first trimester.

The available evidence indicates that gestational length varies with ethnicity. Research suggests that the normal gestational length is shorter in women of Asian and African descent, with fetal maturation occurring earlier as compared to white Caucasian women. A study comparing gestational lengths amongst a cohort of white Caucasian, Asian, and Black nulliparous women with singleton live fetuses at the time of spontaneous labour reported that the median gestational age at delivery was 40 weeks in white Europeans and 39 weeks in Asians and Blacks [4].

The WHO Multinational Longitudinal Study undertaken to establish growth charts for developing countries, reported the **median gestational age at birth in India to be 38 weeks and 4 days**, an observation that must be factored in the identification, monitoring, and management of late term and postterm pregnancies [5].

DIAGNOSIS OF POSTTERM PREGNANCY

A pregnancy is diagnosed to be **late term** when it is between 41 and 42 weeks and **postterm** when it is at or after 42 weeks of gestation. The diagnosis is based on the clinician's most accurate estimate of the woman's EDD.

Ultrasound-based pregnancy dating has become an important part of modern obstetric care. The LMP is used to determine EDD if the ultrasound-based EDD is within 5–7 days of the LMP-based EDD. However, if the ultrasound-based EDD differs from that calculated from the LMP, the EDD should be corrected based on an ultrasound examination as has been described in the section below on the *Role of ultrasound dating*.

In pregnancies with known dates of conception or implantation, such as pregnancies resulting from vitro fertilisaton, the EDD is calculated using the age of the embryo and the date of transfer. For example, for a day-5 embryo, the EDD would be 261 days from the embryo replacement date. Similarly, the EDD for a day-3 embryo would be 263 days from the embryo replacement date.

PREVALENCE OF LATE TERM AND POSTTERM BIRTHS

The reported prevalence of postterm birth is up to 10% worldwide. Large differences exist between and within countries depending on the diversity of the populations studied.

In resource-rich countries, the overall incidence of postterm birth has decreased with the increased use of first-trimester ultrasound and the resultant improved dating of pregnancies. There has also been a decrease in numbers due to the widespread practice of inducing labour once pregnancies reach 41 weeks in a specific effort to avoid the delivery of postterm infants [6]. In LMICs, the available data are unclear, but preterm deliveries are commoner than postterm deliveries.

Key Point

In pregnancies dated by first-trimester ultrasound examination, the prevalence of postterm pregnancy is approximately 2%, with fewer inductions performed for postterm pregnancy than in pregnancies dated by LMP [6].

Role of Ultrasound Dating

Ultrasonographic dating early in pregnancy can improve the reliability of the EDD. If the calculated ultrasonographic gestational age varies from the LMP by more than the respective range of error, it is used instead of the LMP to establish the final EDD.

It is preferable not to date the pregnancy before 8 weeks, which is when the crown–rump length (CRL) can be accurately measured. It is best to date pregnancies in the first trimester between 8 and 13 weeks' gestational age.

Depending on the period of gestation at which the scan is done, the measurement used and the margin of deviation can vary. In the absence of an earlier scan, dating pregnancy in the late second and third trimester is not very accurate due to the large range of error.

Once the pregnancy is correctly dated, it is not changed in subsequent scans.

Margin of deviation

Gestational age assessment based on measurement of the crown–rump length (CRL) has an accuracy of ±5–7 days, up to and including 13+6 weeks of gestation.

Between 14+0 weeks (when the fetus is ≥84 mm) and 20 weeks of gestation, the fetal head circumference (HC) is preferred for dating as it becomes slightly more precise than the biparietal diameter (BPD) [7]. The EDD is changed depending on the discrepancy between ultrasound dating and LMP dating. The guidelines for reassignment of EDD based on ultrasound imaging are presented in Table 31.1.

Table 31.1 Guidelines for reassigning EDD based on discrepancy between LMP-based gestational age and ultrasound-based gestational age

Gestational age	Measurement used	Margin of discrepancy that supports reassignment of EDD
8+6 weeks	CRL	>5 days
9+0–13+6 weeks	CRL	>7 days
14+0–21+6 weeks	HC, BPD, AC, FL	>7–10 days
22+0–27+6 weeks	HC, BPD, AC, FL	>14 days
>28+0 weeks	HC, BPD, AC, FL	>21 days

AC, abdominal circumference; *BPD*, biparietal diameter; *CRL*, crown-rump length; *EDD*, estimated date of delivery; *FL*, femur length; *HC*, head circumference

Key Point

The importance of accurate pregnancy dating, taking into account the gestational age at which ultrasound is done, cannot be overemphasised. Not doing this correctly may have significant consequences as an induction for a 'term' baby could actually result in a preterm birth. Equally, delaying delivery can result in a postterm birth.

Factors Affecting Prevalence

- **Increase in prevalence:** Parity is an important factor that affects the prevalence of late term and postterm pregnancies. **Nulliparous women** are more likely to give birth postterm. **Obesity and maternal age >30 years** also increase the risk of postterm pregnancy [8].
- **Lowering of prevalence:** Factors that lower the prevalence of postterm birth include a high incidence of spontaneous preterm birth, pregnancy complications leading to indicated preterm birth, and obstetric practice norms in a region, such as a high rate of planned cesarean birth, and routine labour induction at 39–40 weeks.

ETIOLOGY OF LATE TERM AND POSTTERM PREGNANCIES

The majority of late term and postterm pregnancies have no known etiology. Maternal or fetal genetic influences on the initiation of parturition cause between a third to half of postterm and late term births. Epigenetic changes may also play a role in the increased incidence of late and postterm births [9].

Maternal Genetic Factors

Maternal, and not paternal, genetic factors influence the rate of late term and postterm pregnancies, accounting for the etiology in as many as 30% of these pregnancies. A Danish study of monozygotic and dizygotic twin pairs who went on to become parents found that late term and postterm gestation was higher in monozygotic twin pairs when compared to dizygotic twin pairs, indicating a genetic effect [10].

Maternal Obesity

Obesity is a recently described risk factor. High maternal BMI in the first trimester and a significant increase in BMI during pregnancy are both associated with late term and postterm pregnancy [11].

Fetal Hormonal Defects

Defects in the production of fetal hormones involved in parturition may cause late term pregnancy. Disorders associated with placental sulphatase deficiency (e.g., X-linked ichthyosis) result in extremely low estriol levels and other hormonal changes as compared to normal pregnancies, with the mean duration of pregnancies being one week longer than pregnancies without this disorder [12].

Fetal Abnormalities

Anencephaly, which results in the absence or hypoplasia of the hypothalamus and pituitary, with adrenal hypoplasia, often result in postterm pregnancy, even when polyhydramnios is present. Since anencephaly is generally detected by antenatal ultrasound in current obstetrics, and terminated or induced, few cases reach the third trimester. Hence, this is now a rare cause of postterm pregnancy [13].

RISK FACTORS FOR LATE TERM AND POSTTERM PREGNANCY

Women at the highest risk (with a significant relative risk) of postterm pregnancy are those who have had a **previous postterm pregnancy**. The risk of a second postterm pregnancy is increased two- to four-fold and is even higher after two prior postterm pregnancies.

More modest risk factors (with a low relative risk) include the following [14]:

- Nulliparity
- Obesity
- Older maternal age
- Maternal history of postterm birth
- Maternal race (with Asians at the lowest risk)
- Male fetus

Key Point

A previous postterm pregnancy is the most important risk factor for late term and postterm pregnancies and must be elicited as an important part of obstetric history.

MORBIDITY AND MORTALITY IN POSTTERM PREGNANCIES

Postterm pregnancy is associated with maternal, fetal, and neonatal complications. Many of these complications are either the result of excessive fetal growth or related to uteroplacental insufficiency associated with the ageing placenta. It is advisable that the management of pregnancies that progress past their EDD should include counselling regarding the maternal and perinatal risks of increasing gestational age, and the available management options.

Maternal Complications

Late term and postterm pregnancies often involve larger fetuses and longer and more difficult labours. This increases the risks of maternal peripartum complications in pregnancies beyond 40 weeks' gestation [15]. The odds ratios (OR) of developing different complications are listed in Table 31.2.

Risk of advancing maternal age

In a national cohort study, it was found that women aged ≥40 have an increased risk of adverse perinatal and maternal outcomes when the pregnancy goes beyond 41 weeks. In such cases, it is important to counsel the woman and advise planned induction between 39 and 40 weeks. In all age categories, the risk of adverse pregnancy outcomes was found to be higher for nulliparous than for multiparous women [16].

Table 31.2 The odds ratios of various maternal complications

Maternal complications	Odds ratio of developing complications
Third- or fourth-degree perineal laceration	1.1
Operative vaginal delivery	1.1
Primary cesarean delivery	1.2
Postpartum hemorrhage	1.2
Chorioamnionitis	1.3
Endomyometritis	1.4
Cesarean delivery for cephalopelvic disproportion	1.6
Cesarean delivery for non-reassuring fetal heart rate	1.8

Key Point

The risk of adverse pregnancy outcomes increases with advancing maternal age when pregnancies continue beyond 41 weeks. These women must be counselled and monitored accordingly.

Perinatal Complications

Fetal macrosomia

Because of the longer duration of intrauterine growth, postterm fetuses tend to be larger than term fetuses and have a higher incidence of macrosomia [17].

Macrosomia increases the risk of the following interventions and adverse outcomes:

- Assisted instrumental vaginal birth
- Cesarean birth
- Abnormal labour progression
- Postpartum hemorrhage
- Shoulder dystocia
- Maternal, fetal, or newborn birth injury
- Neonatal metabolic problems

See **Chapter 34**, *Management of labour with fetal macrosomia*, for further details.

Fetal dysmaturity

Not all postterm fetuses continue to follow a normal growth trajectory. Up to 20% develop **fetal dysmaturity** or **postmaturity syndrome**, terms used to describe fetuses with the characteristics of chronic intrauterine malnutrition. These fetuses are at an increased risk of the following perinatal complications [18]:

- Umbilical cord compression due to oligohydramnios
- Abnormal antepartum or intrapartum fetal heart rate patterns due to uteroplacental insufficiency or cord compression
- Meconium passage, which is related to physiologic maturation of the gut, fetal hypoxia, or both

Dysmature neonates have a long, thin body and long nails, and are small for gestational age. Their skin is dry (with decreased or absent vernix caseosa), meconium-stained, parchment-like, and peeling. The skin appears loose because of the loss of subcutaneous fat, especially over the thighs and buttocks and has prominent creases. Lanugo hair is sparse or absent, and scalp hair is increased. These neonates are at risk of various morbidities associated with growth restriction (see **Chapter 33**, *Management of labour with a growth-restricted fetus*):

- Hypoglycemia
- Polycythemia
- Perinatal asphyxia
- Meconium aspiration
- Persistent pulmonary hypertension
- Neurodevelopmental complications including seizures and cerebral palsy

Neonatal morbidity

Postterm pregnancies are associated with a two-fold increase in admission to the neonatal intensive care unit (NICU), hypoglycemia, infections, and respiratory morbidity over both full term and late term pregnancies [19].

Meconium-stained amniotic fluid, which is a sign of fetal maturity, has been reported to be significantly more common in both preterm and term Asian and Black infants as compared to white European infants, with a corresponding increase in neonatal morbidity [4].

Perinatal mortality

The perinatal mortality rate in postterm pregnancy is twice the rate in term pregnancy, increasing four-fold at 43 weeks and five- to seven-fold at 44 weeks. Neonates born after 41 weeks of gestation experience a one-third greater risk of neonatal mortality than term neonates born before 40 weeks of gestation [20,21].

Stillbirth

Even when the background incidence and absolute rate of fetal or neonatal death are low, there is a significant increase in stillbirths in postterm pregnancies. The reported rate of stillbirth at different gestational ages after term increases on a week-to-week basis [22] (Table 31.3).

Table 31.3 Rate of stillbirth at progressive gestational ages

Gestational age in weeks	Risk of stillbirth
Between 40 and 41	0.86 to 1.08 per 1000 ongoing pregnancies
Between 41 and 42	1.2 to 1.27 per 1000 ongoing pregnancies
Between 42 and 43 weeks	1.3 to 1.9 per 1000 ongoing pregnancies
After 43 weeks	1.58 to 6.3 per 1000 ongoing pregnancies

A systematic review and meta-analysis of cohort studies of 15 million pregnancies [23] concluded that there is a significant additional risk of stillbirth with no corresponding reduction in neonatal mortality when term pregnancies continue to 41 weeks and beyond. The review included studies only from high-income countries with a low baseline of stillbirths. This finding might be more significant in low- and middle-income countries where the majority of stillbirths occur. The incidence of a stillbirth postterm is higher in nulliparous when compared to multiparous women and in women >40 years of age [24,25].

MANAGEMENT OF LATE TERM AND POSTTERM PREGNANCIES

The management of late term and postterm pregnancies includes singleton, cephalic fetuses in otherwise uncomplicated pregnancies. Multiple gestations, non-cephalic presentations, and pregnancies with medical or obstetric complications are generally delivered before 41 weeks.

Induction Versus Expectant Management

Low-risk pregnancies that reach 41 weeks of gestation can either be managed by the induction of labour (IOL) or expectantly with ongoing fetal assessment. An intervention is undertaken if spontaneous labour does not occur by a predefined gestational age or if the fetal assessment is not reassuring.

In the low-risk postterm woman, both of these approaches are associated with low absolute rates of adverse outcomes. Women should be counselled about the maternal and fetal benefits and risks of both approaches and their opinions should be taken into consideration [26].

Induction of labour

The multi-centre ARRIVE trial evaluated the planned induction of labour between 39 and 39 weeks and 4 days of gestation versus expectant management in over 6100 low-risk nulliparous women with the following results [27]:

- Reduced risk of cesarean birth (17.3% at 39 weeks, 22% at 40 weeks, and 37.5% at 42 weeks)
- Lower rate of a composite adverse perinatal outcome (5.1% at 39 weeks, 5.9% at 40 weeks, and 8.2% at 41 to 42 weeks of gestation)

Adverse perinatal outcomes include a low five-minute Apgar score of 3 or less, hypoxic–ischemic encephalopathy (HIE), birth trauma, and intracranial hemorrhage, neonatal seizures, sepsis, meconium aspiration syndrome, and even death.

Key Point

Systematic reviews suggest that induction at an earlier gestational age, at 39–40 weeks, may have similar benefits and no increased risk over later inductions or expectant management.

Induction between 40 weeks and 41 weeks of gestation is generally favoured given that intervention at this time reduces both perinatal morbidity and mortality while reducing cesarean birth rates. This approach is supported by clinical guidelines that suggest that routine induction reduces perinatal morbidity and mortality [23,27,28].

A systematic review of the Cochrane Database compared a policy of induction of labour shortly after 41 completed weeks of gestation with a policy of expectant management. Induction of labour was found to be more favourable due to a significant reduction in several perinatal outcomes [8]:

- Perinatal mortality by 70% (0.4 versus 3.0 per 1000)
- Stillbirth by 50% (1 versus 2 per 1000)
- Cesarean birth by 10% (167 versus 186 per 1000)
- Neonatal intensive care unit admissions by 12% (83 versus 95 per 1000)
- Macrosomia (>4000 g) by 28% (23 versus 74 per 300 infants)
- Meconium aspiration syndrome by 25%

Membrane stripping

Membrane stripping (also called sweeping; see **Chapter 14**, *Induction of labour*) is known to reduce the proportion of women who remain undelivered at 42 weeks. A systematic review of the Cochrane Database found that sweeping of the membranes at term (38–41 weeks) reduced the frequency of pregnancies requiring formal induction of labour [29]. Interestingly, it was also found that women reacted positively to membrane sweeping and felt that its benefits outweighed the harms.

Cervical ripening

Agents such as dinoprostone (PGE2 gel or pessary) or a balloon (Foley) catheter are used in women with an unfavourable cervix (see **Chapter 14**). A comparison of vaginal dinoprostone with a balloon catheter for cervical ripening in pregnancies at and after 41 weeks found that the rates of cesarean birth for non-reassuring fetal status, maternal morbidity, and neonatal morbidity were similar [30].

> **Key Point**
>
> For pregnancies that are ongoing after the EDD, induction between 40 and 41 weeks of gestation is favoured irrespective of cervical status, given that intervention at this time reduces perinatal mortality without increasing perinatal morbidity while reducing cesarean birth rates.

Expectant management

Expectant management is the alternative to the induction of labour. Expectant management of pregnancies includes a twice-weekly assessment of fetal health, beginning at 41 weeks. Intervention leading to delivery is indicated for the following:

- Abnormal fetal surveillance testing or
- If labour does not spontaneously occur by a defined cut-off date

There may be a role for expectant management with fetal monitoring since the absolute rate of perinatal death is relatively low at 41 weeks. When comparing expectant management with induction, data from high-resource countries show 3 perinatal deaths/1000 pregnancies with expectant management and 0.4 perinatal deaths/1000 pregnancies with labour induction [31]. However, keeping in mind the earlier gestational age at delivery for Indian women, this data should be applied with caution to our population.

> **Key Point**
>
> Expectant management is a valid option if a woman expresses a desire to wait for spontaneous labour. However, a policy of labour induction is associated with a 50% reduction in perinatal mortality and stillbirth [8]—this should be emphasised to the couple.

Fetal surveillance

Though fetal surveillance is routinely performed in postterm pregnancies to try and predict fetal compromise, there is a paucity of data from RCTs on the type, timing of initiation, and frequency of tests to be performed. However, it seems reasonable to undertake the following schedule:

- Twice weekly **non-stress test** (NST) using electronic fetal heart rate monitoring (EFM), starting at 40 weeks' gestation
- Twice weekly **amniotic fluid volume assessment** from 40 weeks because amniotic fluid can rapidly reduce within 24–48

hours in the presence of placental insufficiency [32]

Monitoring the postterm fetus with **Doppler ultrasonography** of the umbilical artery and evaluation of pulsatility indices of the uterine arteries, middle cerebral artery, descending aorta, ductus venosus, or inferior vena cava has no proven benefit [33].

Key Point

After 40 weeks, antenatal testing to monitor fetal well-being should include a twice-weekly non-stress test (NST) to diagnose acute hypoxia and an ultrasound assessment of amniotic fluid to identify placental insufficiency. Doppler ultrasonography has no proven benefit.

Timing of delivery in expectantly managed pregnancies

It is important to explain to the woman that the risk of cesarean delivery, admission to the neonatal intensive care unit, and stillbirth increases if the pregnancy continues beyond 41+0 weeks.

Based on this data, NICE guidelines [28] advise induction of labour at 41+0 weeks for postterm pregnancies. They also caution that the risk of stillbirth is 50% higher in Asian women, as shown by the 2020 MBRRACE-UK report on perinatal mortality [34]. In this population, induction may be considered earlier.

Key Point

Considering that the average age of delivery of Indian babies is 38 weeks+4 days [4,5], and the significantly increased risk of stillbirth when pregnancy continues beyond 41 weeks [6,23,34], it seems clinically sound to induce labour between 40+0 weeks and 41+0 weeks of gestation for Indian women.

Management of Labour in Late Term and Postterm Pregnancies

The placental pathophysiology in postterm postmature pregnancies is not well understood. Due to placental dysfunction, there is an increased risk of placental lesions, fetal hypoxia–asphyxia, and fetal growth restriction [18].

Monitoring of labour

Uterine activity and progress of labour should be closely monitored and augmented with oxytocin infusion when indicated.

Anticipating placental dysfunction

Lateral positioning of the gravida helps to counteract supine hypotension and facilitate fetal oxygen supply. During bearing down efforts, the reserves of the postterm placenta may become further compromised. In such cases, instrumental delivery should be considered.

An emergency cesarean section may be resorted to for fetal distress identified by late decelerations on intrapartum EFM and/or meconium-stained liquor if vaginal delivery is not imminent or feasible.

Umbilical cord clamping should be delayed in order to allow increased blood flow to the fetus and to counteract fetal hypovolemia.

Key Point

Intrapartum management should be cognisant of and anticipate placental insufficiency and take proactive measures to protect fetal well-being.

Summary of Management

The management of late term and postterm pregnancies requires understanding and communication, anticipation and planning, patience and thoughtful proactive intervention [39].

- Confirm the gestational age early in all pregnancies by reliable dating and/or corroboration with an early-dating ultrasound
- Rule out associated medical or obstetric conditions that necessitate early delivery
- Offer and perform membrane stripping if feasible at or after 39 weeks
- Provide information and counselling regarding the maternal and perinatal risks associated with increasing gestational age

- Initiate a daily fetal movement count and twice weekly fetal surveillance from 40 weeks by both NST and amniotic fluid assessment by ultrasound
- Perform a pelvic examination for assessment of Bishop's score
- Induce labour between 40 and 41 weeks in an uncomplicated pregnancy or earlier (after 39 weeks), if requested by the woman
- Proceed with cervical ripening by PGE2 application or a balloon catheter
- Perform early artificial rupture of membranes when in labour to diagnose or rule out meconium in liquor
- Initiate oxytocin infusion by titration to augment labour if required
- Monitor fetal heart rate closely
- Assess for a potentially higher fetal weight and the need for instrumental delivery
- Conduct potentially difficult deliveries in an operation theatre with preparation and willingness to resort to cesarean section, if required, in the second stage
- Anticipate and proactively manage shoulder dystocia using preset drills and protocols

PREVENTION OF LATE TERM AND POSTTERM PREGNANCY

Key Point

The incidence of late term and postterm pregnancy and associated maternal and fetal complications can be significantly reduced by more accurate pregnancy dating and simple obstetric practices such as membrane sweeping and induction of labour to prevent the extension of gestation beyond 41 weeks.

- Early routine ultrasound examination and accurate dating reduces the rate of intervention for postterm pregnancy by approximately 50% [36].
- Membrane sweeping at term can initiate labour and has the potential to prevent late term and postterm pregnancy [29].
- Induction at or after 39 weeks can prevent late term and postterm pregnancies with similar benefits and no increased risk over later inductions or expectant management [8].

RECURRENCE RISK OF LATE TERM AND POSTTERM BIRTH

The risk of postterm pregnancy is highest in women with a previous postterm pregnancy. After one postterm pregnancy, the risk of a second postterm birth doubles [37]. The risk of recurrence is even higher after two prior postterm births.

CONCLUSION

Over the last decade, induction of labour after 39–40 weeks in postterm pregnancies has increased. While studies have shown the medical advantages of postterm IOL, less is known about the perspectives of pregnant women [38]. Women's own expectations for spontaneous labour are often superseded by the healthcare professional's recommendation to undergo induction of labour. Their expectations should be handled with empathy and sensitivity.

REFERENCES

1. Norwitz ER, Snegovskikh VV, Caughey AB. Prolonged pregnancy: When should we intervene?. *Clin Obstet Gynecol.* 2007. 50(2):547-57.
2. ACOG Committee Opinion No 579: Definition of term pregnancy. *Obstet Gynecol.* 2013. 122. 1139-40. Reaffirmed 2022.
3. Bennett KA, Crane JM, O'shea P, Lacelle J, Hutchens D, Copel JA. First trimester ultrasound screening is effective in reducing postterm labor induction rates: A randomized controlled trial. *Am J Obstet Gynecol.* 2004. 190(4).1077-81.
4. Patel RP, Steer P, Doyle P, Little MP, Elliott. Does gestation vary by ethnic group? A London-based study of over 122,000 pregnancies with spontaneous onset of labour. *Int J Epidemiol.* 2004. 33(1):107-13.
5. Kiserud T, Piaggio G, Carroli G, Widmer M, Carvalho J, Jensen LN, et al. The World Health Organization Fetal Growth Charts: A multinational longitudinal study of

ultrasound biometric measurements and estimated fetal weight. *PLoS Med.* 2017. 14(1):e1002220.

6. Caughey AB, Nicholson JM, Washington AE. First- vs second-trimester ultrasound: The effect on pregnancy dating and perinatal outcomes. *Am J Obstet Gynecol.* 2008. 198:703. e1-703.e6.
7. Salomon LJ, Alfirevic Z, Bilardo CM, Chalouhi GE, et al. ISUOG practice guidelines: Performance of first-trimester fetal ultrasound scan. *Ultrasound Obstet Gynecol.* 2013. 41(1):102-13. doi: 10.1002/uog.12342. Erratum in: *Ultrasound Obstet Gynecol.* 2013. 41(2):240. PMID: 23280739.
8. Middleton P, Shepherd E, Morris J, Crowther CA, Gomerscll. Induction of labour at or beyond 37 weeks' gestation. *Cochrane Database Syst Rev.* 2020. 7:CD004945.
9. Oberg AS, Frisell T, Svensson AC, Iliadou AN. Maternal and fetal genetic contributions to postterm birth: Familial clustering in a population-based sample of 475,429 Swedish births. *Am J Epidemiol.* 2013. 177:531-7.
10. Laursen M, Bille C, Olesen AW, Hjelmborg J, Skytthe A, Christensen K. Genetic influence on prolonged gestation: A population-based Danish twin study. *Am J Obstet Gynecol.* 2004. 190(2):489-94.
11. Denison FC, Price J, Graham C, Wild S, Liston WA. Maternal obesity, length of gestation, risk of postdated pregnancy and spontaneous onset of labour at term. *BJOG.* 2008. 115(6):720-5.
12. Taylor NF. Review: Placental sulphatase deficiency. *J Inherit Metab Dis.* 1982. 5:164-76.
13. Milic AB, Adamsons K. The relationship between anencephaly and prolonged pregnancy. *J Obstet Gynaecol Br Commonw.* 1969. 76:102-11.
14. Caughey AB, Stotland NE, Washington AE, Escobar GJ. Who is at risk for prolonged and postterm pregnancy? *Am J Obstet Gynecol.* 2009. 200:683.e1-5.
15. Caughey AB, Stoland NE, Washington E, Escobar GJ. Maternal and obstetric complications of pregnancy are associated with increasing gestational age at term. *Am J Obstet Gynecol.* 2007. 196(2):155.e1-6.
16. Kortekaas JC, Kazemier BM, Kuelen JK, et al. Risk of adverse pregnancy outcomes of late- and postterm pregnancies in advanced maternal age: A national cohort study. *Acta Obstet Gynecol Scand.* 2020. 99(8):1022-30.
17. Spellacy WN, Miller S, Winegar A, Peterson PQ. Macrosomia--maternal characteristics and infant complications. *Obstet Gynecol.* 1985. 66:158-61.
18. Vorherr H. Placental insufficiency in relation to postterm pregnancy and fetal postmaturity. Evaluation of fetoplacental function; management of the postterm gravida. *Am J Obstet Gynecol.* 1975. 123:67-103.
19. Linder N, Hiersch L, Fridman E, Klinger G, Lubin D, Kouadio F, et al. Post-term pregnancy is an independent risk factor for neonatal morbidity even in low-risk singleton pregnancies. *Arch Dis Child Fetal Neonatal Ed.* 2017. 102(4):F286-F290.
20. De Los Santos-Garate AM, Villa-Guillen M, Villanueva-García D, et al. Perinatal morbidity and mortality in late-term and post-term pregnancy. NEOSANO perinatal network's experience in Mexico. *J Perinatol.* 2011; 31:789-93.
21. Bruckner TA, Cheng YW, Caughey AB. Increased neonatal mortality among normal-weight births beyond 41 weeks of gestation in California. *Am J Obstet Gynecol.* 2008. 199:421.e1-7.
22. Lindegren L, Stuart A, Herbst A, Källén K. Stillbirth or neonatal death before 45 post-menstrual weeks in relation to gestational duration in pregnancies at 39 weeks of gestation or beyond: The impact of parity and body mass index. A national cohort study. *BJOG.* 2022. 129:761-68.
23. Muglu J, Rather H, Arroyo-Manzano D, et al. Risks of stillbirth and neonatal death with advancing gestation at term: A systematic review and meta-analysis of cohort studies of 15 million pregnancies. *PLoS Med.* 2019. 16:e1002838.
24. Hilder L, Sairam S, Thilaganathan B. Influence of parity on fetal mortality in prolonged pregnancy. *Eur J Obstet Gynecol Reprod Biol.* 2007. 132:167-70.
25. Haavaldsen C, Sarfraz AA, Samuelsen SO, Eskild A. The impact of maternal age on fetal death: Does length of gestation matter? *Am J Obstet Gynecol.* 2010. 203:554. e1-8.
26. Mandruzzato G, Alfirevic Z, Chervenak F, Gruenebaum, Heimstad R, Heinonen S, et al. Guidelines for the management of postterm pregnancy. *J Perinat Med.* 2010. 38:111-9.
27. Grobman WA, Rice MM, Reddy UM, Tita ATN, Silver RM, Mallett G, et al. Labor induction versus expectant management in low-risk nulliparous women. *N Engl J Med.* 2018. 379(6):513-23.
28. NICE guideline 207. Inducing labour. 2021. www.nice.org.uk/guidance/ng207.
29. Finucane EM, Murphy DJ, Biesty LM, et al. Membrane sweeping for induction of labour. *Cochrane Database of Systematic Reviews.* 2020. Issue 2. Art. No.: CD000451. DOI: 10.1002/14651858.CD000451.pub3. Accessed 10 September 2023.
30. Diguisto C, Le Gouge A, Arthuis C, Diguisto C, Le Gouge A, Arthuis C, et al. Cervical ripening in prolonged pregnancies by silicone double balloon catheter versus vaginal dinoprostone slow release system: The MAGPOP randomised controlled trial. *PLoS Med.* 2021. 18:e1003448.

31. Norwitz ER. Postterm pregnancy. Lockwood CJ (Ed). *UpToDate*. 2023. Waltham, MA.
32. Clement D, Schifrin BS, Kates RB. Acute oligohydramnios in postdate pregnancy. *Am J Obstet Gynecol*. 1987. 157:884-6.
33. Kauppinen T, Kantomaa T, Tekay A, Mäkikallio K. Placental and fetal hemodynamics in prolonged pregnancies. *Prenat Diagn*. 2016. 36:622-7.
34. Draper ES, Gallimore ID, Smith LK, Matthews RJ, Fenton AC, Kurinczuk JJ, Smith PW, Manktelow BN, on behalf of the MBRRACE-UK Collaboration. MBRRACE-UK Perinatal Mortality Surveillance Report, UK Perinatal Deaths for Births from January to December 2020. Leicester: The Infant Mortality and Morbidity Studies, Department of Health Sciences, University of Leicester. 2022.
35. Arjun G. *A Practical Guide to Obstetrics*. 2nd edition. Hyderabad. Universities Press. 2022. 409 p.
36. Kaelin Agten A, Xia J, Servante JA, Thornton JG, Jones NW. Routine ultrasound for fetal assessment before 24 weeks' gestation. *Cochrane Database Syst Rev*. 2021. 8:CD014698.
37. Kortekaas JC, Kazemier BM, Ravelli AC, de Boer K, van Dillen J, Mol BW, et al. Recurrence rate and outcome of postterm pregnancy, a national cohort study. *Eur J Obstet Gynecol Reprod Biol*. 2015. 193:70-4.
38. Lou S, Hvidman L, Uldbjerg N, Neumann RM, Jensen TF, Haben JG, et al. Women's experiences of postterm induction of labor: A systematic review of qualitative studies. *Birth*. 2018. 46(3):400-10.

CHAPTER 32

Late Intrauterine Fetal Death and Stillbirth

A G RADHIKA, RICHA AGGARWAL

INTRODUCTION

There has been a reduction in stillbirths worldwide as antenatal services have become more accessible and utilised. However, the stillbirth rates are substantially higher (22.7 deaths per 1000 births) in low- and middle-income countries (LMICs) than in high-income countries (HICs), where the rate is 3 deaths per 1000 births. Most stillbirths (77%) occur in sub-Saharan Africa and South Asia during labour and childbirth [1]. Differences in definitions, use of birth weight or gestational age for reporting stillbirth, and incomplete data from low-income countries result in difficulties in interpreting the data on stillbirth.

This chapter will briefly discuss the diagnosis and investigations of late fetal death and stillbirth and will focus on maternal care and management.

DEFINITIONS

- **Stillbirth** is defined as fetal demise that occurs after fetal viability, which varies according to individual country norms.
- **Antepartum fetal death** is defined as one that occurs prior to the onset of labour.
- **Intrapartum fetal death** is defined as stillbirth that occurs after the onset of labour. The estimated proportion of intrapartum stillbirths is much higher in LMICs (60% in South Asia) as compared with HICs (10%) [2].

The World Health Organization (WHO) recommends standardising the international stillbirth definition for epidemiological studies utilising a birth weight of >1000 g and/or gestation of >28 weeks. This differs significantly from the WHO's recommendation for in-country national reporting, which urges countries to record stillbirths as those with a birth weight >500 g, gestational age >22 weeks, and a crown–heel length of >35 cm [3].

Though the following definitions are discretionary, they help standardise international data reporting.

The WHO [4]

- **Stillbirth:** A newborn at ≥28 weeks of gestation with no signs of life at birth
- **Fetal death:** Intrauterine death at any time during pregnancy

United States National Centre for Health Statistics [5]

The death or loss of the fetus at ≥20 weeks of gestation and before or during birth, with further classification as:

- **Early stillbirth** (20 to 27 completed weeks)
- **Late stillbirth** (28 to 36 completed weeks)
- **Term stillbirth** (≥37 completed weeks)

This subclassification allows the identification of late stillbirths, which may have been prevented by earlier intervention.

Royal College of Obstetricians and Gynaecologists (RCOG) [6]

- **Late intrauterine fetal death** is defined as the in utero demise of a fetus after 24 completed weeks of pregnancy (singleton fetus).
- **Stillbirth** is defined as a baby delivered with no signs of life after 24 completed weeks of pregnancy.

Ministry of Health and Family Welfare, India (MoHFW) [7]

Under the guidelines established for the country by the WHO, the MoHFW has adopted the following definitions:

- **Early fetal death** is defined as the death of a fetus weighing at least 500 g (or, if birth weight is unavailable, after 20 completed weeks gestation, or with a crown–heel length of ≥25 cm).
- **Late fetal death (stillbirth)** is defined as the death of a fetus weighing at least 1000 g (or at a gestational age of 28 completed weeks or a crown–heel length of ≥35 cm).
- **Fresh stillbirth** or **intrapartum stillbirth** is defined as a stillbirth occurring after the onset of labour and within less than 12 hours before delivery, of a fetus with no skin changes, weighing more than 1000 g, and at >28 weeks of gestation. This definition does not include fetuses with severe, lethal congenital abnormalities.
- **Macerated stillbirth** or **antepartum stillbirth** is a baby born with all the features of a fetus retained in utero after death, when the death occurred before the initiation of labour. A macerated fetus shows skin and soft tissue changes (skin discolouration or darkening, redness, peeling, and breakdown).

Key Point

The WHO recommends standardising the international stillbirth definition for epidemiology studies, utilising a birth weight of >1000 g and/or >28 weeks' gestation. In India, a fetus <28 weeks old is considered not viable; however, the reporting for stillbirths is done from 20 weeks onwards [7].

CAUSES OF LATE FETAL DEMISE IN UTERO AND STILLBIRTHS

Traditionally, the causes of stillbirth have been classified into maternal, fetal, placental, and idiopathic factors. Most conditions that have been linked to stillbirth are associations rather than unequivocal causes.

- **Early fetal mortality** is usually associated with congenital anomalies and underlying maternal medical conditions.
- **Late fetal mortality** is associated with maternal medical conditions and obstetric conditions such as placental abruption, placenta previa, cord prolapse, and other complications during delivery and labour [8].
- **Unexplained fetal death** is one that cannot be attributed to any specific fetal, placental, maternal, or obstetric cause. This constitutes 25–60% of all fetal deaths [8,9]. Unexplained fetal death is more likely to occur near term.

The causes of late fetal demise in utero and stillbirths vary with the availability of resources:

- **Low- and middle-income countries:** The lack of resources such as a skilled birth attendant at birth, basic emergency obstetric care, and antenatal care for the detection and management of hypertensive disorders, diabetes, severe malaria, and growth restriction contribute to stillbirths [10]. Late fetal demise and stillbirths also result from inadequate treatment of obstructed/prolonged labour, preeclampsia, and infection.
- **High-income countries:** The causes include congenital anatomical or chromosomal abnormalities, placental problems resulting in growth restriction, and maternal medical conditions [11].

Established Causes

- **Fetal growth restriction (FGR),** especially when unrecognised, is considered the single largest risk factor for stillbirth [12]. Fetuses with FGR have a five- to seven-fold risk of stillbirth as compared to fetuses with normal growth [13].
- **Medical disorders**, e.g., diabetes, hypertensive disorders, substance abuse, chronic renal disease, and antiphospholipid antibody syndrome increase the risk of fetal demise.
- **Previous stillbirth** increases the risk of stillbirth three-fold in the subsequent pregnancy [14].

- **Postterm pregnancy** carries a significant additional risk of stillbirth with no corresponding reduction in neonatal mortality when term pregnancies continue to 41 weeks compared to delivery at 40 weeks [15] (see **Chapter 31**, *Late term and postterm pregnancy*).
- **Infections** play an important role in the etiology of fetal demise, especially in developing countries. Maternal malaria, hepatitis, herpes simplex, toxoplasmosis, parvovirus, and cytomegalovirus infection are established causes of intrauterine fetal demise. Infection with Zika virus has been associated with stillbirth [16].
- **Cord entanglement** is often blamed for an unexplained fetal death. Nuchal cord occurs in 1 out of 3 pregnancies but very rarely causes fetal death. Nuchal cord or knots in the cord must be considered the cause of fetal death **only after thorough assessment for other etiologies.** A recent study from a high-income country found that cord abnormality (compromised fetal microcirculation, cord entrapment, knots, torsions or stricture, and cord prolapse) occurred in 19% of stillbirths in their cohort [17].

Key Point

Establishing an accurate cause of death is essential both for the parents to understand why their baby died and for the obstetrician to provide informed care in future pregnancies in order to prevent a recurrence. Despite advanced testing and autopsy, a definite etiology cannot be found in a significant proportion of stillbirths.

DIAGNOSIS OF INTRAUTERINE FETAL DEMISE (IUFD)

A woman may present with absent fetal movements or may be undergoing a routine antenatal checkup when the absence of fetal heart tones is first noticed.

If intrauterine demise is suspected, it should be confirmed with a real-time ultrasound examination. Auscultation with a handheld Doppler device or electronic fetal monitoring is not enough to establish such a serious outcome.

Real-time ultrasound imaging allows the direct visualisation of fetal heart movement. **The absence of cardiac activity confirms fetal death.**

Other ultrasound features that may help confirm the diagnosis include the following:

- Collapse of the fetal skull (Spalding sign) with overlapping bones
- Maceration resulting in an unrecognisable fetal mass
- Hydrops
- Intrafetal gas (within the heart, great vessels, joints)—called **Robert's sign**
- Hyperflexion of the spine
- Crowding of the rib shadow

If the woman or the family requests, it is good practice to have an independent operator confirm the absence of fetal heart motions even though the clinician may be very sure of the diagnosis.

COMMUNICATING THE DIAGNOSIS OF FETAL DEMISE

Pregnancy is a time of great happiness and expectations. When a catastrophic event like intrauterine demise occurs, it devastates the couple and their families. Therefore, it must be handled with great sensitivity. The woman should be encouraged to have her partner, another family member, or a companion with her while receiving the news. The communication should preferably be handled by a senior obstetrician and conducted in privacy so that the mother and her partner can grieve, away from onlookers [18]. Enough time should be scheduled to allow the couple to take in the news and be able to receive answers to their questions and doubts. The information should not be imparted in a hurried meeting with a doctor who is impatient or curt.

The art of communicating bad news is not formally taught in professional medical courses, though in recent years, it is being introduced in the medical curriculum. Younger professionals should carefully watch and observe an empathetic and communicative senior physician as they impart difficult news to women. Women and their families are often more upset with the poor communication skills of the physician than with the diagnosis itself [19].

The aim of the meeting with the couple is to explain in clear terms what has occurred, without placing blame on the woman, even by implication. It is important to have two or three meetings so that the woman and her family slowly come to terms with the situation. Unless the woman has a significant medical disorder that resulted in the fetal demise, it is important to reassure the couple that the mother's health is not at risk. All the discussions should aim to support the couple's choices. The following points should be discussed, but it is important not to overwhelm the woman and her family with all the information in one sitting:

- The need to establish the cause of death by evaluation and further investigations
- Mode of delivery
- Timing of delivery
- Complications of waiting for too long to deliver the baby
- Need for autopsy and other tests to evaluate the fetus after it is born
- Management of a subsequent pregnancy

Key Point

Once fetal death has been confirmed by ultrasound, the woman and her partner should be informed of the same in privacy and with great sensitivity. Communicating bad news is a skill that can be learned and for which training should be included in the medical curriculum. It is not a natural ability; physicians should practice this conversation to become proficient in conveying difficult diagnoses in a sympathetic manner.

WORK-UP OF A WOMAN FOLLOWING STILLBIRTH

Though the etiology of the stillbirth may not be found in one-third of women [20], a thorough evaluation should be carried out to ascertain the cause of death. On the other hand, when there is an obvious cause such as cord prolapse, a true knot, or anencephaly, further testing may not be required. Identification of the cause of fetal death requires both maternal and fetal evaluation (see section on *Postdelivery evaluation of the fetus*).

Maternal Evaluation

This includes a thorough history (Table 32.1), a physical examination, ultrasound evaluation of the fetus and placenta, and laboratory investigations. It is advisable to obtain original medical records and documentation whenever possible, and review them.

Laboratory testing

Basic blood investigations such as a complete blood count and blood group and typing should be performed in all women with IUFD. Special tests are ordered only when indicated. The investigations based on clinical indications include the following:

- Screening for **diabetes** should be performed in women who have not been diagnosed with overt diabetes antenatally.
- Screening for **antiphospholipid antibody syndrome** should be performed, especially in the presence of fetal growth restriction or early-onset preeclampsia; elevated levels of anticardiolipin and anti-beta-2-glycoprotein-1 antibodies are associated with a three- to five-fold increase in stillbirth.
- **Indirect Coombs test** should be performed to rule out Rh alloimmunisation as a cause of stillbirth in Rh-negative women.
- **Kleihaur-Betke testing** and flow cytometry should be performed on all women with an unexplained stillbirth, though fetomaternal hemorrhage is an uncommon cause of stillbirth; testing before the induction of labour can prevent falsely elevated Kleihaur-Betke levels after delivery.
- **Thyroid function tests**, **liver function tests**, and **inherited thrombophilia** evaluation are

Table 32.1 **Salient points in history taking in a case of stillbirth**

Obstetric history	Characteristics of current pregnancy	Past medical history	Family history
• Recurrent miscarriages or stillbirth • History of a child born with an anomaly, hereditary condition, or growth restriction • History of a hypertensive disorder in a previous pregnancy • History of gestational diabetes • History of placental abruption	• Maternal age • Gestational age • Multifetal gestation • Obstetric conditions, e.g., intrahepatic cholestasis, preterm labour or rupture of membranes • Gestational diabetes/ hypertensive disorders • Fetal anomalies on ultrasound • Placental abruption • Infections • Abdominal trauma	• History of venous thromboembolism, thrombophilias • Diabetes mellitus • Chronic hypertension • Autoimmune diseases • Heart disease • Substance abuse, medications	• Recurrent spontaneous miscarriages or stillbirth • Congenital anomaly or chromosomal abnormalities • Hereditary syndrome or developmental delay • Venous thromboembolism • Consanguinity

carried out only in women in whom there is a clinical suspicion of a specific underlying disorder.

- **Testing for infections** should be targeted based on fetal autopsy or placental pathology. For example, testing for parvovirus would be indicated in cases of severe fetal anemia and/or non-immune hydrops. There is **no evidence** that routine serology for herpes simplex virus, rubella, cytomegalovirus, or toxoplasmosis (TORCH test) is beneficial.
- **Testing for coagulation disorders** is **not** indicated immediately after the diagnosis of fetal demise since it takes up to 4 weeks for disseminated intravascular coagulopathy (DIC) to manifest after the event. In contemporary obstetrics, women are usually delivered soon after the diagnosis.

MANAGEMENT OF LABOUR AND DELIVERY

The management of labour and delivery must be preceded by counselling, taking into consideration the preferences of the woman and her partner. The couple should be informed about the following:

- 85–90% of women will deliver spontaneously within 3 weeks of IUFD [6]. However, delaying delivery beyond 24–48 hours may aggravate maternal anxiety and anguish [21]. Women and their families are usually distressed by the prospect of carrying on a pregnancy with a dead baby.
- Delaying delivery may also increase the risk of DIC. 10–30% of women develop DIC if they remain undelivered 4 weeks after IUFD [22].
- Vaginal delivery should be attempted unless there are definite obstetric indications for a cesarean birth.

Indications for Immediate Delivery

Women with the following conditions should be delivered immediately to avoid placing them at risk for major morbidity:

- Severe preeclampsia
- Antepartum hemorrhage
- Infection
- Rupture of membranes

Indications for Cesarean Delivery

In general, cesarean births for fetal death should be performed on women who have a high risk of uterine rupture (such as those who have undergone a transfundal or classical hysterotomy in the past), as this is associated with possible maternal morbidity without any fetal benefit.

A cesarean delivery should be considered for obstetric indications including the following:

- Major degree of placenta previa
- Abruption
- Transverse lie
- Two or more scars on the uterus
- Significant macrosomia

Induction of Labour

Oxytocin

Women with a favourable cervix (Bishop's score ≥6) in the late second trimester or in the third trimester may have labour induced with standard doses of oxytocin. See **Chapter 14**, *Induction and augmentation of labour*, for further details.

Misoprostol

The effectiveness of misoprostol depends on the gestational age. It appears to be the most effective technique of induction prior to 26 weeks of gestation, regardless of the cervical Bishop's score [23]. Misoprostol regimens used orally and intravaginally are equally efficacious. Two systematic reviews found that 90% of women deliver within 24 hours of induction and 100% within 48 hours, with minimal complications [24,25].

Dosage and route

Though oral, vaginal, sublingual, and buccal routes have been described, vaginal and oral routes are commonly used. The following are the commonly recommended doses [23,26]:

<26 weeks

- Vaginal misoprostol 100 mcg every 6–12 hours for a total of 4 doses.
- If there are no effective contractions (≥2 contractions in 10 minutes) or no cervical changes within four hours, the subsequent dose is doubled to 200 mcg. The maximum daily misoprostol dosing should not exceed 800 mcg.

>26 weeks

- Vaginal misoprostol 25–50 mcg every 4 hours (up to 6 doses).
- If the first misoprostol dose does not lead to effective contractions or if there are no cervical changes within four hours, the subsequent dose is doubled. The maximum daily misoprostol dosing should not exceed 600 mcg.

The contraction frequency should be maintained at no more than 2 contractions in 10 minutes to avoid the risk of hyperstimulation.

> **Key Point**
>
> Misoprostol administration is **not advised** after 24 weeks' gestation for women who have had a previous cesarean delivery. Mechanical methods such as a Foley catheter may be used for cervical ripening in these women.

Mifepristone and misoprostol

This is useful **between 24 and 28 weeks** of pregnancy. When combined with misoprostol for labour induction in the case of stillbirth, mifepristone (200 or 600 mg orally, 24–48 hours before misoprostol) shortens the labour period as compared to misoprostol alone.

Mifepristone alone may also be used, and can considerably enhance the likelihood of labour within 72 hours (avoiding the use of prostaglandin). The dose advised is 200 mg three times a day for 2 days or 600 mg once daily for two days [6]. Approximately 60% of women will deliver with this regimen.

Labour Analgesia

Analgesia is important in cases of intrauterine fetal demise. Women should have access to all the available modalities, including regional anesthesia and patient-controlled anesthesia.

Women Who Have Had a Previous Cesarean Delivery

Induction of labour is a valid option available for women who have had a previous cesarean delivery. However, they are at a higher risk of uterine rupture when labour is induced. In a large series to study the induction of labour in women with stillbirth and a previous cesarean scar, 91% delivered vaginally, with only 2 cases of uterine rupture [27]. Induction in these women should be conducted in a tertiary-care facility where all the resources required for a safe delivery are available. Women with a scarred uterus should be closely monitored for scar rupture during labour.

Mechanical methods of cervical ripening, such as transcervical Foley catheter, are preferred over misoprostol for cervical ripening, in women in the third trimester. The risk of uterine rupture is lower than with misoprostol [28]. However, in the presence of intrauterine demise, mechanical induction techniques may raise the risk of ascending infection.

Misoprostol may be used at lower dosages (25–50 mcg) for women who have previously undergone a cesarean section. However, this recommendation [24] is based on a low level of evidence and **should be used with extreme caution**.

Key Point

Cervical ripening using a transcervical Foley catheter may be a useful option for women with a prior hysterotomy and with a stillbirth beyond 28 weeks of gestation.

Expectant Management

Women who choose to wait for the spontaneous onset of labour should be tested twice weekly for coagulation disorders, though DIC is uncommon till 4 weeks after fetal demise.

It should also be explained to the couple that expectant management may diminish the value of the postmortem examination due to advanced maceration of the fetus.

Viewing or Holding the Baby After Delivery

An offer to see and hold the baby must be made to all couples. While some may want to view the baby, others may decline. Sometimes, only one parent may want to see the baby. In situations where the couple does not want to immediately see the baby, the offer of taking a photograph to view later can be made.

If the mother or the couple wants to see the baby, they should be prepared and counselled. If there is maceration or deformity, it is best to cover those portions of the baby—the couple may be left with very strong negative feelings and psychological trauma if they see a macerated baby. Western literature encourages contact between the parents and the baby to help in the grieving process [29], but two studies [30,31] found that viewing and holding the stillborn baby after delivery resulted in more chances of depression, anxiety, and posttraumatic stress disorder (PTSD) in mothers compared to those who had not.

Key Point

If the couple wants to view the baby, they should be prepared emotionally, and supported in their decision. This step should be tailored to the mother's preferences.

Lactation Suppression after Delivery

Women should be warned about the likelihood of postpartum breast engorgement. Dopamine agonists successfully suppress lactation in a very high percentage of women and are well tolerated by the majority. **Cabergoline** is preferable to bromocriptine. It is given orally as a single dose of 1 mg within 24 hours of delivery or 0.25 mg bid x 2 days to suppress lactation. Women who have preeclampsia or hypertension should not be given cabergoline or bromocriptine.

POSTDELIVERY EVALUATION OF THE FETUS

In addition to fetal autopsy, examination of the placenta, umbilical cord, and membranes and genetic testing should be conducted on stillborn babies.

Examination of the Stillborn Fetus

Estimating the time of death

It is important to estimate the time of death to help in counselling for the next pregnancy. However, estimating the time of fetal death is difficult. The following guidelines have been recommended:

- Brown or red discolouration of the umbilical cord or desquamation of ≥1 cm suggests the fetus has been dead for at least six hours.
- Desquamation of the face, back, and abdomen suggests that the fetus has been dead for at least 12 hours.
- Desquamation of ≥5% of the body or of ≥2 of the body zones suggests the fetus has been dead for at least 18 hours (body zones—scalp, face, neck, chest, back, arms, hand, leg, foot, and scrotum).
- Brown or tan colouration of the skin suggests that the fetus has been dead for at least 24 hours.
- Mummification (i.e., reduced soft tissue volume, leathery skin, deeply brown-stained tissues) suggests the fetus has been dead for at least two weeks.

Physical examination

Stillborn babies should be examined immediately, and their physical parameters should be documented. These include weight, length, and head circumference. Dysmorphic features should be documented in detail [23]. The entire body, the face, extremities, and palms, should be examined. Close-up photos of specific anomalies should be taken and are important in arriving at a diagnosis. These can also be shared with a perinatal pathologist and/or geneticist.

X-rays of the entire body with anterior–posterior and lateral views may uncover an unrecognised skeletal abnormality or further define a grossly apparent deformity.

Fetal postmortem examination

The subject of postmortem examination should be broached with great sensitivity with the couple. It should be explained to them that it is a very important part of the investigation for the etiology of stillbirth and has the highest diagnostic yield [6,23]. The examination is of even more significance in the presence of abnormalities such as dysmorphic features, irregular growth measurements, anomalies, hydrops, or growth restriction.

In India, people tend to refuse postmortem examinations for various reasons such as cultural norms and beliefs, disfigurement concerns, concerns that the child will not be handled with respect, and a belief that an autopsy may not help. Though the postmortem examination should not be forced on a couple, they usually will agree to the suggestion if it is clearly explained that it may help prevent a recurrence.

The postmortem should ideally be performed by a specialised perinatal pathologist [5]. If facilities are not available, the fetus or fetal organs can be sent to a centre where these facilities are available. Histological examination of the placenta may yield findings of clinical relevance.

If the parents do not agree to a postmortem, the following may be performed though they are not substitutes for a complete autopsy:

- Photographs of the fetus
- Whole body radiography
- Ultrasonography
- Magnetic resonance imaging (MRI)
- Needle biopsies

> **Key Point**
>
> A fetal autopsy is the single most useful diagnostic test to identify the possible reason for stillbirth. In addition to the identification of birth defects and morphologic abnormalities suggesting genetic or developmental abnormalities, autopsy can determine and/or confirm numerous other causes of stillbirth including infection, anemia, hypoxia, and metabolic abnormalities.

Disposition of the baby's remains

Following the autopsy, some parents may want to follow rituals specific to their culture or religion. If they want to leave the disposition to the hospital, local laws governing cremation or burial should be followed.

Chromosomal and genetic abnormalities

The karyotype of a stillbirth can be abnormal in 6–13% of cases [22]. In one large series, chromosomal abnormalities were found to be 4.6% in normally-formed fetuses but exceeded 20% in fetuses with anatomic abnormalities. Common karyotypic abnormalities noted in stillbirths include trisomy 21 (31%), monosomy X (22%), trisomy 18 (22%), and trisomy 13 (8%) [32].

The recommended sample for fetal karyotyping is amniotic fluid collected by amniocentesis at the time of diagnosis of demise. There is a much higher rate of successful tissue culture after invasive testing (85%) performed before delivery than with postnatal fetal tissue sampling (28%) [32].

Karyotyping should be performed on fetuses with abnormalities, anomalies, hydrops, growth restriction, and dysmorphic characteristics. If a parent has a balanced chromosomal rearrangement (such as a translocation or inversion) or a mosaic karyotype, the karyotype plays an important role. A microarray analysis is more likely to provide a genetic diagnosis than karyotype analysis due to its success with non-viable tissue.

Key Point

Genetic analyses are ideally performed in all cases of stillbirth after appropriate parental permission is obtained. Amniocentesis and chorionic villi sampling for fetal karyotyping have the highest yield and are particularly valuable if delivery is imminent. Acceptable cytogenetic specimens postnatally include an umbilical cord segment or an internal fetal tissue specimen that thrives under low-oxygen tension such as costochondral or patellar tissue. Fetal skin is least preferred for cytogenetic evaluation.

Examination of the placenta

A thorough gross and microscopic examination of the placenta, umbilical cord, and fetal membranes should be performed by a qualified pathologist as part of the evaluation. The following findings may indicate a possible cause of stillbirth:

- **Placenta**
  - Retroplacental clots suggestive of abruption
  - Placental infarction which may be associated with FGR
  - Chorionicity should be confirmed, and vascular anastomoses should be recognised in multi-fetal gestation
  - Leukocyte infiltration due to chorioamnionitis
  - Velamentous attachment of the cord
  - Vasa previa
- **Cord**
  - True knot with signs of umbilical cord thrombosis

Key Point

Placental and cord samples must not be placed in formalin. They should be sent to the lab in a sterile tissue medium of lactated Ringer's solution [23].

FOLLOW-UP VISIT AFTER DELIVERY

It may be necessary to schedule a follow-up visit early (in two to four weeks) depending on the woman's emotional needs. This may be followed by another one for discussing the reports of tests done, when they become available.

The second postnatal visit should be used to discuss the relevant results of the investigations. Modifiable risk factors should be reviewed, and plans can be made for a subsequent pregnancy. In LMICs, it is particularly important to emphasise the importance of regular antenatal visits to avoid a recurrence.

Key Point

The cause or possible causes of the stillbirth, risk of recurrence, and, if desired, a plan for the next pregnancy is discussed. The information should be provided in clear and non-medical terms and in a language understood by the couple. The information may be repeated if required.

CARE IN SUBSEQUENT PREGNANCY FOLLOWING STILLBIRTH

It is well-documented that a history of stillbirth increases the risk of another stillbirth. However, this is more significant in women with medical disorders such as diabetes or hypertension and those who have obstetric complications such as placental abruption. The risk of stillbirth in the setting of a previously unexplained stillbirth is more difficult to quantify [23].

The risk of recurrence influences both the woman and her caregiver, though there is currently not enough evidence to form clear guidelines for the management of pregnancies following a stillbirth.

The risk of preterm birth, low birth weight, and placental abruption is higher in women with a history of stillbirth.

Increased Antenatal Surveillance

It is common to provide more frequent antenatal check-ups to women with a previous stillbirth. The monitoring of fetal growth by ultrasound imaging is also recommended for women with a stillbirth associated with fetal growth restriction.

Antenatal fetal surveillance with **non-stress testing** or **biophysical profile** is usually initiated two weeks before the gestational age at which the previous stillbirth occurred [23,33].

Key Point

Pregnancies following stillbirth have an increased risk of adverse outcomes, including a 4.8-fold increased risk of stillbirth. Antenatal care in a subsequent pregnancy after stillbirth should ideally be provided by a multidisciplinary team to ensure continuity of medical and emotional support.

The benefit of educating women about **daily fetal movement count** and its effect on decreasing stillbirth is controversial. A systematic review of the Cochrane Database [34] was unable to conclusively prove its benefit for clinical practice, but a study from Norway showed a decrease in stillbirth with the management of decreased fetal movement [35].

Early Delivery

Induction of labour and elective cesarean delivery are frequently requested by the couple and recommended by obstetricians, regardless of other obstetric issues [36]. Keeping in mind the drawbacks of birth prior to 39 weeks, early term (37–39 weeks) birth may be recommended in select cases. However, in the absence of maternal or fetal complications, there is no evidence to support delivery before 37 weeks based on the risk factor of stillbirth alone [37].

Interventions to Improve Outcomes

Improved placental function is the goal of medical treatments meant to lower the chance of stillbirth. However, a recent systematic review of the Cochrane Database did not find enough evidence to recommend either low-dose aspirin or low-molecular-weight heparin (LMWH) for the prevention of stillbirth [35].

Emotional Support

Families who have experienced a stillbirth require emotional support. Pregnancies after stillbirth are linked to a number of negative psychological problems. In addition to providing psychological evaluation, focused follow-up, referrals, and therapy should be provided not just to the couple but to the family as a whole.

CONCLUSION

Stillbirth is a devastating pregnancy complication. It is traumatic for the couple and can also be stressful for the caregiver. Management of late term intrauterine death and stillbirth must be handled with great sensitivity and empathy. The aim is to guide the woman through the termination of pregnancy in the safest way possible. All attempts should be made to arrive at a cause for the stillbirth to be able to counsel the couple for a subsequent pregnancy.

REFERENCES

1. Hug L, You D, Blencowe H, Mishra A, Wang Z, Fix MJ, et al. Global, regional, and national estimates and trends in stillbirths from 2000 to 2019: A systematic assessment. *Lancet*. 2021. 98(10302):772–85.
2. Lawn JE, Blencowe H, Waiswa P, Amouzou A, Mathers C, Hogan D, et al. Stillbirths: Rates, risk factors, and acceleration towards 2030. *Lancet*. 2016. 387: 587–603.
3. World Health Organization. Neonatal and perinatal mortality: Country, regional and global estimates. *World Heal Organization*. 2006. 99:1–75. Available on http//:www.who.int.
4. World Health Organization (WHO). Stillbirths. https://www.who.int/maternal_child_adolescent/epidemiology/stillbirth/en/. Accessed September 2023.
5. What is stillbirth? Centers for Disease Control and Prevention. Available at: https://www.cdc.gov/ncbddd/stillbirth/facts.htm. Accessed September 2023.
6. RCOG Green-top Guideline No.55. Late intrauterine fetal death and stillbirth. 2010.
7. Operational Guidelines for Establishing Sentinel Stillbirth Surveillance System. Child Health Division, Ministry of Health and Family Welfare, Government of India. Developed for Ministry of Health & Family Welfare by World Health Organization Country Office for India. 2016.
8. Hoyert DL, Gregory ECW. National Vital Statistics Reports. Volume 69, Number 4. Cause-of-death—data From the fetal death file: 2015–2017. 2020. 69(4). Available from: https://www.cdc.gov/nchs/products/index.htm.
9. Silver RM, Dudley DJ, Conway D, Aufdemorte K, Rodriguez A, Pina M, et al. Eunice Kennedy Shriver National Institute of Child Health and Human Development, National Institutes of Health: *JAMA*. 2011. 306(22):2459–68.
10. Bhutta ZA, Yakoob MY, Lawn JE, et al. No stillbirths: What difference can we make and at what cost? Title. Lancet. 2011;(377):1523.
11. EM McClure, M Nalubamba-Phiri, RL Goldenberg, Stillbirth in developing countries. *International Journal of Gynecology & Obstetric*. Volume 94. Issue 2. 2006. 82–90.
12. Gardosi J, Madurasinghe V, Williams M, et al. Maternal and fetal risk factors for stillbirth: Population-based study. *BMJ*. 2013. 346:f108.
13. Bukowski R, Hansen NI, Willinger M, et al. Fetal growth and risk of stillbirth: A population-based case-control study. *PLoS*. 2014. 11:e1001633.
14. Lamont K, Scott NW, Jones GT BS. Risk of recurrent stillbirth: Systematic Review and Meta-analysis. *BMJ*. 2015. 350(h3080).
15. Muglu J, Rather H, Arroyo-Manzano D, et al. Risks of stillbirth and neonatal death with advancing gestation at term: A systematic review and meta-analysis of cohort studies of 15 million pregnancies. *PLoS Med*. 2019. 16:e1002838.
16. Sarno M, Sacramento GA, Khouri R, et al. Zika virus infection and stillbirths: A case of hydrops fetalis, hydranencephaly and fetal demise. *PLoS Negl Trop Dis*. 2016. 10:e0004517.
17. Hammad IA, Blue NR, Allshouse AA, Silver RM, Gibbins KJ, Page JM, Goldenberg RL, Reddy UM, Saade GR, Dudley DJ, Thorsten VR, Conway DL, Pinar H, Pysher TJ. NICHD Stillbirth Collaborative Research Network Group. Umbilical Cord Abnormalities and Stillbirth. *Obstet Gynecol*. 2020.
18. Ribeiro LSDC, D'Abreu BF, Santiago AE, Cândido EB, Romão GS, De Sá MFS, et al. Breaking bad news in obstetrics and gynecology: We must talk about it. *Rev Bras Ginecol e Obstet*. 2022. 44(6):621–8.
19. Nuzum D, Meaney S, O'Donohue K. Communication skills in Obstetrics: What can we learn from bereaved parents? *Ir Med J*. 2017. 110(02):512.
20. Stillbirth Collaborative Research Network Writing Group. Causes of death among stillbirths. *JAMA*. 2011. 306(22):2459-68.
21. Rådestad I, Steineck G, Nordin C, Sjögren B. Psychological complications after stillbirth—influence of memories and immediate management: Population-based study. *BMJ*. 1996. 312:1505–8.
22. Parasnis H, Raje B, Hinduja IN. Relevance of plasma fibrinogen estimation in obstetric complications. *J Postgrad Med*. 1992. 38:183–5.
23. Management of stillbirth. ACOG Obstetric Care Consensus No. 10. American College of Obstetricians and Gynecologists. *Obstet Gynecol*. 2020. 135:e110–32.
24. Gómez Ponce de León R, Wing DA. Misoprostol for termination of pregnancy with intrauterine fetal demise in the second and third trimester of pregnancy—a systematic review. *Contraception*. 2009. 79:259.
25. Dodd JM, Crowther CA. Misoprostol for induction of labour to terminate pregnancy in the second or third trimester for women with a fetal anomaly or after intrauterine fetal death. *Cochrane Database Syst Rev*. 2010. Issue 4. Art. no:CD004901.
26. Gómez Ponce de León R, Wing D, Fiala C. Misoprostol for intrauterine fetal death. *Int J Gynaecol Obstet*. 2007. 99 Suppl 2:S190.
27. Boyle A, Preslar JP, Hogue CJ, Silver RM, Reddy UM, Goldenberg RL, et al. Route of delivery in women with stillbirth: Results from the Stillbirth Collaborative Research Network. *Obstet Gynecol* 2017. 129: 693– 8.
28. Grunebaum A, Chervenak FA. Stillbirth: Maternal care. Lockwood CJ (Ed), UpToDate 2023, Waltham, MA.
29. Kingdon C, Givens JL, O'Donnell E, Turner M. Seeing and *Holding Baby*: Systematic Review of Clinical

management and parental outcomes after stillbirth. *Birth*. 2015. 42:206.

30. Hughes P, Turton P, Hopper E, Evans CD. Assessment of guidelines for good practice in psychosocial care of mothers after stillbirth: A cohort study. *Lancet*. 2002. 360:114.
31. Turton P, Evans C, Hughes P. Long-term psychosocial sequelae of stillbirth: Phase II of a nested case-control cohort study. *Arch Womens Ment Health*. 2009. 12:35.
32. Korteweg FJ, Bouman K, Erwich JJ, Timmer A, Veeger NJ, Ravise JM, et al. Cytogenetic analysis after evaluation of 750 fetal deaths: proposal for diagnostic workup. *Obs Gynecol*. 2008. 111:865–74.
33. Ladhani NNN, Fockler ME, Stephens L, Barrett JFR, Heazell AEP. No. 369-Management of Pregnancy Subsequent to Stillbirth. *J Obstet Gynaecol Can*. 2018. 40(12):1669-1683.
34. Mangesi L, Hofmeyr GJ, Smith V, Smyth RM. Fetal movement counting for assessment of fetal wellbeing. *Cochrane Database Syst Rev*. 2015. Issue 10. Art. no. CD004909.
35. Tveit JVH, Saastad E, Stray-Pedersen B, et al. Reduction of late stillbirth with the introduction of fetal movement information and guidelines – a clinical quality improvement. *BMC Pregnancy Childbirth*. 2009. https://doi.org/10.1186/1471-2393-9-32.
36. Robson SJ, Leader LR. Management of subsequent pregnancy after an unexplained stillbirth. *J Perinatol* [Internet]. 2010. 30(5):305–10.
37. Wojcieszek AM, Shepherd E, Middleton P, Lassi ZS, Wilson T, Murphy MM, Heazell AE, Ellwood DA, Silver RM, Flenady V. Care prior to and during subsequent pregnancies following stillbirth for improving outcomes. *Cochrane Database Syst Rev*. 2018. 12(12):CD012203.

CHAPTER 33

Management of Labour With a Growth-Restricted Fetus

TONY TAN

INTRODUCTION

A fetus is considered small-for-gestational age (SGA) when its abdominal circumference (AC) or estimated fetal weight (EFW) is less than the 10th percentile for the selected fetal biometric chart. This would include fetuses that are **growth-restricted** as well as those that are **normal but constitutionally small**.

- **An SGA fetus** is small but not at an increased risk of perinatal morbidity.
- **A growth-restricted fetus** is usually small with evidence of placental dysfunction and is at a higher risk of perinatal morbidity.

Therefore, it is important to identify these small babies and appropriately label them to ensure optimal care.

Fetal Growth Charts

Biometric charts are fundamental to the identification of the SGA/growth-restricted fetus. The selection of the chart can be made from the individual centres' fetal biometric charts specific to the local population [1], customised fetal growth charts [2], or international non-customised fetal growth charts, e.g., the WHO growth charts [3] or INTERGROWTH-21st fetal growth charts [4].

International non-customised fetal growth charts like the WHO and Intergrowth-21st charts were conceived with the idea that the fetuses of pregnant women in ideal conditions have similar growth rates but the fetuses of women in less ideal conditions (e.g., short women or women belonging to lower socio-economic status with poorer nutrition), have suboptimal fetal growths and may have constitutionally small fetuses that are not necessarily growth restricted. The WHO study showed that there are significant differences in biometric measurements and growth rates in different countries [5].

Population-based nomograms remain the most used in clinical practice as these are more easily implemented in currently available ultrasound fetal software packages.

> **Key Point**
>
> An SGA fetus is defined as a fetus with its AC/EFW <10th percentile. In the absence of Doppler abnormalities, this fetus is considered small but not at increased risk of perinatal morbidity. A growth-restricted fetus additionally has abnormal Doppler findings, indicating placental dysfunction, and is at increased risk of perinatal morbidity.

CLASSIFICATION OF SGA FOR THE MANAGEMENT OF LABOUR AND DELIVERY

Constitutionally Small Fetus

A normal SGA fetus with no evidence of structural abnormalities, chromosomal abnormalities, genetic syndromes or fetal infections, or abnormal Doppler indices of maternal and/or fetal vessels, may be managed as a constitutionally small baby and be delivered at term. This SGA fetus is at low risk of fetal acidemia and hypoxemia.

Abnormal SGA Fetus

An abnormal SGA fetus may have one or more of the following:

- Structural abnormalities
- Chromosomal abnormalities
- Genetic syndromes
- Fetal infections

These may be identified at the time of the first- or second-trimester scan and will require a complete evaluation as well as counselling for the couple. If the abnormal SGA fetus does not show abnormal Doppler changes, it should be delivered at term, if the fetal condition permits. A preterm abnormal SGA fetus faces additional risks of prematurity and hence, more risks than a term abnormal SGA fetus.

> **Key Point**
>
> Both normal and abnormal SGA fetuses may go on to develop growth restriction later during pregnancy and, therefore, should be scanned at least fortnightly.

Fetal Growth Restriction (FGR)

A growth-restricted fetus, on the other hand, is one where the fetus fails to achieve its genetic and/or biological growth potential. Such a conceptual definition is easy to grasp but difficult to diagnose clinically as the genetic and biological growth potential is difficult to define for each fetus. The clinical definitions widely accepted are the following:

- The fetus is very-small-for-gestational age (VSGA)—<3rd percentile
- SGA—3rd to <10th percentile—with certain abnormal Doppler indices of maternal and fetal vessels

Defined as such, the growth-restricted fetus should be monitored very closely to time the delivery before anticipated stillbirth and/or irreversible consequences from fetal acidemia/hypoxemia.

CLASSIFICATION OF FGR

Once the diagnosis of FGR is established, differentiating it into **early-** and **late-onset FGR** is useful. It distinguishes two clear phenotypes with differences in the following parameters:

- Severity
- Association with preeclampsia
- The natural history of fetal deterioration

This classification helps identify a fetus that requires fetal surveillance and is most likely to be compromised. It also helps direct the utilisation of the most appropriate surveillance modalities and decide on the timing of delivery based on the findings of antenatal surveillance.

Management of FGR and the decision to deliver aims at an optimal balance between minimising fetal injury or death against the risks of iatrogenic preterm delivery.

> **Key Point**
>
> Early- and late-onset FGR represent two distinct clinical phenotypes of placental dysfunction and differ significantly in clinical progression. The definitions are applicable only to fetuses without congenital abnormalities.

In 2016, an international panel of experts on FGR established the criteria for the diagnosis of early- and late-onset FGR in the Delphi consensus [6].

Early-onset FGR

Early-onset FGR represents 20–30% of all FGR and is associated with gestational hypertension and/or preeclampsia in up to 70% of cases.

It is associated with high-impedance utero-placental perfusion, which in turn, leads to elevated umbilical artery blood flow resistance once villous damage exceeds 30%. A systematic review of the Cochrane Database [7] confirmed that evaluation of placental function by umbilical artery (UA) Doppler studies is the clinical standard for identifying early-onset FGR and that its use in these pregnancies improves a number of obstetric care outcomes and reduces perinatal deaths.

Diagnosis of early-onset FGR

Early-onset FGR is easy to diagnose as the symphysial fundal height (SFH) is reduced and/or easy-to-perform UA Doppler is abnormal [8].

Early-onset FGR is diagnosed at **≤32 weeks' gestation** in the absence of fetal anomalies when the following criteria are met [6] (Fig. 33.1):

- AC and/or EFW is <3rd percentile (also known as very SGA or VSGA)
- Umbilical artery (UA) Doppler shows absent or reversed end-diastolic flow
- AC and/or EFW is <10th percentile combined with:
  - Uterine artery (UtA) pulsatility index (PI) >95th percentile and/or
  - UA–PI >95th percentile

Management of early-onset FGR

Early-onset FGR is difficult to manage as it requires close multimodal surveillance with ultrasound scans, biophysical profile, and if available, computerised cardiotocographic analysis (cCTG) by experts, with delivery delayed until well-described endpoints of monitoring are reached in order to achieve optimum fetal maturity.

Late-onset FGR

As compared to early-onset FGR, only 10% of late-onset FGR are associated with hypertensive disorders of pregnancy [9].

Diagnosis of late-onset FGR

Late-onset FGR is diagnosed at **>32 weeks' gestation** in the absence of fetal anomalies when the following criteria are met [6,10]:

- AC/EFW is <3rd percentile (or VSGA) **or**
- At least two of the following findings are present:
  - AC/EFW <10th percentile
  - AC/EFW dropping by >50 percentile on non-customised growth charts between consecutive ultrasound scans
  - Cerebroplacental ratio (CPR) <5th percentile or UAPI >95th percentile

Management of late-onset FGR

Late-onset FGR is difficult to diagnose but easier to manage [8]. Many cases of late-onset FGR would be missed if routine or frequent third-

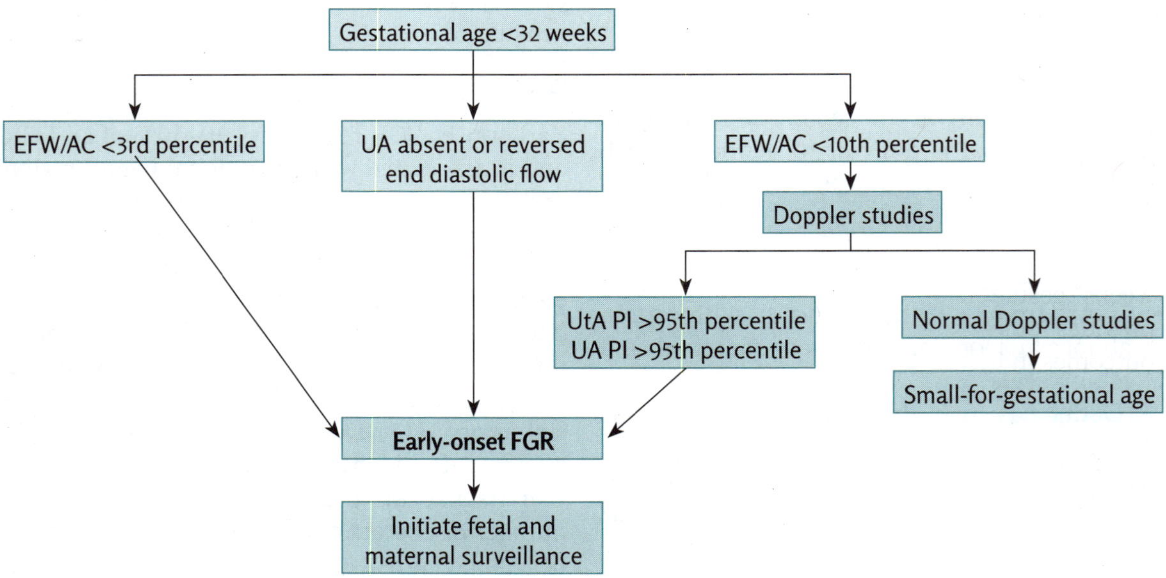

Fig. 33.1 Diagnosis of early-onset FGR

AC, abdominal circumference; *EFW*, estimated fetal weight; *FGR*, fetal growth restriction; *SGA*, small-for-gestational age; *UA—PI*, umbilical artery—pulsatility index

trimester growth scans with Doppler studies of the middle cerebral artery (MCA) were not performed. Serial SFH measurements would miss many cases of SGA fetuses with reduced growth velocities and those with decreased cerebroplacental ratios (CPRs) [11]. Once diagnosed, the decision to deliver at term or near term is easy to undertake.

Cerebroplacental ratio

The cerebroplacental ratio (CPR) is calculated as the simple ratio between the middle cerebral artery pulsatility index (MCA–PI) and the umbilical artery pulsatility index (UA–PI). CPR is an extremely important diagnostic index. It becomes abnormal even when its individual components are still within the normal ranges.

Low CPR (a fetal hypoxemic response) is related to the following:

- Impaired placental perfusion
- Placental dysfunction
- Poor fetal growth

At term, CPR is more diagnostic of placental insufficiency and fetal compromise than birth weight. A decreased CPR (<5th percentile) in the third trimester may be associated with higher rates of adverse perinatal outcomes and perinatal deaths in SGA fetuses [12]. Though a low CPR shows an increase in obstetric intervention due to fetal distress, it is a poor predictor of adverse perinatal outcomes [13]. Moreover, a prospective observational study of 47,211 singleton pregnancies [14] found that at 35–37 weeks' gestation, routine measurement of CPR provides poor prediction of adverse perinatal outcomes in both SGA and AGA fetuses.

> **Key Point**
>
> There is no robust evidence to recommend the routine performance of CPR in the third trimester as a predictor of poor perinatal outcome.

Routine third trimester scanning

The issue of whether routine third-trimester scans should be implemented as standard obstetric care is controversial. Whilst there is evidence that routine third-trimester growth scans in low-risk populations would allow the detection of late-onset structural abnormalities in 1 in 300 women (with previous normal routine second-trimester scans) [15] and increase the detection of SGA fetuses (even if serial SFH measurements were normal) [16,17], **there is little evidence that they reduce adverse perinatal outcomes** [18,19,20].

The majority of current national guidelines **do not recommend routine third-trimester scan** for SGA screening **in low-risk populations** [21]. However, women with **major risk factors** should receive serial scanning in the third trimester.

When performing a third-trimester scan to optimise the detection of late-onset FGR, it is better to time the third-trimester scan at 36 weeks rather than 32 weeks [22].

MODE AND TIMING OF DELIVERY

In suspected SGA pregnancies, umbilical artery Doppler studies are universally advised to guide management [21]. In late-onset fetal growth restriction (≥32 weeks), the general consensus is to use cerebral Doppler studies to steer fetal surveillance and guide the timing of delivery.

SGA Fetuses (AC or EFW Between 3rd–10th Percentile) with Normal Doppler Studies

An SGA fetus with normal Doppler studies should be managed like a fetus that has appropriate growth.

SGA neonates whose birth weights are between the 3rd and 10th percentile with CPR >10th percentile have lower risks of adverse perinatal outcomes compared with SGA neonates with CPR <10th percentile [23].

It would be appropriate to consider induction of labour at 38–39 weeks to reduce the risk of stillbirth [24].

Women should be counselled that the chance of vaginal delivery with induction of labour of

SGA fetuses at term is similar to that for non-SGA fetuses [25]. Retrospective data show that the use of prostaglandins for cervical priming in SGA fetuses (compared to non-SGA fetuses) does not increase the risk of cesarean section [26].

- **Timing of delivery:** 38–39 weeks
- **Mode of delivery:** Vaginal delivery, induction of labour with prostaglandins; cesarean for other obstetric indications

Key Point

In pregnancies with an SGA fetus with normal Doppler studies, induction of labour may be offered at 38–39 weeks.

Very SGA (VSGA) Fetuses

EFW <3rd percentile is the only sonographic weight-related parameter that is found to be consistently associated with adverse outcomes. When this is associated with worsening UA Doppler indices, the perinatal mortality is highest [27]. The rates of adverse perinatal outcomes for VSGA neonates where the birth weights were <3rd percentile were similar to that of SGA fetuses with CPR <10th percentile, whether the VSGA fetus' CPRs were normal or not [28].

Induction of labour

Neonates with birth weights <5th percentile who have been delivered after induced labour have higher rates of NICU admission and acidosis than those delivered by elective cesarean section [28]. When these pregnancies are induced, emergency section is required in 71% and 55% of fetuses with birth weights <1st percentile and from the 1st–2.5th percentiles respectively [23].

Pregnant women with suspected VSGA fetuses should be offered elective cesarean section at 38–39 weeks [29]. In a retrospective cohort study, the risk of fetal death at 39 weeks was estimated to be 32 per 10,000 ongoing pregnancies for fetal weight <3rd percentile, when compared to 2 per 10,000 ongoing pregnancies for fetal weight ≥10th percentile [30].

- **Timing of delivery**: 38–39 weeks (or earlier if maternal or fetal condition deteriorates)
- **Mode of delivery:** Elective cesarean section

Key Point

VSGA fetuses have a high risk of adverse pregnancy outcomes, and the woman should be offered elective cesarean section at 38–39 weeks' gestation (or earlier if maternal or fetal condition deteriorates).

Early-onset FGR

Early-onset FGR is usually associated with maternal hypertensive disease. In fetuses with severe FGR and fetal compromise on evaluation, the aim is to delay delivery till 34 completed weeks, when the chances of fetal survival are better.

Key Point

After 26 weeks' gestation, the fetus should be delivered when the risk of further placental ageing whilst remaining in utero exceeds the risks of prematurity if delivered. In resource-limited settings, 28 weeks would a salvageable gestational age to plan delivery.

The **absolute indications** for delivery, regardless of gestational age, are as follows:

- Worsening of maternal condition, for example, preeclampsia with severe features
- Obstetric emergencies (e.g., abruption) requiring delivery
- Evidence of fetal compromise as indicated by fetal surveillance testing (NST is non-reactive or shows late decelerations, or single deepest pocket of amniotic fluid is ≤2 cm)

Timing of delivery

- **Decreased** UA end-diastolic flow (UA–EDF) or increased UA pulsatility index >95th percentile: **Delivery by 36+0 to 37+6 weeks' gestation**
- **Absent** UA end-diastolic flow (UA-EDF): **Delivery by 32–34 weeks**
- **Reversed** end diastolic flow: **Delivery by 30–32 weeks**

- In LMICs and in resource-poor settings, the neonatal prognosis is poor at **<28 weeks**. Though international recommendations and tertiary NICU settings use 26 weeks as the cut-off for resuscitation, it may not be realistic. The expectant parents should be counselled about the outcome based on the local NICU facility.
- At <26 weeks, perinatal survival is <50% with 80% of the neonates having major complications. Indications for delivery at this early gestational age are chiefly to safeguard the mother (see above).
- **At 26–32 weeks**, ductus venosus Doppler helps in the identification of a fetus with cardiovascular deterioration. The TRUFFLE trial showed that early-onset FGR babies should be delivered based on late ductus venous Doppler changes and abnormal computerised CTG changes, and that delivery should not be based on cerebral Doppler changes alone [31]. This approach was associated with the highest chance of survival without infant neurodevelopmental impairment at two years of age.
    - Immediate delivery is indicated with **absent** or **reversed 'a' wave** on ductus venosus Doppler even if the fetus is <32 weeks.
    - If the ductus venosus Doppler is normal, the fetus can be delivered within a week, after a course of steroids.

- **At ≥34 weeks**, delivery is indicated. A course of steroids may be administered to the mother.
- **Abnormal computerised CTG indices**: European centres follow the TRUFFLE study recommendations which are as follows:
    - Decreased short-term baseline fetal heart rate variation (persisting when repeated after 8 hours) is an indication for immediate delivery if it is:
        - <2.6 milliseconds at 26–28 weeks
        - <3.0 milliseconds at 29–31 weeks
        - <3.5 milliseconds at ≥32 weeks
        - <4.5 milliseconds at ≥34 weeks
    - Unprovoked spontaneous decelerations are an indication for delivery

> **Key Point**
>
> Most centres in India and indeed many parts of the world do not have computerised CTG. In such situations, spontaneous decelerations and reduced variability would be indications for immediate delivery.

Mode of delivery

Cesarean delivery is the optimal route of delivery for early-onset FGR, especially with the following conditions [32]:

- Absent or reversed end-diastolic flow in the UA
- Abnormal Doppler studies in the DV
- Abnormal biophysical profile (BPP)
- Severe maternal condition

Antenatal steroids for pulmonary maturation

A single course of corticosteroids should be offered (if not previously given) 1–7 days before a planned or unscheduled preterm delivery (between 24 to 34 weeks' gestation). See **Chapter 30**, *Preterm labour and prelabour rupture of membranes*, for further details.

Magnesium sulphate for neuroprotection

Magnesium sulphate should be offered to women at risk of preterm delivery between 24 and 32 weeks of gestation to reduce the risk of cerebral palsy [33]. See **Chapter 30** for further details.

The suggested management and timing of delivery for early-onset FGR is presented as an algorithm in Fig. 33.2.

> **Key Point**
>
> Elective cesarean section is recommended for early-onset FGR.

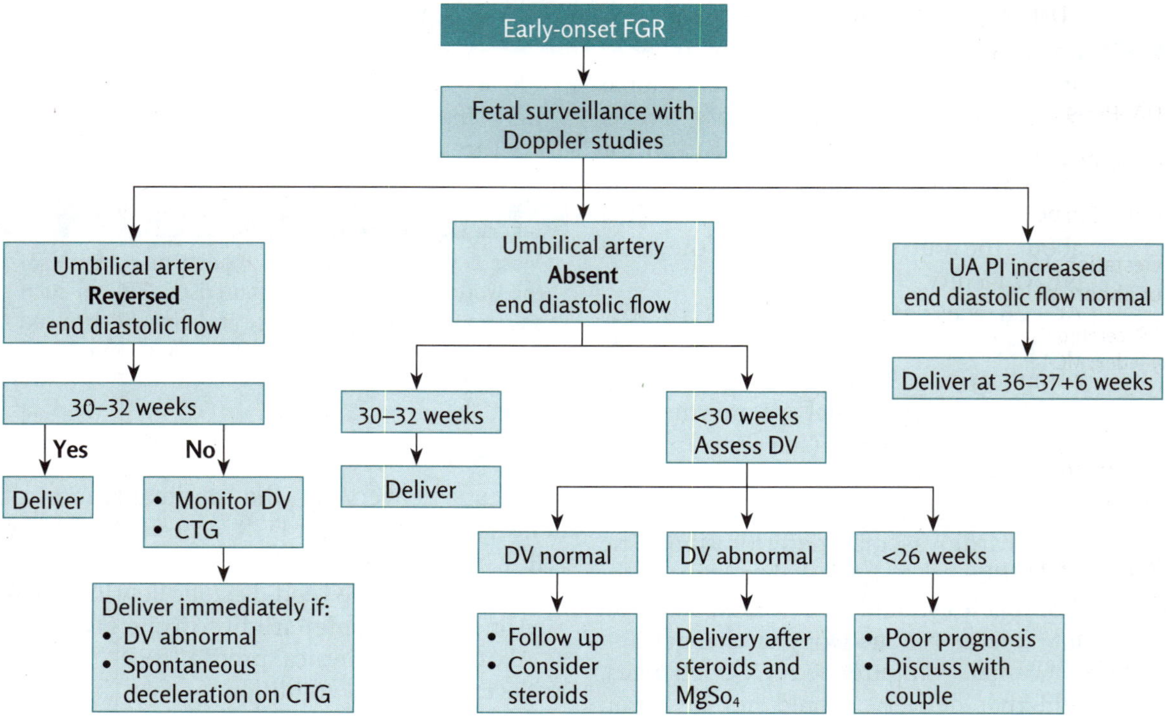

Fig. 33.2 Management algorithm for early-onset FGR
DV, ductus venosus; *UA—PI*, umbilical artery—pulsatility index

Late-onset FGR

The fetus should be delivered when the continuation of pregnancy increases the risk of fetal compromise.

MCA Doppler abnormalities

In late-onset FGR, MCA Doppler abnormalities predict deterioration and stillbirth, in contrast to early-onset FGR, where UA Doppler abnormalities arise first. MCA Doppler findings determine the frequency of fetal surveillance [10]. Even in the absence of UA Doppler abnormalities, 'brain sparing' as denoted by MCA Doppler indices should alert the clinician to the risk of sudden late stillbirth after 37 weeks.

MCA–PI <5th percentile is indicative of hypoxia. Since placental reserve is already minimal, sudden severe deterioration may occur. The term-mature fetus is much more susceptible to hypoxia than the preterm fetus. There is a high risk of intrauterine fetal death after 37 weeks in these cases.

Timing of delivery

There is no international consensus on the timing of delivery in late-onset FGR, with highly variable end points in various national guidelines [21]. Delivery may be induced at 37–38 weeks, though robust evidence on optimal delivery timing is lacking (Table 33.1).

> **Key Point**
>
> In late-onset FGR, MCA Doppler abnormalities predict deterioration and stillbirth, in contrast to early-onset FGR, where UA Doppler abnormalities arise first.

Table 33.1 Delivery timing based on clinical findings

Clinical finding	Timing of delivery
UA–PI >95th percentile	36–37+6 weeks
MCA–PI >5th percentile	37–38 weeks
CPR <5th percentile	37–38 weeks
Gestational age 37–38 weeks or abnormal BPP	Immediate delivery

CPR, cerebroplacental ratio; *UA—PI*, umbilical artery—pulsatility index; *MCA-PI*, middle cerebral artery pulsatility index

Mode of delivery

Spontaneous vaginal delivery

Vaginal delivery may be allowed if the woman goes into labour spontaneously. In late-onset FGR, there is a good chance of successful vaginal delivery even in the presence of Doppler changes. CPR is a poor prognostic predictor of adverse perinatal outcomes in late-onset FGR, though there is an increase in operative delivery rates with reducing CPR [34].

Induction of labour (IOL)

IOL, as opposed to expectant management for late-onset FGR, is associated with similar rates of composite adverse neonatal outcomes and cesarean section rates [24]. Expectant management of late-onset FGR is associated with increased maternal vascular malperfusion and chorioamnionitis [37].

Induction of labour is a reasonable option in the following circumstances:

- UA–PI >95th percentile but without progression to absent or reversed end-diastolic flow—up to 90% may successfully deliver vaginally [35]
- CPR <5th percentile—up to 75% chance of vaginal delivery
- The cervix is unfavourable but CPR is normal—up to 60% chance of vaginal delivery [35,36]

Cervical ripening: Cervical priming with mechanical methods like Foley catheter or hygroscopic dilators is preferred over medical methods like dinoprostone as they may result in a higher rate of vaginal delivery (80% vs. 60%) and a lesser degree of adverse perinatal outcomes [36].

Key Point

In late-onset FGR, induction of labour after 38 weeks is a safe option and does not increase the risk of adverse outcomes. The presence of UA/CPR changes should not prevent an attempt at vaginal delivery.

Cesarean section

Cesarean delivery is performed for standard obstetric indications such as the following:

- There is an urgent maternal or obstetric indication to deliver, e.g., maternal severe preeclampsia, placental abruption, malpresentation
- The risk of fetal distress with vaginal delivery is anticipated to be high, and a joint decision has been made to maximise the outcome for the baby, e.g., spontaneous recurrent unprovoked decelerations on CTG, absent or reversed end-diastolic flow in the UA [38]
- The risk of failed induction of labour is high, e.g., a combination of unfavourable cervix, nulliparity, advanced maternal age with increased body mass index, or CPR <5th percentile

CONDUCTING LABOUR IN PREGNANCIES WITH FGR

The special considerations for the management of labour in pregnancies with FGR include the following:

- **Continuous intrapartum CTG monitoring** is highly recommended (if available) as the risk of fetal distress is higher than the baseline, and growth-restricted fetuses have lower reserves than non-growth-restricted fetuses
- When there is an **anticipation of a higher risk of intrapartum fetal compromise,** clear instructions should be provided to the delivery suite staff on how to deal with the

situation (see **Chapter 15**, *Identification and management of fetal distress,* for further details)

- **Judicious use of oxytocin**
- **Close monitoring** by experienced labour ward staff
- **Optimum pain relief** with early access to epidural analgesia

CONCLUSION

The management of labour in a pregnancy with an SGA fetus or with FGR requires close coordination with the fetal medicine team and the general obstetric team. It requires close monitoring and rapid responses. Though the consensus on the precise timing of delivery for the growth-restricted fetus is lacking, there is a general consensus on how to monitor and conduct labour.

REFERENCES

1. Daniel-Spiegel E, Mandel M, Nevo D, et al. Fetal biometry in the Israeli population: New reference charts. *Isr Med Assoc J*. 2016. 18(1):40-4. PMID: 26964279.
2. Gardosi J, Chang A, Kalyan B, et al. Customised antenatal growth charts. *Lancet.* 1992. 39(8788):283-7. doi: 10.1016/0140-6736(92)91342-6. PMID: 1346292.
3. Kiserud T, Piaggio G, Carroli G, et al. The World Health Organization Fetal Growth Charts: A Multinational Longitudinal Study of Ultrasound Biometric Measurements and Estimated Fetal Weight. *PLoS Med.* 2017. 14(1):e1002220. doi: 10.1371/journal.pmed.1002220.
4. Papageorghiou AT, Kennedy SH, Salomon LJ, et al. International Fetal and Newborn Growth Consortium for the 21(st) Century (INTERGROWTH-21(st)). The INTERGROWTH-21st fetal growth standards: Toward the global integration of pregnancy and pediatric care. *Am J Obstet Gynecol.* 2018. 218(2S):S630-S640.
5. Kiserud T, Benachi A, Hecher K, et al. The World Health Organization fetal growth charts: Concept, findings, interpretation, and application. *Am J Obstet Gynecol.* 2018. 218(2S):S619-S629. doi: 10.1016/j.ajog.2017.12.010. PMID: 29422204.
6. Gordijn SJ, Beune IM, Thilaganathan B, et al. Consensus definition of fetal growth restriction: A Delphi procedure. *Ultrasound Obstet Gynecol.* 2016. 48(3):333-9. doi: 10.1002/uog.15884. PMID: 26909664.
7. Alfirevic Z, Stampalija T, Dowswell T. Fetal and umbilical Doppler ultrasound in high-risk pregnancies. *Cochrane Database Syst Rev.* 2017. Issue 6. Art. No.: CD007529.
8. Lees CC, Romero R, Stampalija T, et al. Clinical Opinion: The diagnosis and management of suspected fetal growth restriction: An evidence-based approach. *Am J Obstet Gynecol.* 2022. 226(3):366-378.
9. Unterscheider J, Daly S, Geary MP, et al. Optimizing the definition of intrauterine growth restriction–results of the multicenter prospective PORTO study. *AJOG.* 2013. 208(4): 290.
10. Figueras F, Caradeux J, Crispi F, et al. Diagnosis and surveillance of late-onset fetal growth restriction. *Am J Obstet and Gynec.* Volume 218. Issue 2. 2018. S790–802. e1.
11. Sovio U, White IR, Dacey A, et al. Screening for fetal growth restriction with universal third trimester ultrasonography in nulliparous women in the Pregnancy Outcome Prediction (POP) study: A prospective cohort study. *Lancet.* 2015. 386(10008):2089-2097. Erratum in: *Lancet.* 2015 Nov 21;386(10008):2058.
12. Conde-Agudelo A, Villar J, Kennedy SH, Papageorghiou AT. Predictive accuracy of cerebroplacental ratio for adverse perinatal and neurodevelopmental outcomes in suspected fetal growth restriction: Systematic review and meta-analysis. *Ultrasound Obstet Gynecol.* 2018. 52(4):430-441.
13. Dall'Asta A, Ghi T, Rizzo G, et al. Cerebroplacental ratio assessment in early labor in uncomplicated term pregnancy and prediction of adverse perinatal outcome: Prospective multicenter study. *Ultrasound Obstet Gynecol.* 2019. 53(4):481-487. doi: 10.1002/uog.19113. Epub 2019 Mar 4. PMID: 29900608.
14. Akolekar R, Ciobanu A, Zingler E, et al. Routine assessment of cerebroplacental ratio at 35-37 weeks' gestation in the prediction of adverse perinatal outcome. *Am J Obstet Gynecol.* 2019. 221(1):65.e1-65.e18. doi: 10.1016/j.ajog.2019.03.002. Epub 2019 Mar 13. PMID: 30878322.
15. Drukker L, Bradburn E, Rodriguez GB, et al. How often do we identify fetal abnormalities during routine third-trimester ultrasound? A systematic review and meta-analysis. *BJOG.* 2021. 128(2):259-269.
16. Sovio U, White IR, Dacey A, et al. Screening for fetal growth restriction with universal third trimester ultrasonography in nulliparous women in the Pregnancy Outcome Prediction (POP) study: A prospective cohort study. *Lancet.* 2015. 386(10008):2089-2097. Erratum in: *Lancet.* 2015. 386(10008):2058. PMID: 26360240; PMCID: PMC4655320.
17. Wanyonyi SZ, Orwa J, Ozelle H, et al. Routine third-trimester ultrasound for the detection of small-for-gestational age in low-risk pregnancies (ROTTUS study): Randomized controlled trial. *Ultrasound Obstet Gynecol.* 2021. 57(6):910-916.
18. Henrichs J, Verfaille V, Jellema P, et al. IRIS study group. Effectiveness of routine third trimester ultrasonography to reduce adverse perinatal outcomes in low-risk

pregnancy (the IRIS study): Nationwide, pragmatic, multicentre, stepped wedge cluster randomised trial. *BMJ*. 2019. 367:l5517.

19. Aderoba AK, Ioannou C, Kurinczuk JJ, et al. Oxford Growth Restriction Identification Programme (OxGRIP) Group. The impact of a universal late third-trimester scan for fetal growth restriction on perinatal outcomes in term singleton births: A prospective cohort study. *BJOG*. 2023. doi: 10.1111/1471-0528.17395. Epub ahead of print. PMID: 36660877.
20. Al-Hafez L, Chauhan SP, Riegel M, et al. Routine third-trimester ultrasound in low-risk pregnancies and perinatal death: A systematic review and meta-analysis. *Am J Obstet Gynecol MFM*. 2020. 2(4):100242.
21. McCowan LM, Figueras F, Anderson NH. Evidence-based national guidelines for the management of suspected fetal growth restriction: Comparison, consensus, and controversy. *Am J Obstet Gynecol*. 2018. 218(2S):S855-S868.
22. Roma E, Arnau A, Berdala R, et al. Ultrasound screening for fetal growth restriction at 36 vs 32 weeks' gestation: A randomized trial (ROUTE). *Ultrasound Obstet Gynecol*. 2015. 46(4):391-7. doi: 10.1002/uog.14915. PMID: 26031399.
23. Karge A, Lobmaier SM, Haller B, et al. Value of cerebroplacental ratio and uterine artery doppler as predictors of adverse perinatal outcome in very small for gestational age at term fetuses. *J Clin Med*. 2022. 11(13):3852.
24. Boers KE, Vijgen SM, Bijlenga D, et al. DIGITAT study group. Induction versus expectant monitoring for intrauterine growth restriction at term: Randomised equivalence trial (DIGITAT). *BMJ*. 2010. 341:c7087.
25. Rhoades JS, Rampersad RM, Tuuli MG, et al. Delivery outcomes after term induction of labor in small-for-gestational age fetuses. *Am J Perinatol*. 2017. 34(6):544-549. doi: 10.1055/s-0036-1593972. Epub 2016 Nov 4. PMID: 27824403.
26. Rosenbloom JI, Rhoades JS, Woolfolk CL, et al. Prostaglandins and cesarean delivery for non-reassuring fetal status in patients delivering small-for-gestational age neonates at term. *J Matern Fetal Neonatal Med*. 2021. 34(3):366-372.
27. Unterscheider J, O'Donoghue K, Daly S, et al. Fetal growth restriction and the risk of perinatal mortality – case studies from the multicentre PORTO study. *BMC Pregnancy Childbirth*. 2014. 14: 63.
28. Maslovitz S, Shenhav M, Levin I, et al. Outcome of induced deliveries in growth-restricted fetuses: Second thoughts about the vaginal option. *Arch Gynecol Obstet*. 2009. 279(2):139-43. doi: 10.1007/s00404-008-0685-5. Epub 2008 May 28. PMID: 18506461.
29. Kazemier BM, Voskamp BJ, Ravelli AC, et al. Optimal timing of delivery in small for gestational age fetuses near term: A national cohort study. *Am J Perinatol*. 2015. 30(2):177-86.
30. Pilliod RA, Cheng YW, Snowden JM, et al. The risk of intrauterine fetal death in the small-for-gestational-age fetus. *Am J Obstet Gynecol*. 2012. 207:318.e1.
31. Frusca T, Todros T, Lees C, Bilardo CM. TRUFFLE Investigators. Outcome in early-onset fetal growth restriction is best combining computerized fetal heart rate analysis with ductus venosus Doppler: Insights from the trial of umbilical and fetal flow in Europe. *Am J Obstet Gynecol*. 2018. 218(2S):S783-S789. doi: 10.1016/j.ajog.2017.12.226. PMID: 29422211.
32. Lees CC, Stampalija T, Baschat A, et al. ISUOG Practice Guidelines: Diagnosis and management of small-for-gestational-age fetus and fetal growth restriction. *Ultrasound Obstet Gynecol*. 2020. 56(2):298-312. doi: 10.1002/uog.22134. PMID: 32738107.
33. Wolf HT, Huusom LD, Henriksen TB, et al. Magnesium sulphate for fetal neuroprotection at imminent risk for preterm delivery: A systematic review with meta-analysis and trial sequential analysis. *BJOG*. 2020. 127(10):1180-1188.
34. Villalain C, Galindo A, Di Mascio D, et al. Diagnostic performance of cerebroplacental and umbilicocerebral ratio in appropriate for gestational age and late growth restricted fetuses attempting vaginal delivery: A multicenter, retrospective study. *J Matern Fetal Neonatal Med*. 2022. 35(25):6853-6859.
35. Pinton A, Lemaire Tomzack C, Merckelbagh H, Goffinet F. Induction of labour with unfavourable local conditions for suspected fetal growth restriction after 36 weeks of gestation: Factors associated with the risk of caesarean. *J Gynecol Obstet Hum Reprod*. 2021. 50(7):101996.
36. Villalain C, Quezada MS, Gómez-Arriaga P, et al. Prognostic factors of successful cervical ripening and labor induction in late-onset fetal growth restriction. *Fetal Diagn Ther*. 2020. 47(7):536-544.
37. Feenstra ME, Schoots MH, Plösch T, et al. More maternal vascular malperfusion and chorioamnionitis in placentas after expectant management vs. immediate delivery in fetal growth restriction at (near) term: A further analysis of the DIGITAT Trial. *Front Endocrinol* (Lausanne). 2019. 10:238.
38. Garcia-Simon R, Figueras F, Savchev S, et al. Cervical condition and fetal cerebral Doppler as determinants of adverse perinatal outcome after labor induction for late-onset small-for-gestational-age fetuses. *Ultrasound Obstet Gynecol*. 2015. 46(6):713-7.

CHAPTER 34

Management of Labour with Fetal Macrosomia

MANISHA MADHAI BECK, NITIN ALEXANDER ABRAHAM

INTRODUCTION

The common definition of **macrosomia**—an infant birth weight of ≥4000 g—does not take into consideration gestational age, sex, or country-/region-specific differences in mean birth weight and maternal body weight [1]. This definition cannot be applied to Asian countries, where 60% of the world's population lives. Data from the WHO's Global Survey on Maternal and Perinatal Health showed that only 0.5% of babies in India are born weighing ≥4000 g as compared to 5–20% in high-income countries [2].

Large-for-gestational age (LGA), defined as birth weight >90th percentile for the given population, is a more sensitive measure as it considers gestational age and sex. It is better suited for making informed decisions based on the population that is under treatment. It is important to remember that the weight cut-off varies not only between countries but also within countries, as the definition of LGA may differ between the urban and the rural populations and between different socio-economic classes.

The World Health Organization [4] and the International Fetal and Newborn Growth Consortium for the 21st Century (Intergrowth-21 project) have published weight tables that should be applicable worldwide [5].

Macrosomia is associated with an increased risk of cesarean section and both maternal and fetal trauma. It has been shown that both clinical and ultrasonographic prediction of macrosomia are prone to error. When macrosomia is suspected, elective cesarean section and early induction of labour have both been associated with a high number of unnecessary procedures.

This chapter will focus on the following:

- The effect of suspected macrosomia on decisions regarding the mode of delivery
- The effect of macrosomia on the progress of labour
- The effect of macrosomia on maternal and neonatal morbidity and mortality

PREVALENCE

The prevalence of macrosomia is approximately 9% worldwide. In India, LGA occurs in 6–12% of pregnancies [1,3]. Variations in prevalence are attributed to differences in the definitions used. The incidence of macrosomia is on the rise as more pregnancies are now complicated by diabetes and obesity.

Key Point

Given that macrosomia is best defined by birth weight >90th percentile, in India, a fetus weighing ≥3500 g at term may be defined as having macrosomia [2].

SPECTRUM OF FETAL GROWTH DISORDERS

Fetal growth disorders can result in a small baby due to **fetal growth restriction** (FGR) or a large baby due to **fetal growth acceleration** (FGA) and **excessive fetal weight gain**. When the estimated fetal weight (EFW) of the fetus is <10th percentile, it is considered to be **small for gestational age (SGA).** On the other end of the size spectrum, the fetus can also experience growth acceleration, and when the **EFW** is >90th percentile, it is considered to be **large for gestational age (LGA).** Fetuses between these two extremes are considered to be **appropriate for gestational age (AGA**; Fig. 34.1).

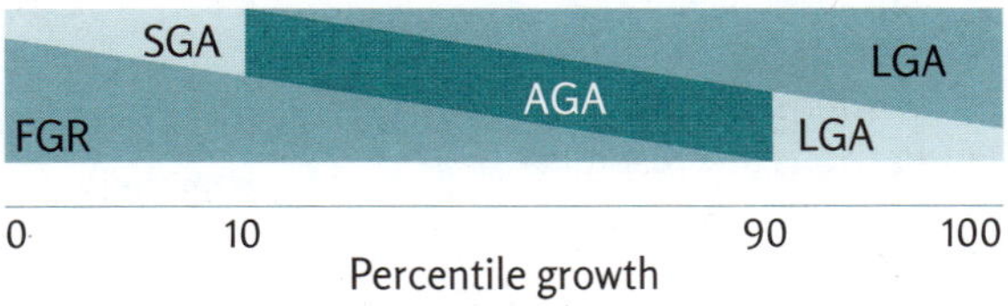

Fig. 34.1 Spectrum of fetal growth disorders
AGA, appropriate for gestational age; *FGR*, fetal growth restriction; *FGA*, fetal growth acceleration; *LGA*, large for gestational age; *SGA*, small for gestational age

Though poor growth leading to SGA and FGR is well-studied, excessive fetal weight gain is often overlooked. Methods are lacking to distinguish healthy large fetuses from overgrown fetuses or to identify overgrown fetuses with appropriate weight, especially in the absence of maternal diabetes [6]. Overgrowth leads to macrosomia and large-for-gestational age babies. No consensus definition for macrosomia exists [6].

Definition of Macrosomia and LGA

Macrosomia: In high-income countries, macrosomia is defined as an EFW above a fixed cut-off, irrespective of gestational age. Arbitrary cut-offs vary between 4000 and 4500 g [7]. The risks of fetal morbidity and mortality increase proportionately with increasing birth weights, being significantly higher at a weight of >5000 g. These cut-offs are used to categorise macrosomia and the associated perinatal risk (Table 34.1).

Large for gestational age: LGA, in contrast, is when the EFW is >90th percentile for a particular gestational age. This definition is based on the average birth weight at each gestational age and is country-specific. This helps in identifying the overgrown fetus, even when it is preterm. Though >90th percentile is taken as a measure of overgrowth, >95th and >97th percentiles are also used to define LGA [7]. It is better to use weight percentiles rather than a fixed cut-off to make clinical decisions.

Table 34.1 Categories of macrosomia (adapted from ACOG Practice Bulletin 216 [7])

Macrosomia	Weight	Perinatal risk
Category I	4000–4499 g	No difference
Category II	4500–4999 g	Morbidity and mortality (stillbirth) significantly increased
Category III	>5000 g	Highest risk

As per the INTERGROWTH 21 charts [8], which are applicable to the Indian subcontinent, cut-offs for LGA at 37 and 40 weeks are 3326 g and 3858 g respectively [9].

Key Point

Though high-income countries define macrosomia as a fetus whose estimated weight is >4000 g, it is sensible to use the definition of LGA for uniformity. An LGA fetus has an estimated weight >90th percentile for the given gestational age.

PATHOPHYSIOLOGY AND RISK FACTORS FOR MACROSOMIA

The Pederson hypothesis [10] states that maternal hyperglycemia, as seen in cases of gestational diabetes (GDM) or pregestational diabetes, can lead to fetal hyperglycemia if it is not well controlled—as a result of placental transfer of glucose. This, in turn, leads to fetal hyperinsulinemia and the production of the insulin-like growth factor-1 (IGF-1), resulting in fetal fat deposition and macrosomia. In obese non-diabetic women, there is a state of insulin resistance too, which leads to intermittent maternal hyperglycemia, setting up a cascade which finally leads to macrosomia (Fig. 34.2).

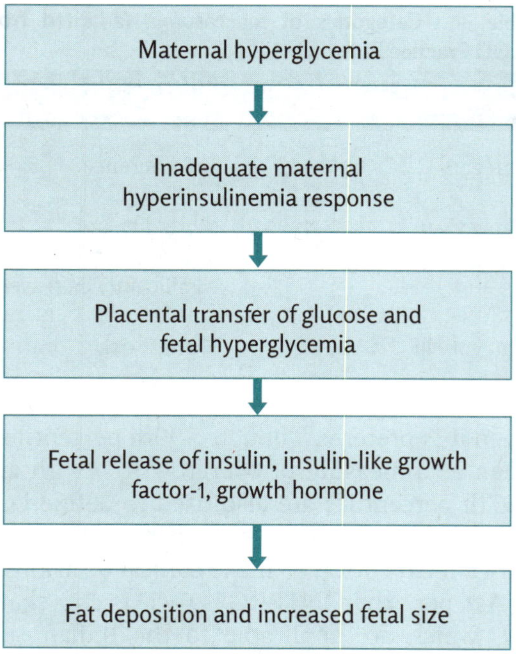

Fig. 34.2 Pathophysiology of fetal macrosomia

Maternal and fetal hyperglycemia alone cannot explain all cases of macrosomia. Inadequate physical activity, increased uteroplacental blood flow, increased placental size, nutrient concentration gradients, and placental ability to transfer them also contribute to the same.

The risk factors for fetal macrosomia are listed in Table 34.2.

Key Points

Macrosomia in fetuses caused by glucose intolerance is different from macrosomia that results from other causes. Babies born to diabetic women tend to have an increased risk of shoulder dystocia because of the following factors:

- Greater total body fat
- Greater shoulder and upper extremity circumferences
- Chest circumference much larger than the head
- Altered fetal body shape—barrel-chested infant with a short neck and broad shoulders

Table 34.2 Risks factors of macrosomia

Maternal	Fetal
• Diabetes* • Obesity* • Excessive gestational or inter-pregnancy weight gain* • Advanced age • Multiparity • Postterm pregnancy • Previous macrosomia** • Maternal macrosomia at birth	• Male fetus • Genetic disorders

* Highest risk of macrosomia
** 10% risk of recurrence

PREDICTION OF MACROSOMIA FOR THE MANAGEMENT OF LABOUR

The ability to predict significant macrosomia before birth is an imprecise science. Both physical examination and ultrasound perform poorly in accurate diagnosis.

Clinical Assessment

Maternal examination to determine uterine size using symphysio-fundal height (SFH) is often inaccurate in diagnosing fetal macrosomia. Palpation through the abdominal wall is made difficult by the following factors:

- Increased quantity of amniotic fluid (polyhydramnios)
- Maternal body fat (in overweight and obese women)
- Multiparity leading to a lax abdominal wall

Ultrasound Estimation of Macrosomia

USG estimation of EFW is based on published formulas that incorporate measurements of fetal head circumference (HC), abdominal circumference (AC), and femur length (FL). However, ultrasound accuracy decreases with increasing fetal weight beyond 4000 g [7].

In a meta-analysis of 41 studies evaluating the role of universal third-trimester USG screening for macrosomia in >100,000 pregnancies, it was found that its sensitivity for diagnosing macrosomia was only 53% and 58% when the EFW was >4000 g and >4500 g respectively [11].

> **Key Point**
>
> Suspected LGA is strongly predictive of the risk of delivering a large infant in low- and mixed-risk populations but only weakly predictive of shoulder dystocia [10].

Similarly, a study found that women undergoing ultrasound examination within two weeks of delivery in an attempt to predict macrosomia and who are found to have an EFW of ≥4000 g are more likely to have a baby with **overestimated** birth weight. Obstetricians should be cautious about intervening based on sonographic EFW alone [12].

> **Key Point**
>
> USG estimation of EFW is the same as the clinical estimate for diagnosing macrosomia. Hence, it should be used for **ruling out** rather than **ruling in** macrosomia [7].

SUSPECTED MACROSOMIA AND DECISIONS REGARDING MODE OF DELIVERY

When macrosomia or LGA is suspected by clinical or ultrasound examination, it raises concerns about vaginal delivery and the consequences for the woman and neonate. Communicating these concerns to the woman and her family may lead to an increase in the rates of induction of labour and elective cesarean rates [7,13].

Decisions regarding the mode and timing of delivery should take into consideration the following:

- **Maternal height and weight:** Taller women (≥160 cm) and women with a higher BMI tend to have larger babies but also have larger pelvises that favour a successful vaginal delivery.
- **Engagement of the head:** When the head is well-engaged, before or at the beginning of labour, the chances of a successful vaginal delivery are higher.
- **History of a successful vaginal delivery of an LGA baby:** This increases the chances of a successful delivery in the present pregnancy. However, a history of shoulder dystocia in a previous pregnancy is a relative contraindication to attempting vaginal delivery.

Induction of Labour (IOL)

With the continuation of pregnancy or expectant management, the concern is that the fetus will continue its accelerated growth, with a possible increase in operative birth or cesarean section. The baby is also at an increased risk of shoulder dystocia and trauma, in particular, fractures and brachial plexus injury. It has been postulated that the induction of labour before term may reduce these risks by decreasing the birth weight. However, induction may result in longer labour and an increased risk of cesarean section.

Though some studies have reported the benefit of IOL, others have not found significant benefit; rather, they reported a higher risk of complications with elective IOL at term.

A recent systematic review of the Cochrane Database [14] reported that the induction of labour for suspected fetal macrosomia results in a lower mean birth weight and fewer birth fractures and shoulder dystocia. However, it should be borne in mind that the number of labour inductions required to prevent a fracture in one baby is 60.

Timing of induction

If the woman and her obstetrician reach a shared decision regarding induction, the American College of Obstetricians and Gynecologists recommends delivery no earlier than 39+0 weeks of gestation in the absence of a medical indication [7]. It is not clear that a reduction in shoulder dystocia would be seen with induction of labour after 39 0/7 weeks of gestation [14].

Key Point

Currently, suspected macrosomia or LGA is not an indication for induction of labour before 39+0 weeks of gestation because the harms of early delivery outweigh the benefits of reducing the risk of shoulder dystocia [7].

When macrosomia is associated with maternal diabetes that is well-controlled with diet and exercise/medication (A1/A2 GDM), IOL is offered at or after 39 weeks. If GDM is poorly controlled, delivery can be planned any time between 37 and 38+6 weeks [15].

Elective Cesarean Section

In the presence of clinically suspected macrosomia or LGA, the clinician must make a decision that will result in a safe delivery and prevent maternal and fetal morbidity. However, most LGA and macrosomic babies have uncomplicated births. In an analysis comparing expectant management to induction of labour or cesarean section, expectant management was found to be the most cost-effective in non-diabetic women with suspected macrosomic fetuses [16].

Cesarean section decreases but does not eliminate the risk of shoulder dystocia and brachial plexus injury. In Western literature, the greatest benefit of cesarean was reported in babies weighing ≥5000 g born to women without diabetes and babies weighing at least 4500 g among women with diabetes. Considering that in Indian babies, LGA is defined as ≥3500 g, cesarean section would be beneficial with an EFW of 4500 g in non-diabetic women and 4000 g in diabetic women. However, there are no RCTs to support or refute this recommendation. This recommendation is based on consensus and expert opinion (Level C) to guide practice and is presented in Table 34.3.

Table 34.3 Indications for elective LSCS in suspected macrosomia*

Western recommendations	Indian women
No diabetes complicating pregnancy and estimated fetal weight >5000 g	No diabetes complicating pregnancy and estimated fetal weight >4500 g
Diabetes complicating pregnancy and estimated fetal weight >4500 g	Diabetes complicating pregnancy and estimated fetal weight >4000 g
Previous shoulder dystocia and estimated fetal weight >4000 g	Previous shoulder dystocia and estimated fetal weight >3500 g

*The woman's height and weight should be taken into consideration while making this decision.

Key Point

In a large study of women with suspected macrosomia who underwent induction of labour or a planned cesarean section, only 20% gave birth to a newborn weighing 4000 g or more, showing that suspected macrosomia is associated with a higher number of interventions [17].

The decision for a cesarean delivery should be a shared one and individualised to each case because 50% of women with shoulder dystocia have no identifiable risk factors; moreover, the prediction of macrosomia is inaccurate, and brachial plexus injury can occur in the absence of macrosomia, shoulder dystocia, and even during cesarean section (see **Chapter 28**, *Shoulder dystocia: prevention and management*).

Key Point

3695 cesareans would have to be performed to prevent a permanent brachial plexus injury in a macrosomic baby born to a non-diabetic woman. 443 cesareans would have to be performed to prevent an injury in an LGA baby born to a diabetic woman [18,19].

THE EFFECT OF MACROSOMIA ON THE PROGRESS OF LABOUR

Prolonged First and Second Stages of Labour

In the presence of macrosomia, the risk of abnormalities in the progression of labour increases. This is often due to cephalopelvic disproportion, fetal malposition, malpresentation, and abnormal lie.

Protracted or arrested first stage of labour: Large fetal size is one of the risk factors for protracted or arrested first stage of labour (see **Chapter 11**, *Abnormalities in the latent phase and the first stage of labour*).

Prolonged second stage of labour: The second stage may also be prolonged in the case of a macrosomic baby. If the woman has been pushing for more than two hours and the head has not descended, this might indicate the possibility of shoulder dystocia or increased risk of emergency cesarean section (see **Chapter 12**, *Abnormalities in the second stage of labour*). In this situation, the woman should be assessed by a senior obstetrician. If the fetal head is above +2 station, a cesarean section should be performed.

> **Key Point**
>
> In an LGA/macrosomic fetus, the head does not become engaged until the active stage is reached. As a result, the bag of membranes is not well applied to the presenting part and often prone to rupture early in labour, increasing the risk of cord prolapse, chorioamnionitis, and prolonged first stage of labour.

Operative Vaginal Delivery in the Presence of Suspected Macrosomia

A difficult operative vaginal delivery should always be avoided in cases of fetal macrosomia as it may lead to severe maternal and fetal morbidity. These include the following:

- Maternal complications
  - Third- or fourth-degree perineal lacerations
  - Postpartum hemorhage (PPH)
- Perinatal complications
  - Severe perinatal asphyxia
  - Shoulder dystocia
  - Obstetric brachial plexus injury (OBPI) and other forms of birth injuries to the baby

The risk of shoulder dystocia is 4–9% with operative vaginal delivery versus spontaneous delivery [20]. While some studies found an increased rate of shoulder dystocia with vacuum extraction in comparison to forceps [21], others have not found any difference in the method of operative vaginal delivery used [22].

The risk of shoulder dystocia at the time of operative vaginal delivery increases with the presence of more than one risk factor. Hence, in a case of macrosomia, if there also has been prolongation of the first or second stage of labour or both, and the woman is a diabetic, the risk of shoulder dystocia is higher in comparison to only macrosomia/LGA being present as a risk factor [7].

> **Key Point**
>
> Operative vaginal delivery in cases of fetal macrosomia is associated with significant maternal and fetal morbidity and should be undertaken cautiously, especially when multiple risk factors are present, as this increases the risk of shoulder dystocia.

Increased Risk of Cesarean Delivery

When compared to women with appropriately grown babies, the risk of LSCS is twice as high in women labouring with macrosomic babies. Intrapartum LSCS is attributed to labour dystocia either in the first or second stage of labour. Second-stage LSCS should be considered in preference over a difficult operative vaginal delivery, especially when the fetal head is at or above the +2 station.

Second-stage LSCS is challenging in these cases due to the presence of a deeply-impacted, large fetal head. There is an existing component of fetal compromise in such cases, and a difficult delivery at LSCS will worsen the fetal condition.

SPECIAL SITUATIONS

External Cephalic Version (ECV)

Although fetal macrosomia is not an absolute contraindication to offering ECV, the procedure may be less likely to be successful if attempted. There is insufficient evidence to show whether ECV should be offered to women with LGA fetuses; the principle of shared decision making should be applied [23].

Vaginal Birth After Cesarean (VBAC)

Macrosomia is not an absolute contraindication to attempting VBAC. However, the success rate of VBAC declines and the risk of uterine rupture increases in women attempting VBAC with an EFW ≥4000 g. Nevertheless, the success rate may be >50% in women who have had a previous successful vaginal delivery or VBAC [24].

Shoulder Dystocia

Shoulder dystocia is defined as failure of spontaneous delivery of the shoulders following the delivery of the fetal head. This results from the anterior shoulder getting hinged below the pubic symphysis. The odds of shoulder dystocia are seven times more in macrosomia in comparison to AGA babies. The risk of shoulder dystocia is higher in cases of macrosomia associated with maternal diabetes due to the abnormal fat distribution.

The risk of injuries related to shoulder dystocia is increased in the presence of fetal macrosomia—there is a 10-fold increase in fracture of the clavicle and an 18–21-fold increase in brachial plexus injury.

See **Chapter 28** for further details.

NEONATAL COMPLICATIONS

Complications in a macrosomic neonate may be secondary to a difficult delivery, related to macrosomia itself, maternal diabetes, or a combination of factors.

- **Hypoglycemia** is the most common complication and occurs due to the withdrawal of high maternal glucose levels from the fetal circulation postdelivery. Since the neonate continues to have high circulating levels of insulin, neonatal hypoglycemia ensues.
- **Metabolic acidosis** is often due to a difficult delivery superimposed on a state of chronic hypoxia in these fetuses.
- **Polycythemia** is secondary to chronic hypoxia seen in macrosomic babies, especially those born to diabetic women.
- **Respiratory distress** is due to delayed lung maturation seen in infants born to diabetic women.
- **Long-term complications** associated with macrosomia which manifest in adulthood include the following:
  - Obesity
  - Impaired glucose tolerance
  - Metabolic syndrome
  - Cardiac remodelling

CONCLUSION

When macrosomia is suspected in the third trimester, it should be remembered that a single ultrasound estimate between 29 and 34 weeks of gestation has very poor predictive value for birth weight at term. More babies are likely to be classified as macrosomic with the increasing use of third-trimester ultrasound. The sensitivity and specificity of ultrasound estimation of fetal weight and its correlation with the risk of shoulder dystocia is poor at weights >4000 g. The presence or absence of maternal hyperglycemia and the woman's previous obstetric history, especially that of the vaginal delivery of a large baby, will influence decision making regarding the mode of delivery. Though operative delivery may be required for a proportion of these babies, careful counselling to ensure that the woman understands the risks and benefits, along with careful monitoring of labour progress can result in a successful vaginal delivery.

REFERENCES

1. Harvey L, van Elburg R, van der Beek EM. Macrosomia and large for gestational age in Asia: One size does not fit all. *J Obstet Gynaecol Res*. 2021. 47(6):1929–45.
2. Koyanagi A, Zhang J, Dagvadorj A, et al. Macrosomia in 23 developing countries: An analysis of a multicountry, facility-based, cross-sectional survey. *Lancet*. 2013. 381: 476–83.
3. Jeyaseelan L, Yadav B, Silambarasan V, et al. Large for gestational age births among south Indian women: Temporal trend and risk factors from 1996 to 2010. *J Obstet Gynaecol India*. 2016. 66(Suppl 1):42–50.
4. Kiserud T, Piaggio G, Carroli G, et al. The World Health Organization fetal growth charts: A multinational longitudinal study of ultrasound biometric measurements and estimated fetal weight. *PLoS Med*. 2017. 14(1): e1002220.
5. Stirnemann J, Villar J, Salomon LJ, et al. International estimated fetal weight standards of the INTERGROWTH-21st Project. *Ultrasound Obstet Gynecol*. 2017.
6. Damhuis SE, Ganzevoort W, Gordijn SJ, et al. Abnormal fetal growth small for gestational age, fetal growth restriction, large for gestational age: Definitions and epidemiology. *Obstet Gynecol Clin N Am*. 2021. 48.267–279
7. Macrosomia. ACOG Practice Bulletin No. 216. American College of Obstetricians and Gynecologists. *Obstet Gynecol*. 2020;135:e18–35.
8. Papageorghiou AT, Ohuma EO, Altman DG, et al. International standards for fetal growth based on serial ultrasound measurements: the Fetal Growth Longitudinal Study of the INTERGROWTH-21st Project. *Lancet*. 2014. 384(9946):869–79.
9. Stirnemann J, Villar J, Salomon LJ, et al. International Fetal and Newborn Growth Consortium for the 21st Century (INTERGROWTH-21st). International estimated fetal weight standards of the INTERGROWTH-21st Project. *Ultrasound Obstet Gynecol*. 2017. 49(4):478-486.
10. Pedersen J. *The pregnant diabetic and her newborn: Problems and management,* by Farquhar J. The Williams and Wilkins Company Baltimore. 1968.
11. Moraitis AA, Shreeve N, Sovio U, et al. Universal third-trimester ultrasonic screening using fetal macrosomia in the prediction of adverse perinatal outcome: A systematic review and meta-analysis of diagnostic test accuracy. *PLoS Med*. 2020. 17(10):e1003190.
12. Zafman KB, Bergh E, Fox NS. Accuracy of sonographic estimated fetal weight in suspected macrosomia: The likelihood of overestimating and underestimating the true birth weight. *J Matern Fetal Neonatal Med*. 2020. 33(6):967-972.
13. Sadeh-Mestechkin D, Walfisch A, Shachar R, et al. Suspected macrosomia? Better not tell. *Arch Gynecol Obstet*. 2008. **278**, 225–230. https://doi.org/10.1007/s00404-008-0566-y.
14. Boulvain M, Thornton JG. Induction of labour at or near term for suspected fetal macrosomia. *Cochrane Database Syst Rev*. 2023. Issue 3. Art. no.:CD000938.
15. ACOG Practice Bulletin No. 190: Gestational Diabetes Mellitus. *Obstet Gynecol*. 2018. 131(2):e49.
16. Herbst MA. Treatment of suspected fetal macrosomia: a cost-effectiveness analysis. *Am J Obstet Gynecol*. 2005.193: 1035–9.
17. Cheng ER, Declercq ER, Belanoff C, et al. Labor and delivery experiences of mothers with suspected large babies. *Matern Child Health J*. 2015. 19: 2578– 86.
18. Rouse DJ, Owen J, Goldenberg RL, Cliver SP. The effectiveness and costs of elective cesarean delivery for fetal macrosomia diagnosed by ultrasound. *JAMA*. 1996; 276: 1480–6. (Level III).
19. Rouse DJ, Owen J. Prophylactic cesarean delivery for fetal macrosomia diagnosed by means of ultrasonography—a Faustian bargain? *Am J Obstet Gynecol*. 1999. 181: 332– 8. (Level III).
20. Bouchghoul H, Hamel JF, Mattuizzi A, et al. Predictors of shoulder dystocia at the time of operative vaginal delivery: A prospective cohort study. *Sci Rep*. 2023. 13:2658.
21. Dall'Asta A, Ghi T, Pedrazzi G, Frusca T. Does vacuum delivery carry a higher risk of shoulder dystocia? Review and meta-analysis of the literature. *Eur J Obstet Gynecol Reprod Biol*. 2016; 204: 62–8.
22. Overland EA, Vatten LJ, Eskild A. Risk of shoulder dystocia: Associations with parity and offspring birth weight. A population study of 1 914 544 deliveries. *Acta Obstet Gynecol Scand*. 2012. 91: 483– 8.
23. Diagnosis and management of suspected fetal macrosomia. 2021. RANZCOG. Available at https://ranzcog.edu.au/wp-content/uploads/2022/05/Diagnosis-and-management-of-suspected-fetal-macrosomia.pdf.
24. Elkousy MA, Sammel M, Stevens E, et al. The effect of birth weight on vaginal birth after cesarean delivery success rates. *Am J Obstet Gynecol*. 2003. 188(3):824–30.

CHAPTER 35

Malpositions and Malpresentations (Other Than Breech)

JYOTHI UNNI

INTRODUCTION

Malpositions and malpresentations commonly result in abnormal labour. Malpresentations of the fetus complicate labour in about 5% of pregnancies, and malpositions, especially the occipitoposterior position, complicate another 20%. Malpositions and malpresentations lead to an increase in perinatal complications and maternal morbidity and mortality. To improve maternal and neonatal outcomes, it is important to anticipate and identify the problem early and intervene appropriately.

At the beginning of labour, the fetus may be in a longitudinal, transverse, or oblique lie. In 96–97% of cases, the fetus is in the **cephalic presentation** [1] and, in the vast majority, in the **occipitoanterior position**, which is the position that is considered normal.

This chapter will deal with malpositions and malpresentations other than breech presentation.

MALPOSITIONS

When the vertex presents with the occiput in the right or left posterior quadrant of the pelvis, it is referred to as a **malposition.** A malposition could be left occipitoposterior position (LOP) or right occipitoposterior position (ROP). See **Chapter 2,** *Mechanics of labour,* for details.

Occipitoposterior (OP) Position

This is the most common abnormal position. There is an increased risk of operative deliveries when the fetus remains in this position. The OP position accounts for about 5% of cephalic presentations in labour [2]. Sometimes, a fetus that was in the occipitoanterior (OA) or occipitotransverse (OT) position may move into the occipitoposterior position.

Occipitoposterior positions lead to prolonged first and second stages of labour. Women often have more backache than with anterior positions. Since there is a prolongation of labour in the OP position, there is a higher likelihood of intervention such as oxytocin augmentation and operative births. There is also a higher chance of cesarean birth with an OP position [3].

Key Point

The OP position, seen in about 5% of labour, may result in the prolongation of the first or second stage of labour or it may cause arrest of labour in the second stage.

Risk factors

The most common causes of OP position include nulliparity, an android pelvis anterior placenta, cephalopelvic disproportion, and epidural analgesia.

Diagnosis

On abdominal palpation, the head may be deflexed. The anterior fontanelle is felt anteriorly on vaginal examination. There is usually significant caput, and there may be asynclitism. It is sometimes difficult to identify the position in the presence of a large caput. If a diagnosis of OP position is made in the first stage of labour, no intervention is required as many fetuses rotate to OA later in the first stage.

Ultrasound examination helps to confirm the diagnosis and is recommended particularly before embarking on an operative vaginal delivery [4]. See **Chapter 20**, *Role of ultrasound in the labour room*, for further details.

Mechanism of labour

In most cases, the head rotates through 135^0 (long arc) from the ROP to the OA position (Fig. 35.1), and the delivery occurs as usual.

Sometimes, the head malrotates posteriorly through 45° (Fig. 35.2a), assuming the direct OP (**persistent occiput posterior**) position (Fig. 35.2b). The delivery then takes place **face-to-pubis** (Fig. 35.2c). The birth of the head occurs by a combination of flexion and extension. After the occiput is delivered by flexion, the nose, mouth, and chin are delivered by extension [5].

Occasionally, there is no rotation, and the head remains in an ROP position. Rotation may also be arrested in the occiput transverse (OT) position (**deep transverse arrest**). In these cases, management depends on the station of the head and fetal status (see **Chapter 12**, *Abnormalities in the second stage of labour*).

Management

If there is persistent OP position in the second stage, watchful expectancy is advocated as long as fetal and maternal conditions are satisfactory. The woman can be asked to kneel forward or lie on the side of the occiput to help rotation [5].

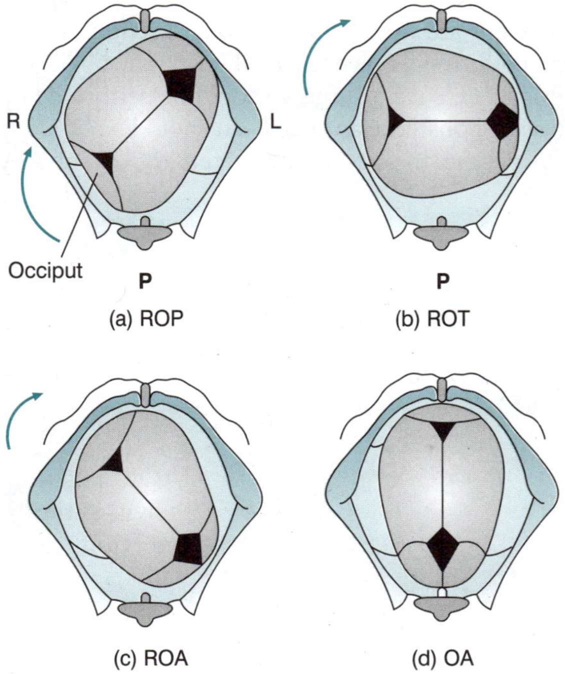

Fig. 35.1 Long arc rotation (135°) in occiput posterior position: (a) The occiput is lying in the right posterior quadrant of the pelvis, (b) it undergoes rotation to reach the right occiput transverse position, and (c) passing through the right anterior quadrant, reaches the occiput anterior (OA) position (d)

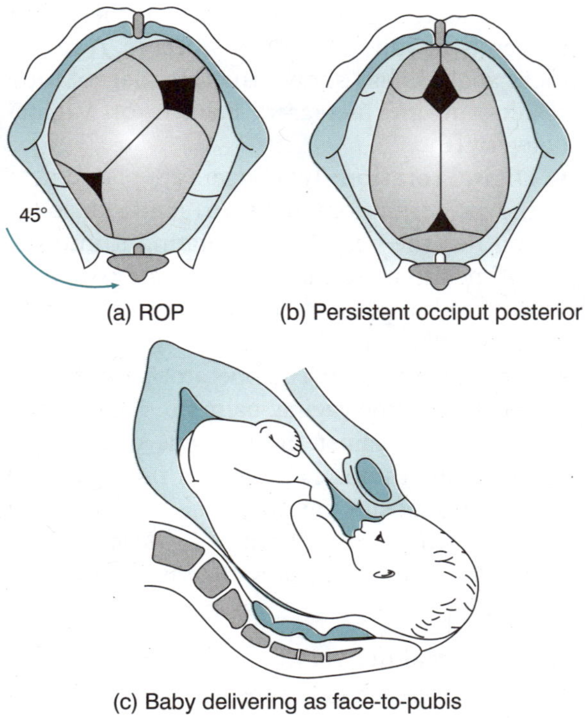

Fig. 35.2 Mechanism of labour in short arc rotation (45^0): (a) The occiput, which is lying in the right posterior quadrant, rotates through 45° to (b) persistent occiput posterior position and (c) the baby delivers face-to-pubis

Oxytocin augmentation

If the contractions are not adequate, a low-dose oxytocin infusion may be commenced. Artificial rupture of the membranes may be performed if there is undue delay in the progress of labour.

If rotation does not occur, despite the delay in descent, the fetus is often delivered safely as face-to-pubis. In this situation, episiotomy is usually required to avoid third- and fourth-degree perineal tears as the larger diameters of the fetal skull negotiate the perineum.

Digital or manual rotation

If the descent slows down, manual rotation to OA may be performed, and the second stage is allowed to progress. The rotation is performed during a contraction, with the woman pushing down so that the digital rotation assists the physiological rotation of the head. Quite often, as soon as the rotation is achieved, the vertex descends rapidly, and delivery occurs. A recent meta-analysis has shown that manual rotation results in an increased chance of vaginal delivery [6].

- **Digital rotation**: Two fingers are placed near the posterior fontanelle to gently dislodge and flex the head before rotating it into the OA position. It may be necessary to hold the head in place for the next contraction to ensure that it does not rotate back.
- **Manual rotation:** The operator's right hand is placed in the vagina, palm up. Four fingers are placed against the left side of the fetal head. The thumb is placed on the right side of the opposite parietal bone, and rotation is performed. See **Chapter 4,** *Management of the first and second stages of normal labour,* for details.

Instrumental delivery

In some cases, when the second stage is unduly prolonged or there is maternal exhaustion, forceps or ventouse can be applied. One must remember that in the presence of a significant caput, ventouse may fail.

It is important to confirm that there is no more than one-fifth of the head palpable abdominally and that the station is at 0 or below [7]. When in doubt, the position can be confirmed by ultrasound (see **Chapter 20**). The instrument may be applied with the head in the OP position, and the baby can be delivered as face-to-pubis (Fig. 35.3).

Rotation by forceps may be attempted if the operator is skilled in the procedure. If rotational forceps such as Kielland's forceps are used, the delivery can be performed directly after rotation. If not, the forceps are removed after rotation and reapplied for delivery as OA.

Rotation to OA may occur spontaneously during delivery by ventouse. See **Chapter 21,** *Operative vaginal delivery,* for further details.

Cesarean section

If the criteria for safe vaginal or operative vaginal delivery are not met, a cesarean section should be performed. Since the fetal head may be deeply impacted, such a surgery should be performed by a senior obstetrician. The head should be brought up to the incision and rotated to OT or OA

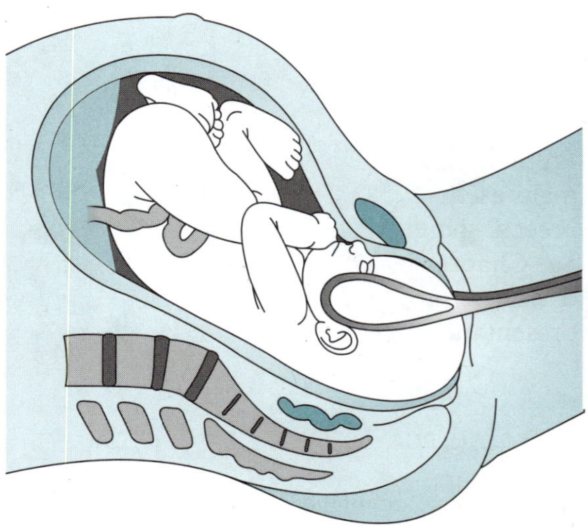

Fig. 35.3 Forceps application for persistent occipitoposterior position—the baby is delivered as face-to-pubis

before being delivered. Occasionally, an assistant may need to elevate the fetal head by introducing their fingers or hand into the woman's vagina and applying upward pressure (see **Chapter 22**, *Cesarean section: Procedure and technique*).

> **Key Points**
>
> - Most OP positions will spontaneously rotate to occipitoanterior and deliver as such.
> - Manual rotation is an important obstetric skill that can help resolve persistent OP position. If that fails, face-to-pubis delivery may be conducted safely.

Occipitotransverse Position

Usually, if the head is in an occipitotransverse position, it will rotate into the OA or, occasionally, to the OP position. Management should be as for OA or OP position.

However, in some cases, there is **deep transverse arrest**. In such cases, the management will depend on the station of the head, parity, and fetal well-being. If the head is not low enough for manual rotation or rotation by an instrument to be performed safely, a cesarean section may be required (see **Chapter 12**, *Abnormalities in the second stage of labour*).

MALPRESENTATIONS

Presentations other than vertex are called malpresentations. These include face, brow, breech, shoulder, and compound presentations. See **Chapter 27,** *Breech delivery (including external cephalic version)*, for details of managing breech presentation.

Brow Presentation

Brow presentation is rare—it occurs in 1 in 500 to 1 in 1400 cases [8]. Partial extension makes the head present as a brow, and the presenting part of the fetus is from the anterior fontanelle to the brow (Fig. 35.4a). The **presenting diameter is the verticomental**, which is 13.5 cm.

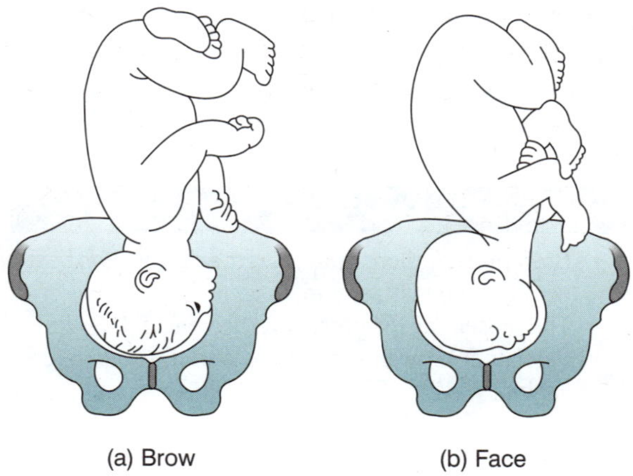

Fig. 35.4 Brow and face presentations: (a) Brow presentation is a position of partial extension, halfway between complete flexion and complete extension and (b) face presentation results when the head is hyperextended, with the occiput touching the fetal back

Diagnosis

On abdominal palpation, the head is not engaged. On vaginal examination, the anterior fontanelle is easily felt, but the sagittal suture is not [9]. The supraorbital ridges may be felt while the mouth and chin are not; this confirms the diagnosis. As the feel of the vertex and brow are similar, there is often a delay in the diagnosis. Ultrasound is a more accurate way of confirming the diagnosis [10]. If there is undue delay in the progress of labour, malpresentation should be suspected and the possibility of a brow presentation should be kept in mind.

Management of labour

Brow presentation may be a transitional presentation. When diagnosed early in labour, 60–70% of cases convert spontaneously to a more favourable presentation that will allow for vaginal delivery. If diagnosed in the second stage, 50% convert to the face or occipitoposterior position while 50% remain as brow. **Persistent brow presentation cannot be delivered vaginally.**

Delay in diagnosis causes extensive moulding, traumatic delivery, fetal morbidity, and mortality. Once diagnosed in the second stage, it is best to proceed with a cesarean delivery.

Key Points

- Brow presentation is rare, and the diagnosis is best confirmed by ultrasound.
- The presenting diameter is verticomental (13.5 cm).
- Persistent brow presentation cannot be delivered vaginally.

Face Presentation

The incidence of face presentation is low, accounting for approximately 1 in 600 presentations [10]. Face presentation results when the head is hyperextended, with the occiput touching the fetal back (Fig. 35.4b). **In face presentation, all parts of the face, from the chin to the glabella** (the smooth area between the eyebrows just above the root of the nose), **present in the pelvis.**

The **presenting diameter is submentobregmatic, measuring 9.5 cm**. In >50% of cases, the chin or mentum is anterior, and over 75% will deliver vaginally [11]. The rest may present as mentum posterior (30%) or mentum transverse (20%).

Diagnosis

On abdominal palpation, the back and the occiput are on the same side due to the extension of the head. Vaginal examination reveals the absence of the hard vertex. The fontanelles are not felt. A soft, irregular structure is felt, which may be confused with the breech. One can palpate the orbital ridge and orbits, saddle of the nose, mouth, and chin. Identifying the eyes or mouth helps to clinch the diagnosis. Ultrasound is useful when there is uncertainty [9].

Management of labour

- **Mentoanterior presentation:** Face presentation is often diagnosed late in labour. Both the first and second stages of labour are prolonged. Membranes usually rupture early in labour. Labour may progress in a mentoanterior position, where the chin delivers under the symphysis pubis, and the rest of the head is born by flexion (Fig. 35.5a–e) [12]. In a mentotransverse position, delivery is possible if it rotates to mentoanterior. Fetal heart rate abnormalities are more common in face presentation [13]. If there is a delay in delivery, it is prudent to perform a cesarean section. There are usually more perineal lacerations, and the baby's face appears swollen and misshapen at birth.

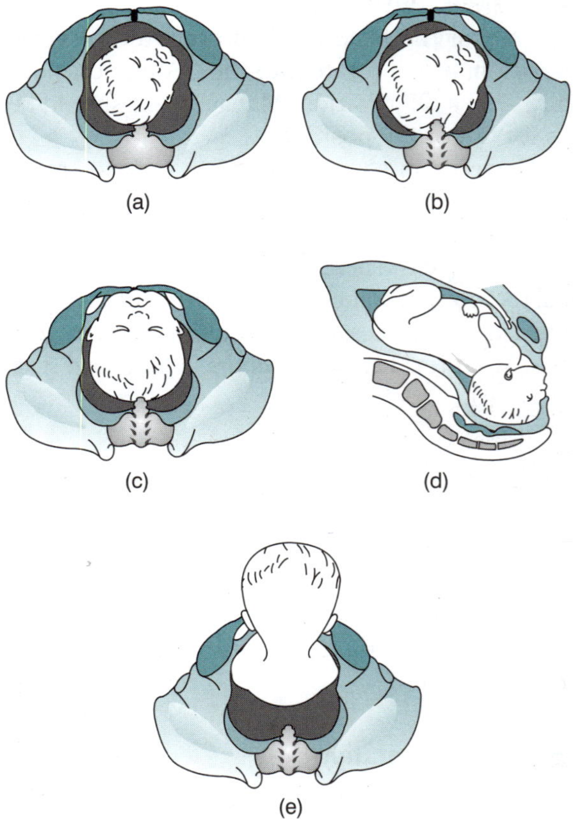

Fig. 35.5 Mechanism of labour in face presentation: (a) Left mentoanterior at onset of labour; (b) extension and descent; (c) internal rotation to mentoanterior; (d) lateral view of mentoanterior, with chin hitched under the symphysis pubis and (e) head delivering by flexion

- **Mentoposterior presentation:** Vaginal delivery is only possible with rotation to a menoanterior position. If that does not occur, a cesarean section should be performed. **There is no mechanism of labour for a persistent mentoposterior position**, as the neck is already maximally extended and cannot extend any further to allow the occiput to negotiate and pass below the symphysis pubis.

Key Points

- Face presentation occurs when the fetal head is fully extended.
- Vaginal delivery is possible if the chin (mentum) is anterior, and the head is born by flexion. Mentoposterior face presentation cannot be delivered vaginally and will require cesarean delivery.

TRANSVERSE LIE OR SHOULDER PRESENTATION

Transverse lie occurs when the long axis of the fetus is perpendicular to the long axis of the woman (Fig. 35.6). It is rare and accounts for about 1 in 300 cases [14]. The shoulder is usually the presenting part; however, it could also be the arm, back, or abdomen. Some of the risk factors include prematurity, grand multiparity, polyhydramnios, placenta previa, and multiple pregnancy. It is most common to see a transverse lie early in pregnancy, which usually converts to a cephalic or breech presentation as pregnancy advances. By term, most fetuses are in a longitudinal lie.

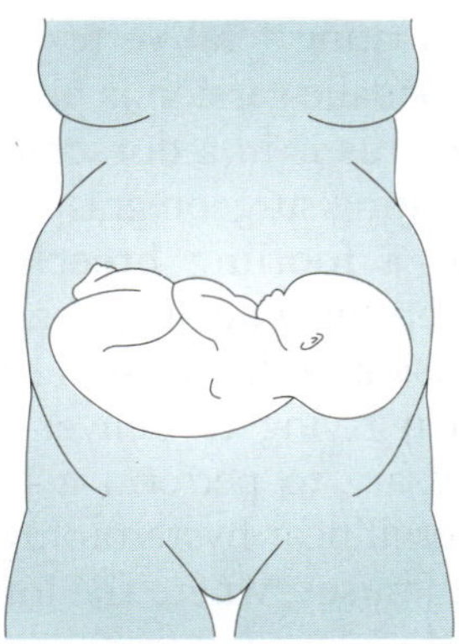

Fig. 35.6 Transverse lie—the long axis of the fetus is perpendicular to the long axis of the mother

Diagnosis

Diagnosis is made by abdominal palpation and should be suspected when the presenting part is not felt in the lower abdomen on pelvic grip. The fetal head may be felt in either flank. Ultrasound is used to confirm the diagnosis and ascertain the position of the fetus.

There are two possible positions based on the curvature of the spine:

- **Dorsoinferior**, where the curvature of the spine is downwards ('back down') and the shoulder is the presenting part (Fig. 35.7a)
- **Dorsosuperior,** where the curvature of the spine is upwards ('back up'), and the cord or small parts are the presenting part (Fig. 35.7b)

Key Point

If a transverse lie is diagnosed in the antenatal period (after 37 weeks) or in early labour before the membranes have ruptured, external cephalic version may be attempted.

Management of Labour

When the diagnosis is made in the late third trimester, women should be informed that a cesarean delivery may be required if the fetus continues in the transverse lie. They should be advised to report to the hospital as soon as there are any signs of labour or membrane rupture, as hand prolapse or cord prolapse may occur as labour advances.

Before the onset of labour

If the woman presents before the onset of labour, external cephalic version (ECV) may be attempted after 37 weeks [15]. See the section on ECV in **Chapter 27**, *Breech delivery*, for details of the technique.

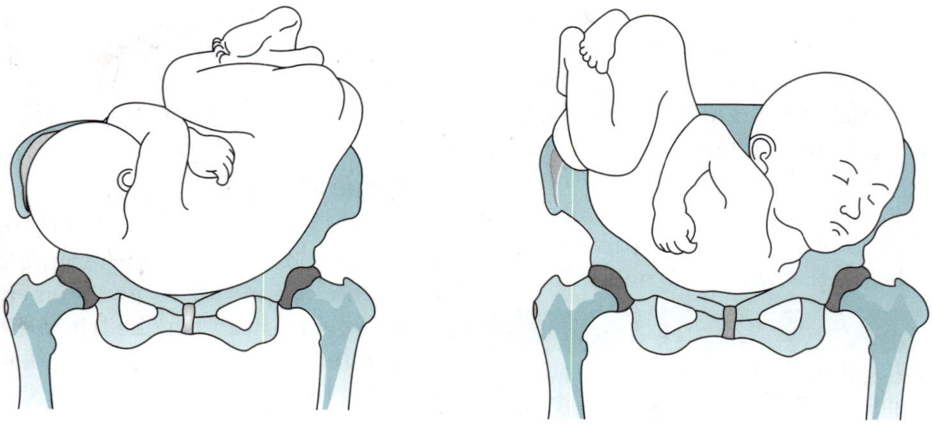

Fig. 35.7 (a) Dorsoinferior ('back down') left shoulder presentation and (b) dorsosuperior ('back up') presentation

In women in whom ECV is successful, but the fetus reverts to transverse lie, it may be appropriate to perform an ECV at 38–39 weeks followed by elective induction when the fetus is still cephalic. In women who decline ECV, an elective cesarean delivery at 39 weeks is discussed.

In early labour

In women who present in early labour with intact membranes, ECV can be attempted after counselling. If ECV is successful, spontaneous progression of labour can be allowed. However, if ECV is not successful or if the woman declines ECV, a cesarean section should be performed. ECV is not offered in the presence of ruptured membranes, even if the woman is in early labour.

In established labour

In women who present in established labour or with ruptured membranes after 34 weeks' gestation, delivery should be by prompt cesarean section. Under 34 weeks, if there is PPROM but no spontaneous contractions, one can wait for a course of antenatal steroids to be completed. However, the risk of cord prolapse is high, and therefore, the facility should be equipped and staffed for an emergency cesarean section at any time.

Management at Cesarean Section

There can be challenges in the delivery of a transverse lie by cesarean section.

During cesarean section, after the abdomen is opened and before an incision is made on the uterus, an attempt may be made to convert the lie to a longitudinal one so that extraction of the fetus is easier. This is particularly valuable in a **dorsoinferior position** as it is much harder to grasp the feet when the back is down. Although cephalic or podalic version can be performed, breech extraction is technically easier in the setting of a floating fetal vertex presentation, and hence, a podalic version is preferred.

When the fetus is in a **dorsosuperior position**, the operating surgeon grasps the fetal feet and performs a **footling breech extraction.** One must keep in mind that there is a possibility of extension of the incision into the broad ligament when trying to deliver the fetus. It may be necessary to perform a J or T extension of the curvilinear hysterotomy incision. In very preterm fetuses, where the lower segment is not formed, a low vertical incision may be necessary.

Neglected Transverse Lie

This may occur due to a failure to diagnose a transverse lie. The cervix may dilate slowly to begin with. Membranes tend to rupture early due to an ill-fitting presenting part. As the contractions get stronger, the fetal shoulder enters the pelvis and gets impacted.

A neglected transverse lie is an obstetric emergency, and delivery should be by cesarean section. If this is not immediately done, uterine rupture may ensue. If uterine inertia occurs, and the woman is left unattended, sepsis may ensue, and there is a high risk of fetal and maternal mortality [16].

Key Point

Women who present in established labour with a transverse lie should be delivered by cesarean section. A neglected transverse lie is an obstetric emergency, and a cesarean should be performed without delay to prevent uterine rupture.

Second Twin

After the delivery of the first twin, if the second twin is in a transverse lie, an internal podalic version can be performed, and the fetus can be delivered by breech extraction. If this is not successful, a cesarean section should be performed for the delivery of the second twin (see **Chapter 17,** *Management of labour with multiple pregnancy*).

Labour Before Viability

In this situation, the small fetus may fold on itself and deliver vaginally.

OBLIQUE LIE

When the long axis of the fetus is at an angle to the long axis of the uterus, the lie is said to be oblique. This is usually transient and will often convert to a longitudinal or transverse lie early in labour and can be managed as such. Women who are diagnosed to have an oblique lie close to term should be counselled to report to the hospital as soon as any signs of labour begin because the risk of early membrane rupture and cord prolapse is high. In the event of persistent oblique lie in established labour, a cesarean section may be required.

CONCLUSION

Malpresentations and malpositions complicate a small proportion of labour. Identification is the key to appropriate management. In presentations in which labour cannot progress such as transverse lie, brow, and mentoposterior face presentation, cesarean section is offered early. In the occipitoposterior and mentoanterior positions, skilled management of labour can result in a safe vaginal delivery.

REFERENCES

1. Posner GD. Fetopelvic Relationships. In Posner GD, Dy J, Black A, Jones GD. *Oxorn-Foote Human Labor and Birth*. 6th Ed. 2013. New York. Mc-Graw Hill Publishers, New York.
2. Hjartardottir H, Lund SH, Benediktsdottir S, Geirsson RT, Eggebo M. When does fetal head rotation occur in spontaneous labor at term: Results of an ultrasound-based longitudinal study in nulliparous women. *Am J Obstet Gynecol.* 2021. 224(5):514.e1-e9.
3. Sizer AR, Nirmal DM. Occipitoposterior position: Associated factors and obstetric outcome in nulliparas. *Obstet Gynecol.* 2000. 96(5 Pt 1):749-52.
4. Malvasi A, Tinelli A, Barbera A, Eggebø TM, Mynbaev OA, Bochicchio M, Pacella E, Di Renzo GC. Occiput posterior position diagnosis: Vaginal examination or intrapartum sonography? A clinical review. *J Matern Fetal Neonatal Med.* 2014. 27(5):520-6. doi: 10.3109/14767058.2013.825598. Epub 2013 Sep 13. PMID: 23865738.
5. Dy J and El-Chaar D. Abnormal Cephalic Presentations. In Posner GD, Dy J, Black A, Jones GD. *Oxorn-Foote Human Labor and Birth.* 6th Ed. 2013. Mc-Graw Hill Publishers, New York.
6. Bertholdt C, Morel O, Zuily S, Ambroise-Grandjean G. Manual rotation of occiput posterior or transverse positions: A systematic review and meta-analysis of randomized controlled trials. *Am J Obstet Gynecol.* 2022. 226(6):781-793
7. RCOG Green-Top Guideline No 26. Assisted Vaginal Birth. 2020

8. Gardberg M, Leonova Y, Laakkonen E. Malpresentations--impact on mode of delivery. *Acta Obstet Gynecol Scand.* 2011. 90(5):540-2.
9. Bellussi F, Ghi T, Youssef A, Salsi G, Giorgetta F, Parma D et al. The use of intrapartum ultrasound to diagnose malpositions and cephalic malpresentations. *Am J Obstet Gynecol.* 2017. 217(6):633-641.
10. Lau WL, Leung WC, Chin R. Intrapartum translabial ultrasound demonstrating brow presentation during the second stage of labor. *Int J Gynaecol Obstet.* 2009. 107(1):62-3. doi: 10.1016/j.ijgo.2009.05.024. Epub 2009 Jul 3. PMID: 19577235.
11. Duff P. Diagnosis and management of face presentation. *Obstet Gynecol.* 1981. 57:105.
12. Cruikshank DP, Cruikshank JE. Face and brow presentation: A review. *Clin Obstet Gynecol.* 1981. 24:333.
13. Benedetti TJ, Lowensohn RI, Truscott AM. Face presentation at term. *Obstet Gynecol.* 1980. 55(2):199-202. PMID: 7352081.
14. Gemer O, Segal S. Incidence and contribution of predisposing factors to transverse lie presentation. *Int J Gynaecol Obstet.* 1994. 44:219.
15. Strauss RA, Herrera, CA. Transverse fetal lie. Berghella V (Ed). *UpToDate.* 2023. Waltham, MA.
16. Tauragi G. Transverse Lie. In Posner GD, Dy J, Black A, Jones GD. *Oxorn-Foote Human Labor and Birth.* 6th Ed. 2013. Mc-Graw Hill Publishers, New York.

CHAPTER 36

Management of Labour in Women With Fibroids

GITA ARJUN

INTRODUCTION

Myomas (fibroids) are the most common benign smooth muscle tumours of the uterus. Though their prevalence is hard to evaluate because of the paucity of longitudinal studies, it has been estimated that they occur in over 70% of women by the onset of menopause [1]. Fibroids affect approximately 35–77% of reproductive-age women [2]. Moreover, 25% of women of reproductive age have clinically apparent fibroids [3].

Uterine fibroids are less frequently seen in pregnant women as compared to the general population. The reported incidence of fibroids in pregnancy ranges from 0.1 to 10.7% of all pregnancies [4]. Fibroids during pregnancy are more likely to be encountered in women who are 35 years of age and older and in nulliparas [5]. Ultrasound plays a major role in the detection of fibroids in pregnancy.

Pregnant women as well as their healthcare providers have concerns about the potential effects of fibroids on pregnancy and the possible effects of pregnancy on fibroids. Obstetricians and midwives should be aware of the behaviour of fibroids in pregnancies, the associated complications, and the management of these complications in pregnancy.

It is a reassuring fact that the majority of women with uterine fibroids will have normal pregnancy outcomes [6,7].

Key Point

The majority of women with uterine fibroids will have normal pregnancy outcomes.

BEHAVIOUR OF FIBROIDS IN PREGNANCY

A common misconception is that fibroids always increase in size during pregnancy. However, several studies using ultrasonographic monitoring of fibroids during pregnancy have shown that this is not true [8,9]. Data from these studies suggest that fibroid size remains stable (<10% change) through pregnancy in 50–60% of cases, increases in 22–32%, and decreases in 8–27% (Table 36.1). Very few fibroids will increase more than 25% in volume.

A recent prospective cohort study [10] concluded that the total fibroid volume **declined on average** through the course of pregnancy. If fibroids in pregnancy are stratified by size at first detection in pregnancy (<1 cm [small], 1 to <3 cm [medium], or ≥3 cm [large] in diameter), it is easier to prognosticate whether they will grow or not. The volume of fibroids was found to increase by 2% per week in small fibroids and decrease by 0.5 and 2.2% in medium and large fibroids [10]. Larger fibroids (>5 cm in diameter) have a greater chance of growing than smaller ones [11].

Table 36.1 Change in size in fibroids during pregnancy as noted with ultrasound follow-up [8,9]

Change in fibroid size during pregnancy	Percentage of fibroids (%)
Stable, with <10% change	50–60
Increases	22–32
Decreases	8–27

Postpartum Regression

The majority (90%) of fibroids detected in the first trimester will undergo regression within 3–6 months after delivery. 10% may show an increase in size. Postpartum regression may be reduced in women who use progestin-only contraception.

> **Key Point**
>
> Fibroids that do grow tend to grow most in the first trimester, with very little further growth in the second and third trimesters [12].

POTENTIAL EFFECTS OF FIBROIDS ON PREGNANCY

Uterine fibroids, by themselves, do not adversely affect pregnancy in the majority of women [6]. In those affected, pain is the most common problem.

A causative relationship between fibroids and early pregnancy loss is questionable. The risk may be increased in the presence of multiple submucous fibroids and possibly, with large intramural fibroids, but this risk is not associated with subserosal or pedunculated fibroids [4,6].

There may be slightly increased risks of placenta previa, placental abruption, and abnormal fetal position, chiefly due to the mechanical impact of multiple and/or large fibroids. Cesarean section and preterm birth rates are also probably increased in the presence of fibroids.

> **Key Point**
>
> Uterine fibroids by themselves do not adversely affect pregnancy in the majority of women.

Pain

The most commonly reported complaint associated with uterine fibroids during pregnancy is pain, which occurs most often in women with large fibroids (>7–10 cm). Pain from fibroids in pregnancy can be due to an increase in size, red degeneration or rarely, torsion of a pedunculated fibroid.

Increase in size

The **rapid growth** of a fibroid causes ischemia with resultant pain [4]. In such cases women are usually admitted with pain in the **late first** or **early second trimester**, which corresponds to the time at which fibroids are most likely to grow rapidly.

Red degeneration

Acute pain during pregnancy can arise because of **red degeneration**. This type of degeneration is found usually, but not exclusively, during pregnancy and is associated with pain, fever, and leucocytosis [13]. Degenerating fibroids may have a complex appearance on ultrasound, with areas of cystic change [14].

Three theories have been proposed to explain the severe pain associated with red degeneration:

- Rapid fibroid growth results in the tissue outgrowing its blood supply, leading to tissue anoxia, necrosis, and infarction.
- Even in the absence of fibroid growth, the growing uterus results in a change in the architecture (kinking) of the blood supply to the fibroid, leading to ischemia and necrosis.
- The pain results from the release of prostaglandins from cellular damage within the fibroid [15]. This is supported by the observation that ibuprofen and other prostaglandin synthetase inhibitors effectively and rapidly control pain associated with red degeneration.

Torsion

Rarely, pain arises because of the **torsion** of a subserous pedunculated fibroid.

Pain management

Pain due to fibroids during pregnancy is usually managed conservatively with bed rest, hydration, and simple analgesics like paracetamol. If there is no improvement, ibuprofen (400 mg 6–8 hourly) usually provides good relief. When NSAIDs are used for more than 48 hours, it may be prudent to monitor for oligohydramnios by ultrasound imaging.

Severe pain may necessitate inpatient admission, additional pain medication (narcotic analgesia), or in rare instances, epidural analgesia. In cases of intractable pain due to the torsion of a subserous pedunculated fibroid, a **myomectomy** can be performed.

Spontaneous Miscarriage

In an analysis of more than 20,000 pregnant women [16], it was found that the presence of fibroids was **not associated** with an increased risk of spontaneous miscarriage. This is an important finding and is reassuring for pregnant women with fibroids as well as their obstetricians/midwives. However, evidence suggests that multiple fibroids may increase the miscarriage rate as compared to a single fibroid [17].

Location of fibroid and its effect on miscarriage risk

Subserosal and pedunculated fibroids clearly have no effect on the risk for miscarriage. The effect of **intramural fibroids** is debated, but early miscarriage may be more common in women with large fibroids located in the uterine corpus than in the lower uterine segment [18].

Submucosal fibroids may interfere with placentation and the development of normal uteroplacental circulation [4]. Large submucosal fibroids that distort the cavity may cause infertility, but if implantation does occur, the risk of early miscarriage is higher.

> **Key Point**
>
> Early pregnancy loss is more common in women with large submucosal fibroids that distort the cavity.

Bleeding in Early Pregnancy

The location of the fibroid determines the risk of bleeding. Bleeding in early pregnancy is significantly more common (60%) if the placenta implants close to the fibroid as compared to pregnancies in which there is no contact between the placenta and fibroid (9%) [19].

Placental Abruption

Though there are conflicting reports, the risk of placental abruption is increased three-fold in women with fibroids [20]. The highest risk of abruption is with retroplacental fibroids, submucosal fibroids, and fibroids measuring >7–8 cm in diameter [4].

> **Key Point**
>
> Retroplacental fibroids, submucosal fibroids, and fibroids >7–8 cm diameter are independent risk factors for placental abruption [4].

Placenta Previa

Most studies have not shown any association between fibroids and placenta previa, though there may be a slight increase in risk in the presence of large and/or multiple fibroids [6].

Malpresentation

The risk of breech presentation is slightly increased in pregnancies with fibroids. The risk of malpresentation increases with a large submucosal fibroid, multiple fibroids, a fibroid located behind the placenta or in the lower uterine segment, or a large fibroid (>10 cm in diameter) [4].

Preterm Labour

Fibroids may increase the risk of preterm labour [20] if they are large, if there are multiple fibroids, or if placentation occurs next to or overlying a fibroid. The presence of fibroids alone is not an indication to use ultrasound to monitor cervical length for shortening during pregnancy. Fibroids **do not** appear to be a risk factor for preterm premature rupture of membranes (PPROM).

Fetal Growth Restriction

Fibroids have **not** been shown to have any effect on fetal growth [20,4].

Fetal Demise

Rates of fetal demise are **not** increased in pregnancies complicated by uterine fibroids. The couple should be reassured about this [21].

MANAGEMENT OF LABOUR IN A PREGNANCY WITH FIBROIDS

Vaginal Delivery

Most women with fibroids will have a successful vaginal delivery [21]. A trial of labour should be offered unless there is a clear obstetric indication for a cesarean delivery, e.g., failure to progress, breech or transverse presentation.

When women with large fibroids enter labour with a cephalic presentation, their likelihood of having a successful vaginal delivery remains high [22].

> **Key Point**
>
> Most women with fibroids will have a successful vaginal delivery. Even large fibroids (>5 cm) need not be regarded as a contraindication to a trial of labour [21].

Dysfunctional labour

It has been proposed that the presence of fibroids in the myometrium may decrease the force of uterine contractions or disrupt the coordinated spread of the contractile wave, thereby leading to dysfunctional labour and cesarean birth. However, studies have been conflicting in their conclusions and it is not certain whether the presence of fibroids leads to dysfunctional labour [4]. Even women with leiomyomata 10 cm or larger could have a 70% chance of achieving a vaginal delivery [5].

Cesarean Delivery

Cesarean section should be reserved for women with obstetric indications. However, several studies have reported that uterine fibroids are associated with an increased risk of cesarean birth [5,21,23,24]. The risk increases when the fibroids are located in the lower uterine segment. Multiple factors may contribute to this increased rate, such as a higher risk of malpresentation (especially breech presentation), obstruction of the birth canal by a large fibroid, and placental abruption.

Elective cesarean delivery may be indicated in women with a large fibroid (cervical or lower uterine segment) located between the fetal head and the cervix close to term, which may potentially obstruct the descent of the fetal head.

Technical issues at cesarean section

- **Location of fibroids:** In the third trimester, a good quality ultrasound is essential to map the location of the fibroids. This is particularly important in the case of large fibroids and helps in the planning of the cesarean, be it elective or an emergency.
- **Skin incision:** A vertical skin incision may sometimes be required if a large fibroid is occupying the lower uterine segment.
- **Hysterotomy**: To avoid large fibroids located in the lower uterine segment, the hysterotomy may have to be placed either in the upper segment (classical incision), or in rare cases, on the posterior uterine surface.

Women who have had a prior myomectomy

Elective cesarean may also be indicated in women who have undergone **an extensive or complicated myomectomy** due to an increased risk of **uterine rupture**, similar to women who have had a previous classical cesarean incision. These women are best delivered at 36+0 to 37+0 weeks of gestation since pregnancies with fibroids may be at risk of preterm labour [20].

A systematic review [25] concluded that the overall risk of uterine rupture during birth after a prior myomectomy was <1%. A trial of labour in a woman with a prior myomectomy was associated with <0.5% risk of uterine rupture. It is important to note that in this review, six of the seven ruptures occurred in women who had a prior **laparoscopic myomectomy.** This may probably be due to the technical difficulties of achieving good apposition of the edges with laparoscopic suturing [26]. The rate of rupture following abdominal myomectomy is extremely low [27].

Prior hysteroscopic removal of a submucosal fibroid may increase the risk of abnormal placentation, especially **placenta accreta**, though the risk is low. In such a case, it is recommended that ultrasound evaluation for possible placenta accreta be performed in the late second or early third trimester [4].

Trial of labour with a prior myomectomy

Women who have had an intramyometrial myomectomy can be offered a trial of labour if the following criteria are met:

- Documentation is available about the myomectomy that could have significantly compromised the myometrium—deep or shallow incision, large or small fibroid, location, any postoperative complications
- Availability of continuous intrapartum fetal monitoring
- The ability to perform an emergency cesarean delivery within 30 minutes, if it becomes necessary; this includes the immediate availability of anesthetic services and access to a blood bank

Myomectomy at cesarean section

A systematic review and meta-analysis [28] found that women undergoing myomectomy during a cesarean section had a greater reduction in hemoglobin levels and a higher risk of blood transfusion as compared to women who did not.

Myomectomy at the time of cesarean delivery should only be performed in the following circumstances:

- If the fibroid is along the site of the uterine incision or makes it difficult to access the incision
- To facilitate the safe delivery of the fetus
- To facilitate closure of the hysterotomy

In a series of 60 cases of fibroids in pregnancy [29], it was found that **pedunculated subserosal fibroids** could be safely removed at the time of cesarean delivery. However, the removal of non-pedunculated fibroids resulted in severe hemorrhage, leading to the risk of hysterectomy.

POSTPARTUM COMPLICATIONS

Pregnant women with uterine fibroids are at an increased risk of postpartum hemorrhage (PPH) [30]. This is most likely caused by decreased uterine contractility in women with fibroids. The rates of PPH are significantly higher with increasing size of the uterine fibroid and its location, with large intramural fibroids having the highest risk of PPH.

CONCLUSION

The majority of women with uterine fibroids in pregnancy have uncomplicated pregnancies with good outcomes. The size and location of the fibroid determine the risks in pregnancy. Large fibroids, especially in the lower segment, can increase the chances of malpresentation, preterm births, and dysfunctional labour. Most women can achieve a vaginal delivery despite fibroids. However, based on size and location, delivery may be complicated. Therefore, these cases require diligent management.

REFERENCES

1. Flake GP, Andersen J, Dixon D. Etiology and pathogenesis of uterine leiomyomas: A review. *Environ Health Perspect*. 2003. 111.1037–54.
2. Cramer SF, Patel A. The frequency of uterine leiomyomas. *Am J Clin Pathol* 1990. 94:435–8.
3. Stewart EA, Cookson CL, Gandolfo RA, Schulze-Rath R. Epidemiology of uterine fibroids: A systematic review. *BJOG*. 2017. 124: 1501– 1512.
4. Ouyang DW, Norwitz ER. Pregnancy in women with uterine leiomyomas (fibroids). Lockwood CJ (Ed). *UpToDate*. 2023. Waltham, MA.
5. Qidwai G, Caughey A, Jacoby A. Obstetric outcomes in women with sonographically identified uterine leiomyomata. *Obstet Gynecol*. 2006. 107:376–82.
6. Segars JH, Parrott EC, Nagel JD, et al. Proceedings from the Third National Institutes of Health International Congress on Advances in Uterine Leiomyoma Research: Comprehensive review, conference summary and future recommendations. *Hum Reprod Update*. 2014. 20:309.
7. Parker WH. Etiology, symptomatology, and diagnosis of uterine myomas. *Fertil Steril*. 2007. 87:725.
8. Neiger R, Sonek JD, Croom CS, Ventolini G. Pregnancy-related changes in the size of uterine leiomyomas. *J Reprod Med*. 2006. 51:671.
9. Rosati P, Exacoustòs C, Mancuso S. Longitudinal evaluation of uterine myoma growth during pregnancy. A sonographic study. *J Ultrasound Med*. 1992. 11:511.
10. Mitro SD, Peddada S, Chen Z, et al. Natural history of fibroids in pregnancy: National Institute of Child Health and Human Development Fetal Growth Studies—Singletons cohort. *Fertil Steril*. 2022. 118:656.
11. Strobelt N, Ghidini A, Cavallone M, et al. Natural history of uterine leiomyomas in pregnancy. *J Ultrasound Med*. 1994. 13:399.
12. Ciavattini A, Delli Carpini G, Clemente N, et al. Growth trend of small uterine fibroids and human chorionic gonadotropin serum levels in early pregnancy: An observational study. *Fertil Steril*. 2016. 105:1255.
13. Parker WH. Etiology, symptomatology, and diagnosis of uterine myomas. *Fertil Steril*. 2007. 87:725.
14. Wilde S, Scott-Barrett S. Radiological appearances of uterine fibroids. *Indian J Radiol Imaging*. 2009. 19(3): 222–231.
15. De Carolis S, Fatigante G, Ferrazzani S, et al. Uterine myomectomy in pregnant women. *Fetal Diagn Ther*. 2001.16:116.
16. Sundermann AC, Velez Edwards DR, Bray MJ, et al. Leiomyomas in pregnancy and spontaneous abortion: A systematic review and meta-analysis. *Obstet Gynecol*. 2017. 130:1065.
17. Benson CB, Chow JS, Chang-Lee W, et al. Outcome of pregnancies in women with uterine leiomyomas identified by sonography in the first trimester. *J Clin Ultrasound*. 2001. 29:261–264.
18. Lee HJ, Norwitz ER, Shaw J. Contemporary management of fibroids in pregnancy. *Rev Obstet Gynecol*. 2010. 3(1):20–27.
19. Winer-Muram HT, Muram D, Gillieson MS. Uterine myomas in pregnancy. *J Can Assoc Radiol*.1984. 35:168–170.
20. Klatsky PC, Tran ND, Caughey AB, et al. Fibroids and reproductive outcomes: A systematic literature review from conception to delivery. *Am J Obstet Gynecol*. 2008. 198:357–366.
21. Coronado GD, Marshall LM, Schwartz SM. Complications in pregnancy, labor, and delivery with uterine leiomyomas: A population-based study. *Obstet Gynecol*. 2000. 95(5):764.
22. Vergani P, Locatelli A, Ghidini A, et al. Large uterine leiomyomata and risk of cesarean delivery. *Obstet Gynecol*. 2007. 109:410-4
23. Zhao R, Wang X, Zou L, et al. Adverse obstetric outcomes in pregnant women with uterine fibroids in China: A multicenter survey involving 112,403 deliveries. *PLoS One*. 2017. 12:e0187821.
24. Choudhary A, Inamdar SA, Sharma U. Pregnancy with uterine fibroids: Obstetric outcome at a tertiary care hospital of central India. *Cureus*. 2023. 15(2):e35513.
25. Gambacorti-Passerini Z, Gimovsky AC, Locatelli A, Berghella V. Trial of labor after myomectomy and uterine rupture: A systematic review. *Acta Obstet Gynecol Scand*. 2016. 95(7):724-34. Epub 2016 May 25.
26. Nezhat C. The 'cons' of laparoscopic myomectomy in women who may reproduce in the future. *Int J Fertil Menopausal Stud*. 1996. 41:280.
27. Miller CE. Myomectomy. Comparison of open and laparoscopic techniques. *Obstet Gynecol Clin North Am*. 2000. 27:407-420.
28. Pergialiotis V, Sinanidis I, Louloudis IE, et al. Perioperative complications of cesarean delivery myomectomy: A meta-analysis. *Obstet Gynecol*. 2017. 130:1295.
29. Hasan F, Arumugam K, Sivanesaratnam V. Uterine leiomyomata in pregnancy. *Int J Gynaecol Obstet*. 1991. 34:45–48.
30. Zhao R, Wang X, Zou L, et al. Adverse obstetric outcomes in pregnant women with uterine fibroids in China: A multi-center survey involving 112,403 deliveries. *PLoS One*. 2017. 12:e0187821.

CHAPTER 37

The Hypertensive Woman in Labour

NUZHAT AZIZ, SAILAJA DEVI KALLUR

INTRODUCTION

Hypertensive disorders in pregnancy are a major cause of maternal morbidity and mortality [1]. Hypertension (HTN) can be present before pregnancy (**chronic hypertension**) or may develop during pregnancy (**gestational hypertension**) [2,3].

Pregnancy-induced hypertension is present in 6–8% of all pregnant women and is responsible for a major proportion of maternal deaths and a large proportion of the maternal morbidity that women suffer during pregnancy. Long-term cardiovascular effects in later life add to the concerns about the management of this disorder [2].

Labour is a challenging time for any woman; hypertensive disorders add to these challenges as they are associated with the possibility of adverse outcomes for both mother and baby. Labour management of a hypertensive woman includes not only maternal and fetal monitoring and pain relief, but also the control of hypertension and the prevention of complications related to both labour and hypertension.

The aim of clinical management is to minimise morbidity associated with hypertension. Early identification, early transfer to a tertiary centre, appropriate interventions, and timed delivery will contribute to better outcomes for both the mother and the baby.

This chapter is limited to the evaluation, monitoring, and management of a woman with hypertension admitted for labour and delivery.

CLASSIFICATION OF HYPERTENSIVE DISORDERS IN PREGNANCY

Hypertensive disorders are classified into chronic hypertension, chronic hypertension with superimposed preeclampsia, gestational hypertension, preeclampsia with or without severe features, and eclampsia (Table 37.1).

Severe hypertension is regarded as systolic blood pressure (BP) of >160 mmHg or diastolic blood pressure of >110 mmHg [1].

Preeclampsia may rapidly become a major threat to the mother and fetus. Classifying it into mild or severe may mislead a less experienced obstetrician. The ACOG has eliminated the diagnosis of severe preeclampsia and instead, classified it as preeclampsia with or without severe features [4].

Preeclampsia with severe features includes the following:

- BP of ≥160/110 mmHg
- Symptoms of cerebral irritation (headache, blurring of vision, vomiting, blindness, convulsions)
- Renal or liver dysfunction, or thrombocytopenia, or hemolysis, or a combination of organ dysfunction
- HELLP (hemolysis, elevated liver enzymes, low platelets syndrome), or multi-organ dysfunction

Eclampsia is diagnosed when convulsions develop in a woman with a hypertensive disorder [1,2,3].

In addition to these, the International Society for the Study of Hypertension in Pregnancy (ISSHP) includes 'white coat hypertension' and

Table 37.1 Classification of hypertensive disorders in pregnancy—adapted from The International Society for the Study of Hypertension in Pregnancy (ISSHP) [3]

Category	Diagnosis and clinical characteristics	Outcomes
Chronic HTN	Hypertension predating pregnancy or diagnosed before 20 weeks of pregnancy	Associated with adverse maternal and fetal outcomes
White coat HTN	Elevated BP (≥140/90 mmHg) in the presence of a physician or nurse, but normal BP measured at home or work (<135/85 mmHg)	• Has higher adverse outcomes and is not a benign condition • Associated with an increased risk of preeclampsia
Masked HTN	• More difficult to diagnose • BP is normal at clinic and office but increased at other times • Diagnosis is made based on ambulatory BP recording for 24 hours or automated BP recording at home	Associated with higher rates of preeclampsia with severe features on admission for delivery [5]
Gestational HTN	Hypertension arising de novo after 20 weeks' gestation without proteinuria, or biochemical or hematological abnormalities	• Outcomes good in the majority • 25% of women with gestational HTN will progress to preeclampsia and may have poorer outcomes
Preeclampsia	Diagnostic criteria are the presence of de novo hypertension after 20 weeks' pregnancy accompanied by proteinuria and/or evidence of maternal acute kidney injury, neurological features, liver dysfunction, thrombocytopenia, hemolysis, or fetal growth restriction	Preeclampsia can deteriorate rapidly and without warning and result in maternal and fetal morbidity and mortality
HELLP syndrome	Hemolysis, elevated liver enzymes, low platelets syndrome is a severe manifestation of preeclampsia	Associated with maternal and fetal morbidity and mortality
Eclampsia	Defined as HTN with new-onset tonic–clonic, focal, or multifocal seizures in the absence of other causative conditions	Associated with maternal mortality, especially in low-resource settings

BP, blood pressure; *HTN*, hypertension; *HELLP*, hemolysis, elevated liver enzymes, low platelet count

'masked hypertension', both of which are associated with adverse outcomes [3,5].

STRUCTURED ASSESSMENT AT ADMISSION

The management of a hypertensive woman in labour begins with detailed history taking, gathering of relevant information, current diagnosis and concerns, diagnostic evaluation, and the assessment of the maternal and fetal condition.

Key Points

- Preeclampsia is a multisystem disorder with varying severity and rates of disease progression.
- Classification into different hypertensive disorders of pregnancy and evaluation of organ function helps to prognosticate, call for a multidisciplinary team, determine the need for transfer to the labour ward, high dependency unit (HDU), or intensive care unit (ICU), the frequency of lab testing and the need for early delivery.

Risk Assessment at Admission for Delivery

Systematic documentation of the woman's history, antenatal care, investigations, and evaluation of both the woman and the fetus along with a summary of pregnancy complications and concerns helps in performing a rapid review without missing out on important information. The risk assessment summary can be documented in the form of a dashboard with clear communication in times of emergency. An example is presented in Table 37.2.

> **Key Point**
>
> Review and documentation of the woman's clinical information helps in optimising care. Good communication prevents errors and improves outcomes.

Clinical Assessment at Admission

Clinical examination

A detailed clinical examination must be performed at admission to the labour ward. The process must include an introduction of the care provider's team, review of symptoms, recording of vital signs, clinical examination of all organ systems, obstetric examination and documentation and summarisation of findings.

A uniform documentation format for a hypertensive woman at the time of admission to the labour room along with appropriate prompts for admission orders can prevent errors. Fig. 37.1 is an example of such a checklist.

The **seven symptoms** that must be asked for pertaining to hypertensive disorders are headache, nausea, vomiting, blurring of vision (cerebral irritation, raised intracranial tension), epigastric pain (liver involvement), decreased urine output (impaired renal function), and perception of fetal movements.

The **seven signs** that must be documented are level of alertness, all the vital signs, neurological assessment (focal deficit may be a sign of intracranial bleed), lung crepitations (by auscultation), jugular venous pressure (JVP), deep tendon reflexes, and obstetric examination for fetal well-being and to rule out abruption. Table 37.3 lists the symptoms and signs that should be documented.

Review of investigations

The investigations chart must include baseline antenatal investigations and those pertaining to the medical disorder. Many complications of preeclampsia are diagnosed by laboratory testing and trends of change reflect worsening organ function. The rationale and range of laboratory investigations recommended in a hypertensive woman are enumerated in Table 37.4.

Table 37.2 Example of risk assessment at admission to the labour room in the form of a dashboard

Name	Obstetric formula	Gestation	Antenatal risk factors	SGA risk factors
Mrs S	Primigravida	37 w 1 d	• BMI >30 Kg/m^2 • Hypothyroid	• Low PAPP-A • 0.28 MoM
VTE risk factors	**PPH risk factors**	**Other concerns**		
BMI >30 Kg/m^2	None	• SGA—7th percentile, normal Dopplers • Preeclampsia—severe features; severe HTN • Urine protein 3+ • Induction of labour with PGE2 gel		

BMI, body mass index; *HTN*, hypertension; *MoM*, multiples of median; *PAPP-A*, pregnancy-associated plasma protein-A; *SGA*, small-for-gestational age; *VTE*, venous thromboembolism

Admission Checklist
HYPERTENSIVE WOMAN IN LABOUR

Name Mrs S
ID No AAA123
Date 6.4.2023
Time of Admission 1:20 am

Complaints:

Obstetric Formula: Primigravida
Gestation 37 weeks

Diagnosis

Category	Tick	Mention diagnostic criteria
Chronic HTN		
Gestational HTN		
Preeclampsia without severe features		
Preeclampsia with severe features	✓	BP 170/110
Eclampsia		
Chronic HTN superimposed preeclampsia		

Proteinuria		Important Symptoms			
- Dipstick urine protein	3+	Headache	-	Epigastric pain	-
- Urine spot protein creatinine ratio		Nausea/vomiting	-	Decreased fetal movements	-
- Urine 24 hours protein		Blurred vision	-	Decreased urine output	-

Clinical Examination

Vital Signs	Findings	System examination	Findings
Alertness	Alert	Neurological system	Normal
Heart rate	88/min	Respiratory system	Normal
Resp rate	20/min	CVS	Normal
Blood pressure	146/100 mmHg	Hepatic	Normal
MAP	115	Hematological	Normal
SpO_2	99%	Deep tendon reflexes	Normal
Temperature	98.4 F	Edema	2+

Obstetric exam	Findings	Vaginal exam	Findings
Uterus SFH	34 cm	Cx length	1 cm
Contractions	2/10 min	Effacement	50%
Multifetal	No	Consistency	Soft
Lie	Longitudinal	Position	Central
Presenting part	Cephalic	Station	-2
FHR	156/min	Membranes	Present
Other findings	Head palpable 2/5	Other findings	

Medications

Drug Name	Dose	Last Dose
IV Labetalol		
Oral Labetalol	200 mg 8th hourly	11 pm
Cap Nifedipine		
Tab SR Nifedipine	10 mg 8th hourly	9 pm
Magnesium sulphate		
antenatal steroids		

Lab Tests Checklist

Test	Findings
Blood Group/Rh	B+ve
HIV	Non-reactive
HBsAg	Non-reactive
Hemoglobin	10.2
WBC	10,200
Platelets	94,000
MCV	83
Urine - protein	3+
Urine - pus cells	2-3
Urine - sugar	Nil
TSH	2.8
S Creatinine	1.0
S Bilirubin	0.8
S LDH	450
SGPT	56
OGTT	76/150/98
Urine culture	Sterile
S Electrolytes - Na	
S Electrolytes - K	
S Electrolytes - Cl	
ABG-pH	
ABG-base deficit	

Doctor ____________________ Signature ____________________

Fig. 37.1 Admission checklist for a hypertensive woman in labour

Table 37.3 The seven symptoms and signs that should be looked for and documented at admission to the labour room

Symptoms	Signs
Headache	Level of alertness
Nausea	Vital signs
Vomiting	Neurological assessment (focal deficit may be a sign of intracranial bleed)
Blurring of vision (cerebral irritation, raised intracranial tension)	Lung crepitations (by auscultation)
Epigastric pain (liver involvement)	Jugular venous pressure (JVP)
Decreased urine output (impaired renal function)	Presence or absence of deep tendon reflexes
Perception of fetal movements	Obstetric examination for fetal well-being and to rule out abruption

Table 37.4 Laboratory investigations in a hypertensive woman and their clinical relevance [4]

Test	Rationale	Clinical significance
Urine protein	Diagnosis of proteinuria	Urine protein dipstick 1+ or more suggests proteinuria
Spot urine protein: creatinine ratio	Diagnosis of proteinuria	Ratio >0.3 suggests significant proteinuria
24-hour urine protein estimation	Diagnosis of proteinuria	Significant proteinuria is >300 mg in 24 hours
Hemogram	Diagnosis of thrombocytopenia, fragmented RBCs for evidence of hemolysis	• Platelets <100,000/mm^3 indicates thrombocytopenia, can be a part of HELLP syndrome • Hemoglobin may be higher due to hemoconcentration • New-onset anemia may be due to hemolysis
Serum creatinine	Renal function	• Serum creatinine >1.2 mg/dL is diagnostic of renal dysfunction • Acute renal failure is defined as an increase in creatinine by 0.3 mg/dL above a baseline value, if available
Liver function tests	Liver function	• Elevated transaminases are a diagnostic criterion for HELLP syndrome • Any value >72 IU/L for transaminases (AST/ALT) is a concern (or three times the reference range) • Serum bilirubin >1.2 mg/dL also signifies hemolysis
Lactate dehydrogenase	Evidence of hemolysis	LDH >600 is the diagnostic cut-off for HELLP syndrome
Serum electrolytes	Abnormal electrolyte levels	• Hyponatremia is a common finding in preeclampsia • Hyperkalemia may be associated with renal dysfunction
Other tests as indicated	Serum amylase, lipase	May show evidence of pancreatic involvement as preeclampsia is a multi-organ disorder
	Arterial blood gases	Acid–base maintenance is affected by multi-organ dysfunction due to cardiorespiratory dysfunction

Identifying HELLP syndrome

The diagnosis of HELLP syndrome is important as it represents a rapidly progressive complication of preeclampsia disorders. It requires early recognition and diagnosis (Table 37.4) to prevent associated morbidity and mortality [4]. The Mississippi classification of HELLP syndrome [6] additionally uses the degree of thrombocytopenia and has three classes, of which class 1 is the most severe:

- **Class 1:** <50,000 platelets/microL
- **Class 2:** 50,000 to 100,000 platelets/microL
- **Class 3:** 100,000 to 150,000 platelets/microL

The identification and categorisation of HELLP syndrome allows prognostication and defines the need for organ monitoring and support.

MANAGEMENT OF LABOUR IN THE HYPERTENSIVE WOMAN

Delivery is the first line of treatment of preeclampsia. All other treatments are only to stabilise the maternal condition and to prolong pregnancy safely to gain fetal maturity.

The components of the management of labour remain the same. The primary aim is to have a healthy outcome for both mother and baby. The monitoring of the maternal condition, fetal condition, and progress of labour for a hypertensive woman in labour is focused on the early identification and prevention of the complications of preeclampsia.

The three major interventions that are added to the labour management of a hypertensive woman are as follows [1]:

- Control of hypertension
- Prophylaxis for prevention of seizures
- Monitoring for organ dysfunction in preeclampsia

Immediate Delivery vs. Expectant Management

The decision to deliver or manage expectantly depends on the gestational age at the time of diagnosis of preeclampsia with severe features. The World Health Organization recommends the following [7]:

- **Fetus not viable or unlikely to achieve viability within one or two weeks:** Immediate induction of labour is strongly recommended.
- **Viable fetus <34 weeks of gestation:** Expectant management is recommended, with close monitoring of the maternal and fetal condition. Uncontrolled maternal hypertension, increasing maternal organ dysfunction, or fetal distress should be absent.
- **Viable fetus between 34 and 36+6 days weeks of gestation:** Expectant management may be recommended with close monitoring. Uncontrolled maternal hypertension, increasing maternal organ dysfunction or fetal distress are indications for immediate delivery.
- **≥37 weeks of gestation:** Induction of labour is recommended for immediate delivery. A cesarean delivery is only performed for obstetric indications.

Timing of Delivery

Preterm delivery

Delivery may be planned at any gestation if there are life-threatening complications such as uncontrolled refractory hypertension, HELLP syndrome, acute renal failure, pulmonary edema, intracranial hemorrhage, eclampsia, abruption, or fetal death. Delivery may also be planned for fetal compromise and non-reassuring fetal status after fetal viability. Preeclampsia is a multi-organ multisystem disorder, and organ dysfunction is the main factor that influences the timing of delivery in preterm gestations. Pre-viable termination may be necessary when severe features of preeclampsia appear at <24 to 26 weeks of gestation [1,2,3].

Term delivery

Dilemmas for timing of delivery start when the disease remains mild and stable till term. The HYPITAT trial (hypertension and preeclampsia interventional trial at term) [8] compared the outcomes of planned induction for women with gestational hypertension or mild preeclampsia, at different weeks starting from 37 weeks. They found improved maternal outcomes in women beyond 37 weeks. The maternal and fetal outcomes were better **for induced delivery at 37–38 weeks' gestation** as there is a possibility of disease worsening with expectant management.

The HYPITAT trial also concluded that induction of labour did not increase the cesarean section rates or worsen perinatal outcomes [8].

Planning a birth before 37 weeks in cases of stable disease (gestational hypertension, chronic hypertension without superimposed preeclampsia, and preeclampsia without severe features) will increase neonatal morbidity [1,2,4,8,9]. Decisions should be based on a balance of maternal risks associated with continued pregnancy versus fetal risks of preterm birth [4].

Preeclampsia with severe features and chronic hypertension with superimposed preeclampsia are at the severe end of the disease spectrum and require delivery when there is a complication that threatens maternal or fetal life. Severe hypertension (blood pressure ≥160/110 mmHg) is the only one among all severe features of preeclampsia which can be controlled and stabilised to allow the progress of pregnancy for better fetal survival. Expectant management is suggested with a close watch for disease progression till 34 weeks' gestation. All the remaining severe features represent organ dysfunction and are indications to proceed with delivery [1,2,4,9].

Mode of Delivery

Vaginal birth: The recommendations for mode of delivery favour vaginal delivery over cesarean section. Cesarean delivery is performed for obstetric indications. Induction of labour and the time taken for delivery in induced labour do not increase maternal and neonatal morbidity and mortality when compared to immediate cesarean delivery.

Cesarean delivery: Immediate cesarean in preeclampsia with severe features does not seem to confer any benefits [10].

Cesarean section rates are higher in all hypertensive disorders compared to normotensive women [11]. The higher rates are related to the lower gestational ages, fetal growth restriction, severe disease, and organ dysfunction. A fetus with abnormal Doppler studies with absent end-diastolic flow or reversal of flow in the umbilical artery will not tolerate labour and will benefit from a planned cesarean birth [1,5] (see **Chapter 33**, *Management of labour with a growth-restricted fetus*, for further details).

> **Key Point**
>
> The decision for cesarean delivery should be individualised, based on the anticipated probability of vaginal birth, severity of preeclampsia, and rate of progression of disease in preterm gestations.

Second and third stages of labour

The management principles for the second and third stages of labour remain the same for a woman with a hypertensive disorder who is stable (see **Chapter 4**, *Management of the first and second stages of normal labour* and **Chapter 5**, *Management of the third stage of labour*).

Preeclampsia with severe features may require individualisation of care protocols. The recommendations for special situations are as follows:

- Women with pulmonary edema, eclampsia, or cerebral complications may require assisted vaginal birth to cut short the second stage of labour.
- Traumatic delivery should be avoided in the presence of HELLP syndrome and coagulopathy.
- Coagulopathy confirmed by laboratory investigations should be corrected before a surgical intervention. Blood products should be reserved, and a multidisciplinary team should be available for the management of catastrophic

bleeding (see **Chapter 13**, *Abnormalities in the third stage of labour: Postpartum hemorrhage and retained placenta*).

  — Cesarean section may require drains, and closure of the abdominal wall with mattress sutures.

- Oxytocin is the drug of choice for the active management of the third stage of labour. Methyl ergometrine is **contraindicated** as it may cause an acute rise of blood pressure and seizures in these women [1].

Pain Relief Options for Hypertensive Women in Labour

Labour analgesia is a crucial component of the management of labour in women with preeclampsia and its complications. Pain induces a stress response which results in the release of stress hormones like catecholamines, cortisol and adrenocorticotrophins. These hormones further increase the vasoconstriction, resulting in an acute elevation of blood pressure and a decrease in uteroplacental circulation.

The pain relief options remain the same with no contraindication for opioids, nitrous oxide, or epidural analgesia (see **Chapter 9**, *Labour analgesia*).

Epidural analgesia is contraindicated in the presence of thrombocytopenia or coagulopathy. A platelet count of ≥70,000 cells/microL is the cutoff for safe epidural placement or operative cesarean delivery. It is mandatory to get a platelet count before the procedure [12]. Preloading with intravenous fluids prior to epidural is **not recommended** in women with hypertensive disorders.

Fetal Monitoring in Labour

Hypertensive disorders are a major risk factor for fetal growth restriction due to placental insufficiency. A woman with a growth-restricted fetus requires targeted fetal surveillance in labour (see **Chapter 33**, *Management of labour with a growth-restricted fetus*). Assessing the amniotic fluid volume, and a baseline non-stress test may help decide if the fetus will tolerate labour.

Continuous CTG during labour is recommended for preeclampsia and chronic hypertension with superimposed preeclampsia. If a CTG is not available, fetal heart rate monitoring should be done with a handheld Doppler. The presence of fetal growth restriction is an important risk factor for fetal heart rate abnormalities with the onset of uterine contractions.

Maternal Monitoring With the Use of Early Warning Systems

Preeclampsia can progress rapidly and result in maternal mortality. Early warning systems have been developed to alert clinicians about worsening clinical maternal condition, and to set in motion investigations and interventions to protect the mother. Studies have shown that maternal morbidity and mortality in hypertensive diseases in pregnancy can be reduced through the planned implementation of standardised guidelines and treatment protocols [13,14]. However, these tools should be easy to use if they are to be adopted by labour and delivery staff, including those working in low-resource settings.

Modified early obstetric warning scores (MEOWS)

This was one of the first systems described and most widely used across the world. An alert must lead to an appropriate, expected response for reducing morbidity and mortality. Subsequent systems changed the alert criteria to reduce the number of triggers for intervention [15].

Maternal early warning trigger tool (MEWT)

This tool was developed to introduce response pathways for four of the major causes of maternal morbidity and mortality [16]. The hypertension pathway clearly provides alerts for investigations, treatment, and seizure prophylaxis, with a watch on respiratory rate and oxygen saturation indicative of pulmonary edema (Fig. 37.2).

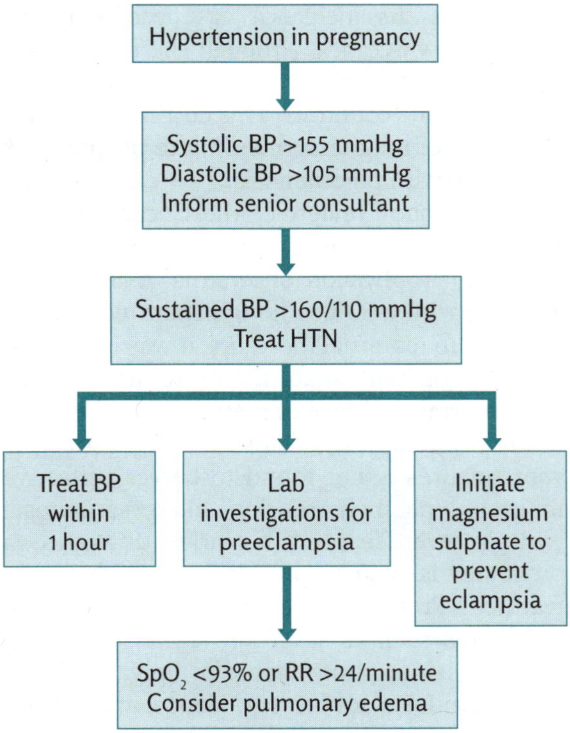

Fig. 37.2 The hypertension pathway in the Maternal Early Warning Trigger tool (MEWT) [16]

BP, blood pressure; *HTN*, hypertension; *RR*, respiratory rate

CONTROL OF HYPERTENSION IN THE LABOURING WOMAN

Labour is a time of stress and pain. This leads to fluctuations in BP and cardiac output. An emphasis on rapid management of acute elevations of blood pressure significantly decreases maternal morbidity [16].

In the labouring woman, the same medications, at the same dosage that she was on for hypertension should be continued. The aim is to minimise the occurrence of a hypertensive crisis.

Management of Hypertensive Crises

An acute elevation of systolic blood pressure **(≥160 mmHg)** and diastolic blood pressure **(≥110 mmHg)** may occur during labour. If this persists for **>15 minutes**, it is considered a **hypertensive emergency**. Management of severe hypertension aims to reduce the risk of stroke, intracranial hemorrhage, eclampsia, and abruption. Every obstetric unit should have an evidence-based protocol for managing hypertensive crises. Protocol-based treatment has been shown to reduce maternal mortality [13,17].

The concept of five 'Rs': **Recognition, Responding, Responsibility, Reviewing, and Realising** was introduced by Moodley and Ngene from South Africa [17]. They showed that the implementation of clinical protocols and checklists have standardised care and management of hypertensive crises (Table 37.5).

Care must be taken to monitor fetal well-being because uteroplacental blood flow may be compromised in the presence of sudden hypotension resulting from antihypertensive therapy.

Drugs of choice for hypertensive crises

Oral nifedipine

Both immediate release oral nifedipine [18,19] and sustained release oral nifedipine [20] have proven effective in the management of an acute

Table 37.5 The five 'Rs' team approach for optimising the management of hypertension in pregnancy [17]

Recognition	Responding	Responsibility	Reviewing	Realising
Acute-onset severe hypertension (BP ≥160/110 mmHg) in pregnancy is a MAJOR alerting trigger	Notify or seek advice from most appropriate health professional or specialist	For initiating early antihypertensive therapy, monitoring and stabilising the woman	Entire clinical situation is reviewed after hypertension is stabilised	• BP control is not the treatment of preeclampsia • Expediting delivery and implementing post-delivery care should be considered

hypertensive emergency. Oral nifedipine has been shown to lower blood pressure more quickly than intravenous labetalol [19]. In low-resource settings, oral nifedipine is the first-line drug of choice.

Recommended dosage [18]

- 10 mg orally, and record BP after 20 minutes.
- If BP is still >160/100 mmHg, administer 20 mg of nifedipine every 20 minutes till target blood pressure of 150/100 mmHg is achieved.
- If the target BP is not achieved **within an hour**, switch to intravenous labetalol.

Key Point

Nifedipine capsules should be administered orally and should not be punctured or administered sublingually.

Intravenous labetalol

Intravenous labetalol may be used either as the first-line drug for treatment of acute, severe hypertension in pregnancy or after failed treatment with oral nifedipine [1,4,18].

Recommended dosage [18]

- An initial dose of 20 mg intravenously (IV) given over 2 minutes
- If the target BP is not achieved in 10 minutes, administer 40 mg IV over 2 minutes
- If the target BP is not achieved in the next 10 minutes, administer 80 mg IV over 2 minutes
- If the target BP is not achieved, switch to nifedipine

Monitoring after achieving target blood pressure

After achieving the target BP of ≤150/100 mmHg, BP should be documented every 10 minutes for 1 hour, then every 15 minutes for 1 hour, then every 30 minutes for 1 hour, and then every hour for 4 hours.

PROPHYLAXIS FOR PREVENTION OF SEIZURES

Eclampsia is a complication of preeclampsia, and the incidence varies across countries and institutions. Its incidence has decreased over the past few decades, although the reduction is greater in high-income countries when compared to low-income countries. This decrease is related to the use of **magnesium sulphate prophylaxis** in women with preeclampsia.

A systematic review of the Cochrane Database [21] on the benefits of using magnesium sulphate prophylaxis showed a reduction in eclampsia by >50%. Though there was also a decrease in maternal mortality, it was not statistically significant. Maternal morbidity or perinatal mortality showed no effect.

Prophylactic magnesium sulphate to prevent seizures is not found to be very effective in gestational hypertension and preeclampsia without severe features. A marked difference in outcomes is seen in preeclampsia with severe features. Prophylaxis is most effective when symptoms such as severe headache, vomiting, blurred vision, photophobia or epigastric pain or hyperreflexia are present. Hence, magnesium sulphate prophylaxis is recommended for preeclampsia with severe features or eclampsia, and individualised decisions are recommended for other categories of the hypertensive spectrum [21,22].

Magnesium sulphate has been found to be a better drug when compared to other anticonvulsants like phenytoin or diazepam in preventing or treating convulsions in pregnancy. Other antiepileptics are considered only if magnesium sulphate is contraindicated or not available.

There is no evidence of the ideal dose of magnesium sulphate or the most ideal therapeutic blood concentration that has the maximum benefit and least adverse effects. Magnesium sulphate can be administered intravenously or intramuscularly (if there is difficulty in establishing IV access or an infusion pump is not available).

Recommended Dosage of Magnesium Sulphate

The dosage of magnesium sulphate for the prevention and treatment of eclampsia is described in Table 37.6. The infusion should be continued

Table 37.6 Dosage of magnesium sulphate for the prevention and treatment of eclampsia

Route	Dosage	Timing
Intramuscular	• **Loading dose** 10 g of 50% solution (5 g IM in each buttock) • **Followed by** 5 g of 50% solution every 4 hours, alternate buttocks (may be mixed with 1 mL of 2% xylocaine to reduce pain)	• **Cesarean delivery** (before onset of labour):Initiate before surgery, continue during surgery, maintain for 24 hours afterwards • **Vaginal delivery:** Continue for 24 hours after delivery • **If convulsions recur:** Additional 2 g of 20% solution IV over 3–5 minutes
Intravenous (with infusion pump)	• **Loading dose** 4 g diluted in 100 mL of IV fluid over 20–30 minutes • **Followed by** a maintenance dose of 1 g/hour	

IM, *intramuscular*; IV, *intravenous*

in the intrapartum period, and during surgery if an operative intervention is necessary. The infusion is stopped 24 hours after delivery [22].

Monitoring magnesium sulphate administration

Magnesium sulphate concentrations are affected by **impaired renal clearance** as the drug is excreted by the kidneys. Reducing the maintenance dose to half is recommended when the urine output is <0.5 mL/Kg body weight per hour or when there is impaired renal function with serum creatinine >1.2 mg/dL.

A body mass index of > 35 Kg/m^2 is known to have an effect on therapeutic levels and may require frequent assessment of magnesium levels to ensure optimal results.

Magnesium toxicity results in the disappearance of deep tendon reflexes first, then respiratory depression, and finally, cardiorespiratory arrest. Hence, all women on magnesium sulphate therapy should be monitored every hour to check their vitals, tendon reflexes, and urine output.

The **antidote for magnesium toxicity** is an injection of calcium gluconate 10 g intravenous over 3 minutes as magnesium sulphate is a smooth muscle relaxant.

Management of Eclampsia

In the presence of seizures, the priority is to maintain airway patency and prevent aspiration. Once that is achieved, the focus is on terminating the seizures, preventing maternal hypoxia and trauma, controlling severe hypertension and prevention of recurrence. Stabilisation is followed by complete assessment of the maternal and fetal condition to plan prompt delivery. Apart from the obstetric team, neonatologists, anesthetists, maternal–fetal medicine specialists, nephrologists, and cardiologists should be involved. The ICU should be alerted.

Key Point

An eclampsia tray or box with all the equipment and medicines required for emergency management should be present in the labour room.

MONITORING FOR ORGAN DYSFUNCTION IN PREECLAMPSIA

Diagnosis of organ dysfunction in preeclampsia requires frequent clinical and laboratory testing to alert clinicians to any developing complication. A multidisciplinary team should care for the woman, and anesthesia and critical care teams should be informed.

A woman with preeclampsia with severe features can be monitored in a high-dependency unit within the labour and delivery complex if complications are limited to one organ. If multiorgan dysfunction occurs, then shifting to ICU is a better option to provide organ support if necessary.

Urine Output and Appearance

Urine output is a clinical indicator of renal function and all women with hypertensive disorders should have an intake/output chart. A urine output of <0.5 mL/Kg/hour is regarded as decreased output and may be due to inadequate intake or acute kidney injury. Adding a urometer allows the accurate assessment of urine output.

Smoky or cola-coloured urine is a marker for hemolysis, bloodstained urine for thrombocytopenia, and deep yellowish colour for bilirubinuria.

Signs and Symptoms of Worsening Disease

Headache, nausea, and vomiting may be signs of raised intracranial pressure. Epigastric pain may direct the clinician towards tests to rule out hepatic hematoma. Breathlessness, fall in oxygen saturation and orthopnea are signs of pulmonary edema. Sudden blindness, seizures, and neurological deficit represent neurological complications of preeclampsia requiring appropriate imaging to confirm the diagnosis.

Key Point

Complications of preeclampsia can worsen rapidly and these can only be diagnosed by repeating the tests at regular intervals.

Laboratory Testing

A baseline panel of tests is done at the onset of labour to detect the following:

- Thrombocytopenia
- Elevated liver enzymes
- Renal dysfunction
- Hemolysis
- HELLP syndrome

These tests may be repeated in labour if there are deranged baseline tests, or there is acute worsening of maternal condition such as decreased urine output, symptoms of cerebral irritation (severe headache, photophobia, irritability, vomiting, blurred vision) or epigastric pain. Arterial blood gas analysis should be requested if there is multiorgan derangement.

Key Point

HELLP syndrome is a multiorgan syndrome that needs very frequent laboratory testing to detect worsening.

POSTPARTUM FOLLOW-UP

Medications

Antihypertensives are continued in the same dose in the immediate postpartum period. Labetalol and nifedipine can be continued without any concerns about drug levels in breast milk as the levels are very low [1,5]. Alpha-methyldopa may need to be changed to another drug as it has an association with postpartum depression. Enalapril or calcium channels blockers such as amlodipine can be added if a second line of drug is required. **The target is to maintain BP below 140/90 mmHg.** If a woman was not on any antihypertensives, then 150/100 mmHg BP is taken as a cut-off to start antihypertensives in the postnatal period. The dosage should be reviewed if the BP falls below 130/80 mmHg.

Monitoring

Women with gestational hypertension, chronic hypertension and preeclampsia without severe features can be discharged after 24 hours with instructions on which symptoms and signs should be reported to the team. Blood pressure should be monitored at least twice a day, with a scheduled review after a week.

The risk of an acute elevation of blood pressure in the postnatal period is greatest between the 3rd and 5th postnatal days. Even women without severe features of preeclampsia might develop postpartum eclampsia or stroke.

Overwhelming evidence is available on the risk of cardiovascular disease as a late sequel of hypertension in pregnancy [2,23,24]. The odds of developing hypertension, myocardial infarction, congestive heart failure, cerebrovascular events (stroke), peripheral arterial disease, and cardiovascular mortality are doubled. These women should be counselled about lifestyle modifications to better manage risk factors for cardiovascular disease.

Key Point

All women should be counselled about the recurrence risks in the next pregnancy, prevention of sequelae and the need for follow-up in later life.

CONCLUSION

Hypertensive women in labour need focused care and management for the best outcome for them and their babies. Hypertensive disorders are the second leading cause of maternal mortality. All obstetric care providers should watch for complications, and involve a multidisciplinary team (obstetricians, maternal–fetal medicine specialists, neonatologists, nephrologists, cardiologists, anesthesiologists, nurses, and midwives). In severe cases, the woman should be transferred to a tertiary unit to reduce the morbidity and mortality for both mother and baby.

REFERENCES

1. Hypertension in pregnancy: Diagnosis and management. London: National Institute for Health and Care Excellence (NICE). 2019. NICE Guideline. No. 133.
2. Garovic VD, Dechend R, Easterling T, et al. On behalf of the American Heart Association Council on Hypertension. Council on the Kidney in Cardiovascular Disease, Kidney in Heart Disease Science Committee. Council on Arteriosclerosis, Thrombosis and Vascular Biology; Council on Lifestyle and Cardiometabolic Health; Council on Peripheral Vascular Disease; and Stroke Council. Hypertension in pregnancy: Diagnosis, blood pressure goals, and pharmacotherapy: A scientific statement from the American Heart Association. *Hypertension*. 2022.79:e21–e41.
3. Brown MA, Magee LA, Kenny LC, Karumanchi SA, McCarthy FP, Saito S, Hall DR, Warren CE, Adoyi G, Ishaku S. International Society for the Study of Hypertension in Pregnancy (ISSHP). Hypertensive Disorders of Pregnancy: ISSHP Classification, Diagnosis, and Management Recommendations for International Practice. *Hypertension*. 2018.72(1):24-43.
4. Gestational hypertension and preeclampsia. ACOG Practice Bulletin No. 222. American College of Obstetricians and Gynecologists. *Obstet Gynecol*. 2020.135:e237–60.
5. Mussarat N, Biggio J Jr, Martin J, Morgan J, et al. Masked pregnancy-associated hypertension as a predictor of adverse outcomes. *Am J Obstet Gynecol* MFM. 2023.5(7):100976.
6. Martin JN, Jr, Rose CH, Briery CM. Understanding and managing HELLP syndrome: the integral role of aggressive glucocorticoids for mother and child. *Am J Obstet Gynecol*. 2006.195:914–934.
7. WHO recommendations: policy of interventionist versus expectant management of severe pre-eclampsia before term ISBN 978-92-4-155044-4. World Health Organization. 2018.
8. Koopmans CM, Bijlenga D, Groen H, et al. HYPITAT study group. Induction of labour versus expectant monitoring for gestational hypertension or mild preeclampsia after 36 weeks' gestation (HYPITAT): a multicentre, open-label randomised controlled trial. *Lancet*. 2009.374:979–988.
9. Yuce T, Keskin M, Seval MM, Söylemez F. Effect of the timing of delivery on perinatal outcomes at gestational hypertension. *Interv Med Appl Sci*. 2015.7(2):59-62.
10. Coppage KH, Polzin WJ. Severe preeclampsia and delivery outcomes: Is immediate caesarean delivery beneficial? *Am J Obstet Gynecol*. 2002.186(5):921–923.
11. Pacher J, Brix E, Lehner R. The mode of delivery in patients with preeclampsia at term subject to elective or emergency caesarean section. *Arch Gynecol Obstet*. 2014.289(2):263–267.
12. Bauer ME, Arendt K, Beilin Y, Gernsheimer T, et al. The Society for Obstetric Anesthesia and Perinatology Interdisciplinary Consensus Statement on Neuraxial Procedures in Obstetric Patients with Thrombocytopenia. *Anesth Analg*. 2021.132(6):1531-1544.
13. O'Brien L, Duong J, Winterton T, et al. Management of Hypertension on the Labour and Delivery Unit: Delivering Care in the Era of Protocols and Algorithms. *Perm J*. 2018.22:17-170.
14. Menzies J, Magee LA, Li J, et al. Preeclampsia Integrated Estimate of RiSk (PIERS) Study Group. Instituting surveillance guidelines and adverse outcomes in preeclampsia. *Obstet Gynecol*. 2007.110(1):121-7
15. Robbins T, Shennan A, Sandall J. Modified early obstetric warning scores: A promising tool but more evidence and standardization is required. *Acta Obstet Gynecol Scand*. 2019.98:7–10.
16. Shields LE, Wiesner S, Klein C, Pelletreau B, Hedriana HL. Use of Maternal Early Warning Trigger tool reduces

maternal morbidity. *Am J Obstet Gynecol.* 2016.214(4):527.e1-527.e6.

17. Moodley J, Ngene NC. Severe hypertension in pregnancy: Using dynamic checklists to save lives. *S Afr Med J.* 2016.106(8):767-70.
18. Emergent Therapy for Acute-Onset, Severe Hypertension During Pregnancy and the Postpartum Period: ACOG Committee Opinion, Number 692. *Obstetrics & Gynecology.* 2017.129(4):p e90-e95.
19. Shekhar S, Sharma C, Thakur S, Verma S. Oral nifedipine or intravenous labetalol for hypertensive emergency in pregnancy: a randomized controlled trial. *Obstet Gynecol.* 2013.122:1057–63.
20. Easterling T, Mundle S, Bracken H, Parvekar S, Mool S, Magee LA, von Dadelszen P, Shochet T, Winikoff B. Oral antihypertensive regimens (nifedipine retard, labetalol, and methyldopa) for management of severe hypertension in pregnancy: An open-label, randomised controlled trial. *Lancet.* 2019.394(10203):1011.
21. Duley L, Gülmezoglu AM, Henderson-Smart DJ, Chou D. Magnesium sulphate and other anticonvulsants for women with pre-eclampsia. *Cochrane Database of Systematic Reviews.* 2010. Issue 11. Art. No.: CD000025.
22. Sibai BM. Magnesium sulfate prophylaxis in preeclampsia: Lessons learned from recent trials. *Am J Obstet Gynecol.* 2004.190:1520–6.
23. McDonald SD, Malinowski A, Zhou Q, Yusuf S, Devereaux PJ. Cardiovascular sequelae of preeclampsia/eclampsia: A systematic review and meta-analyses. *Am Heart J.* 2008.156:918–30.
24. Ray JG, Vermeulen MJ, Schull MJ, Redelmeier DA. Cardiovascular health after maternal placental syndromes (CHAMPS): Population-based retrospective cohort study. *Lancet.* 2005.366:1797–803.

CHAPTER 38

Management of Labour in a Woman with Diabetes

LAKSHMI SHANMUGASUNDARAM, UMA RAM

INTRODUCTION

Hyperglycemia in pregnancy (HIP) is one of the most common medical disorders in pregnancy. About 12–17% of pregnancies are complicated by hyperglycemia, 84% of which are due to gestational diabetes mellitus (GDM) [1]. In India, GDM complicates approximately 4 million pregnancies annually, which places a large subset of the population at high risk of adverse perinatal morbidity and mortality unless the condition is managed appropriately [2]. HIP is associated with several short- and long-term complications for the woman and her baby. Good glycemic control (both during the antenatal and intrapartum period), appropriate timing of delivery, and vigilant intrapartum monitoring can significantly reduce adverse outcomes.

The labour care plan should be based on the woman's individual medical circumstances while respecting her right to make an informed choice. Educating the woman in the antenatal period about the additional intrapartum monitoring required and the risks that may arise can help her be better prepared. Adequate support, ensuring companionship and communication (see **Chapter 3**, *Respectful obstetric care and the role of a birth companion*), along with documentation of clinical records are vital components of intrapartum care.

Multidisciplinary perinatal care is paramount for all women with HIP. A written policy/guideline, agreed upon by a multidisciplinary diabetes care team, is very important, especially in pregestational diabetics, as it helps with timely and uniform implementation of standard care by all the intrapartum care providers. Periodic training for all healthcare professionals on relevant aspects of pregnancy and diabetes such as current intrapartum guidelines, recent updates, insulin types, safe administration of medication, and use of equipment will help to ensure safe intrapartum care.

INTRAPARTUM COMPLICATIONS OF HIP

Intrapartum complications in women with HIP include the following:

- Preterm delivery
- Operative delivery
- Infection
- Obstetric anal sphincter injury (OASI)
- Hypoglycemia or diabetic ketoacidosis (DKA)/end-organ involvement
- Complications related to comorbid conditions

Neonatal risks include the following:

- Neonatal hypoglycemia (occurs in up to 50% of neonates born to mothers with pregestational diabetes, and between 5% and 20% of women with gestational diabetes)
- Macrosomia or LGA
- Shoulder dystocia and birth trauma
- Fetal acidemia
- Stillbirth and perinatal death
- Delayed transition and respiratory distress
- Poor feeding

The intrapartum, fetal, and and neonatal complications of HIP are summarised in Table 38.1.

Table 38.1 Intrapartum and neonatal complications associated with hyperglycemia in pregnancy (HIP)

Maternal risks	Fetal and neonatal risks
• Preterm delivery • Operative delivery • Infection • Obstetric anal sphincter injury (OASI) • Glycemic complications: Hypoglycemia/ DKA/end-organ involvement • Complications related to comorbid conditions	• Large for gestational age (LGA) • Shoulder dystocia • Birth trauma • Fetal acidemia • Stillbirth and perinatal death • **Neonatal:** Hypoglycemia, transient tachypnea, hypocalcemia, hypothermia, respiratory distress, poor feeding

DKA, diabetic ketoacidosis

AIM OF INTRAPARTUM CARE

The aim of enhanced vigilance for women with diabetes is to minimise adverse outcomes. This chapter will address the following:

- Intrapartum complications for woman and child
- Timing of birth
- Route of birth
- Glycemic monitoring and control during labour and birth
- Immediate care of the neonate

TIMING OF BIRTH

While making a decision about delivering a woman with diabetes, the risk of intrauterine fetal death must be weighed against the risks of preterm birth. Pregestational diabetes is associated with more frequent pregnancy complications than GDM [3].

The chief driver for planned delivery in women with diabetes is the increased risk of **stillbirth** and **macrosomia** (see sections on *Stillbirth and Macrosomia*). Historically, increased stillbirth has been observed in untreated and undiagnosed gestational diabetes. The Australian Carbohydrate Intolerance Study in Pregnant Women (ACHOIS) trial [4] underlined the significant benefit of management of hyperglycemia antenatally to prevent fetal death, shoulder dystocia, bone fracture, and nerve palsy.

Guidelines vary in their recommendations for the timing of birth in well-controlled GDM. The evidence for these recommendations comes from small, single-centre or national data that may not be applicable universally. In practice, most women with GDM deliver (or are induced) by 39–40 weeks and hence, data on birth after 40 weeks too has limited clinical applicability.

Stillbirth

Studies have reported a 4–6 times higher risk of stillbirth in the presence of diabetes than in the absence of it; 4% of all stillbirths are attributable to HIP [5]. Women with type 2 DM may be more affected due to the presence of comorbidities such as obesity, advanced maternal age, and hypertension.

The risk of stillbirth in women with GDM varies with the method of diagnosis, glycemic management and control, maternal comorbidities, and ethnicity. This could be the reason for conflicting data on the impact of management on stillbirth in GDM. The risk of stillbirth is impacted by gestational age and fetal size and increases over time to exceed the risk of expectant management at 39 weeks [6].

Macrosomia and Shoulder Dystocia

Observational studies have shown that elective induction before 38 weeks does not necessarily reduce the risk of macrosomia or shoulder dystocia. However, some of these studies were underpowered and did not address the risk of stillbirth [2].

A recent meta-analysis suggests that induction reduces macrosomia and perineal trauma but does not impact cesarean rates and perinatal or neonatal morbidity [8]. However, the overall quality of the studies was stated as low to very low, including only three RCTs, one of which was nearly 30 years old. Clearly, there is a need for good-quality studies to guide decision-making in this important area. Until then, for women with diabetes, there is a need for careful individualised care to plan the timing of delivery considering the type of HIP, comorbidities, and obstetric history [9].

Timing of Delivery in Pregestational Diabetes

The decision to deliver a woman with pregestational diabetes is influenced by the following:

- Gestational age
- Estimated fetal weight
- Maternal glycemic control and comorbidities (e.g., vascular disease)
- Prior stillbirth

Women with type 1 or type 2 diabetes with poor glycemic control have higher rates of cesarean sections, instrumental delivery, low Apgar scores, seizures, and hypoxic–ischemic encephalopathy [10].

- **For women with well-controlled glucose levels and no vascular disease**, delivery is recommended at 39+0 to 39+6 weeks. Expectant management beyond 40+0 weeks is not recommended [11,12,13].
- **For women with uncontrolled hyperglycemia** or **vascular disease**, delivery is recommended at 36+0 to 38+6 weeks (or even earlier if the severity of complications warrants earlier delivery) [11,12,13].

Timing of Delivery in Gestational Diabetes

There is substantial controversy in the literature and in clinical practice regarding the optimal time to deliver a woman with GDM to minimise the risks to her fetus. It is appropriate to base the decision on whether the hyperglycemia is controlled with diet and exercise alone (A1GDM) or if it is well-controlled with the addition of medication (A2GDM) [14].

Induction of labour vs. expectant management

There are no robust RCTs to recommend induction over expectant management in GDM. However, smaller studies and systematic reviews have shown the following:

- A prospective RCT by Kjos [15] in 1993 supported the induction of labour at 38 weeks in women with insulin-dependent GDM.
- In another study involving women with insulin-dependent GDM, induction of labour at 38–39 weeks reduced the incidence of shoulder dystocia and did not increase the incidence of cesarean delivery. Shoulder dystocia was reported in 10% of those in the expectant management group after >40 weeks of gestation versus 1.4% in the group that underwent labour induction [16].
- A systematic review suggested that active rather than expectant management of labour at term for women with GDM may reduce the rates of macrosomia and related complications [17].
- A study that compared induction of labour before 40 weeks of gestation with expectant management among women with GDM found a reduction in the incidence of cesarean delivery in the induced group [18].
- A simulated study that looked at the optimal gestational age to deliver women with A1GDM found that delivery at 38–38+6 weeks of gestation reduced the chances of IUFD without increasing the risk of neonatal morbidities from preterm delivery [19].

The various recommendations from professional obstetric bodies are summarised in Table 38.2. The following recommendations may be followed:

- **For women with well-controlled A1GDM (well-controlled with exercise and medical nutrition therapy [MNT])**, delivery should not be performed before 39 weeks of gestation

Table 38.2 **Timing of birth in women with diabetes in pregnancy (recommendations from various guidelines)**

Organisation	Recommended gestational age for delivery (weeks)				
	Pregestational diabetes (Type 1 or 2) (Without complications)	Pregestational diabetes (Type 1 or 2) (With complications)	A1GDM (Well-controlled)	A2GDM (Well-controlled)	GDM (Poor glycemic control)
NICE [9]	Induced labour or (if indicated) cesarean section at 37–38+6 days	Before 37 weeks	Deliver by 40+6	Deliver by 40+6	Between 34 and 39+6 weeks
ACOG and SMFM [11, 14]	39–39+6 weeks (with fetal surveillance)	36–38+6 weeks or even earlier	39+0–39+6	39+0–39+6	36+0–38+6
FOGSI [21] and Government of India guidelines [22]	–	–	At or after 39 weeks	At or after 39 weeks	To be individualised by the obstetrician
SOGC [23]	Between 38 and 40 weeks	Between 38 and 40 weeks	Between 38 and 40 weeks	Between 38 and 40 weeks	38–39 weeks

A1GDM, gestational diabetes managed with exercise and medical nutrition therapy; *A2GDM*, gestational diabetes managed with medication; *GDM*, gestational diabetes mellitus

unless otherwise indicated. In such women, expectant management up to 40+6 weeks of gestation is generally appropriate. However, these women should be monitored carefully with recommended fetal surveillance [14,20].

- **For women with A2GDM (well-controlled with medication)**, delivery is recommended between 39+0 weeks and 39+6 weeks of gestation [14,20].
- **For women with poor glycemic control**, delivery is recommended between 34 and 39+6 weeks of gestation [9]. The ACOG recommends hospitalisation and close fetal surveillance with delivery between 37 weeks and 38+6 weeks [14].

Key Point

It is important to adopt a protocol for choosing the timing of delivery based on the local availability of facilities, the average gestational age of delivery in the population, the control of hyperglycemia in the individual woman, and her obstetric history.

An algorithm for the timing of delivery in women with HIP is presented in Fig. 38.1.

ROUTE OF BIRTH

Vaginal Delivery

Induction of labour and vaginal delivery are appropriate for women with gestational diabetes with good glycemic control. Though women with pregestational diabetes (type 1 or type 2) and good glycemic control may be allowed to have a vaginal delivery, cesarean delivery is more common in women with pregestational diabetes than in women with GDM [2].

Assisted vaginal delivery

In diabetic women with suspected macrosomia, a prolonged second stage may be a warning sign for the possibility of shoulder dystocia. In such a case, it would be reasonable to proceed with a cesarean section (see **Chapter 28**, *Shoulder dystocia: Prevention and management*).

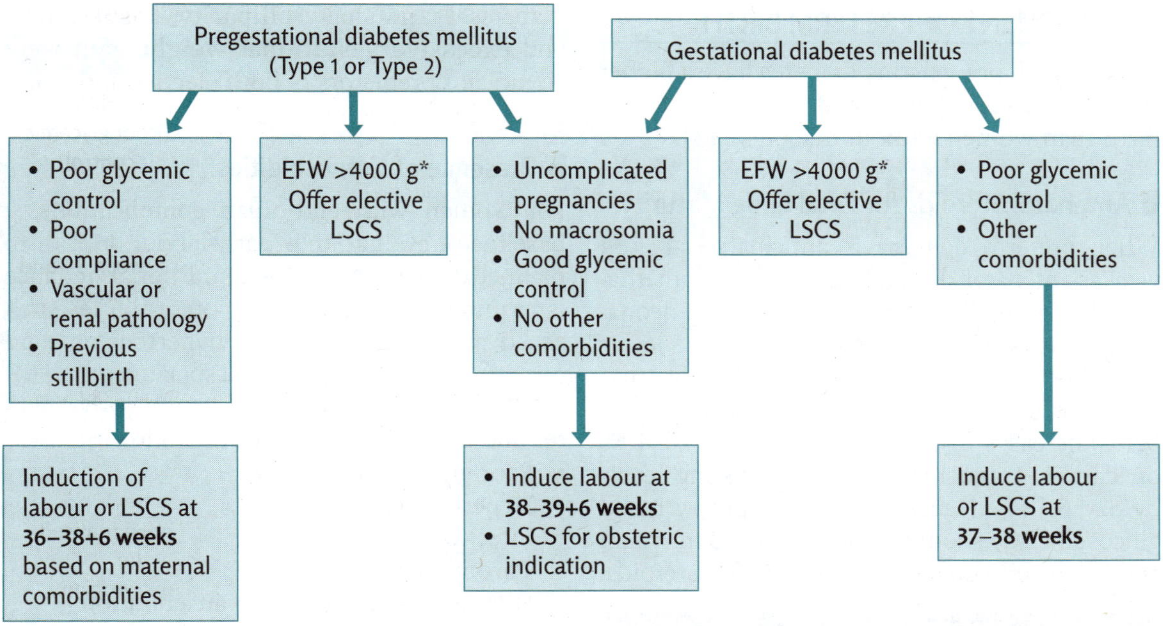

Fig. 38.1 An algorithm for the timing of delivery based on the type of diabetes, the presence of comorbidities, fetal macrosomia, and glycemic control [9,11,14,21,22,23]

*Though ACOG recommends an elective cesarean for EFW of ≥4500 g, in Indian women, ≥4000 g would be a more appropriate cut-off

EFW, estimated fetal weight; *LSCS*, lower segment cesarean section

Cesarean Section

Diabetes, by itself, is not an indication for cesarean delivery in the absence of any other obstetric indication [13].

- **Suspected macrosomia:** In diabetic women, especially those with pregestational diabetes, macrosomia can be an indication for cesarean birth due to the risk of morbidity from shoulder dystocia (see **Chapter 34**, *Management of labour with fetal macrosomia*). Fetuses of diabetic women have greater shoulder and chest-to-head disproportion than macrosomic infants of non-diabetic women. The ACOG recommends prophylactic cesarean birth to prevent brachial plexus injury when the EFW is greater than 4500 g in women with diabetes [11]. In Indian women, it would be reasonable to proceed with an elective cesarean for an EFW of ≥4000 g. While using these cut-offs, we must be aware that the ultrasound prediction of macrosomia is imprecise.
- **History of shoulder dystocia:** A history of a previous delivery complicated by shoulder dystocia and a previous instance of neonatal injury as well as EFW have a bearing on the decision about the route of delivery.
- **A trial of labour after a previous cesarean birth (TOLAC)**: Though maternal diabetes is not a contraindication to a trial of labour after a previous cesarean birth, the success rate may be lower than it is in women without diabetes (see **Chapter 26,** *Vaginal birth after a previous cesarean delivery*).

MANAGEMENT OF PRETERM BIRTH

Women with pre-existing diabetes have a higher risk of both spontaneous and indicated preterm birth than women without diabetes [13].

Antenatal Steroids for Fetal Lung Maturity

When preterm delivery is anticipated at <34 weeks, antenatal dexamethasone or betamethasone has a significant role in improving neonatal outcomes. However, maternal glucose levels should be monitored carefully. The use of antenatal corticosteroids in women with type 1 diabetes increases insulin requirement by 20–40% on days 1–4 and returns to pre-existing levels by day 6 [24]. Hence, maternal capillary blood glucose (CBG) should be monitored to maintain good glycemic control on days 1–5 after steroids.

> **Key Point**
>
> If preterm delivery occurs within six days of steroid administration, extra vigilance for neonatal hypoglycemia is required.

Tocolysis

The use of beta-mimetic agents for tocolysis is associated with the risk of hyperglycemia and should be avoided. Calcium channel blockers such as nifedipine and oxytocin antagonists may be used for tocolysis.

MATERNAL SURVEILLANCE IN LABOUR

Documenting Progress of Labour

To provide a comprehensive overview of labour, a partograph or the WHO Labour Care Guide may be used (see **Chapter 6**, *Monitoring labour: Partograph to Labour Care Guide*). In women with diabetes, early recognition of slow progress of labour aids in making a decision for active labour management. Failure to progress in labour is more common in women with HIP. Studies have highlighted operator bias resulting in a lower threshold for cesarean in women with HIP. A risk score that was developed to predict the risk of cesarean in women with gestational diabetes found that **nulliparity**, **insulin use**, and **excessive gestational weight gain** were significant predictors of both elective and emergency cesarean delivery [25].

Presence of Comorbidities

For women with end-organ complications, a baseline re-evaluation in early labour or prior to planned delivery is required. Additional vigilance is required for women with comorbidities such as advanced maternal age, hypertension, and obesity, that are commonly associated with HIP.

Obesity is a common association with diabetes and increases the risk of the following:

- Poor glycemic control
- Hypertension
- Infection
- Thromboembolism
- Difficulty with fetal heart auscultation
- Difficulty in access for regional analgesia

While focusing on diabetes care, it is important to not miss out on other standard aspects of care. An example of this is routine antibiotic prophylaxis and mechanical aids for venous thromboprophylaxis during cesarean delivery in an obese woman. Body weight-based heparin dosing and early ambulation should be utilised for postpartum thromboprophylaxis.

> **Key Point**
>
> It would be prudent for all women with comorbidities to be assessed by an anesthetist in the antenatal period. This allows for anesthetic risk assessment and helps with birth planning.

Glycemic Control During Labour and Delivery

In general, the need for insulin decreases in labour due to reduced intake and increased expenditure of calories from physical exertion. Achieving glycemic control is one of the key aspects of intrapartum diabetes care. The factors that affect glycemic control in labour include:

- The metabolic demands of labour
- Dextrose-containing IV fluids
- Food restriction in active labour

Fetal and neonatal concerns

In women with pregestational diabetes, maternal hyperglycemia has been linked to major fetal complications—**fetal hypoxemia, perinatal asphyxia** [26], and **neonatal hypoglycemia**. It is, therefore, important to ensure euglycemia during labour.

Fetal hypoxemia

Maternal hyperglycemia leads to fetal hyperglycemia and hyperinsulinemia, which increase fetal oxygen consumption and can lead to fetal hypoxemia, acidemia, and (if severe enough) death. The hypoxemia may manifest as late decelerations, prolonged fetal bradycardia, or 1-minute Apgar <6. This effect is heightened in women with poorly controlled diabetes as demonstrated by high antenatal HbA1C.

Neonatal hypoglycemia

Hyperinsulinemia, triggered by maternal hyperglycemia, leads to neonatal hypoglycemia. It is the most common neonatal adverse outcome and occurs in half of the babies born to women with pre-existing diabetes and in 5–20% of women with gestational diabetes.

> **Key Point**
>
> Intrapartum blood glucose monitoring and maintenance of maternal glucose levels between 72 and 126 mg/dL is recommended to minimise the risk of fetal distress and neonatal hypoglycemia [9,11,14].

A1GDM (well-controlled on medical nutrition therapy [MNT])

Women with blood glucose levels well-controlled with diet alone are managed similarly to non-diabetic women. Care providers should document HIP as a risk factor in the partograph so that heightened maternal and fetal care can be continued.

A2GDM (well-controlled on insulin or oral medication)

Latent phase of labour

In the latent phase, the metabolic demand is not altered much. So, the woman can continue to follow the same glycemic control methods and diet she followed in the antenatal period.

Oral hypoglycemics can be continued in the latent phase of labour. **Insulin** can be maintained in the woman's usual subcutaneous dose during the latent phase of labour, and while she is able to eat normally. Capillary glucose levels should be monitored hourly.

Active labour

Oral hypoglycemics are stopped at the onset of active labour. Periodic assessment of capillary blood glucose is advised to ensure that the values are within range; insulin cover should be provided if needed.

Insulin administration is switched to sliding scale/variable rate intravenous insulin infusion (VRIII) in active labour. Hourly capillary monitoring is continued for all diabetics during active labour. The use of continuous glucose monitoring (CGM) is best avoided as capillary testing is more accurate, particularly when changes are rapid. Women using continuous subcutaneous insulin infusion pumps can continue using this in labour, provided the target levels are achieved [27].

Sliding scale/variable rate intravenous insulin infusion (VRIII): Hyperglycemia in labour should be managed with the help of an endocrinologist who is involved in the care of the woman.

- Two separate IV lines are set up, one for maintenance intravenous fluids (if oral hydration is not permitted for clinical reasons) and another one for insulin infusion.
- **Maintenance IV fluids** are given in the form of 500 mL of 5% glucose in 0.9% saline with 0.3% of potassium chloride per bag. This solution is infused at the rate of 50 mL/hour and increased depending on the need [27].
- **The indications for VRIII** include the following [27]:
    - *Women with type 1 diabetes*: VRIII is commenced when established labour is confirmed (either spontaneous or induced) or at 7 am on the day of the elective cesarean.

- *Women with type 2 diabetes and GDM who required a large dose of insulin* antenatally (>80 units): VRIII is commenced when labour is established or at 6 am on the day of the elective cesarean.
- *Two consecutive CBGs are >126 mg/dL* (with the second within 30 minutes of the first CBG >126 mg/dL to prevent any delays): VRIII should be commenced immediately.

- **Administration of VRIII** should always be through a syringe pump. The solution is prepared with 50 units of soluble insulin (Actrapid®) in 49.5 mL normal saline, giving a concentration of 1 unit per mL (Table 38.3). **The IV line used for insulin must not be used for any other medications.**
- **Hypoglycemia** (blood glucose level <72 mg/dL) is managed by stopping the infusion for 20 minutes. If the glucose level is still low, the woman can be given appropriate food or drink. If she is being maintained nil per orum (NPO), 5% dextrose in normal saline maintenance infusion should be started.
- **Diabetic ketoacidosis** is more common in women with type 1 diabetes. It is important to always involve the medical/diabetes team and follow a structured protocol for monitoring and management of DKA. Continuous CTG is necessary to monitor the fetal status until recovery from DKA.

Table 38.3 Sliding scale/variable rate intravenous insulin infusion (VRIII) for women requiring insulin in labour

CBG mg/dL	Standard infusion rate (units/hour=mL/hour)	Increase rate if hyperglycemia not controlled (units/hour=mL/hour)
<72	• Stop insulin infusion • Manage hypoglycemia	0
73–126	1	2
127–198	2	4
199–270	4 exclude DKA	6
271–360	5 exclude DKA	7
361–504	6 exclude DKA	8
>505	8 exclude DKA	10

CBG, capillary blood glucose; *DKA*, diabetic ketoacidosis

Special precautions with elective cesarean delivery

In women who need an elective cesarean section, surgery is planned in the morning as first on the list. The bolus dose of insulin is omitted on the morning of cesarean, and any long-acting basal insulin is continued but reduced by 20–50%. Blood glucose is monitored with a fasting sample and rechecked one hour before the time of the planned cesarean. VRIII is initiated if target values are not met.

IMMEDIATE POSTPARTUM MANAGEMENT

Blood glucose monitoring should be continued. After the delivery of the fetus and the placenta, the requirement for insulin will drop abruptly.

Pregestational Diabetes Type 1

The woman should receive 25–50% of her pregnancy dose of insulin. Her blood glucose levels should be monitored regularly, and the dosage should be adjusted. The insulin requirement is 15–20% lower in breastfeeding women [28].

Pregestational Diabetes Type 2

If the woman was started on insulin during pregnancy, the insulin can be stopped immediately after delivery. Blood sugar should be monitored, and metformin may be restarted.

Gestational Diabetes

With the delivery of the baby and the placenta, insulin resistance rapidly disappears. These women can be managed without any medications.

Breastfeeding proffers metabolic advantages in preventing the development of type 2 diabetes in women with gestational diabetes [29].

MANAGEMENT OF NEONATAL COMPLICATIONS

Fetal Acidemia

Continuous cardiotocography (CTG) in active labour is recommended along with vigilance for other features of fetal compromise such as fresh meconium and scanty or excess liquor. Intrapartum stillbirth and the risk of fetal acidosis is increased in HIP. The presence of a normal fetal CTG pattern is associated with a low risk of acidosis.

Many women with HIP undergo induced labours and therefore, may require continuous CTG monitoring. The role of CTG in reliably detecting acidemia has limitations (see **Chapter 8**, *Fetal surveillance in labour*, for further details).

Neonatal Hypoglycemia

Early breastfeeding is very important to minimise hypoglycemia and other newborn complications. Hence, the woman should receive good lactational support, starting at birth. The newborn's care must be adequately supervised and should include protocol-based neonatal monitoring for hypoglycemia.

CONCLUSION

Maintaining normoglycemia, both in the antenatal and intrapartum periods, the timing of delivery based on individual circumstances, active management of labour, and the availability of a multidisciplinary team are important aspects of labour care for women with HIP. Antenatal discussions about the timing and mode of delivery and the associated benefits and risks should be documented in clinical records.

REFERENCES

1. Hod M, Kapur A, Sacks DA, Hadar E, Agarwal M, Di Renzo GC, Cabero Roura L, McIntyre HD, Morris JL, Divakar H. The International Federation of Gynecology and Obstetrics (FIGO) Initiative on gestational diabetes mellitus: A pragmatic guide for diagnosis, management, and care. *Int J Gynaecol Obstet*. 2015. 131 Suppl 3:S173-211.
2. Guariguata L, Linnenkamp U, Beagley J, Whiting DR, Cho NH. Global estimates of the prevalence of hyperglycaemia in pregnancy. *Diabetes Res Clin Pract*. 2014. 103:176–85.
3. Malaza N, Masete M, Adam S, et al. A systematic review to compare adverse pregnancy outcomes in women with pregestational diabetes and gestational diabetes. *Int J Environ Res Public Health*. 2022. 19(17):10846.
4. Crowther CA, Hiller JE, Moss JR, et al. Effect of treatment of gestational diabetes mellitus on pregnancy outcomes for the Australian Carbohydrate Intolerance Study in Pregnant Women (ACHOIS) trial group. *N Engl J Med*. 2005. 352: 2477-2486.
5. Starikov R, Dudley D, Reddy UM. Stillbirth in the pregnancy complicated by diabetes.*Curr Diab Rep*. 2015. 15(3):11.
6. Rosenstein MG, Cheng YW, Snowden JM, et al. The risk of stillbirth and infant death stratified by gestational age in women with gestational diabetes. *Am J Obstet Gynecol*. 2012. 206(4):309 e1-7.
7. Alberico S, Erenbourg A, Hod M, et al. Immediate delivery or expectant management in gestational diabetes at term: The GINEXMAL randomised controlled trial. *BJOG*. 2017. 124(4): 669-77.
8. Luo R, Wen W, Corsi DJ, et al. Comparison of adverse maternal and perinatal outcomes between induction and expectant management among women with gestational diabetes mellitus at term pregnancy: A systematic review and meta-analysis. *BMC Pregnancy Childbirth*. 2023. 23(1):509.
9. NICE Guideline No. 3. Diabetes in pregnancy: management from preconception to the postnatal period. London: National Institute for Health and Care Excellence (NICE). 2020. Available from: https://www.ncbi.nlm.nih.gov/books/NBK555331/.
10. Ornoy A, Becker M, Weinstein-Fudim L, Ergaz Z. Diabetes during pregnancy: A maternal disease complicating the course of pregnancy with long-term deleterious effects on the offspring. A Clinical Review. *Int J Mo Sci*. 2021. 22, 2965.
11. American College of Obstetricians and Gynecologists' Committee on Practice Bulletins—Obstetrics. ACOG Practice Bulletin No. 201: Pregestational Diabetes Mellitus. *Obstet Gynecol*. 2018. 132:e228. Reaffirmed 2023.
12. American College of Obstetricians and Gynecologists' Committee on Obstetric Practice, Society for Maternal-Fetal Medicine. Medically Indicated Late-Preterm and Early-Term Deliveries: ACOG Committee Opinion. Number 831. *Obstet Gynecol*. 2021. 138:e35.

13. Ecker JL, Powe CE. Pregestational (preexisting) diabetes mellitus: Obstetric issues and management. Werner EF (Ed). *UpToDate*. 2022. Waltham, MA.
14. American College of Obstetricians and Gynecologists. Gestational Diabetes Mellitus. ACOG Practice Bulletin No. 190. *Obstet Gynecol*. 2018. 131. e49–e64.
15. Kjos SL, Henry OA, Montoro M, Buchanan TA, Mestman JH. Insulin-requiring diabetes in pregnancy: A randomized trial of active induction of labor and expectant management. *Am J Obstet Gynecol*. 1993. 169:611–615.
16. Luri S, Insler V, Hagay ZJ. Induction of labor at 38 to 39 weeks of gestation reduces the incidence of shoulder dystocia in gestational diabetic patients class A2. *Am J Perinatol*. 1996. 13:293–6.
17. Witkop CT, Neale D, Wilson LM, et al. Active compared with expectant delivery management in women with gestational diabetes: A systematic review. *Obstet Gynecol*. 2009. 113:206–17.
18. Melamed N, Ray JG, Geary M, et al. Induction of labor before 40 weeks is associated with lower rate of cesarean delivery in women with gestational diabetes mellitus. *Am J Obstet Gynecol*. 2016. 214:364.e1–8.
19. Niu B, Lee VR, Cheng YW, Frias AE, Nicholson JM, Caughey AB. What is the optimal gestational age for women with gestational diabetes type A1 to deliver? *Am J Obstet Gynecol*. 2014. 211(4):418.e1-6.
20. Li X, Li TT, Tian RX, et al. Gestational diabetes mellitus: The optimal time of delivery. *World J Diabetes*. 2023. 14(3):179-187.
21. FOGSI Endocrinology Committee guidelines on Gestational Diabetes. March 2021.Available at https://www.fogsi.org/wp-content/uploads/committee-2020-activities/vol-17-endocrinology-committee-newsletter.pdf.
22. Diagnosis & Management of Gestational Diabetes Mellitus Technical Guidelines. Maternal Health Division. MoHFW, Government of India. Available at https://nhm.gov.in/New_Updates_2018/NHM_Components/RMNCH_MH_Guidelines/Gestational-Diabetes-Mellitus.pdf.
23. SOGC Clinical Practice Guideline| No. 393. Diabetes in Pregnancy. 2019 (replaces No. 334, July 2016). JOGC. Volume 41. Issue 12, P1814-1825.E1.
24. Matheisen ER, Christensen AB, Hellmuth E, et al. Insulin dose during glucocorticoid treatment for fetal lung maturation in diabetic pregnancy: Test of an algorithm. *Acta Obstet Gynecol Scand*. 2002. 81:835-9.
25. Phaloprakarn C, Tangjitgamol S. Risk score for predicting primary cesarean delivery in women with gestational diabetes mellitus. *BMC Pregnancy Childbirth*. 2020. 20, 607.
26. Mimouni F, Miodovnik M, Siddiqi TA, Khoury J, Tsang RC. Perinatal asphyxia in infants of insulin-dependent diabetic women. *J Pediatr*. 1988. 113(2):345-53.
27. Management of glycaemic control in pregnant women with diabetes on obstetric wards and delivery units. Joint British Diabetes Societies for inpatient care guideline (JBDS-IP). 2017.
28. Ringholm L, Stougaard EB, Nørgaard SK, et al. Diabetes management during breastfeeding in women with type 1 diabetes. *Curr Diab Rep*. 2020. 20:34.
29. Ley SH, Chavarro JE, Li M, et al. Lactation duration and long-term risk for incident type 2 diabetes in women with a history of gestational diabetes mellitus. *Diabetes Care*. 2020. 43:793.

CHAPTER 39

Other Medical Disorders

Cardiac Disorders, Antiphospholipid Syndrome, Hepatic Disorders, and Epilepsy

TARAKESWARI S

INTRODUCTION

The process of labour and delivery affects maternal physiology in a number of ways that must be given due consideration while managing women with medical disorders. Upgraded diagnostic modalities and improved treatment plans have resulted in an increase in the cohort of pregnant women with identified medical comorbidities. It is essential to know how to provide intrapartum care for this vulnerable group.

Women with cardiac disease, known cases of antiphospholipid antibody syndrome (APS), women with hepatic disorders, and women with epilepsy (WWE) form the majority of complicated pregnancies encountered in practice. A management plan should be in place in each institution to handle such pregnancies. Communication with the couple should be clear and transparent, and they should be involved in the decision-making process.

This chapter outlines the management principles in labour and delivery for women with the above-mentioned disorders.

CARDIAC DISORDERS

CARDIAC DISEASE AND PHYSIOLOGY OF LABOUR

Women with underlying cardiac diseases may tolerate the hemodynamic changes of pregnancy poorly. During pregnancy, there are several gradual changes in the performance of the heart and circulation. However, the intrapartum period and early postpartum period (including the first hours and days after birth) can result in changes that can lead to a sudden deterioration in cardiac function. It is important that investigations are undertaken and acted upon immediately.

Changes in Cardiac Output in Labour

During labour, cardiac output (CO) progressively increases due to pain, anxiety, and autotransfusion. With each contraction, the stroke volume (SV) and heart rate (HR) rise and fall, with peaks as high as 30–50% above prelabour values. Further, during the second stage of labour, with maternal bearing down efforts, there is increased intrathoracic pressure, resulting in decreased venous return, decreased preload, and decreased CO.

Immediately after delivery, whether vaginal or cesarean, CO peaks as the pressure of the pregnant uterus on the inferior vena cava is relieved. The evacuated uterus contracts, and blood from the myometrial veins is autotransfused into the systemic venous system, resulting in greater venous blood return to the heart, which increases the stroke volume [1].

INTRAPARTUM MANAGEMENT

Managing a pregnant woman with cardiovascular disease requires a cardio-obstetric team involving obstetricians, cardiologists, anesthesiologists, maternal–fetal medicine specialists, and neonatologists, preferably at a tertiary–care centre [2].

It is best to discuss the delivery plan with the woman and her partner between 20 and 30 weeks of pregnancy. The cardio-obstetric team should be involved in the decision-making process so that the chosen plan is the safest for the woman [3]. If necessary, plans should be made to transfer the woman to a tertiary-care centre closer to term.

The delivery plan should include additional planning for emergency cesarean delivery, emergency preterm delivery, postpartum hemorrhage, and management of cardiopulmonary complications or cardiac arrest. As pregnancy progresses, the plan should be updated according to evolving factors such as fetal growth and maternal adaptation to pregnancy.

The key management issues in a woman with heart disease are as follows:

- Risk assessment
- Timing of delivery: Induction vs. spontaneous
- Mode of delivery: Vaginal birth vs. cesarean
- Managing anticoagulation
- Effective analgesia
- Optimising hemodynamics: Reducing the effect of tachycardia and increased cardiac output in labour
- Endocarditis prophylaxis
- Management of the third stage: Postpartum hemorrhage (PPH) prophylaxis and management

Risk Assessment

For women with heart disease, the intrapartum risk should be reassessed regularly during pregnancy and the intrapartum period using all of the following modalities [1]:

- Comprehensive clinical assessment, including history and physical examination
- The modified World Health Organization (WHO) classification of risk, which is considered the best predictive model for cardiovascular risk (Table 39.1)
- The New York Heart Association (NYHA) functional class (Table 39.2)

Table 39.1 The modified World Health Organization classification of maternal cardiovascular risk

Class	Risk
Class I	Very low
Class II	Low to moderate
Class III	High risk
Class IV	Extremely high risk

Table 39.2 The New York Heart Association (NYHA) Functional Classification based on limitations of physical activity

Class	Symptoms
I	No limitation of physical activity. Ordinary physical activity does not cause undue fatigue, palpitation, or shortness of breath.
II	Slight limitation of physical activity. Comfortable at rest. Ordinary physical activity results in fatigue, palpitation, shortness of breath, or chest pain.
III	Marked limitation of physical activity. Comfortable at rest. Less than ordinary activity causes fatigue, palpitation, shortness of breath, or chest pain.
IV	Symptoms of heart failure at rest. Any physical activity causes further discomfort.

Timing of Birth

The timing of delivery should be individualised after weighing maternal, obstetric, and fetal risks, and should include inputs from the cardio-obstetrics team. For pregnant women with stable cardiac disease, the ACOG recommends elective induction of labour between 39 and 40 weeks of gestation if there are no other associated maternal/fetal comorbidities [3].

For pregnant women with a mechanical heart valve and no other complication, the Society for Maternal-Fetal Medicine (SMFM) recommends a planned delivery between 37 and 38 weeks of gestation [4].

For women with WHO class IV cardiac conditions, the timing of delivery should be decided on a case-by-case basis by the cardio-obstetric team.

Spontaneous labour versus induction of labour

For most women with heart disease who are functionally normal or well-controlled, spontaneous onset of labour is preferred over induced labour [5]. When induction of labour is considered due to concerns about the functional adequacy of the heart and circulation, it should be carried out under controlled conditions. Cervical ripening with PGE2 or mechanical means can be followed by oxytocin augmentation. The induction should be planned so that the delivery occurs during the day with all the team members being available.

Mode of Birth

In general, vaginal delivery is the preferred mode of delivery unless there is an obstetric or specific cardiac indication for cesarean section. It should be determined beforehand which women are not candidates for vaginal delivery and those who will require an assisted second stage of labour.

In the case of **mechanical heart valves**, planned cesarean section or induction of labour should be offered in order to minimise the time without anticoagulation. However, this also needs to be balanced with the risks of bleeding around the time of birth [1].

Vaginal delivery

Management of the first stage of labour

Women with significant cardiovascular disease should be placed in a semi-recumbent position with a lateral tilt during the intrapartum period. Vital signs should be assessed frequently. Cardiac decompensation may mandate the initiation of intensive medical management.

Fluid management and hemodynamic monitoring

The management plan for monitoring should be drawn up in the antenatal period. Changes in blood pressure, blood volume, and fluid shifts during labour and birth, and the type of monitoring needed to manage these should be given due consideration. The American Society of Anesthesiologists recommends the following [6]:

- Intake of moderate amounts of clear fluids throughout labour to avoid dehydration
- Maintaining adequate intravascular volume (preload)

Women with mild heart disease (modified WHO I and NYHA class I): The intrapartum hemodynamic monitoring would be the same as for any other woman [1].

Women with modified WHO III and IV heart disease: Intrapartum hemodynamic monitoring should include the following:

- Hourly monitoring of fluid intake and output (or at least 4-hourly)
- Vitals—blood pressure, pulse, respiratory rate, and oxygen saturation to be monitored intensively
- Continuous electrocardiogram (ECG)
- Continuous intra-arterial blood pressure monitoring
- Cardiac output monitoring with non-invasive techniques
- Serial echocardiography

Anesthesia and analgesia

Effective regional analgesia is an important element in the management plan to enhance hemodynamic stability (minimising catecholamine release and resultant cardiac output fluctuations) [6].

- Women with milder forms of cardiac disease such as the modified WHO I or II risk category, should be offered labour analgesia/anesthesia as per routine protocols for other healthy women.
- Regional anesthesia/analgesia should be given preference for women with modified WHO class III and IV heart disease.
- Women with left ventricular outflow tract obstruction or cyanotic congenital heart disease must be given modified neuraxial anesthesia due to the risk of cardiovascular decompensation related to the reduction of systemic vascular resistance [3].

- For a woman on anticoagulation with low-molecular-weight heparin (LMWH), the timing of regional analgesia, including the insertion and removal of a catheter, is summarised in Table 39.3.

Management of the second stage of labour

Maternal pushing efforts must be avoided since they are associated with unwanted circulatory effects. The advantage of epidural analgesia for women with cardiac disease is the descent of the fetal head due to uterine contractions alone, without active maternal pushing efforts. The second stage should be cut short by a low or outlet operative vaginal delivery (either forceps or vacuum extraction) when the fetal head reaches the pelvic floor.

Key Point

Maternal pushing efforts must be avoided, and the second stage should be cut short with the help of an assisted vaginal birth.

Table 39.3 **Timing of regional analgesia for a woman on anticoagulation [4]**

Action	Low-molecular-weight heparin (LMWH)	Timing to avoid epidural hematoma
Regional analgesia initiation	Prophylactic dose	≥12 h after the last dose
	Therapeutic dose	≥24 h after the last dose
Epidural catheter removal	On LMWH	10–12 h after the last dose
Resuming anticoagulation	Next dose	• 4 h after removal • Therapeutic dose of LMWH should not be administered while epidural catheter is in place

Management of the third stage of labour

Uterotonics: Oxytocin decreases the mean arterial pressure and total peripheral vascular resistance and possibly causes a slight increase in pulmonary artery pressure [8]. It should not be administered IV **as a bolus** in women with cardiovascular disease, especially cardiovascular lesions with limited or fixed low cardiac output or preload-dependent circulation (as in cases of aortic stenosis, hypertrophic obstructive cardiomyopathy, ischemic heart disease, or aortic aneurysm with risk of dissection) [9].

Carboprost tromethamine is to be avoided in women with an intracardiac shunt because it causes bronchospasm which may increase shunting and alterations in the ventilation/perfusion ratio, resulting in hypoxemia and decreased cardiac output [10].

Methergine is contraindicated in women with any cardiac disease [11] because it causes vasoconstriction leading to sudden systemic hypertension. It can also cause coronary vasospasm as well as an increase in pulmonary arterial pressure.

Cesarean delivery

Cesarean delivery is performed for obstetric indications. Cardiac conditions where cesarean section is recommended as the best option for delivery include the following [1,12]:

- Aortic root dilatation—progressive enlargement or >4.5 cm
- Severe peripartum cardiomyopathy/severe left ventricular dysfunction
- Aortic dissection
- NYHA class III or IV heart disease
- Pulmonary arterial hypertension

Key Point

To avoid sudden hemodynamic changes, in the postpartum period, a slow infusion of oxytocin (at a rate of 2.5–7.5 IU/hour for elective cesarean delivery or 7.5–15 IU/hour for intrapartum cesarean delivery) is recommended.

Bacterial Endocarditis Prophylaxis

Infective endocarditis prophylaxis is **not recommended** for women with acquired or congenital structural heart disease for either vaginal or cesarean delivery according to the guidelines issued by the American Heart Association and the American College of Cardiology [7]. The small subset of women who require prophylaxis for bacterial endocarditis are those with:

- Cyanotic cardiac disease
- Prosthetic valves

If a woman is already receiving intrapartum antibiotic therapy for another indication that would also provide coverage against endocarditis, separate antibiotic coverage for endocarditis is not required.

Special Situations

Women with mechanical heart valves

In a woman with a mechanical heart valve, the anticoagulation management is a double-edged sword. She is prone to thrombosis if inadequately anticoagulated, but vulnerable to excessive bleeding if she receives too much anticoagulation. Either can lead to devastating and potentially fatal incidents for the woman and her baby. It is, therefore, important that planning for the management of anticoagulation during the intrapartum period starts when pregnancy is confirmed. The following are the general recommendations for managing anticoagulation.

- **Women on warfarin** in the second and third trimesters of pregnancy [4]:
  - Transition to dose-adjusted LMWH at 35–36 weeks of gestation (with planned delivery at 37–38 weeks of gestation)
  - Bridge anticoagulation with IV unfractionated heparin (UFH) in an inpatient setting 36–48 hours before planned delivery
- **Women on dose-adjusted LMWH** in the second and third trimesters of pregnancy [4]:
  - Transition to IV UFH in an inpatient setting 36–48 hours before planned induction/delivery
  - IV UFH is usually started 12 hours after the discontinuation of LMWH
    - Continued until 4–6 hours before a planned cesarean section
    - Continued until active labour (6 cm cervical dilation in most cases) and then stopped in the case of a vaginal delivery

Anticoagulation immediately postdelivery

The European Society of Cardiology (ESC) guidelines recommend reintroducing therapeutic anticoagulation 4–6 hours after birth [13]. The risk of peripartum mechanical heart valve thrombosis is higher in pregnancy and is of greater consequence than the increased risk of uterine hemorrhage with earlier reintroduction of anticoagulation. A switch over to warfarin should be considered not before 5–7 days after birth [13].

Anticoagulation reversal in emergency situations

In the event of an urgent need to deliver a fully anticoagulated woman, **warfarin** may be reversed with prothrombinase complex concentrates and vitamin K, and **heparin** and **LMWH** with protamine sulphate. Protamine sulphate only partially reverses the anticoagulant effect of LMWH [14,15].

In cases of therapeutic anticoagulation with warfarin within the last two weeks in women who need urgent delivery, a cesarean delivery is recommended to avoid fatal complications related to therapeutic anticoagulation with warfarin [4].

Women with acute myocardial infarction

Myocardial infarction (MI) is the irreversible necrosis of the heart muscle secondary to prolonged ischemia. In pregnancy, there is a 3- to 4-fold increase in the risk of myocardial infarction (MI) compared with non-pregnant women of comparable age.

- In women with a recent history of percutaneous coronary intervention (PCI), details of the revascularisation procedure with regard to lesion location, stent type (drug-eluting or bare-metal), and date of intervention should be documented.

- Dual antiplatelet drugs (aspirin and clopidogrel) that are mandatory following acute MI require modification before labour.
- It is always better to delay delivery for at least 2–3 weeks after acute MI [16].
- The mode of delivery should be individualised depending on obstetric and clinical factors. In women on clopidogrel and women with intractable heart failure, a cesarean delivery is preferred. In the first 48 hours of the postpartum period, monitoring should be conducted in a coronary care unit.

Heart failure in the intrapartum period

Symptoms suggestive of heart failure (in the absence of another likely cause) include the following:

- Breathlessness when lying down (after ruling out aortocaval compression) or at rest
- Unexplained cough, particularly when lying down or when it produces frothy, pink sputum
- Paroxysmal nocturnal dyspnea—being woken from sleep by severe breathlessness and coughing, which may produce pink, frothy sputum and is improved by moving to an upright position
- Palpitation (awareness of persistent fast heart rate at rest)

Signs suggestive of heart failure include the following:

- Paleness, sweating, agitation with cool peripheries
- Heart rate persistently >110 beats per minute at rest
- Respiratory rate persistently >20 breaths per minute at rest
- Hypotension (systolic blood pressure <100 mmHg)
- Oxygen saturation <95% on air
- Elevated jugular venous pressure
- Added murmur or heart sound
- Reduced air entry, basal crackles, or wheezing on listening to the chest

When clinical examination raises the suspicion of heart failure, imaging and blood tests are needed to assist the review by a cardiologist or the most senior available clinician to make a definitive diagnosis.

ANTIPHOSPHOLIPID SYNDROME (APS)

IMPLICATIONS FOR LABOUR AND DELIVERY

Antiphospholipid syndrome is an autoimmune, systemic disorder characterised by the presence of clinical features of vascular thrombosis (venous or arterial) and/or specific adverse pregnancy outcomes in the presence of specified levels of circulating antiphospholipid antibodies (APLA).

There are two major categories of APS from the management point of view:

- APS without prior thrombosis
- APS with prior thrombosis

The key challenges in the management of APS in labour and delivery are the following:

- Timing, mode, and management of delivery
- Anticoagulation
- Analgesia

Like with many medical conditions in pregnancy, a multidisciplinary approach involving a rheumatologist, an obstetrician experienced in high-risk care, and a fetal medicine specialist, is necessary for a successful pregnancy outcome in a woman with APS. The involvement of a nephrologist in case of associated comorbidities such as systemic lupus erythematosus (SLE) nephritis, or a pediatric cardiologist in cases of fetal heart block, is recommended.

This chapter will deal exclusively with the management of a woman with APS in labour and delivery.

TIMING AND MODE OF DELIVERY

Timing

In a pregnancy with APS, the management plans should be individualised. With uncomplicated APS, planned delivery (induction or cesarean) can be considered at term (at 39 weeks of gestation). This allows sufficient time to reverse the effects of anticoagulation.

However, women who have had a previous pregnancy loss due to APS may be delivered at any time after 37 weeks if there are no complications in the current pregnancy. Earlier delivery may be considered in women with complications such as the following:

- Preeclampsia
- Fetal growth restriction (FGR)
- Oligohydramnios
- Chronic hypertension
- Connective tissue disorder
- Renal disease
- Previous history of thrombosis

Mode of Delivery

Vaginal delivery is the preferred mode of delivery because a cesarean section would add to the risk of venous thromboembolism (VTE). Cesarean section should be reserved for obstetric indications or for women who present in an emergency while on full anticoagulation.

INTRAPARTUM MANAGEMENT OF ANTICOAGULATION

The approach to the management of anticoagulation in labour and delivery is dependent on the indication for anticoagulation and the type of anticoagulant medication.

Therapeutic Low-Molecular-Weight Heparin (LMWH)

This is also referred to as the weight-adjusted, full-treatment dose and is administered to women with a previous history of arterial or venous thrombosis, **with or without APS-defining pregnancy morbidity.** These women are at a high risk of recurrent thrombosis [17]. The risk of hemorrhage resulting from anticoagulation is low.

Either of the following drugs may be used:

- **Enoxaparin** 1 mg/Kg every 12 hours
- **Dalteparin** 200 units/Kg once daily **or** 100 units/Kg every 12 hours

Women receiving therapeutic anticoagulation

Women receiving therapeutic LMWH are generally switched to therapeutic doses of UFH at 36–37 weeks' gestation since UFH has a shorter half-life. This allows for the administration of neuraxial anesthesia and minimises delivery-related bleeding if spontaneous labour occurs in the late preterm or early term period.

- Anesthesia guidelines recommend at least a 24-hour interval between the last dose of therapeutic dose LMWH and the placement of an epidural catheter (Table 39.3).
- Therapeutic UFH therapy is discontinued 24 hours before labour and delivery to allow for the administration of neuraxial anesthesia and minimise delivery-related bleeding. A normal aPTT should be verified prior to administering an epidural.
- This approach generally ensures that women with prior thrombosis are not off anticoagulants for more than 48 hours.

Prophylactic LMWH

The following doses are recommended:

- **Enoxaparin** 40 mg SC once daily
- **Dalteparin** 5000 units SC once daily

These doses may need to be modified at the extremes of body weight.

Management of women receiving prophylactic anticoagulation

Woman with a previous adverse pregnancy outcome

In these circumstances, LMWH can be discontinued at 34–37 weeks' gestation unless there are risk factors for venous thromboembolism, in which case, it can be discontinued 12 hours prior to planned induction or cesarean, or at the onset of labour.

Woman with APS with other risk factors for VTE and no history of arterial or venous thrombosis

These women may be advised to discontinue LMWH 12 hours prior to planned induction or cesarean, or at the onset of labour. This ensures that for planned delivery, there is at least a 12-hour window to allow for the siting of regional anesthesia or analgesia.

If this plan is adopted, particularly in a multiparous woman in whom the onset of spontaneous labour is awaited, she may not be able to receive epidural analgesia if she goes into labour within 12 hours of her last dose of LMWH. This possibility should be discussed with the woman if she has planned to receive epidural analgesia in labour.

If a cesarean is required <12 hours after the last dose of LMWH, it will need to be performed under general anesthesia instead of regional block to avoid the risk of bleeding.

Analgesia for women on anticoagulation

For a woman on anticoagulation with LMWH, the timing of regional analgesia, including the insertion and removal of the catheter, is the same as that in women with artificial valves on anticoagulation (Table 39.3).

POSTPARTUM MANAGEMENT OF ANTICOAGULATION

Women With No Risk Factors for VTE

Anticoagulation can be discontinued after delivery for women with APS who have no risk factors for VTE, no previous history of VTE, and no inherited thrombophilia.

Women With Risk Factors for VTE or History of Thrombotic Event

Anticoagulation can generally be resumed 4–6 hours after vaginal delivery or 6–12 hours after cesarean delivery unless there is significant bleeding or a risk for significant bleeding. If heparin is contraindicated because of heparin-induced thrombocytopenia (HIT), which occurs rarely in pregnancy, then danaparoid or fondaparinux are reasonable options [18].

For women with APS who have had a previous thrombotic event, prophylactic anticoagulation with heparin should be continued till six weeks postpartum [19]. This prophylaxis can be safely accomplished with vitamin K antagonists such as warfarin [20].

For long-term management postpartum, women with APS should be referred to a physician with expertise in the treatment of the syndrome, such as an internist, hematologist, or rheumatologist.

Key Point

LMWH should be restarted within 4–6 hours postpartum and continued for six weeks in the case of previous VTE, hereditary thrombophilia with a family history, or sickle cell disease [12].

SPECIAL CONSIDERATIONS

APS with Thrombocytopenia

The prevalence of thrombocytopenia is between 30 and 46% among women with APS [21]. The mechanism of thrombocytopenia in APS is not clearly known; it is thought to result from the binding of antiphospholipid antibodies to platelets and the formation of thrombus by the promotion of platelet activation and aggregation along with the immune-mediated clearance of platelets.

Thrombocytopenia associated with APS is usually mild and is typically associated not with hemorrhagic complications, but with thrombotic events. Other causes of thrombocytopenia should be excluded. As thrombocytopenia in APS predicts thrombosis at a later time, women may be given platelet aggregation inhibitors and/or anticoagulant therapy. Thromboprophylaxis should be stopped only in cases of severe thrombocytopenia.

HEPATIC DISORDERS

IMPACT OF HEPATIC DISEASE ON PREGNANCY

Hepatic diseases in pregnancy have a varied spectrum ranging from the asymptomatic elevation of liver enzymes to severe deterioration of liver function that can result in maternal and fetal morbidity and mortality.

Many of the physiological and hormonal changes that occur in pregnancy mimic those seen in women with cirrhosis and portal hypertension. The clinical consequences of these changes are the development of de novo or worsening varices, ascites, or hepatic encephalopathy which will impact intrapartum care and management plans.

As with other medical comorbidities in pregnancy, a multidisciplinary approach is essential, including maternal–fetal medicine specialists, anesthetists, neonatologists, and hepatologists. A thorough evaluation including a detailed history, physical exam, and focused serological workup should be performed as indicated by the clinical presentation.

This section will deal with the following:

- Hepatic diseases unique to pregnancy
  - — Intrahepatic cholestasis of pregnancy (ICP)
  - — Acute fatty liver of pregnancy (AFLP)
  - — Preeclampsia with severe features/ HELLP (hemolysis, elevated liver enzymes, low platelet count) syndrome
- Coincident hepatic diseases
  - — Acute viral hepatitis A and E
- Chronic hepatic diseases exacerbated by pregnancy
  - — Hepatitis B
  - — Hepatitis C
  - — Cirrhosis and portal hypertension
  - — Fulminant hepatic failure in pregnancy

HEPATIC DISEASES UNIQUE TO PREGNANCY

Intrahepatic Cholestasis of Pregnancy (ICP)

ICP is a multifactorial condition, affecting 0.4–10% of pregnancies [22]. It is characterised by generalised pruritus, most severe in the palms and soles, in the absence of a primary skin condition, with abnormal maternal bile acid concentrations [23,24].

Management of delivery in a woman with ICP

Studies have shown an association between raised total bile acid concentrations and adverse outcomes and stillbirth. The risk of stillbirth increases with increasing serum total bile acid levels, especially at ≥100 micromol/L [25].

Timing of delivery

Planned delivery between 36+0 weeks and 38+6 weeks of gestation

Early delivery is recommended to reduce the risk of stillbirth and to relieve the woman of severe pruritus [26]. The timing of delivery can be decided based on the total bilirubin concentration (Table 39.4).

Indications for delivery before 36 weeks

In some cases of ICP, delivery prior to 36 weeks may be indicated if:

- Maternal pruritus is extremely distressing and is not responding to medication
- Jaundice is present
- Fetal demise occurred in a previous pregnancy before 36 weeks due to ICP
- Total serum bile acid concentration is ≥100 micromol/L

Table 39.4 Recommended timing of delivery based on total bilirubin concentration

Total bilirubin concentration	Timing of delivery	Monitoring during labour
<40 micromol/L	Planned birth at 37+0 to 38+6 weeks of gestation	Intrapartum care can follow institutional policy
40–99 micromol/L and no other risk factors	Planned birth at 36+0 to 37+0 weeks of gestation	Intrapartum care can follow institutional policy
≥100 micromol/L	Planned birth at ≤36+0 weeks of gestation	Continuous electronic fetal monitoring should be offered, if available

Mode of delivery

Vaginal delivery may certainly be attempted in cases of cholestasis in pregnancy. ICP by itself is not an indication for elective cesarean section, which is performed only for obstetric indications [23,24,25].

> **Key Point**
>
> Women with moderate and severe ICP are more likely to have meconium-stained liquor. This will influence the need for continuous electronic monitoring in labour.

The rest of the intrapartum management, including analgesia and management of the second and third stages of labour, should follow routine protocols.

Special considerations

Follow-up

Women with ICP should be followed-up for at least four weeks postpartum. This is recommended to confirm the resolution of liver function test abnormalities. In the presence of persistent symptoms or gross liver function derangement, the follow-up should be sooner [22].

Contraception

- Estrogen–progestin contraceptives with low-dose estrogen may be prescribed to women with a history of ICP since the contraceptive rarely results in recurrent cholestasis [26]. Liver function tests should be performed after three to six months of such contraception.
- Progestin-only pills may be prescribed to women who develop pruritus or cholestasis after using combined estrogen-containing contraceptives.

Acute Fatty Liver of Pregnancy (AFLP)

This is considered an obstetric emergency that may result in severe morbidity and possible mortality for both the mother and the fetus. It is characterised by maternal liver dysfunction which may lead to fulminant hepatic failure.

Early recognition, prompt delivery, and supportive care are essential to optimise maternal and fetal prognosis. If hepatic function does not rapidly improve, in rare situations, the woman may need to be evaluated for liver transplantation, which may be the best chance for her survival.

Management of delivery

When the diagnosis of acute fatty liver of pregnancy is confirmed, immediate delivery should be planned.

Route of delivery

This depends on the rate and degree of maternal/fetal decompensation and the probability of successful vaginal birth.

Vaginal delivery may be attempted, and labour can be induced if the following conditions are met:

- Fetal status is reassuring
- Vaginal birth is likely to be accomplished within 24 hours
- The disease is not rapidly progressing within that time frame

Cervical ripening agents can be used for an unfavourable cervix.

Cesarean delivery is indicated in the following situations:

- A successful vaginal birth is unlikely within 24 hours
- There is rapidly progressing maternal/fetal decompensation

A recent review found the cesarean delivery rate to be 66.7% in AFLP [27]. A multidisciplinary team in a tertiary centre should be involved in this situation. The woman's condition should be stabilised before surgery, with special attention given to correcting any coagulopathy.

Postpartum management

The postpartum clinical course depends on the interval between the onset of symptoms and the termination of pregnancy. The infant should be monitored for manifestations of deficiency of long-chain 3-hydroxyacyl-coenzyme A dehydrogenase, including hypoketotic hypoglycemia and fatty liver.

Preeclampsia with Severe Features/ HELLP Syndrome

See **Chapter 37,** *The hypertensive woman in labour,* for further details.

COINCIDENT HEPATIC DISEASES

Acute Hepatic Viral Infections A and E

The incidence of viral hepatitis A is the same in pregnancy as it is for the general population, but the incidence of hepatitis E is much higher in pregnancy.

Hepatitis A infection is caused by the hepatitis A virus (HAV) and per se is not an indication for delivery. However, it has been associated with preterm labour and premature rupture of membranes [22]. Labour management is supportive, with adherence to routine protocols. Women should be tested for HAV-IgM since vertical transmission of HAV has been reported, even leading to outbreaks within neonatal care units. HAV immunoglobulin treatment is recommended for the neonate if the maternal HAV infection occurs within two weeks of delivery [22].

Hepatitis E infection is caused by hepatitis E virus (HEV). It is more easily acquired and has more adverse effects in pregnancy than in the non-pregnant state. Mortality is high among HEV-positive pregnant women due to diminished cellular immunity and a high level of endogenous steroid hormones. However, this will not change the decision regarding the timing or mode of delivery. Treatment is supportive. There is a risk of progression to acute liver failure and the need for liver transplantation evaluation in some cases.

CHRONIC HEPATIC DISEASES, CIRRHOSIS, AND LIVER TRANSPLANTATION

Hepatitis B

Pregnancy provides an important opportunity to identify hepatitis B virus (HBV)-infected women and implement measures to prevent mother-to-child transmission (MTCT). Hence, testing for hepatitis B surface antigen (HbsAg) is a part of routine antenatal screening, and is performed even if the woman has been vaccinated [28].

Timing and mode of delivery

Chronic hepatitis B has little influence on the course of pregnancy. The timing and mode of delivery would be as per obstetric indications. Cesarean section should not be performed electively in HBV-positive mothers for the sole purpose of preventing MTCT.

> **Key Point**
>
> A woman infected with HBV is highly infectious to anyone handling her bodily fluids. Standard universal precautions should be taken to prevent contamination and acquired infection.

Reducing the risk of MTCT

Women who are HbsAg-positive and have a high HBV DNA load have an increased risk of MTCT. The greatest risk factor for MTCT is the presence of maternal HbeAg.

Quantification of HBV DNA should be done in the second trimester, and if maternal HBV DNA is >200,000 IU/mL, antiviral therapy should be started between 28 and 32 weeks' gestation [29]. Starting antiviral treatment with tenofovir disoproxil fumarate (TDF) in the third trimester reduces MTCT from 18% to 5%.

Immunoprophylaxis for infants

Perinatal transmission is prevented by providing active and passive immunoprophylaxis to all infants born to HBV-infected mothers. This includes the administration of hepatitis B immunoglobulin (HBIG) and hepatitis B vaccination immediately after birth (within 12 h), followed by two additional doses of the vaccine within 6–12 months, thus preventing transmission in 95% of babies.

Breastfeeding

There is no contraindication to breastfeeding, even in the presence of cracked or bleeding nipples as the infant is protected by immunoprophylaxis [22].

Hepatitis C (HCV)

HCV testing is not a part of routine screening in pregnant women. Only those with risk factors such as previous blood transfusions, history of injectable drug abuse, and high-risk professions such as healthcare providers need to be screened.

Delivery and prevention of MTCT

The timing and mode of delivery should be as per obstetric indications. Cesarean section is not indicated electively in HCV-positive women for the sole purpose of preventing fetal infection. The risk of MTCT in HCV is 3–10% at the time of birth with the risk being higher in women with HIV coinfection. However, there is no treatment strategy to mitigate this risk.

Intrapartum management should avoid the prolonged rupture of membranes (>6 hours), invasive fetal monitoring, and unindicated episiotomies [30].

Breastfeeding is not contraindicated in HCV infection. However, it should be avoided when the potential risk for exposure is higher, e.g., in the presence of cracked nipples or skin breakdown [22,30].

Cirrhosis and Portal Hypertension

Pregnancy is not common in women with cirrhosis. However, when it does occur, it is associated with a higher risk of pregnancy-related complications. The most common etiology of cirrhosis in the childbearing age is non-alcohol-associated fatty liver disease (NAFLD) [31].

The following are the key concerns in these women:

- Variceal bleeding
- Thrombocytopenia
- Anticoagulation treatment adjustments

To ensure a good outcome, a multidisciplinary team including a maternal–fetal medicine specialist, hepatologist, and vascular surgeon should be available.

Timing and mode of delivery

The decisions regarding delivery should be guided by obstetric indications [22].

- The increase in intra-abdominal pressure during vaginal delivery might increase portal pressure and the risk of variceal rupture. Assisted vaginal delivery to minimise straining and shorten the second stage of labour can reduce this risk.
- Cesarean delivery may increase the risk of bleeding from direct injury to abdominal wall varices and the risk of postpartum ascites [32]. For cesarean delivery, platelet counts should generally be >50,000/mL. In some cases where there is uncontrolled bleeding from the collaterals, vascular surgical assistance may be needed.
- Active management of the third stage of labour will prevent postpartum hemorrhage.

Variceal bleeding

Variceal bleeding is the most frequent and feared complication of portal hypertension during pregnancy, with an increased risk at delivery. Pregnant women with suspected portal hypertension should undergo screening with upper endoscopy for esophageal varices in the second trimester. Those found to have large esophageal varices should be treated with beta-blockers and/or band ligation [22].

Fulminant Hepatic Failure in Pregnancy

Fulminant hepatic failure refers to the development of severe acute impairment of synthetic function (INR of ≥1.5) and an encephalopathy within eight weeks of the appearance of the first symptoms in a woman without a pre-existing liver disease.

Intrapartum management

The preferred mode of delivery is vaginal. In the presence of deranged coagulation, the INR should be kept at <2. Fresh frozen plasma (FFP) is given as a dose of 15 mL/Kg body weight (usually 3–4 units) stat followed by 2 units every eight hours till at least 24 hours after delivery. Massive FFP transfusion should be avoided.

EPILEPSY

Epilepsy is the most common neurological condition in pregnancy and is characterised by excessive neuronal discharge resulting in recurrent, unprovoked seizures [33]. The risk of intrapartum seizures in epilepsy is around 3.5% [42]. The primary goal in treating women with epilepsy (WWE) is adequate seizure control. The care of women with epilepsy in pregnancy and childbirth is of utmost importance [34].

Key Point

The risk of mortality for pregnant women with epilepsy is greater than any other single pre-existing medical condition and almost ten times higher than that of the general population [34].

RISK ASSESSMENT

Accurate documentation of the type of seizures and their frequency will help to identify any provoking factors and plan management [35].

TIMING AND MODE OF DELIVERY

There is no robust evidence on the optimal timing and mode of delivery for women with epilepsy [35].

In order to prevent convulsions during labour, proper seizure control should be achieved during the third trimester. Adequate analgesia, good hydration, compliance with antiepileptic drugs (AEDs), and avoidance of stress and hyperventilation are the principles of labour management in WWE [47].

Vaginal Birth

Vaginal birth at term is preferred. Epilepsy, per se, is not an indication for the induction of labour. However, there is an increased risk of fetal growth restriction in women on polytherapy with AEDs, and induction of labour may be indicated as per the protocols of the institution. There are no known contraindications to the use of any induction agents for women taking AEDs [35].

Management of the first stage

Psychological, hormonal, and pharmacokinetic changes in pregnancy and labour may escalate seizure activity. Seizures in labour lead to maternal hypoxia, resulting in fetal hypoxia and acidosis secondary to uterine hypertonus. Thus, seizures in labour need to be prevented. If they do occur, seizures must be treated promptly.

Women with epilepsy should be admitted in early labour and will require intravenous access. The labour and delivery room environment should be optimised with the lowering of light to encourage sleep. There should be one-to-one support by a labour companion to reduce the woman's stress.

Cesarean Delivery

Cesarean birth should be reserved for obstetric indications. In a small proportion of women with significant deterioration of seizures (recurrent and prolonged) and those who are at high risk of status epilepticus, elective cesarean section may be considered.

Analgesia and Anesthesia

Transcutaneous electrical nerve stimulation (TENS), nitrous oxide and oxygen (Entonox®) and regional analgesia (epidural, spinal, combined spinal–epidural) are all suitable and safe methods of analgesia in labour for women with epilepsy [35].

An epidural can be considered early in labour to minimise precipitating factors for seizures during labour such as hyperventilation, sleep deprivation, pain, and emotional stress. In fact, under epidural, the woman can be encouraged to sleep, especially during early labour.

Diamorphine should be used in preference to pethidine for analgesia in labour. Pethidine should be avoided or used with caution.

If general anesthesia becomes necessary, it is prudent to avoid anesthetic agents such as ketamine, pethidine, and sevoflurane. The first two are known to lower seizure threshold and the third may have epileptogenic potential [35].

AED Medications

Antiepileptic medications should be continued without missing a dose in the intrapartum stage. In case of excessive vomiting, parenteral alternatives must be considered.

Women at a very high risk of seizures can be managed with an additional benzodiazepine such as **clobazam** [36]. Prophylactic clobazam should be considered in the following cases:

- Recent convulsive seizures
- Recent history of seizure provocation by stress or sleep deprivation
- History of seizures in previous labour

The benefit of seizure prevention from clobazam needs to be balanced against the risks such as respiratory depression in the newborn.

Management of Seizures in Labour

Any seizure lasting more than five minutes is unusual and represents a high risk of progressing to convulsive status epilepticus, a life-threatening medical emergency which affects around 1% of pregnancies in women with epilepsy [49].

> **Key Point**
>
> Every obstetric unit should have written guidelines on the management of seizures in labour.

Maternal stabilisation

The following steps should be followed:

- Left lateral tilt (or manual displacement of the uterus) to reduce the risk of supine hypotension
- Oxygen administration to prevent hypoxia
- Prevention of aspiration by raising the head end of the table
- Tocolytic drugs may be administered if there is persistent uterine hypertonus
- Medications to control seizures
  - Lorazepam is the drug of choice in status epilepticus. It is given intravenously at the dose of 0.1 mg/Kg (usually a 4 mg bolus, with a further dose after 10–20 minutes).
  - Diazepam 5–10 mg administered slowly intravenously is an alternative. If there is no intravenous access, diazepam 10–20 mg may be administered rectally, and repeated once 15 minutes later.
  - If there is a continued risk of status epilepticus, midazolam 10 mg is administered as a buccal preparation.
  - If seizures are not controlled, the administration of phenytoin or fosphenytoin should be considered. The loading dose of phenytoin is 10–15 mg/Kg by intravenous infusion, with the usual dosage for an adult being approximately 1000 mg.

Management once the woman is stabilised

- Continuous electronic fetal monitoring should be maintained.
- Delivery should be considered if the fetal heart rate does not begin to recover within five minutes of the seizure or if the seizures are recurrent. This may require a cesarean delivery if vaginal delivery is not imminent.

Neonatal Care

The neonatal team should be kept informed of cases involving women with epilepsy, as there is a risk of neonatal withdrawal syndrome with the maternal use of benzodiazepines and AEDs [37]. All babies born to women taking enzyme-inducing AEDs should be given 1 mg of intramuscular vitamin K to prevent hemorrhagic disease of the newborn.

CONCLUSION

Women with cardiac disease, antiphospholipid antibody syndrome (APS), hepatic disorders, or epilepsy form the majority of complicated pregnancies encountered in practice. The joint efforts of a multidisciplinary team are essential to reduce the morbidity and mortality for both the woman and her baby.

REFERENCES

1. Intrapartum care for women with existing medical conditions or obstetric complications and their babies. National Institute for Health and Care Excellence (NICE), London. 2019. PMID: 31194308.
2. Mehta LS, Warnes CA, Bradley E, Burton T, Economy K, Mehran R, et al. Cardiovascular considerations in caring for pregnant women: A scientific statement from the American Heart Association. *Circulation*. 2020. 141:e884–e903.
3. ACOG Practice Bulletin No. 212: Pregnancy and Heart Disease. *Obstetrics & Gynecology*. 2019. 133(5):p e320-e356.
4. Pacheco LD, Saade G, Shrivastava V, et al. Publications Committee. Society for Maternal–Fetal Medicine Consult Series #61: Anticoagulation in pregnant women with cardiac disease. *Am J Obstet Gynecol*. 2022. 227(2):B28-B43.
5. European Society of Gynecology (ESG), Association for European Paediatric Cardiology (AEPC), German Society for Gender Medicine (DGesGM), et al. ESC Guidelines on the management of cardiovascular diseases during pregnancy: The Task Force on the Management of Cardiovascular Diseases during Pregnancy of the European Society of Cardiology (ESC). *Eur Heart J*. 2011. 32:3147.
6. Practice Guidelines for Obstetric Anesthesia. An Updated Report by the American Society of Anesthesiologists Task Force on Obstetric Anesthesia and the Society for Obstetric Anesthesia and Perinatology. *Anesthesiology*. 2016. 124:270–300.
7. Nishimura RA, Otto CM, Bonow RO, et al. AHA/ACC focused update of the 2014 AHA/ACC guideline for the management of women with valvular heart disease: A report of the American College of Cardiology/American Heart Association Task Force on Clinical Practice Guidelines. *Circulation*. 2017. 135:e1159–195.
8. Weis FR Jr, Markello R, Mo B, Bochiechio P. Cardiovascular effects of oxytocin. *Obstet Gynecol*. 1975. 46(2):211-4.
9. Heesen M, Carvalho B, Carvalho JCA, Duvekot JJ, Dyer RA, Lucas DN, et al. International consensus statement on the use of uterotonic agents during caesarean section. *Anaesthesia*. 2019. 74(10):1305-1319.
10. O'Leary AM. Severe bronchospasm and hypotension after 15-methyl prostaglandin F(2alpha) in atonic postpartum haemorrhage. *Int J Obstet Anesth*. 1994. 3(1):42-4.
11. Abouleish E. Postpartum hypertension and convulsion after oxytocic drugs. *Anesth Analg*. 1976. 55(6):813-5.
12. Dhanjal M, Nelson-Piercy C. Labour in women with medical disorders. Warren R, Arulkumaran S (eds). *Best Practice in Labour and Delivery*. 2nd Edition. Cambridge: Cambridge University Press. 2016. page 264–79.
13. Regitz-Zagrosek V, Roos-Hesselink JW, Bauersachs J, Blomström-Lundqvist C, Cífková R, De Bonis M, et al. ESC Scientific Document Group. 2018 ESC Guidelines for the management of cardiovascular diseases during pregnancy. *Eur Heart J*. 2018. 39(34):3165-3241.
14. Harenberg J, Gnasso A, de Vries JX, Zimmermann R, Augustin J. Inhibition of low molecular weight heparin by protamine chloride in vivo. *Thromb Res*. 1985. 38(1):11-20.
15. Massonnet-Castel S, Pelissier E, Bara L, Terrier E, Abry B, Guibourt P, et al. Partial reversal of low molecular weight heparin (PK 10169) anti-Xa activity by protamine sulfate: In vitro and in vivo study during cardiac surgery with extracorporeal circulation. *Haemostasis*. 1986;16(2):139-46.
16. Jyotsna M, Garre I, Acute myocardial infarction during pregnancy. *Indian Journal of Cardiovascular Disease in Women* WINCARS. Vol. 3. 2018. No. 2-3.
17. Tektonidou MG, Andreoli L, Limper M, et al. EULAR recommendations for the management of antiphospholipid syndrome in adults. *Ann Rheum Dis*. 2019. 78:1296.
18. Chaudhary RK, Nepal C, Khanal N, Pathak R, Giri S, Bhatt VR. Management and outcome of heparin-induced thrombocytopenia in pregnancy: A systematic review. *Cardiovasc Hematol Agents Med Chem*. 2015. 13(2):92-7.
19. ACOG Practice Bulletin No. 132: Antiphospholipid Syndrome. *Obstet Gynecol*. 2012 (reaffirmed 2021). 120(6):1514-21.
20. Cáliz Cáliz R, Díaz Del Campo Fontecha P, Galindo Izquierdo M, López Longo FJ, Martínez Zamora MÁ, Santamaría Ortiz A, et al. Recommendations of the Spanish Rheumatology Society for Primary Antiphospholipid Syndrome. Part I: Diagnosis, Evaluation and Treatment. *Reumatol Clin* (Engl Ed). 2020. 16(2 Pt 1):71-86.
21. Tomasello R, Giordano G, Romano F, Vaccarino F, Siragusa S, Lucchesi A, Napolitano M. Immune

thrombocytopenia in antiphospholipid syndrome: Is it primary or secondary? *Biomedicines*. 2021. 9. 1170.

22. Sarkar M, Brady CW, Fleckenstein J, Forde KA, Khungar V, Molleston JP, et al. Reproductive health and liver disease: Practice Guidance by the American Association for the Study of Liver Diseases. *Hepatology*. 2021 Jan;73(1):318-365.
23. Girling J, Knight CL, Chappell L. On behalf of the Royal College of Obstetricians and Gynaecologists. Intrahepatic cholestasis of pregnancy. *BJOG*. 2022. 129(13): e95–e114.
24. Mitchell AL, Ovadia C, Syngelaki A, Souretis K, Martineau M, Girling J, et al. Re-evaluating diagnostic thresholds for intrahepatic cholestasis of pregnancy: Case-control and cohort study. *BJOG*. 2021.128(10):1635-1644.
25. Ovadia C, Seed PT, Sklavounos A, Geenes V, Di Ilio C, Chambers J, et al. Association of adverse perinatal outcomes of intrahepatic cholestasis of pregnancy with biochemical markers: Results of aggregate and individual woman data meta-analyses. *Lancet*. 2019. 393(10174):899-909.
26. Lindor KD, Lee RH. Intrahepatic cholestasis of pregnancy. Lockwood CJ (Ed). *UpToDate*. 2023. Waltham, MA.
27. Nelson DB, Byrne JJ, Cunningham FG. Acute fatty liver of pregnancy. *Clin Obstet Gynecol*. 2020. 63:152.
28. Terrault NA, Lok ASF, McMahon BJ, Chang KM, Hwang JP, Jonas MM, et al. Update on prevention, diagnosis, and treatment of chronic hepatitis B: AASLD 2018 hepatitis B guidance. *Hepatology*. 2018. 67(4):1560-1599.
29. Pan CQ, Duan Z, Dai E, Zhang S, Han G, Wang Y, et al. China study group for the mother-to-child transmission of hepatitis B. Tenofovir to prevent hepatitis B transmission in mothers with high viral load. *N Engl J Med*. 2016.374(24):2324-34.
30. Cottrell EB, Chou R, Wasson N, Rahman B, Guise JM. Reducing risk for mother-to-infant transmission of hepatitis C virus: A systematic review for the U.S. Preventive Services Task Force. *Ann Intern Med*. 2013.158(2):109-13.
31. Flemming JA, Mullin M, Lu J, et al. Outcomes of pregnant women with cirrhosis and their infants in a population-based study. *Gastroenterology*. 2020. 159:1752.
32. Wood AM, Grotegut CA, Ronald J, Pabon-Ramos W, Pedro C, Knechtle SJ, et al. Identification and Management of Abdominal Wall Varices in Pregnancy. *Obstet Gynecol*. 2018. 132(4):882-887.
33. Harden CL, Meador KJ, Pennell PB, et al. American Academy of Neurology. American Epilepsy Society. Practice parameter update: Management issues for women with epilepsy—focus on pregnancy (an evidence-based review). Teratogenesis and perinatal outcomes: report of the Quality Standards Subcommittee and Therapeutics and Technology Assessment Subcommittee of the American Academy of Neurology and American Epilepsy Society. *Neurology*. 2009. 14;73(2):133-41.
34. Sveberg L, Svalheim S, Taubøll E. The impact of seizures on pregnancy and delivery. *Seizure*. 2015. 28:35-8.
35. Royal College of Obstetricians and Gynaecologists. Epilepsy in pregnancy. Green-top Guideline No. 68. London. *RCOG*. 2016.
36. Kevat D, Mackillop L. Neurological diseases in pregnancy. *J R Coll Physicians Edinb*. 2013. 43:49–58.
37. Hernández-Díaz S, Smith CR, Shen A, Mittendorf R, Hauser WA, Yerby M, et al. North American AED Pregnancy Registry; North American AED Pregnancy Registry. Comparative safety of antiepileptic drugs during pregnancy. *Neurology*. 2012.78(21):1692-9.

CHAPTER 40

SARS-CoV-2

SOPHIE RELPH, PAT O'BRIEN

INTRODUCTION

SARS-CoV-2 (severe acute respiratory syndrome-coronavirus-2) is the strain of coronavirus that caused the **COVID-19** pandemic. It was first identified in Wuhan City, China, in 2019 and subsequently spread across the world, causing the World Health Organization (WHO) to declare it a public health emergency in January 2020 and a pandemic in March 2020. By the end of 2022, over 700 million cases and 6.7 million deaths had been attributed to COVID-19 and reported to the WHO [1].

The COVID-19 pandemic has had a major impact on healthcare systems and care pathways, motivated by a need to prevent population transmission, to prioritise services to people admitted to the hospital with the severe effects of COVID-19, and to protect vulnerable people from the infection.

Adverse maternal outcomes due to COVID infection such as the need for critical care admission, mechanical ventilation, and death are more prevalent amongst pregnant women than in women who are not pregnant. Among pregnant women, adverse perinatal outcomes such as preterm birth and stillbirth are more common among those who are infected as compared to the uninfected.

This chapter deals with specific evidence-based considerations and recommendations for the care of pregnant women admitted for labour and birth with suspected or confirmed COVID-19.

TRANSMISSION

SARS-CoV-2 has been isolated from respiratory droplets and secretion, feces, and exposed fomites (other surfaces). Transmission most commonly occurs through close contact with an infected person.

> **Key Point**
>
> Vertical transmission (from an infected woman to her fetus) has been occasionally reported but is not common.

Pregnant women appear no more likely than the general population to be infected with SARS-CoV-2 [2], although its diagnosis during hospital attendance is more prevalent amongst pregnant women with obesity, pre-existing diabetes mellitus, or gestational diabetes requiring insulin than amongst pregnant women without these characteristics [3].

Mask-wearing and physical distancing are two measures that have been demonstrated to reduce the transmission of SARS-CoV-2. Handwashing has also been advocated as a transmission-reducing practice, although its benefit is less certain [4].

> **Key Point**
>
> Pregnant women are no more likely than the general population to be infected with SARS-CoV-2 [2].

MORBIDITY AND MORTALITY DUE TO SARS-COV-2 INFECTION IN PREGNANCY

Systematic reviews and meta-analyses of the rapidly building literature [5] have demonstrated the following:

- Pregnant women have worse outcomes than non-pregnant women when they are infected with the SARS-CoV-2 virus.

- Pregnant women with SARS-CoV-2 infection have worse outcomes than pregnant women without this infection.

On comparing pregnant women with SARS-CoV-2 infection to non-pregnant women with SARS-CoV-2 infection, it is evident that pregnant women are more likely to:

- Require mechanical ventilatory support
- Be admitted to an intensive care unit
- Die from COVID-19

Compared to pregnant women who are uninfected with this virus, pregnant women with SARS-CoV-2 infection are also at greater risk of adverse outcomes including the following [6]:

- All-cause mortality
- Admission to an intensive care unit
- Preterm birth
- Cesarean birth

The fetus or neonate of such a woman is at greater risk of the following:

- Stillbirth
- Admission to a neonatal unit
- Neonatal death

In a systematic review [5], there was no change in the overall rates of gestational syndromes (preeclampsia or diabetes), induced labour or modes of birth, or neonatal complications (neonatal death, low birth weight, neonatal unit admission, or low Apgar score) among pregnant women who were infected with COVID-19.

Age, BMI, ethnicity, socio-economic class, and vaccination status are some of the factors that increase the risk of developing severe SARS-CoV-2 infection (Box 40.1).

Box 40.1 Women at risk of severe COVID-19

The following groups of women are at the greatest risk of severe COVID-19 [5,6]:

- Those unvaccinated against SARS-CoV-2
- Those aged 35 years or above
- Those who have a body mass index (BMI) of 30 Kg/m^2 or above
- Those of non-Caucasian ethnicity
- Those who are socio-economically deprived
- Those who are at risk of occupational exposure (e.g., healthcare workers)
- Those who have a comorbidity of any kind (but particularly chronic hypertension or gestational or pre-existing diabetes)

Stillbirth

The COVID-19 pandemic led to an overall increase in the rates of stillbirth. The inability to access institutional care due to lockdowns resulted in an increase in stillbirths in many LMICs [7].

Preterm Birth

A study comprising almost 2500 women [8] found the incidence of preterm birth among symptomatic women with COVID-19 to be 19%, in contrast to 8.8% among asymptomatic and 7.1% among uninfected women. The higher rate of preterm birth can largely be attributed to iatrogenic early delivery performed to support maternal ventilatory requirements. However, other systematic reviews found no difference [5]; in fact, a decrease in preterm births was noted in high-income countries [5].

Maternal Death

SARS-CoV-2 infection at any time during pregnancy increases the risk of maternal death. A systematic review with data from 12 countries showed that as compared with uninfected pregnant women, infected pregnant women were at significantly increased risk of maternal mortality [9]. However, maternal death was only reported from studies in LMICs.

SUSPECTING AND DIAGNOSING SARS-COV-2 INFECTION

Signs and Symptoms

The majority of pregnant women with SARS-CoV-2 infection are asymptomatic [10], and are identified due to policies of routine testing during the pandemic. Most of those who have symptoms experience only mild to moderate disease. On an average, it takes 5–6 days from transmission until symptoms become evident, although it can take up to 14 days. Pregnant women are most likely to be admitted to the hospital with symptomatic COVID-19 in the third trimester of pregnancy [11].

> **Key Point**
>
> The majority of pregnant women with SARS-CoV-2 infection are asymptomatic [5], and most of those with symptoms experience mild-to-moderate disease.

With regards to mild symptoms, the classic triad of COVID-19 symptoms are fever, cough, and a loss of taste or smell. Other common mild to moderate symptoms include fatigue, myalgia, headache, and sore throat. This symptom profile of COVID-19 has, however, changed over the course of the pandemic with the advent of new strains of the virus. The prevalence of loss of taste and smell has reduced, and symptoms such as sore throat and sneezing have become more common [12].

> **Key Point**
>
> The symptom profile of COVID-19 has changed over the course of the pandemic. The prevalence of loss of taste and smell has reduced, and symptoms such as sore throat and sneezing have become more common [12].

More severe but less common symptoms include difficulty in breathing, chest pain, loss of speech or mobility, and confusion [12]. In the most severe cases, people with COVID-19 may exhibit septic shock, respiratory failure, and multi-organ failure. Other established complications include arterial and venous thromboses, myocarditis, acute coronary syndrome, and acute thrombotic stroke. Following recovery, some individuals experience post-COVID or long-COVID syndrome, which most commonly includes ongoing breathlessness, cognitive dysfunction, and fatigue.

Diagnostic Tests

Nucleic acid amplification tests (NAATs)

The gold-standard diagnostic test for SARS-CoV-2 infection is the testing of a respiratory sample (e.g., nose and/or throat swab) by nucleic acid amplification testing (NAAT), e.g., reverse transcriptase-polymerase chain reaction (RT-PCR) [1]. This method tests for viral ribose nucleic acid (RNA), which is usually detectable 1–2 days before the onset of symptoms. It is the most accurate test available and may remain positive for weeks, and in some cases, even up to 2–3 months following clinical recovery.

Antigen-detecting rapid diagnostic tests (Ag-RDTs)

Lateral flow tests (LFTs) are rapid (can provide a result within 30 minutes) and more convenient, providing an option for community testing in areas where there is no easy access to laboratory facilities. Unfortunately, LFTs have lower sensitivity (73.0%) in symptomatic individuals but similar specificity (99%) as RT-PCR tests [13].

Antibody tests are not recommended to diagnose acute infection because it takes time for the body to develop antibodies to the infection. Furthermore, it is not known how long the antibody tests remain positive after the acute infection, but when positive, they are more useful to indicate past rather than current infection [1].

A repeat RT-PCR test may be indicated in the presence of symptoms consistent with the diagnosis but an initially negative swab. Alternative diagnoses should also be considered, and testing offered, e.g., for influenza strains, if the RT-PCR test is negative.

Key Point

The gold-standard diagnostic test for SARS-CoV-2 infection is the testing of a respiratory sample (nose and/or throat swab) by nucleic acid amplification testing (NAAT), e.g., reverse transcriptase polymerase chain reaction (RT-PCR).

PREVENTING TRANSMISSION AND INFECTION

The first pillar of preventing transmission and the serious effects of the disease is **vaccination**. However, given that pregnant women are more vulnerable to the severe effects of COVID-19 and adverse pregnancy outcomes as a result, **preventing transmission and infection to uninfected women** in the maternity unit is a key part of the care of women admitted for labour and birth. It is also important to **protect healthcare workers**.

Vaccination

The development of vaccines against SARS-CoV-2 has been referred to as a 'miracle of modern science'. In less than a year, different types of vaccines were produced by different drug companies, each having been developed and tested through large-scale clinical trials, proving them to be both safe and effective [14]. Vaccine development continues at a pace to keep up with the ever-changing viral strains.

Effectiveness

It is now well established that vaccination against SARS-CoV-2 infection is effective. A meta-analysis including over 100,000 vaccinated pregnant women [15] estimated that it reduced RT-PCR-confirmed COVID-19 by 89.5% seven days after the second dose. This, however, included almost exclusively mRNA-type vaccines. The WHO [16] recommends the use of the Oxford (Astra-Zeneca) vaccine in pregnant women since it is an inactivated vaccine. In LMICs, this vaccine is more easily available and more accessible than the more expensive mRNA vaccines. The efficacy of these vaccines is similar in pregnant and non-pregnant individuals. Astra-Zeneca started withdrawing its vaccine in March 2024, citing a surplus of updated vaccines designed to combat new virus variants.

Key Point

An international population registry study demonstrated the effectiveness of vaccination in preventing admission to critical care because of severe COVID-19. In five of the six included countries, more than 90% of women admitted to critical care because of COVID-19 were unvaccinated [17].

Safety

Vaccines are overall very safe. Vaccination reduces the risk of stillbirth by 15%. Amongst all vaccinated and unvaccinated individuals (not specific to those with SARS-CoV-2 infection), there was no difference in adverse outcomes such as miscarriage, early birth, placental abruption, pulmonary embolism, postpartum hemorrhage, maternal death, intensive care unit admission, low birth weight, and neonatal unit admission [15].

Adverse maternal effects

The minor and common side effects of the SARS-CoV-2 vaccine include pain at the injection site, headache, and fatigue. There is no evidence that this is any different or more common for pregnant women.

Serious side effects of vaccination have been documented but are very rare. These include the **vaccine-induced thrombosis, thrombocytopenia (VITT) syndrome**—which has been associated with the Oxford Astra-Zeneca and Janssen viral vector vaccines—and **vaccine-induced myocarditis** or **myopericarditis**—which has been associated with the Moderna and Pfizer mRNA vaccines. VITT is an unpredictable and idiosyncratic reaction, for which the risk is not increased by traditional venous thromboembolism (VTE) risk factors; specifically, there is no evidence that pregnancy increases the risk.

The risk of vaccine-induced myocarditis is low (~2 per million in women aged 25–40 years and ~4 per million in women aged 18–25 years). It should be balanced against the risk of COVID-19-induced myocarditis, which appears to be higher [10].

Fetal effects

SARS-CoV-2 IgG antibodies have been identified both in neonatal cord blood and in breast milk following maternal infection or maternal vaccination (with mRNA vaccines) during pregnancy [18,19]. According to one multicentre study from the USA, this neonatal immunity provides true protection to the neonate or infant, with as many as 61% fewer hospital admissions of infants aged less than 6 months because of the current COVID-19 [20].

Preventing Transmission and Infection to Uninfected Women

Screening

Case identification is key to preventing nosocomial transmission within healthcare environments, not least when admitted for labour and delivery care. Given that the majority of pregnant women with COVID-19 are believed to be asymptomatic, universal screening, i.e., the screening of both symptomatic and asymptomatic women, is necessary.

Case isolation

A key strategy to prevent transmission around the time of labour and birth is the isolation of people currently infected with SARS-CoV-2. Ideally, infected persons should isolate at home unless hospital admission is required for urgent or emergency care.

When women are in active labour or need admission either for obstetric reasons or because of being ill from COVID-19 infection, they should ideally be cared for in a single, well-ventilated room. When case numbers are high and there are insufficient side-rooms available, infected people may need to be cared for in cohorted wards.

Limiting time in the hospital and labour ward without compromising the woman's safety also helps reduce transmission, as does limiting visitors.

Protecting Healthcare Workers

Handwashing

Handwashing is a long-established means of reducing the transmission of infection. Hands should be washed using the widely described **seven-step technique** with either an alcohol-based solution (containing between 60–80% alcohol) or soap and water in each of the following scenarios:

- Before touching a patient
- Before performing clean or aseptic procedures
- After being exposed to body fluids
- After touching a patient or her surroundings

Personal protective equipment (PPE)

PPE aims to reduce, but does not completely eliminate, exposure to SARS-CoV-2. The use of PPE protects workers and service users within healthcare settings from viral transmission. It can also be extended to protect the community through widespread adoption. The WHO has different recommendations for the type of PPE to be used according to exposure risk [21]. These recommendations apply to women admitted for labour and birth (Table 40.1).

Respiratory emissions during labour and delivery

During labour, deep respiratory efforts in the active phase, and pushing in the second stage are all aerosol-generating events (AGPs) [22]. This may contribute to the increased risk of respiratory transmission of SARS-CoV-2. Healthcare workers should use both contact and droplet precautions with eye protection and airborne precautions (i.e., N95 mask or powered air purifying respirator).

Table 40.1 PPE recommendations for different clinical situations

Clinical situation	PPE
Preliminary screening procedures without patient contact	• Physical distancing methods with clear glass or plastic screens to separate the healthcare worker from the woman • Continuous wearing of a medical mask
Providing direct care in labour or birth to women with confirmed COVID-19 without an aerosol-generating procedure (AGP)	Medical mask, gown, gloves, and eye protection (goggles or face shield)
Providing direct care to women in labour/ birth with confirmed COVID-19 with AGPs	A respiratory mask (e.g., FFP3 or N95), a fluid-resistant gown (or gown with underlying apron), gloves, and eye protection
Performing a surgical procedure	Fluid-resistant medical mask OR respiratory mask if AGP is anticipated + a fluid-resistant gown (or gown with underlying apron), gloves, and eye protection

CARE OF PREGNANT WOMEN INFECTED WITH COVID-19

The care of women infected with COVID-19 includes antenatal care, intrapartum care, and postpartum care.

Antenatal Care

Several professional bodies released guidelines for the management of antenatal visits during the COVID-19 pandemic [10,23]. A combination of fewer visits with the addition of novel types of care delivery models (video or telephone calls) was instituted for low-risk antenatal women. With the waning of the pandemic, some of these care delivery models have continued to be useful in dealing with infected women till their isolation period is over.

Care of women with mild COVID-19 infection

Community care

Women with mild COVID-19 can often be managed at home but should be advised to self-isolate, remain hydrated, and mobilise to reduce their risk of VTE. Women discharged to go home with mild COVID-19 should be advised about what to look out for and how to seek help if the symptoms deteriorate. Where available, home monitoring of oxygen saturation should be considered as it is helpful to monitor any deterioration.

Venous thromboprophylaxis

International guidelines for the care of pregnant women with COVID-19 vary in their recommendations for women self-managing at home. Whilst some guidelines recommend universal low-molecular-weight heparin (LMWH) **thromboprophylaxis** for women with milder disease until symptoms alleviate, others recommend hydration and mobilisation, with LMWH thromboprophylaxis reserved for those with other significant risk factors [24]. The consensus is that asymptomatic women do not require anticoagulation unless there are other risk factors [25].

> **Key Point**
>
> It is recommended that pregnant women who are receiving anticoagulant or antiplatelet therapies for underlying conditions continue these medications after they are diagnosed with COVID-19 [25,26].

Intrapartum Care

Pregnant women presenting in labour or for planned birth (induction of labour or cesarean section) with symptoms suggestive of COVID-19 should be investigated and treated as if they were not pregnant unless there is a clear reason not to. This includes offering radiological investigations (e.g., chest X-ray or CT scan) and medical treatments unless there is an established and substantial risk to the fetus and an equally acceptable alternative, particularly when the woman is severely or critically unwell.

Initial assessment

When a woman presents to maternity services with symptoms consistent with possible COVID-19, her systematic evaluation should include a detailed history, with due attention to possible exposures and risk factors for severe disease, assessment of vital signs, and examination to rule in or out differential diagnoses.

At the very minimum, the examination should include chest auscultation and abdominal palpation. Speculum or vaginal examination should also be performed if there is possible uterine activity, ruptured membranes, or vaginal bleeding. For a pregnancy in the third trimester, and only if the woman is well enough to undergo this, a cardiotocograph (CTG) may be performed to assess fetal well-being. This should not be prioritised over urgent or emergency maternal investigations and treatment.

Investigations

Investigations to determine the cause and severity of pyrexia include the following:

- Specimens for microbiology (vaginal swab, urine, blood cultures)
- Specimens for virology (throat or nasal swab)—to test for influenza during seasonal peaks and RT-PCR test for SARS-CoV-2
- Blood samples—for complete blood count (CBC), renal function, coagulation studies, C-reactive protein, and lactate
- Radiological investigations—including chest X-ray and/or CT scan

Lymphopenia is the classic finding on CBC among women with COVID-19. Neutrophilia on CBC increases the possibility of either primary or secondary (superimposed) bacterial infection. C-reactive protein and ferritin are both acute-phase indicators of inflammation and are usually raised in cases of COVID-19. D-dimers are also usually raised in COVID infections and often with normal pregnancy, and are therefore not useful discriminators of VTE in this context.

Occasionally, COVID-19 can cause disseminated intravascular coagulation (DIC), indicated by low fibrinogen and platelets, sometimes in association with prolonged prothrombin time (PT) and/or activated partial thromboplastin time (APTT).

When chest pain and/or breathlessness predominate, additional investigations to determine potential alternative diagnoses to COVID-19 and its complications might include:

- Additional blood tests, e.g., cardiac-specific troponins, B-natriuretic peptide
- Chest CT (including the option to perform CT pulmonary angiography) or ventilation–perfusion (V/Q) scan (if pulmonary embolus is suspected and chest X-ray is normal)
- Electrocardiogram (ECG)
- Echocardiogram

A suggested approach to the investigation of pregnant women presenting to the hospital in labour or for planned birth with fever and respiratory symptoms consistent with COVID-19 is presented in Fig. 40.1.

Mode of birth

There is no evidence to favour one mode of birth over another in women with COVID-19. The rate of neonatal COVID-19 infection is no greater when the baby is born vaginally than when born by cesarean [27,28]. Therefore, current COVID-19 infections should not affect a woman's planned mode of birth unless urgent birth is required or if she is too unwell to labour and give birth vaginally.

Assisted vaginal birth should be offered as per usual obstetric indications and may also be offered to women in the second stage of labour who are exhausted or hypoxic because of current COVID-19.

The need for the whole team to don PPE prior to an emergency cesarean birth is expected to lengthen the decision-to-birth interval [29,40]. This should be considered when an urgent birth seems likely.

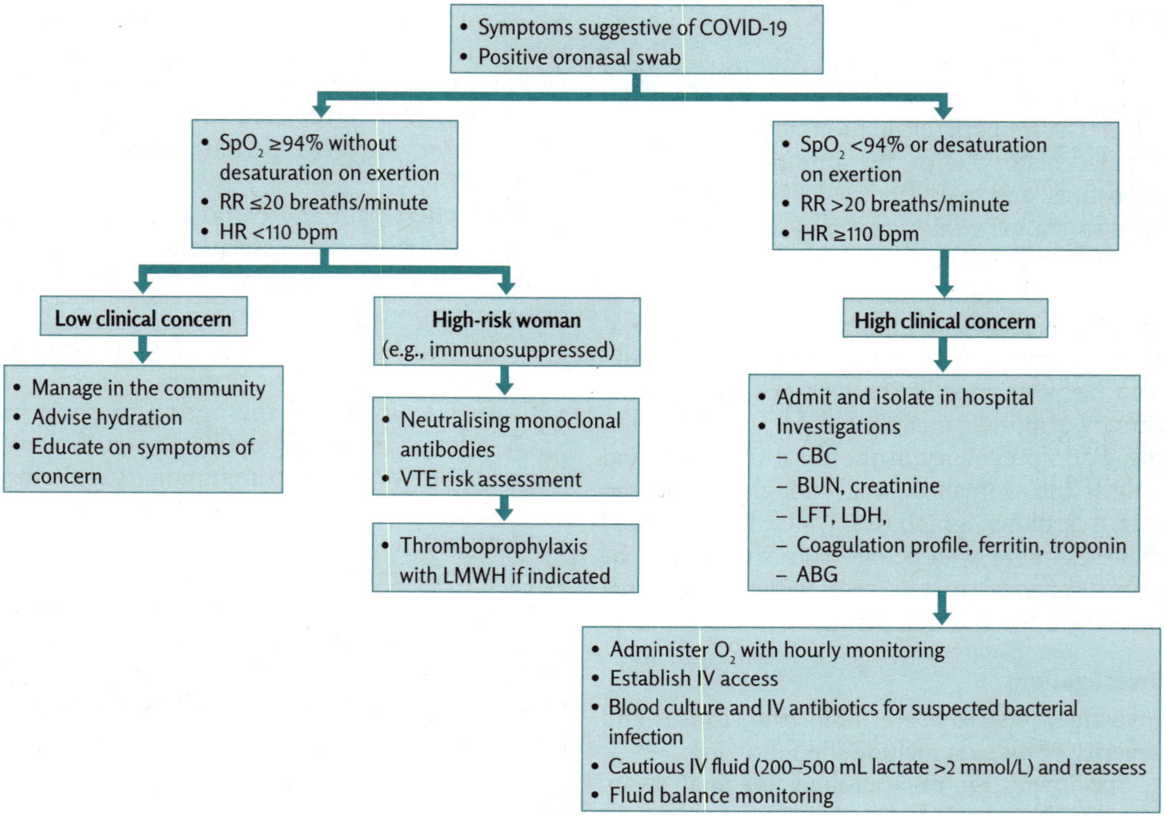

Fig. 40.1 A suggested approach to the investigation of pregnant women presenting in labour or for planned birth with fever and respiratory symptoms consistent with COVID-19

ABG, arterial blood gas; *HR*, heart rate; *IV*, intravenous; *LFT*, liver function test; *LDH*, lactate dehydrogenase, *LMWH*, low-molecular-weight heparin; *RR*, respiratory rate; *VTE*, venous thromboembolism

Water birth is not contraindicated for women who are asymptomatic of COVID-19. However, for infected women who are unwell, labour in water is less suitable because they require closer monitoring and may also require oxygen support.

Key Point

Current COVID-19 should not affect a woman's planned mode of birth unless urgent birth is required or she is too unwell to labour and have a vaginal birth.

Fetal monitoring

Fetal compromise has been reported to be more common in women who are symptomatic of COVID-19 [30–33,45–48] but not in those who are asymptomatic. Continuous electronic fetal monitoring (CEFM) should therefore be offered, at the minimum, to women who are symptomatic of COVID-19. For asymptomatic women, an assessment of the need for CEFM should take into consideration any other risk factors for adverse birth outcomes.

There are no known specific contraindications to the use of a fetal scalp electrode or fetal blood sampling in women infected with COVID-19.

Analgesia and anesthesia for birth

Entonox® (50% nitrous oxide and 50% oxygen) can be safely offered with a standard single-patient microbiological filter. This is not an aerosol-generating procedure (AGP).

There is no evidence that epidural or spinal analgesia or anesthesia is contraindicated in the presence of coronavirus infections [42]. Where available, epidural analgesia should be offered early in labour to women with COVID-19, explaining that this could reduce the risk of them requiring general anesthesia in case of emergency birth. As general anesthesia is an AGP, this carries additional risks for staff and incurs time that is required for the staff to prepare by donning higher-grade PPE before entering the theatre.

Given the small risk of thrombocytopenia associated with COVID-19, a complete blood count should be performed before undertaking neuraxial anesthesia techniques (epidural/spinal/combined spinal–epidural).

Key Point

Entonox and epidural analgesia can be offered safely to women with COVID-19 infection.

Place of birth

Women who are asymptomatic for COVID-19 can be offered the same range of birthplace options that they would ordinarily be offered. Being asymptomatic for COVID-19 is not expected to increase the risk of adverse outcomes for the mother or baby.

In contrast, symptomatic COVID-19 has been associated with adverse outcomes for the mother and fetus (cesarean birth, preterm birth, stillbirth, neonatal unit admission) [43,34], although not when the population is restricted to those giving birth at term [44,35]. Symptomatic women giving birth also need a higher level of monitoring than can safely be offered in low-risk community facilities. Such women should, therefore, be advised to give birth in tertiary care facilities with access to trained medical staff, critical care and neonatal intensive care facilities, and operating theatres.

Timing of birth

Women with mild infection

Whilst the spontaneous onset of labour cannot be controlled, it may be possible to delay elective birth (planned cesarean section or planned induction of labour) until after the period of maximal infectivity. If considering delaying elective birth, it is important to consider the benefits (reduced transmission) as well as the risks (maternal or fetal compromise) associated with delaying birth, particularly where elective birth is indicated because of maternal or fetal morbidity.

Women with moderate or severe infection

First or second trimesters of pregnancy: The majority of investigations and COVID-19 therapies can be safely administered during an ongoing pregnancy. Early birth is unlikely to significantly improve the maternal outcome and carries the significant risk of avoidable extreme prematurity and its associated complications for the fetus.

Third trimester: The gravid uterus may contribute to respiratory compromise and also limits the ability to position the woman prone. An individualised assessment by the multidisciplinary team may be used to determine whether earlier birth of the fetus is expected to improve the ability to provide optimal care to the pregnant woman, improving her chances of recovery. Factors to consider include the severity of COVID-19 illness, the impact that the gravid uterus is having on the woman's condition and treatment, and the gestational stage. An earlier gestation will need to be considered for multiple pregnancies.

If earlier birth is indicated by other obstetric indications (e.g., preeclampsia or fetal growth restriction), then the maternal condition should be stabilised before expediting birth.

Antenatal corticosteroids for fetal lung maturation and magnesium sulphate for fetal neuroprotection are indicated prior to 34 weeks' and 32 weeks' gestation respectively. If dexamethasone or betamethasone have already been given in doses equivalent to (or greater than) those recommended by standard antenatal protocols, but for the treatment of COVID-19, then these do not need to be repeated, especially if they were administered within seven days prior to birth (Fig. 40.2). If, however, the maternal steroid treatment has been with oral prednisolone or IV hydrocortisone, then dexamethasone or betamethasone should be given according to the usual regimen for fetal maturation prior to delivery (see section above on *Corticosteroids*, under *Medical treatment*).

Pregnant women at highest risk of hospitalisation

Definitions of who is at high risk of hospitalisation vary, but generally include unvaccinated adults who have at least one characteristic or comorbidity placing them at greater risk of severe disease; the WHO considers pregnancy to be a risk factor for hospitalisation [36].

The WHO recommends that people at risk of hospitalisation due to COVID-19 be administered nirmatrelvir and ritonavir (the combination is sold as Paxlovid®) as soon as possible after the onset of symptoms. Given that there is no evidence of serious risk and moderate evidence of benefit, this recommendation has been extended to use in pregnant women [36].

The use of nirmatrelvir and ritonavir has been associated with a significant reduction in the odds of hospital admission (OR 0.13, 95% CI 0.04-0.40). Lesser or more uncertain but significantly different effects have also been noted with molnupiravir (OR 0.54, 95% CI 0.30-0.90) and remdesivir (OR 0.25, 95% CI 0.07-0.86) [37].

Care of women with moderate to severe infection

Women who require oxygen to maintain their saturations above 94% should be cared for by a multidisciplinary team within a hospital setting, ideally with access to critical care in case of deterioration.

Multidisciplinary care

For women who are moderately or severely unwell with COVID-19, multidisciplinary teamwork is key to optimising outcomes for the woman and her baby. Care plans should include specialist knowledge from the following specialists:

- Obstetricians and midwives—on antenatal and intrapartum care, including knowledge about the physiology and pathology of pregnancy, specific considerations in pregnancy (including risk of VTE, risks to the fetus, safety of investigations and drugs), and planning the timing and mode of birth
- Obstetric anesthetists—on safe and alternative methods of anesthesia for labour and birth and physiology of pregnancy and critical care of the woman going through labour and/or birth (vaginal or cesarean section)
- Physicians and/or obstetric physician—on non-critical care of people with moderate to severe COVID-19, its complications, or alternative medical diagnoses
- Critical care intensivists and their teams—on the need and availability of critical care, and the additional monitoring and therapies that can be offered in this environment, especially where critical care is indicated or there is a reasonable risk of deterioration
- Neonatologists and neonatal nurses on the risks of prematurity, and availability of services to care for the neonate, in case early birth is indicated
- The woman and/or her next of kin—offering a discussion regarding the woman's wishes with respect to care options

The multidisciplinary team discussion should cover the key priorities for the care of the unwell pregnant woman, particularly around the time of labour and/or birth, the most appropriate location to offer this care (dependent on the availability and familiarity of skilled staff and the required equipment), and concerns amongst the team regarding specific considerations when caring for an unwell pregnant woman.

Monitoring

Following hospital admission for labour or planned birth (induction of labour or cesarean section), ongoing monitoring is essential to observe trends in terms of clinical improvement or deterioration. For women requiring oxygen supplementation to achieve saturations above 94%, hourly vital signs should be recorded. Attention should be paid to the absolute values as well as the overall trends, providing earlier warning of the risk of deterioration. Fit and healthy pregnant women are generally able to compensate for longer than older people but may then deteriorate more quickly when that ability to compensate is lost.

The level of care should be escalated (where possible) if any of the following occur:

- An increase in the fraction of inspired oxygen (FiO_2) required to achieve saturation >94%, particularly if the FiO_2 exceeds 35%
- An increase in the respiratory rate above 25 breaths/minutes or a rapidly rising rate below this level
- A reduction in the urine output
- Development of acute kidney injury (serum creatinine levels above 77 µmol/L or 0.87 mg/dL where there is no known chronic renal disease)
- Drowsiness
- Lung infiltrates >50%

Medical treatment

Oxygen

Oxygen should be up-titrated to achieve saturations of 94–98% (or saturation levels similar to baseline in women with lower baseline rates due to chronic disease) using nasal cannula or face/venturi mask, and escalating to non-invasive positive airway pressure (e.g., continuous PAP), intubation, and intermittent positive pressure ventilation (IPPV).

When adequate oxygenation cannot be achieved through standard ward-based and/or critical care ventilatory protocols, respiratory extracorporeal membrane oxygenation (ECMO) may be the only option.

Corticosteroids

The RECOVERY (Randomised Evaluation of COVID-19 Therapy) trial was a landmark COVID-19 therapies randomised controlled trial that recruited pregnant women amongst its population. For women receiving respiratory support, **dexamethasone administration was associated with a significantly reduced incidence of death** as compared to the usual care group.

> **Key Point**
>
> Corticosteroids are recommended for all individuals with COVID-19 who require oxygen supplementation including pregnant women [38].

Because dexamethasone is known to cross the placenta and repeated doses have been associated with adverse long-term neonatal outcomes [38], the corticosteroid protocol of the RECOVERY trial was modified for pregnant women. Instead of standard dexamethasone, the following are recommended:

- Oral prednisolone 40 mg daily or IV hydrocortisone 80 mg twice daily should be given for 10 days (or until discharge, if sooner).
- IV methylprednisolone is an option for intensive care units more familiar with this preparation (e.g., 1 mg/Kg twice daily for 5–7 days, weaned to 1 mg/Kg once daily for 5–7 days).
- If steroids are indicated for fetal lung maturity, intramuscular dexamethasone can be given (two doses of 12 mg given 24 hours apart) instead of the daily doses of prednisolone or hydrocortisone on those two days followed by the standard regimen recommended above.

Immunomodulators

The WHO has recommended the use of anti-IL-6 agents (e.g., tocilizumab or sarilumab) for individuals with severe or critical COVID-19; this recommendation extends to pregnant women. Both drugs are administered as a single intravenous infusion.

Thromboprophylaxis

Pregnancy is well established as a prothrombotic state. COVID-19 is also associated with an increased risk of VTE, particularly among individuals admitted to an intensive care unit [39].

> **Key Point**
>
> In non-COVID cases, LMWH thromboprophylaxis should be avoided if the woman is bleeding (other than with normal postpartum lochia), if her platelet count falls below 50×10^9/L, or if labour or birth are expected within the next 12 hours (given the potential need for neuraxial anesthesia and the 12-hour window required prior to its administration).

International guidelines for the care of pregnant women with COVID-19 universally recommend the prescription of thromboprophylaxis for women admitted to the hospital with the disease [24].

Additional critical care therapies

Prone positioning has been shown to improve respiratory function in people with severe acute respiratory distress syndrome (ARDS) including in awake and intubated patients with severe COVID-19 [40,41]. It can be used for pregnant women in the first or second trimesters (with cushioned support) or in the postnatal period and sometimes in the early third trimester [42,43].

The treatment, based on severity of infection, is summarised in Fig. 40.2.

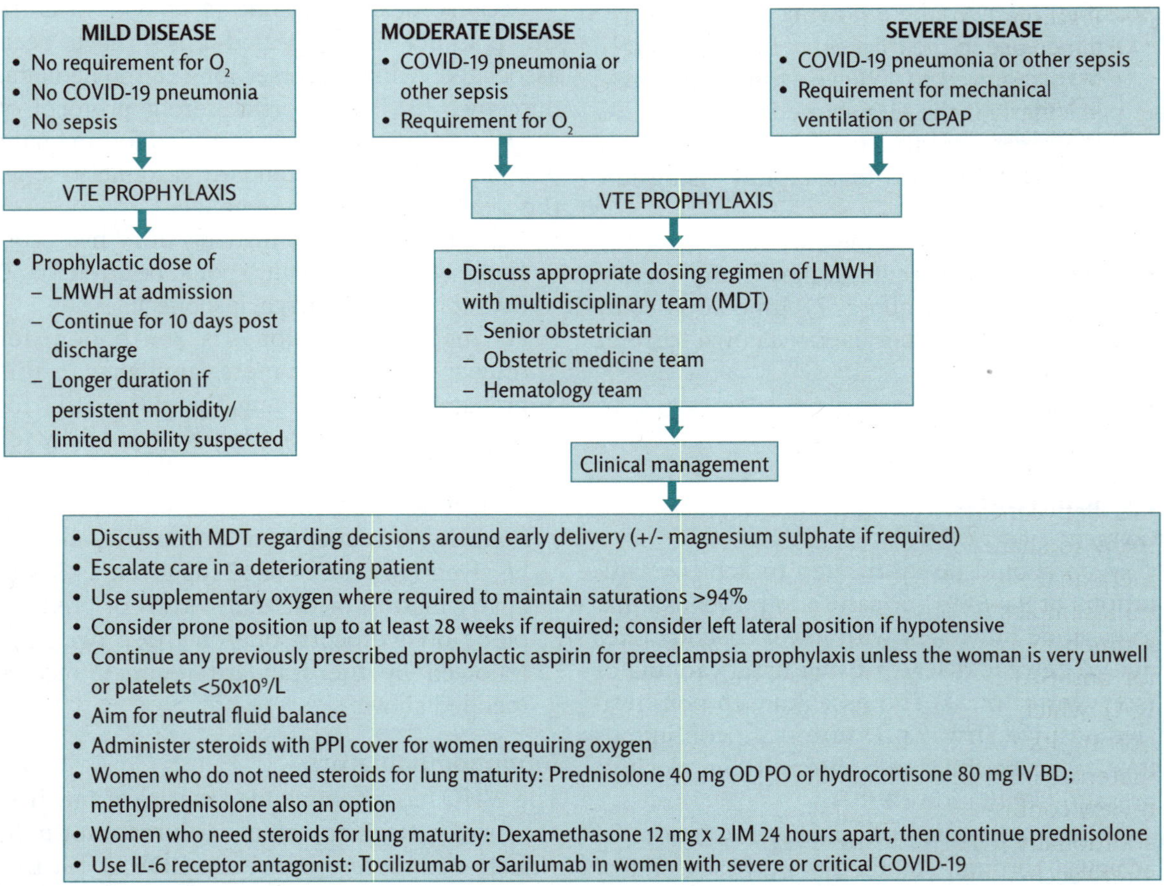

Fig. 40.2 Suggested treatment protocol for women presenting with symptoms of COVID-19
CPAP, continuous positive airway pressure; *BD*, twice daily; *IM*, intramuscularly; *LMWH*, low-molecular-weight heparin; *PPI*, proton pump inhibitors, *OD*, once daily, *PO*, per oral

CARE OF THE NEONATE

Neonatal SARS-CoV-2 infection in the first 28 days of life is rare (its incidence in a large UK population cohort was found to be 5.6/10,000 livebirths, 95% CI 4.3–7.1) and severe neonatal infection is even rarer (2.4/10,000 livebirths, 95% Cl 1.6–3.4) [44].

Women and their babies should therefore be supported to remain together and to practise skin-to-skin/kangaroo care in the immediate postpartum period if they do not otherwise require urgent maternal care or additional neonatal support.

Key Points

- Practising delayed cord clamping and early skin-to-skin contact between the woman and her baby have been shown to not increase the transmission of SARS-CoV-2 to the neonate.
- Neonatal SARS-CoV-2 infection in the first 28 days of life is rare. Hence, women and their babies should be supported to remain together, breastfeed, and practise skin-to-skin/kangaroo care.

Breastfeeding

The long-term benefits of breastfeeding are well-established and highly likely to outweigh any potential risks of transmission of the virus through breast milk [45,46]. The main risk of breastfeeding is postulated to be the close contact between the baby and the mother, who is likely to share infective respiratory droplets. A meta-analysis estimated that only 5% of breast-milk samples test positive for SARS-CoV-2, and a much higher proportion (83%) test positive for anti-SARS-CoV-2 antibody (predominantly IgA) which is passed onto the neonate, supporting its own immunity against exposure to maternal infection [47]. A different systematic review confirmed this finding of antibodies and additionally found that these were also present after vaccination [48].

CONCLUSION

The care of pregnant women with SARS-CoV-2 infection was difficult and challenging across the different waves of the COVID-19 pandemic. While the majority of women who were symptomatic and those who had mild infection could be treated in the community, appropriate triage and escalation of care were required for the more seriously ill women. Vaccination was a big breakthrough and continues to be safe for use in pregnancy. Even now, as SARS-CoV-2 infection prevails, it is important that we remember all the principles of management discussed in this chapter.

REFERENCES

1. COVID-19 dashboard [https://covid19.who.int].
2. Docherty AB, Harrison EM, Green CA, et al. Features of 20133 UK patients in hospital with covid-19 using the ISARIC WHO Clinical Characterisation Protocol: Prospective observational cohort study. *BMJ*. 2020. 369:m1985.
3. Eskenazi B, Rauch S, Iurlaro E, Gunier RB, et al. Diabetes mellitus, maternal adiposity, and insulin-dependent gestational diabetes are associated with COVID-19 in pregnancy: The INTERCOVID study. *Am J Obstet Gynecol*. 2022. 227(1):74.e71-74.e16.
4. Talic S, Shah S, Wild H, Gasevic D, et al. Effectiveness of public health measures in reducing the incidence of covid-19, SARS-CoV-2 transmission, and covid-19 mortality: Systematic review and meta-analysis. *BMJ*. 2021. 375:e068302.
5. Chmielewska B, Barratt I, Townsend R, Kalafat E, et al. Effects of the COVID-19 pandemic on maternal and perinatal outcomes: A systematic review and meta-analysis. *The Lancet Global Health*. 2021. 9(6):e759-e772.
6. Allotey J, Stallings E, Bonet M, Yap M, et al. Clinical manifestations, risk factors, and maternal and perinatal outcomes of coronavirus disease 2019 in pregnancy: Living systematic review and meta-analysis. *BMJ*. 2020. 370:m3320.
7. Mahajan NN, Pophalkar M, Patil S, Yewale B, et al. Pregnancy outcomes and maternal complications during the second wave of coronavirus disease 2019 (COVID-19) in India. *Obstet Gynecol*. 2021. 138: 660–662.

8. Blitz MJ, Gerber RP, Gulersen M, et al. 2021. Preterm birth among women with and without severe acute respiratory syndrome coronavirus 2 infection. *Acta Obstet Gynecol Scand.* 100(12):2253-2259.
9. Smith ER, Oakley E, Grandner GW, et al. Adverse maternal, fetal, and newborn outcomes among pregnant women with SARS-CoV-2 infection: An individual participant data meta-analysis. *BMJ Glob Health.* 2023. 8.
10. Coronavirus (COVID-19) Infection in Pregnancy v16.0 [https://www.rcog.org.uk/media/ftzilsfj/2022-12-15-coronavirus-covid-19-infection-in-pregnancy-v16.pdf]
11. Knight M, Bunch K, Vousden N, Morris E, et al. Characteristics and outcomes of pregnant women admitted to hospital with confirmed SARS-CoV-2 infection in UK: National population based cohort study. *BMJ.* 2020. 369:m2107.
12. Looi M-K: How are COVID-19 symptoms changing? *BMJ.* 2023. 380:p3.
13. Dinnes J, Sharma P, Berhane S, et al. Rapid, point-of-care antigen tests for diagnosis of SARS-CoV-2 infection. *Cochrane Database Syst Rev.* 2022. 7(7):Cd013705.
14. Stokel-Walker C: How are vaccines being adapted to meet the changing face of SARS-CoV-2? *BMJ.* 2022. 377:o1257.
15. Prasad S, Kalafat E, Blakeway H, et al. Systematic review and meta-analysis of the effectiveness and perinatal outcomes of COVID-19 vaccination in pregnancy. *Nat Commun.* 2022. 13(1):2414.
16. Interim recommendations for use of the ChAdOx1-S [recombinant] vaccine against COVID-19 (AstraZeneca COVID-19 vaccine AZD1222 Vaxzevria™, SII COVISHIELD™) WHO reference number: WHO/2019-nCoV/vaccines/SAGE_recommendation/AZD1222/2022.1. © *World Health Organization.* 2022.
17. Engjom H, van den Akker T, Aabakke A, et al. Severe COVID-19 in pregnancy is almost exclusively limited to unvaccinated women—2013; time for policies to change. *The Lancet Regional Health – Europe.* 2022. 13.
18. Flannery DD, Gouma S, Dhudasia MB, et al. Assessment of maternal and neonatal cord blood SARS-CoV-2 antibodies and placental transfer ratios. *JAMA Pediatr.* 2021. 175(6):594-600.
19. Juncker HG, Romijn M, Loth VN, Ruhé EJM, et al. Antibodies against SARS-CoV-2 in human milk: Milk conversion rates in the Netherlands. *Journal of Human Lactation.* 2021. 37(3):469-476.
20. Halasa NB, Olson SM, Staat MA, et al. Effectiveness of maternal vaccination with mRNA COVID-19 vaccine during pregnancy against COVID-19-associated hospitalization in infants aged <6 months - 17 states, July 2021-January 2022. *MMWR Morb Mortal Wkly Rep.* 2022. 71(7):264-270.
21. World Health Organization: Rational use of personal protective equipment for COVID-19 and considerations during severe shortages: Interim guidance. 2020.
22. Mok T, Harris E, Vargas A, et al. Evaluation of respiratory emissions during labor and delivery: Potential implications for transmission of severe acute respiratory syndrome coronavirus 2 (SARS-CoV-2). *Obstet Gynecol.* 2021. 138(4):616-621.
23. Zangmo R, Kumari A, Garg D, Sharma KA. Redesigning routine antenatal care in low-resource settings during the COVID-19 pandemic. *WHO South-East Asia J Public Health.* 2021. 10(Suppl. 1):S36–S40.
24. D'Souza R, Malhamé I, Teshler L, Acharya G, Hunt BJ, McLintock C: A critical review of the pathophysiology of thrombotic complications and clinical practice recommendations for thromboprophylaxis in pregnant patients with COVID-19. *Acta obstetricia et gynecologica Scandinavica.* 2020. 99(9):1110-1120.
25. Antithrombotic Therapy in Patients With COVID-19. COVID-19 Treatment Guidelines Panel. Coronavirus Disease 2019 (COVID-19) Treatment Guidelines. National Institutes of Health. Available at: https://www.covid19treatmentguidelines.nih.gov/therapies/antithrombotic-therapy/ (Accessed in August 2023).
26. RECOVERY Collaborative Group. Aspirin in patients admitted to hospital with COVID-19 (RECOVERY): a randomised, controlled, open-label, platform trial. *Lancet.* 2022. 399 (10320):143-151.
27. Walker KF, O'Donoghue K, Grace N, et al. Maternal transmission of SARS-COV-2 to the neonate, and possible routes for such transmission: a systematic review and critical analysis. *BJOG.* 2020. 127(11):1324-1336.
28. Knight M, Bunch K, Vousden N, Morris E, Simpson N, et al. Characteristics and outcomes of pregnant women admitted to hospital with confirmed SARS-CoV-2 infection in UK: National population based cohort study. *BMJ.* 2020. 369:m2107.
29. Cuerva MJ, Carbonell M, Martin Palumbo G, et al. Personal protective equipment during the COVID-19 pandemic and operative time in cesarean section: A retrospective cohort study. *J Matern Fetal Neonatal Med.* 2020. 1-4.
30. Chen H, Guo J, Wang C, Luo F, et al. Clinical characteristics and intrauterine vertical transmission potential of COVID-19 infection in nine pregnant women: A retrospective review of medical records. *Lancet.* 2020. 395(10226):809-815.

31. Zhu H, Wang L, Fang C, Peng S, et al. Clinical analysis of 10 neonates born to mothers with 2019-nCoV pneumonia. *Transl Pediatr.* 2020. 9(1):51-60.
32. Zimmermann P, Curtis N. COVID-19 in children, pregnancy and neonates: A review of epidemiologic and clinical features. *Pediatr Infect Dis J.* 2020. 39(6):469-477.
33. Yang Z, Wang M, Zhu Z, Liu Y: Coronavirus disease 2019 (COVID-19) and pregnancy: A systematic review. *J Matern Fetal Neonatal Med.* 2020. 1-4.
34. Update to living systematic review on covid-19 in pregnancy. *BMJ.* 2022. 377:o1205.
35. Gurol-Urganci I, Jardine JE, Carroll F, et al. Maternal and perinatal outcomes of pregnant women with SARS-CoV-2 infection at the time of birth in England: national cohort study. *Am J Obstet Gynecol.* 2021. 225(5):522.e521-522.e511.
36. Therapeutics and COVID-19: Living guideline, 13 January 2023. [https://www.who.int/publications/i/item/WHO-2019-nCoV-therapeutics-2023.1.
37. Siemieniuk RA, Bartoszko JJ, Zeraatkar D, et al. Drug treatments for covid-19: Living systematic review and network meta-analysis. *BMJ.* 2020. 370:m2980.
38. Abani O, Abbas A, Abbas F, Abbas M, et al. Casirivimab and imdevimab in patients admitted to hospital with COVID-19 (RECOVERY): A randomised, controlled, open-label, platform trial. *The Lancet.* 2022. 399(10325):665-676.
39. Tan BK, Mainbourg S, Friggeri A, et al. Arterial and venous thromboembolism in COVID-19: A study-level meta-analysis. *Thorax.* 2021. 76(10):970-979.
40. Li J, Luo J, Pavlov I, Perez Y, Tan W, et al. Awake prone positioning for non-intubated patients with COVID-19-related acute hypoxaemic respiratory failure: A systematic review and meta-analysis. *Lancet Respir Med.* 2022. 10(6):573-583.
41. Chua EX, Zahir S, Ng KT, Teoh WY, et al. Effect of prone versus supine position in COVID-19 patients: A systematic review and meta-analysis. *J Clin Anesth.* 2021. 74:110406.
42. Tolcher MC, McKinney JR, Eppes CS, Muigai D, Shamshirsaz A, Guntupalli KK, Nates JL: Prone positioning for pregnant women with hypoxemia due to coronavirus disease 2019 (COVID-19). *Obstet Gynecol.* 2020. 136(2):259-261.
43. Péju E, Belicard F, Silva S, Hraiech S, Painvin B, Kamel T, Thille AW, Goury A, Grimaldi D, Jung B, et al. Management and outcomes of pregnant women admitted to intensive care unit for severe pneumonia related to SARS-CoV-2 infection: The multicenter and international COVIDPREG study. *Intensive Care Med.* 2022. 48(9):1185-1196.
44. Gale C, Quigley MA, Placzek A, Knight M, Ladhani S, Draper ES, Sharkey D, Doherty C, Mactier H, Kurinczuk JJ. Characteristics and outcomes of neonatal SARS-CoV-2 infection in the UK: A prospective national cohort study using active surveillance. *Lancet Child Adolesc Health.* 2021. 5(2):113-121.
45. Breastfeeding and COVID-19 [https://www.who.int/news-room/commentaries/detail/breastfeeding-and-covid-19]
46. Williams J, Namazova-Baranova L, Weber M, et AL. The importance of continuing breastfeeding during coronavirus disease-2019: In support of the World Health Organization statement on breastfeeding during the pandemic. *J Pediatr.* 2020. 223:234-236.
47. Zhu F, Zozaya C, Zhou Q, De Castro C, Shah PS: SARS-CoV-2 genome and antibodies in breastmilk: a systematic review and meta-analysis. *Arch Dis Child Fetal Neonatal Ed* 2021, 106(5):514-521.
48. Pérez-Bermejo M, Peris-Ochando B, Murillo-Llorente MT: COVID-19: Relationship and Impact on Breastfeeding-A Systematic Review. *Nutrients* 2021, 13(9).

CHAPTER 41

Chickenpox

MANDIRA DASGUPTA, BHASKAR PAL

INTRODUCTION

Chickenpox is caused by the varicella-zoster virus (VZV), which is a DNA virus that belongs to the herpesvirus family. It is transmitted as a droplet infection and by direct personal contact. Adults are at risk of more severe disease and have a higher incidence of complications as compared to children. VZV stays dormant in the sensory nerve ganglia as a latent infection. Reactivation of latent infection causes herpes zoster. Recovery from primary varicella infection usually provides immunity for life.

The incidence of chickenpox in pregnancy in temperate countries has been reported to be around 2–3/1000 pregnancies [1]; in these areas, it is a disease of childhood, and 90% of adults are seropositive. In tropical countries, on the other hand, seroconversion occurs in adolescence and adulthood, and only 25–80% of adults are seropositive [2]. This leaves a large number of pregnant women susceptible to the complications of chickenpox. A small study from South India found high varicella susceptibility rates during pregnancy among urban and rural pregnant women [3].

To understand the management of labour with an ongoing chickenpox infection, it is important to first comprehend the pathology and the effect of the disease on the mother and the baby. Like most other viral infections, chickenpox has gestation-specific impact on the mother as well as the baby.

Maternal Complications

Chickenpox is a self-limiting disease with minimal complications. However clinicians should be aware that pregnancy increases the risk of severe morbidities like pneumonia, which may affect approximately 10–20% of pregnant infected women and can result in maternal mortality, estimated to be as high as 40% [4]. It may also result in hepatitis and encephalitis.

Fetal and Neonatal Consequences

The fetus is not affected in most cases. For practical purposes, infection with VZV in the first trimester does not increase the risk of spontaneous miscarriage [5,6]. However, maternal infections before 28 weeks may cause **fetal varicella syndrome** or **varicella infection of the newborn** (previously known as **congenital varicella syndrome [CVS]**) in 0.4–2% of cases, with severe congenital defects affecting eyes, bones, central nervous system, and skin. These babies have a mortality of 30% in the first month of life.

Fetal growth restriction (FGR) occurs in approximately 23% of cases [5], and low birth weight is virtually universal.

A very small proportion (0.8–1.7%) of fetuses exposed to maternal varicella between 13 and 36 weeks of pregnancy manifest zoster in the first two years of life [6]. In pregnancies after 36 weeks, the baby is at the greatest risk of contracting chickenpox, i.e., **neonatal varicella,** which may be a mild disease or progress to a severe, fulminant infection.

Planning the management of labour with chickenpox should take into account the effects of the infection on the mother as well as the baby to ensure a favourable outcome. The appropriate treatment plan should be formulated in consultation with a multidisciplinary team that includes an obstetrician, a fetal medicine specialist, an infectious disease specialist, and a neonatologist. The planning includes the following:

- Treatment of maternal chickenpox
- Planning the date and mode of delivery
- Adoption of measures to protect the baby from the untoward effects of the infection

In this chapter, these components of management will be discussed in detail.

COMPONENTS OF DELIVERY CARE IN WOMEN WITH CHICKENPOX

The components of delivery care of pregnant women suffering from chickenpox involve the following (Fig. 41.1):

- Care of the pregnant woman
  - — Routine antenatal care
  - — Management of varicella infection
    - ▪ General measures
    - ▪ Medical therapy
- Formulating delivery plan
  - — When to deliver
  - — Where to deliver
  - — How to deliver
- Vaginal delivery
  - — Induction/augmentation
  - — Monitoring of labour
  - — AMTSL and monitoring of the third stage
- Cesarean delivery
  - — Cesarean technique
  - — Anesthesia
- Postpartum care
  - — General newborn care
  - — Specific measures to prevent/treat neonatal varicella
  - — Breastfeeding
- Protection of the healthcare provider

CARE OF THE WOMAN

The woman's care should be appropriate for the gestational age and proceed as a continuum

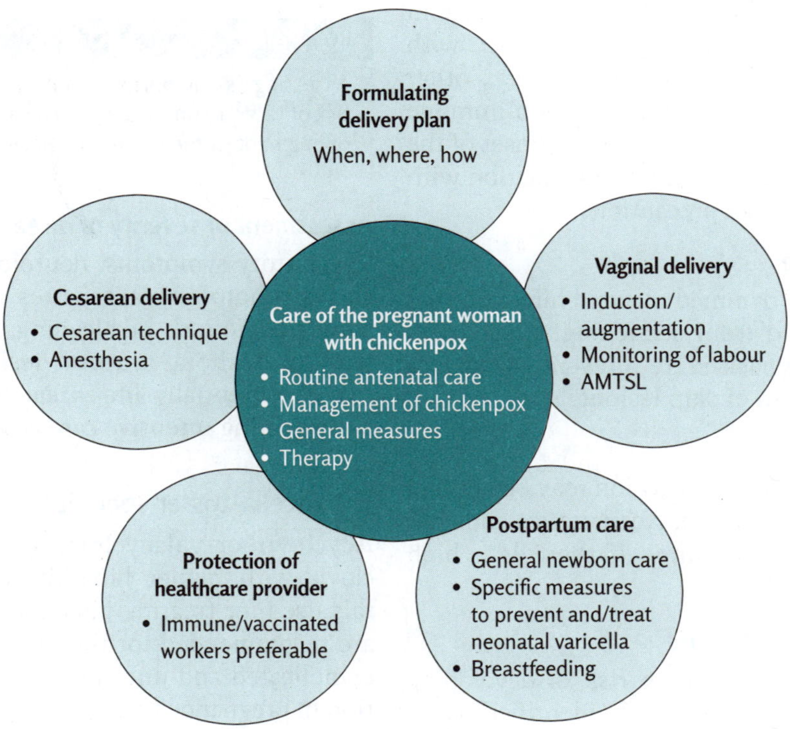

Fig. 41.1 Care of a pregnant woman who has chickenpox at the time of delivery
AMTSL, active management of the third stage of labour

throughout pregnancy, together with specific measures against the varicella-zoster virus. In addition to routine care in labour, aspects of care specific to chickenpox need to be kept in mind.

The management of chickenpox entails general measures, varicella-zoster-specific medications, and the management of complications [7].

General Measures

The principles of general management of a pregnant woman suffering from chickenpox include nursing care in isolation, maintaining hygiene, and providing symptom relief.

An assessment of risk factors and disease severity should be done to identify women who may be at risk of complications necessitating intensive care admission.

Isolation

Chickenpox is highly infectious, especially from 48 hours prior to the onset of rashes until the lesions have crusted over. Infected pregnant women should be kept isolated in the hospital and should avoid contact with potentially susceptible individuals—e.g., other pregnant women, neonates, and non-immune staff—usually for five days after the onset of the rash. They should be cared for in isolation with airborne and contact precautions.

General hygiene

Nails should be trimmed to avoid infection that may be acquired from scratching. Cleanliness should be emphasised to prevent secondary bacterial infection of skin lesions.

Symptom relief

Emollients like calamine lotion may be applied to soothe skin irritation. Antipyretics and cold sponging may be required if there is a high fever.

Assessment of risk factors

Women who are at a high risk of developing varicella pneumonia should be identified based on the risk factors [8]:

- Infection in the third trimester
- ≥100 skin lesions (indicating high viral load) or hemorrhagic lesions
- History of smoking
- Chronic lung disease
- Immunosuppression (including those who have taken systemic corticosteroids in the preceding three months)

A hospital assessment should be considered in these women who are at a high risk of severe or complicated chickenpox even in the absence of symptoms or signs of concern. This assessment should take place in an area where the woman will not come into contact with other pregnant women [8].

Radiologic changes alone do not predict clinically significant pneumonia requiring treatment. Moreover, a chest X-ray immediately after the onset of the rash might not predict later development of varicella pneumonia. Therefore, a routine chest X-ray is not warranted for all pregnant women who develop varicella.

Key Point

Assessing risk factors for complications, especially the risk of VZV pneumonia, is crucial in the management of pregnant women with varicella infection.

Assessment of severity of disease

Respiratory symptoms, neurological symptoms such as photophobia, seizures, or drowsiness, a hemorrhagic rash or bleeding, or a dense rash with or without mucosal lesions are indicative of potentially life-threatening chickenpox necessitating intensive care access [9].

Varicella-zoster-specific Medications

Acyclovir or **valacyclovir** (a prodrug of acyclovir with higher bioavailability) are antivirals used for treating infection with VZV. They are recommended for the management of both complicated and uncomplicated varicella infection in pregnancy [2]. All pregnant women with established chickenpox should receive oral acyclovir or valacyclovir [10].

The RCOG recommends oral acyclovir for pregnant women with chickenpox if they present within 24 hours of the onset of the rash and if they are at 20+0 weeks of gestation or beyond. The use of acyclovir before 20+0 weeks should also be considered [11].

The pros and cons of treatment should be discussed with women with uncomplicated chickenpox before prescribing the medication.

Dosage of antivirals

The following oral dosages are recommended [10]:

- **Acyclovir** 800 mg five times daily for 7 days or
- **Valacyclovir** 1 g three times daily for 7 days

There is a small window of up to 72 hours after the onset of the rash when antivirals may be useful. Compared with placebo, these drugs reduce the duration of fever and symptoms of chickenpox if commenced within 24 hours of rash development.

> **Key Point**
>
> If antivirals are given within 24 hours and up to 72 hours of rash, there may be a reduction in maternal and fetal morbidity and mortality associated with VZV infection [8,12,13].

Safety of antivirals

Acyclovir crosses the placenta and can be found in the amniotic fluid, umbilical cord blood, and other fetal tissues [14], though it does not appear to accumulate in the fetus. However, there is no evidence of fetal benefits with respect to the prevention or amelioration of varicella infection of the newborn or neonatal varicella. As viral replication during maternal viremia is inhibited, it may indirectly reduce transplacental transmission of VZV.

Small studies of valacyclovir use in late pregnancy have found no clinical or laboratory evidence of toxicity in infants followed up to one month or six months of age [15].

Management of Complications

Maternal complications may be severe, and the woman may need hospitalisation and a systematic approach to prevent mortality.

VZV pneumonia

Varicella pneumonia during pregnancy is a medical emergency [7]. It presents with cough, dyspnea, fever, and tachypnea. The chest X-ray findings include a bilateral diffuse or miliary/nodular infiltrative pattern, often in the peribronchial distribution.

While pneumonia has been associated with relative maternal immunosuppression [8], it may also be mechanical, with increasing splinting of the diaphragm as the gravid uterus occupies more space. The effect is more marked in the later weeks of pregnancy [16].

Pregnant women with VZV pneumonia should be monitored intensively and antiviral therapy should be initiated immediately. In the pre-antiviral era, up to 40% of women were reported to need mechanical ventilation [17]. Mortality in severe cases (those who required mechanical ventilation) in the pre-antiviral era was 20–45% but has dramatically decreased after the use of antivirals and is currently being reported to be 14% [13].

> **Key Point**
>
> A pulmonologist and intensive care specialist should be available when a woman with VZV pneumonia is in labour.

Antiviral therapy

Guidelines are unanimous in recommending intravenous acyclovir in cases of severe varicella infection because of higher bioavailability, especially in the second half of pregnancy. The preferred dose is 10–15 mg/Kg of body weight IV every 8 hours for 5–10 days for VZV pneumonia and should be started within 24–72 hours of the appearance of the rash [2,8,10,18].

Key Point

Dosage of IV acyclovir: 10–15 mg/Kg of body weight IV every 8 hours for 5–10 days in pneumonia/severe illness.

FORMULATING THE DELIVERY PLAN

The timing of delivery of the pregnant woman with chickenpox must be individualised. It is good practice to involve the neonatologist and physician/infectious disease specialist in making the care plan for delivery.

When to Deliver

Delivery in the viremia phase with active chickenpox vesicles requires careful management. There may be significant maternal hemorrhage and/or coagulopathy due to changes in liver function or viral thrombocytopenia. There is also a very high risk of peripartum transmission to the newborn, which may progress to fulminant infection with dire consequences [19].

Ideally, delivery is safest if a minimum of seven days has elapsed from the onset of lesions. During this time, supportive treatment is desirable, allowing resolution of the rash, immune recovery, and transfer of protective antibodies from the mother to the fetus. However, the woman may spontaneously go into labour in this critical period or it may be necessary to hasten the delivery of a woman in respiratory failure due to viral pneumonia [11].

Where to Deliver

It is prudent to deliver the woman in a hospital where critical care and neonatal intensive care facilities are available. Delivery may be complicated by maternal hemorrhage. The baby also has a high risk of either congenital or neonatal varicella infection with significant morbidity and mortality. Fetal growth restriction (FGR) occurs in approximately 23% of cases, and low birth weight is virtually universal. The incidence of preterm deliveries is also high, with a spontaneous preterm birth rate of 5.6% in unexposed pregnant women vs. 14.3% for pregnancy with chickenpox [6].

Mode of Delivery

The mode of delivery should also be individualised. After an initial review of the antenatal records and obtaining relevant history regarding the date of the onset of the rash, treatment received, and any other pregnancy complications and a detailed general and obstetric examination, a decision regarding vaginal or cesarean birth should be made.

- **Vaginal delivery**: In stable women, there is no contraindication for vaginal birth outside the seven-day danger period, and augmentation and induction are the same as in normal pregnancies.
- **Cesarean birth**: This option may be preferred in women with the following:
  - Extensive vulvar and vaginal lesions
  - Respiratory failure (to facilitate ventilation)
  - Obstetric indications

Since chickenpox spreads by droplets and fomites, labour should be conducted in isolation after adopting airborne and contact precautions, ideally by personnel immune to varicella.

Airborne precautions should be used for the following:

- Women who have active vesicles at delivery
- Susceptible women who were exposed to varicella and give birth during the mother's incubation period (10–21 days following exposure to varicella)
- Women who develop symptoms of varicella within 3 days of delivery

In any woman or infant with active vesicles, contact precautions should also be used.

Vaginal delivery

While planning and conducting vaginal delivery in women with VZV infection, the following issues need to be addressed.

Induction or augmentation

In planned deliveries, induction and augmentation should be according to local guidelines for a normal pregnancy.

Monitoring of labour

If vaginal delivery is contemplated, labour management follows routine assessment and documentation according to the local protocol. Special precautions are to be taken to prevent dehydration and control febrile episodes, if any.

Active management of the third stage of labour (AMTSL)

Pregnant women who have chickenpox are at risk of postpartum hemorrhage. For this reason, along with AMTSL, a close watch must be kept with rigorous monitoring in the third stage of labour.

Cesarean delivery

Precautions

There are no special guidelines for cesarean section in a woman with a varicella infection. The incision on the skin should preferably be made over a vesicle-free area or an area where few vesicles are present.

Anesthesia

It is important to keep the anesthetic team involved when providing care to a woman with chickenpox in pregnancy.

General anesthesia may cause pneumonia with respiratory compromise. For regional anesthesia, either epidural or spinal, it is recommended that a site free of cutaneous lesions should be chosen for needle placement. There is a theoretical risk of transmitting the virus from the skin to the CNS via the spinal cord.

Epidural may have an edge over spinal anesthesia because it has a lower potential to cause CNS infections as the dura is not penetrated. However, the epidural needle is a wide-bore needle; therefore, there is a theoretical risk of depositing a greater viral load [20].

Key Point

A site free of cutaneous lesions should be chosen for needle placement when epidural or spinal anesthesia is administered to a pregnant woman who has chickenpox.

CARE OF THE NEONATE

Nursing Care for the Newborn and Mother

Following delivery, the newborn and the mother are not separated if the infection occurred remote from the time of delivery.

Severe chickenpox is most likely to occur if the infant is born within seven days of the onset of the mother's rash or if the mother develops the rash up to seven days after delivery [11]. In such cases, it is important to administer varicella-zoster immunologbulin (VZIG) to the baby.

The newborn should remain under airborne precautions for 21 days after the last exposure to the mother's active vesicles. This period should be extended to 28 days if the newborn receives VZIG, since the immunoglobulin can increase the incubation period.

If the newborn develops varicella, airborne and contact precautions should be maintained until the vesicles crust over.

Breastfeeding

Women with chickenpox should be allowed to breastfeed if they wish to and if they are free of complications. In the presence of active chickenpox lesions close to the nipple, breast milk is expressed from the affected breast until the lesions have crusted over. Babies receiving treatment with VZIG and/or acyclovir may be fed on expressed breast milk.

Screening for Varicella Infection of the Newborn

After completing routine newborn care, the baby is examined for the stigma of varicella infection of the newborn, the features of which include the following [6]:

- Skin lesions (70%)
- Limb hypoplasia (46–72%)
- Neurological abnormalities including microcephaly, cortical atrophy, hydrocephaly (48–62%)
- Ocular defects including microphthalmia, chorioretinitis, and cataracts (44–52%)
- Muscle hypoplasia
- Abnormalities of the gastrointestinal and genitourinary tracts, and the cardiovascular system
- Developmental delays and intellectual disability may be long-term effects

A neonatal ophthalmic examination should be performed. Serological testing of the fetal or cord blood for VZV IgM at birth and the persistence of specific IgG after seven months of age confirms the diagnosis.

Most cases of varicella infection of the newborn occur following maternal infection between 8 and 20 weeks' gestation. However, the overall risk of vertical transmission is quite small—approximately 2% in women infected before 20 weeks [7].

Prognosis

Varicella infection of the newborn has a mortality rate of 30% in babies with clinically apparent lesions [7]. There is a 15% risk of developing herpes zoster between the 2nd and 41st month of life [2]. However, despite a poor initial prognosis, the long-term outcome for survivors is good.

Neonatal Varicella

The neonate may acquire the infection transplacentally, by the vaginal route, or as a result of direct contact with lesions during or after delivery.

Neonatal chickenpox in the first 10–12 days of life is caused by intrauterine transmission, whereas after the 13th day, it is likely to be a postnatal infection [2,5]. The newborn can develop infection up to 21 days after birth (or 28 days if VZIG is administered because VZIG may prolong the incubation period).

Spectrum of neonatal varicella

When acquired in utero in the last three weeks of pregnancy, the severity of varicella disease in the newborn is determined by the interval between maternal infection and delivery and the rate of maternal-specific antibody formation and transfer to the fetus [22]. Except for the very premature and low-birth-weight babies (<28 weeks' gestation or <1000 g), varicella infection acquired postnatally during the first month of life will, in the vast majority of cases, lead to mild-to-moderate disease. Irrespective of the timing of acquiring maternal VZV, infected newborns can further develop zoster during the first year of their life [5].

Key Point

Before the availability of neonatal intensive care, VZIG, and antivirals, the mortality rate for neonatal chickenpox was 31% and continues to be 7% in the modern era [21].

The severity of neonatal disease and its correlation to the onset of infection in the mother is summarised in Table 41.1.

Management of the neonate

The management of the exposed newborn involves the prevention of neonatal varicella and/or treating the infection if it eventually develops even after all precautions.

Administration of varicella-zoster immunoglobulin (VZIG)

The prevention of neonatal infection involves the administration of VZIG to exposed newborns. While VZIG may not prevent infection, it may reduce the severity of neonatal infection. However, it is of no benefit once signs of chickenpox manifest [2,22].

Table 41.1 Spectrum of neonatal varicella according to onset of maternal infection [22]

Timing of maternal varicella infection	Neonatal effects	Neonatal mortality
Varicella 5 days before delivery to 2 days after delivery	• Neonatal varicella 20–50% • Severe or fulminant neonatal varicella 30%	20%
20 days to 5 days before delivery	• Neonatal infection 50% • Clinical chickenpox 23%	0–3%

The recommended VZIG dose is as follows:

- 125 U IM for newborn weighing <2 Kg
- 250 U IM for newborn weighing >2 Kg

Administration of acyclovir

As yet, there is no controlled clinical trial that has evaluated the efficacy of acyclovir treatment in neonatal varicella. However, it is the treatment of choice. The neonatal team is involved in the management of these babies.

PROTECTION OF THE HEALTHCARE PROVIDER

Healthcare personnel involved with infected women should preferably be immune against the disease, i.e., they should either have had chickenpox in the past or should have been immunised. If non-immunised, they should be given VZIG and isolated for 28 days.

Vaccination of employees with a negative or uncertain history of varicella is recommended.

Key Point

Healthcare providers who do not have immunity against varicella should ideally not be involved in the intrapartum care of infected women.

CONCLUSION

Medical science has made numerous advances in the last few decades. However, managing and conducting labour in a pregnant woman with chickenpox remains a challenge. It involves a continuum of care of the woman together with the planning and monitoring of labour with appropriate safety precautions for the woman, her baby, and the healthcare personnel responsible for her care. With a good multidisciplinary team approach, a favourable outcome can be achieved.

REFERENCES

1. Miller E, Marshall R, Vurdien JE. Epidemiology, outcome and control of varicella-zoster infection. *Rev Med Microbiol*. 1993. 4:222–30.
2. Lamont RF, Sobel JD, Carrington D, Mazaki-Tovi S, Kusanovic JP, Vaisbuch E, Romero R. Varicella-zoster virus (chickenpox) infection in pregnancy. *BJOG*. 2011. 118(10):1155-62.
3. Inbaraj LR, Chandrasingh S, Arun Kumar N, Suchitra J, Manesh A. High susceptibility to varicella among urban and rural pregnant women in South India: A brief report. *Epidemiol Infect*. 2021. 149:e63.
4. ACOG Practice Bulletin No. 151. Cytomegalovirus, parvovirus B19, varicella zoster, and toxoplasmosis in pregnancy. American College of Obstetricians and Gynecologists. *Obstet Gynecol*. 2015. 125:1510–25.
5. Sauerbrei A, Wutzler P. Herpes simplex and varicella-zoster virus infections during pregnancy: Current concepts of prevention, diagnosis and therapy. Part 2: Varicella-zoster virus infections. *Med Microbiol Immunol*. 2007. 196:95–102.
6. Pastuszak AL, Levy M, Schick B, et al. Outcome after maternal varicella infection in the first 20 weeks of pregnancy. *N Engl J Med*. 1994. 330:901.
7. Riley LE. Prenatal care: Varicella-zoster virus infection in pregnancy. Hirsch MS, Lockwood CJ (Eds). *UpToDate*. 2023. Waltham, MA.
8. Harger JH, Ernest JM, Thurnau GR, Moawad A, Momirova V, Landon MB, et al. Risk factors and outcome of varicella-zoster virus pneumonia in pregnant women. *J Infect Dis*. 2002. 185:422-7.
9. Nathwani D, Maclean A, Conway S, Carrington D. Varicella infections in pregnancy and the newborn.

A review prepared for the UK Advisory Group on Chickenpox on behalf of the British Society for the Study of Infection. *J Infect*. 1998. 36 Suppl 1:59–71.

10. Gardella C, Brown ZA. Managing varicella zoster infection in pregnancy. *Cleve Clin J Med*. 2007. 74(4):290–296.
11. Royal College of Obstetricians and Gynaecologists. Green-top Guideline No. 13. Chickenpox in Pregnancy. 2015. RCOG. London.
12. Mohsen AH, McKendrick M. Varicella pneumonia in adults. *Eur Respir J*. 2003. 21(5):886–891.
13. Smego RA Jr, Asperilla MO. Use of acyclovir for varicella pneumonia during pregnancy. *Obstet Gynecol*. 1991. 78(6):1112–1116.
14. Frenkel LM, Brown ZA, Bryson YJ, Corey L, Unadkat JD, Hensleigh PA, et al. Pharmacokinetics of acyclovir in the term human pregnancy and neonate. *Am J Obstet Gynecol*. 1991. 164(2):569– 576.
15. Ogilvie MM. Antiviral prophylaxis and treatment in chickenpox. A review prepared for the UK Advisory Group on Chickenpox on behalf of the British Society for the Study of Infection. *J Infect*. 1998. 36 (Suppl 1):31–38.
16. Schutte TJ, Rogers LC, Copas PR. Varicella pneumonia complicating pregnancy: A report of seven cases. *Infect Dis Obstet Gynecol*. 1996. 4(6):338–346. [PubMed: 18476122].
17. Cox SM, Cunningham FG, Luby J. Management of varicella pneumonia complicating pregnancy. *Am J Perinatol*. 1990. 7(4):300–301. [PubMed: 2222616].
18. Shrim A, Koren G, Yudin MH, Farine D. Maternal Fetal Medicine Committee. Management of varicella infection (chickenpox) in pregnancy. SOGC Clinical Practice Guideline No. 274. *J Obstet Gynaecol Can*. 2012. 34:287–92.
19. Meyers JD. Congenital varicella in term infants: risks reconsidered. *J Infect Dis*. 1974. 129:215–7.
20. Brown NW, Parsons AP, Kam PC. Anaesthetic considerations in a parturient with varicella presenting for cesarean section. *Anaesthesia*. 2003. 58:1092–5.
21. Miller E, Cradock-Watson JE, Ridehalgh MK. Outcome in newborn babies given anti-varicella-zoster immunoglobulin after perinatal maternal infection with varicella-zoster virus. *Lancet*. 1989. 2(8659):371–373.
22. Sauerbrei A, Wutzler P. Neonatal varicella. *J Perinatol*. 2001; 21(8):545–549. [PubMed: 11774017].

CHAPTER 42

HIV

PALLAVI CHANDRA RAVULA, HEMAMALINI VADLAMANI

INTRODUCTION

There have been significant advances in the prevention, screening, diagnosis, treatment, and follow-up of HIV globally. Over the last few decades, there has been a remarkable reduction in HIV-related morbidity, mortality, and perinatal transmission due to the advent of newer molecules for treatment which are less toxic and more cost-effective.

The goal of HIV management in labour is optimising maternal health and preventing mother-to-child transmission. The National AIDS Control Organisation (NACO), India, was established in 1992 to oversee policies for the prevention and control of HIV infection. The National AIDS Control Programme-III (NACP-III), 2006–2011, focused on reversing the epidemic and achieved the reduction of new infections by 50%. NACP-IV (2012–2017) aimed at improving the integration of HIV care into the general health system. The current phase, NACP-V (2021–2026), focuses on ensuring that people living with HIV lead long and productive lives.

This chapter will discuss the management of HIV-infected women who present in labour. For more information on antiretroviral therapy (ART) during the antenatal period, the reader is referred to other resources.

PREVALENCE

An estimated 37.6 million people are living with HIV as per the UNAIDS 2021 global report [1]. Approximately 1.5 million people acquired HIV worldwide in 2020, of whom an estimated 690,000 lives were lost due to AIDS-related illnesses worldwide in 2020. An estimated 27.4 million were accessing antiretroviral therapy in 2020 globally.

There is a considerable difference in the prevalence of HIV across different countries. In India, HIV infections are declining both in men and women [2] and the prevalence rate of HIV in 2022 in adults aged 15–49 was estimated to be 0.2% [3]. Despite this low prevalence rate, India still has the third highest burden of HIV worldwide [2]. The states with the highest prevalence are Maharashtra, Tamil Nadu, Karnataka, Andhra Pradesh, Manipur, and Nagaland.

Approximately 2.4 million adults in India are living with HIV, of whom 1.1 million are women. 80% of infected women are of childbearing age. Gender inequalities, reduced access to healthcare facilities, and sexual violence increase women's vulnerability to infection.

Key Point

Despite a low prevalence rate, India still has the third highest burden of HIV worldwide [2].

PATHOGENESIS

HIV is a lentivirus that causes **acquired immunodeficiency syndrome (AIDS)**. In AIDS, there is a progressive failure of the immune system. Life-threatening opportunistic infections and cancers flourish in this immunosuppressed state. Without treatment, life expectancy after infection with HIV is estimated to be 9–11 years.

Two types of HIV virus have been identified, HIV-1 and HIV-2.

- **HIV-1** is more virulent and more infective and causes the majority of HIV infections globally. The virus infects CD4+ receptors and starts replicating within them. Infected cells release virions by surface budding or lysis, leading to the infection of additional cells.
- **HIV-2** is prevalent in small foci in Western India. It is less transmissible from mother-to-child (transmission risk 0.4%). The disease is slow-progressing, has a longer asymptomatic stage, a slow decline in the CD4 count, lower viral load, and shows good response to ART. Non-nucleoside reverse transcriptase inhibitors (NNRTIs) such as Efavirenz and Nevirapine are ineffective for the treatment of HIV-2. Hence, neonatal prophylaxis is carried out with Zidovudine syrup rather than Nevirapine syrup.

EFFECT OF PREGNANCY ON HIV

Pregnancy is associated with a depression of cell-mediated immunity and a decline in the CD4 lymphocyte count similar to that seen in HIV infection. Several symptoms of HIV infection such as breathlessness may mimic pregnancy symptoms. In asymptomatic women, pregnancy does not have a major adverse effect on the disease progression. There is no evidence to suggest that pregnancy increases the risk of progression to AIDS or a decline in the CD4 count to less than 200/cubic mm.

EFFECT OF HIV ON PREGNANCY

In advanced HIV infection, there is an increased risk of miscarriage, preterm birth, and fetal growth restriction, especially in developing countries, reflecting the poor nutritional status and access to ART. There is no evidence that suggests an increase in congenital malformations.

SCREENING

Screening for HIV is recommended as standard care for all pregnant women. Women should be offered voluntary HIV testing with informed consent as early as possible in pregnancy. If a woman screens positive, she should be informed about the results in person, with her privacy and confidentiality ensured. She should be given detailed information about HIV infection, further investigations, the need for treatment, and the possible effects of the infection on her and the baby. Interventions to reduce vertical transmission to the child should be initiated immediately.

> **Key Point**
>
> If a woman screens positive, she should be informed about the results in person, while ensuring her privacy and confidentiality.

Repeat Screening in Pregnancy

Women at increased risk of acquiring the infection should be offered testing again in the third trimester, even if the first trimester report was negative. These include women with the following risk factors [4]:

- Residence in high-prevalence areas
- Engagement in sex work
- Employment in healthcare facilities
- Injection drug use
- Multiple sex partners, sex with HIV-positive partners or drug users

Repeat testing is also recommended for women with sexually transmitted diseases in the past year and for those who show signs and symptoms of acute HIV infection (e.g., fever, lymphadenopathy, skin rash, myalgias, arthralgias, headache, oral ulcers, leukopenia, thrombocytopenia, or transaminase elevation).

Woman in Labour with Unknown HIV Status

When a woman presents in labour, it is good practice to document the HIV status from her antenatal screening. Women whose HIV status is unknown should undergo point-of-care HIV testing. Knowing their HIV status allows the initiation of anti-viral prophylaxis before delivery to prevent mother-to-child transmission (MTCT).

Rapid or point-of-care tests

Any woman presenting in labour who has not undergone testing during the antenatal period or who is unaware of her HIV status in the current pregnancy should be screened with a rapid HIV test in the labour room after getting her informed consent.

Rapid tests use a drop of blood from a finger-stick or an oral swab. They can be performed anywhere and do not require laboratory facilities or highly trained staff. Results are obtained in as little as 20 minutes and usually within an hour. The most commonly used rapid tests are based on enzyme immune assay, immunochromatography, immuno-concentration, and particle agglutination. These tests have a sensitivity of more than 99.5% and specificity of more than 98%.

Since these tests check for the presence of antibodies, the test may miss a recent HIV infection **('window period')**.

Window period

It is the period between infection with HIV and the time when HIV antibodies can be detected in blood, which is usually between 6 and 12 weeks. Tests performed during the window period may yield a negative result for HIV antibodies. If the woman is considered to be at high risk for HIV infection, the test should be repeated after 12 weeks.

Management of results from rapid testing in the woman in labour

Reactive rapid test

- Antiretroviral prophylaxis with tenofovir, lamivudine, and dolutegravir (TLD) should be initiated immediately for the mother (Table 42.1).
- Blood should be sent for supplemental testing to confirm the presence or absence of infection with HIV. If the supplemental test comes back non-reactive, antiretroviral prophylaxis should be discontinued.
- If the diagnosis of HIV infection is confirmed by supplementary testing, in the postpartum period, the woman should be offered education on her condition and referred to a specialist in HIV for follow-up care for herself and her neonate.

Rapid tests not available

The untested woman should be managed as if she is HIV infected to prevent possible perinatal HIV transmission. The ART regimen used for such a woman is presented in Table 42.1.

MOTHER-TO-CHILD TRANSMISSION (MTCT)

Perinatal or vertical transmission refers to the transmission of HIV from mother to child during pregnancy, labour, birth, or breastfeeding. In developed countries with ample resources, the vertical transmission of HIV is rare. However, it continues to be a public health challenge in resource-limited settings.

Efforts to increase the use of antiretroviral therapy and better access to comprehensive

Table 42.1 ART regimen in the intrapartum period and during breastfeeding (adapted from NACO guidelines [2])

Maternal status	Intrapartum	Postpartum
Presenting in labour with undocumented HIV status, reactive rapid test, no previous ART	Initiate TLD regimen Tenofovir 300 mg (TDF) + Lamivudine 300 mg (3TC) + Dolutegravir 50 mg (DTG) once daily	Continue TLD regimen TDF (300 mg) + 3TC (300 mg) + DTG (50 mg) once daily

ART, antiretroviral therapy

HIV and pregnancy care services have led to a marked decrease in vertical HIV transmission rates in LMICs such as India. UNICEF data [5] have shown a dramatic 58% decrease in vertical transmission between 2010 and 2022. In 2020, globally, an estimated 85% of HIV-infected pregnant women received antiretroviral therapy for their own health and to prevent vertical transmission of HIV to their infants [6].

In India, the National AIDS Control Organisation launched the National Prevention of Parent-to-Child Transmission (PPTCT) programme [7] with an aim to eliminate vertical transmission of HIV. The PPTCT programme has four elements:

- Primary prevention of HIV among women of childbearing age
- Prevention of unplanned pregnancies among women with HIV
- Prevention of HIV transmission from pregnant women to their children
- Providing care, support, and treatment to women living with HIV and their families and children

Routes of MTCT

Transmission of HIV from the mother to her child may occur in the following ways:

- In utero in the antepartum period
- Through exposure to maternal blood and bodily fluids at the time of birth
- Through breastfeeding

Two-thirds of cases of MTCT occur around birth. Breastfeeding can double the rate of transmission from 15% to 30%.

This chapter will deal with the prevention of MTCT in the intrapartum period and during breastfeeding.

Mechanism of Vertical Transmission

Intrapartum transmission

Two mechanisms are responsible for the transmission of HIV to the fetus or newborn during labour and delivery:

- As the infant passes through the vagina, its mucous membranes come into contact with the virus present in the blood and secretions associated with birth.
- In a woman who is not on ART, membrane rupture >4 hours before delivery has been associated with an increased risk of transmission [8]. However, it is now accepted that the duration of membrane rupture of 4 or more hours is not a risk factor for the perinatal transmission of HIV in women with a viral load <1000 copies/mL receiving combination ART [9]. A viral load of >10,000 copies/mL is considered a risk factor for perinatal transmission if the membranes have been ruptured for >4 hours.
- During labour contractions, maternal infected blood is transfused across the placenta into the fetus.

> **Key Point**
>
> In the presence of ruptured membranes for >4 hours, a viral load of >10,000 copies/mL is considered a risk factor for perinatal transmission.

Breastfeeding and vertical transmission

Though it is clear that HIV is transmitted from mother to child during breastfeeding, the exact mechanism of this has not been clearly understood. HIV-infected cells within breast milk may play an important role in transmission to the infant. Infected breast milk cells may have a greater role in transmission than the cell-free virus [10]. The virus may then enter the child's circulation through the tonsillar or intestinal tissues.

Risk Factors for MTCT

Factors that increase the likelihood of MTCT during labour, delivery, and the postpartum period are the following:

Maternal factors

Antepartum factors

- High viral load
- Low CD4 counts and low CD4:CD8 ratios reflecting poor immunological status

- Advanced disease
- Recent HIV infection
- Seroconversion during pregnancy
- Sexually transmitted infections

Intrapartum factors

- Prolonged rupture of membranes for >4 hours (doubles the risk of transmission with high viral loads)
- Preterm labour
- Assisted vaginal birth
- Invasive procedures during the intrapartum period such as episiotomy and fetal scalp electrode monitoring

Postpartum factors

- Breast-related issues like sore nipples, breast abscess, mastitis

Fetal and neonatal factors

- Prematurity: Gestational age <35 weeks
- Low birth weight
- Mixed feeds
- Oral ulcers or thrush

INTRAPARTUM MANAGEMENT OF HIV-INFECTED WOMEN

Antiretroviral Therapy

Women with HIV should receive ART throughout pregnancy in accordance with the accepted guidelines. Early initiation of combination antiretroviral drug regimens during or before pregnancy (rather than at delivery) is associated with a lower risk of infant transmission.

In the past, treatment in resource-limited settings focused on and demonstrated the efficacy of one- or two-drug regimens (zidovudine, zidovudine/lamivudine, nevirapine) given in the last trimester and around labour/delivery because they were less expensive and more deliverable in resource-limited settings. However, a recent study from Africa and India [11] that compared the one- or two-drug regimens with immediate three-drug ART initiated at diagnosis showed that combination ART is much more effective in preventing MTCT.

Women infected with HIV should receive a combination of at least three ARV drugs for fetal protection even when they are stable and asymptomatic. The combination drugs inhibit the replication of HIV and reduce the viral load to undetectable levels, which in turn, results in the restoration of the immune response with an increase in the CD4 count. The disease progression slows down with fewer chances of opportunistic infections and better quality of life and life span.

Key Point

Immediate initiation of three-drug combination ART at diagnosis is effective in preventing MTCT.

Mode of Delivery

All women should give birth in a healthcare centre that provides access to immediate neonatal care. The decision about the mode of delivery is made based on the woman's viral load near the time of delivery, as the risk of HIV transmission can be predicted by the viral load.

- **Lowest risk:** Undetectable viral load (<50 copies/mL)
    - — May be delivered by the **vaginal route**. In women already receiving ART and with a very low or undetectable viral load, elective cesarean does not offer any advantage.
    - — The need for cesarean delivery is determined by obstetric indications.
- **Low-to-moderate risk:** Detectable viral load (≥50 copies/mL but ≤1000 copies/mL)
    - — Should be delivered based on the obstetric indication.
- **High risk:** >1000 copies/mL near the time of delivery or no ART during pregnancy
    - — Should be delivered by an elective cesarean section at 38 weeks' gestation.

Delivery in low-resource settings

Scheduled cesarean delivery has been shown to be associated with reduced rates of perinatal transmission in resource-rich settings. However, in resource-limited settings, where cesarean section is not always available, the presence and status of HIV infection in the pregnant woman does not affect decisions on the mode of delivery. The national guidelines in India issued by NACO [2] recommend vaginal delivery for all women with HIV, unless there is an obstetric indication for a cesarean delivery.

Key Point

In resource-poor settings, vaginal delivery is the acceptable mode of delivery. Cesarean section is reserved for obstetric indications.

In settings where testing for viral load is not available, decisions regarding the mode of delivery should be based on antenatal ART, the combination of ART used, and adherence to therapy. The risks and benefits of a cesarean section should be considered.

These guidelines are summarised in Table 42.2.

Vaginal delivery

Decreasing the risk of MTCT during vaginal delivery

The risk of HIV transmission during vaginal birth can be reduced by the following:

- Minimising digital vaginal examination
- Avoiding artificial rupture of membranes
- Avoiding invasive procedures such as fetal scalp electrode testing
- Avoiding prolonged labour
- Avoiding instrumental birth
- Avoiding episiotomy
- Practicing standard/universal precautions

Intrapartum ART

- **Vaginal birth:** All women with HIV should receive intravenous zidovudine during labour unless contraindicated. It is given as a loading dose of 2 g/Kg over an hour, followed by 1 g/hour throughout labour while continuing other oral ART [13].

Table 42.2 **Intrapartum management and infant prophylaxis for pregnant women with HIV (based on WHO consolidated guidelines on the use of antiretroviral drugs for treating and preventing HIV infection [12])**

Treatment based on maternal viral load (VL)	Woman on antepartum ART			No antepartum ART
	Undetectable VL (<50 copies/mL) near time of delivery	Detectable: ≥50 copies/mL but ≤1000 copies/mL near time of delivery	>1000 copies/mL near time of delivery	
Risk of HIV transmission	Lowest risk	Low–moderate risk	High risk	High risk
Mode of delivery	• Vaginal delivery • Cesarean section only for obstetric indication	Based on obstetric indication	Elective cesarean delivery* at 38 weeks	Cesarean delivery*
Intrapartum ART	Continue ART the woman was on	In addition, consider IV zidovudine	In addition, administer IV zidovudine	Start triple combination ART
Infant prophylaxis	4 weeks of NVP/ zidovudine	Combination prophylaxis	Combination prophylaxis	Combination prophylaxis for 12 weeks

NVP, nevirapine; *VL*, viral load

*In resource-limited settings, vaginal delivery may be the only option available. In such situations, the presence and status of HIV infection in the mother does not affect decisions on the route of delivery.

- **Elective cesarean delivery:** Intravenous zidovudine should be given at least 3 hours prior to the procedure [14]. **IV zidovudine is currently not available in India.**

Timing of Delivery

Vaginal delivery

Women with a viral load of ≤1000 copies/mL at 36 weeks may be allowed to await spontaneous onset of labour. Elective delivery before 40+0 weeks' gestational age has not been shown to lower the risk of mother-to-child transmission [15].

Elective cesarean delivery

As a medically-indicated procedure, cesarean should be scheduled at 38+0 weeks' gestation to avoid the likelihood of onset of labour or rupture of membranes before delivery.

Prelabour Rupture of Membranes (PROM)

In the era before combination ART, a duration of membrane rupture of ≥4 hours was considered a risk factor for MTCT. For women on ART whose viral loads are ≤1000 copies/mL, there seems to be no association between the duration of rupture of membranes and increase in MTCT [16,17].

Special Scenarios

- In a woman with a previous cesarean birth, trial of labour (TOLAC) can be offered if the viral load is <50 copies/mL as the risk of maternal blood entering the fetal circulation is low.
- In a woman with breech presentation, external cephalic version can be offered if the viral load is <50 copies/mL as the risk of maternal blood entering the fetal circulation is low [18].
- Sero-discordant couple—if the woman is HIV-positive and the man is negative and the couple is planning to conceive, they may use the option of self-insemination or intrauterine insemination (IUI). The man should be on ART as long as the couple is planning to conceive.

POSTPARTUM MANAGEMENT

ART should not be stopped postpartum. Postpartum complications are high among women with HIV. Fever, endometritis, wound infection, and urinary tract infections are more common in women with cesarean birth and in those with advanced disease [19,20].

Contraception

Combination hormonal contraceptives are highly effective in preventing pregnancies. The couple should be encouraged to use condoms to prevent other sexually transmitted diseases. The other options are transdermal or intravaginal hormonal contraceptives. Intrauterine contraceptive devices are safe and effective options. The levonorgestrel IUCD has the added advantage of reducing blood loss during menstruation. For couples who have completed their family, permanent female or male sterilisation should be discussed and encouraged.

Screening for Cervical Cancer

Screening should be performed at the initiation of ART. The test should be repeated within three years. Visual inspection with acetic acid (VIA) or cervical cytology should be performed at three months postpartum.

FOLLOW-UP

Partner screening and testing for other children should be completed if the woman is newly diagnosed with HIV. Long-term follow-up of HIV-infected pregnant women is required.

MANAGEMENT OF HIV-EXPOSED INFANTS

MTCT is the major route of transmission of HIV in 90% of children. Initiating maternal prophylaxis during labour and birth and neonatal prophylaxis within 24 to 48 hours of birth can decrease the rates of infection in infants [21].

The risk of HIV transmission from mother to child is as high as 30–45% if she is not on ART and breastfeeds, and as low as 1% when she is on three ARV drugs and does not breastfeed (Table 42.3).

In India, the MTCT rate showed a sharp decline from 40.6% in 2010 to 24.25% in 2021 [22] due to the use of peripartum ART.

Table 42.3 Risk of MTCT with or without interventions (adapted from the WHO recommendations for ART for pregnant women and preventing MTCT [20])

Antiretroviral therapy (ART)	Risk of MTCT (%)
No ART, breastfeeding	30–45
No ART, no breastfeeding	20–25
Short course of ARV with one drug, breastfeeding	15–25
Short course of ARV with one drug, no breastfeeding	5–15
Short course with two ARV, breastfeeding	5
3-drug ART with breastfeeding	2
3-drug ART without breastfeeding	1

ARV, *antiretroviral drug*

Risks of HIV Exposure for the Infant

HIV-exposed infants are at a higher risk of malnutrition, developmental delay, growth restriction, and recurrent infections. Care of HIV-exposed infants is very important to reduce the risk of HIV transmission. Timely detection and management are required to improve immediate and long-term outcomes. Care of the HIV-exposed infant includes the following:

- Immediate care at birth
- Decisions about infant feeding
- Antiretroviral prophylaxis
- Immunisation
- Vitamin A supplementation
- Follow-up

Immediate Care of the Newborn

Immediate care includes the following:

- Wiping of the mouth and nostrils soon after birth
  — Oral suctioning with DeLee suction trap should be avoided
- Avoiding milking of the cord
- Immediate cord clamping
- Handling the neonate with gloves
- Initiating feeding within an hour

Infant Feeding

The options available for infant feeding should be discussed with the couple in the antenatal period. These options include the following:

- Exclusive breastfeeding
- Exclusive replacement feeding
- Mixed feeding

Information should be provided regarding the advantages of breastfeeding and the possible risk of transmission associated with it. The woman should also be counselled that while breastfeeding, the risk of transmission can be lowered by strictly adhering to combined ART. The woman should make an informed choice about infant feeding options.

The risk of HIV transmission via breast milk in LMICs when the woman is on combination ART is 1.08% at 6 months, and 2.93% at 12 months [24]. In the more recent PROMISE trial, women received combined ART throughout the breastfeeding period, and the transmission rate was 0.3% at 6 months and 0.6% at 12 months [25].

Exclusive breastfeeding grants the infant with the nutritive and immunological benefits of breast milk. Breastfeeding is safe when the woman is receiving ART and the baby is receiving prophylactic ARV therapy. Mothers should be encouraged to exclusively breastfeed their babies for 6 months. Complementary feeds can be introduced after this time. They can continue breastfeeding for as long as 12–24 months.

Exclusive replacement feeding involves formula feeds, unmodified animal milk, or prepacked toned milk. It should be given when the mother opts for it or when exclusive breastfeeding is not possible. While there is no risk of HIV transmission with replacement feeds, there is a risk of infections such as diarrhea and pneumonia. **This model of feeding is not encouraged in LMICs.**

Mixed feeding involves a combination of breastfeeds and replacement feeds. The use of formula feeds and cow's milk increases the chance of infection by causing inflammation in the gut mucosa and making it easier for the transmission of infection.

Infant Antiretroviral Prophylaxis

All infants born to women with HIV should receive postpartum antiretroviral (ARV) prophylaxis to reduce the risk of perinatal transmission. The prophylaxis should be started as soon as possible after birth, preferably within 6 hours of birth.

Exposed infants are categorised as low-risk and high-risk based on the ART received by the mother and her viral load.

- **Low-risk infants** should receive single ARV prophylaxis for at least 6 weeks.
- **High-risk infants** should receive dual ARV prophylaxis for 12 weeks.

Syrup nevirapine and zidovudine are the first line of drugs for ART for infants (Tables 42.4, 42.5, and 42.6). When zidovudine syrup is not available, the alternative is lopinavir/ritonavir (LPV/r) syrup; it should be used 14 days after birth. **Lopinavir/ritonavir should not be used for infants <2 weeks old.** Nevirapine syrup should be administered for the first two weeks followed by LPV/r.

Cotrimoxazole Prophylaxis

Cotrimoxazole prophylaxis is an effective and proven strategy for reducing morbidity and mortality in children with HIV infection. It protects infants and children from various opportunistic infections like *Pneumocystis jirovecii* infection, malaria, diarrhea due to *Isospora* and *Cyclospora*, toxoplasmosis, and other bacterial diseases. All HIV-exposed infants should receive cotrimoxazole prophylaxis at a dose of 5 mg/Kg/day as a single dose from the age of 6 weeks.

Table 42.4 Dosage of nevirapine for infant ARV prophylaxis

Infant age	Infant weight (g)	Nevirapine
Birth to 6 weeks	<2000	2 mg/Kg once daily
	2000–2500	10 mg (1 mL) once daily
	>2500	15 mg (1.5 mL) once daily
6 weeks to 6 months	–	20 mg (2 mL) once daily
6 months to 9 months	–	30 mg (3 mL) once daily
>9 months until breastfeeding is stopped	–	40 mg (4 mL) once daily

Table 42.5 Dosage of zidovudine for infant ARV prophylaxis

Infant weight (g)	Zidovudine
<2000	5 mg (0.5 mL) twice daily for 6 weeks
2000–2500	10 mg/dose (1 mL) twice daily for 6 weeks
>2500	15 mg (1.5 mL) twice daily for 6 weeks

Table 42.6 Dosage of lopinavir/ritonavir for infant ARV prophylaxis

Infant age	Infant weight (g)	Dosage of lopinavir/ritonavir (LPV/r)
2–4 weeks	2000–2999	0.6 mL twice daily
	30000–3999	0.8 mL twice daily
	4000–4999	1 mL twice daily
>4 weeks	3000–5999	1 mL twice daily
	6000–9999	1.5 mL twice daily

Newborn Follow-up

Newborn babies should be followed-up for signs and symptoms of HIV infection. Each follow-up visit should include assessment of feeding, growth, development, and immunisation as per schedule.

Early Infant Diagnosis

Maternal HIV antibodies, which are transferred passively to the infant during pregnancy, usually persist for nearly 9–12 months in the infant. Thus, children born to HIV-infected mothers will test positive for HIV antibodies regardless of their own infection status. A positive ELISA or rapid test that detects antibodies to HIV, therefore, does not necessarily indicate the presence of HIV infection in the infant/child; rather, it indicates exposure to HIV. More reliable indicators of the status of HIV infection of the infant are tests that detect HIV DNA or antigens. The current test of choice is HIV-1 total nucleic acid (TNA) PCR test that detects HIV pro-viral DNA and RNA.

POST-EXPOSURE PROPHYLAXIS (PEP) FOR HEALTHCARE PROFESSIONALS

Standard Universal Precautions

A skin-penetrating injury (e.g., a needlestick or scalpel laceration) is a risk to healthcare providers and may occur at a delivery, whether vaginal or cesarean. Every medical unit should have policies for appropriate care and standard universal precautions against such injuries. The risk of such injury should not affect decision-making regarding the route of delivery.

The various devices associated with injury are needles, scalpels, sharp retractors, and pre-filled syringes. Accidental exposure through a needle or sharp object may occur during usage, before disposal, before disassembling, during disposal, or while recapping. Standard work-place precautions should be taken to prevent accidental exposure, the most important steps of which are to follow universal precautions, use protective gear, maintain safe handling of needles and instruments, and considering all blood samples to be infectious.

If an injury does occur despite taking all precautions, the injury site should be washed thoroughly and followed by postexposure antiviral prophylaxis.

Post-exposure Antiviral Prophylaxis

After accidental exposure, PEP should be started as early as possible but not later than 72 hours after exposure (Table 42.7). The duration of PEP is 28 days regardless of the regimen.

Table 42.7 Recommended post-exposure antiviral prophylaxis for adults

Preferred regimen	Alternative regimens
Tenofovir (300 mg) + lamivudine (300 mg) + dolutegravir (50 mg)	Tenofovir (300 mg) + lamivudine (300 mg) + lopinavir (200 mg)/ ritonavir (50 mg) (two tablets BD) OR Tenofovir (300 mg) + Lamivudine (300 mg) + Efavirenz (600 mg)

Baseline investigations such as HIV, HBsAg, HCV, hemogram, and liver function tests should be performed. HIV, HBsAg, and HCV should be tested for 6 days after accidental exposure, and the tests should be repeated at 6 weeks, 12 weeks, and 24 weeks from the date of exposure if the person is not on PEP.

CONCLUSION

Vertical transmission of HIV during labour and birth is rare in resource-rich settings. However, it continues to occur in resource-limited settings. Efforts to increase the use of antiretroviral therapy (ART) and better access to HIV and pregnancy care services have led to a marked decrease in vertical HIV transmission rates in LMICs.

REFERENCES

1. UN Joint Programme on HIV/AIDS (UNAIDS) (2021) Global AIDS update-2021: Confronting inequalities. Available at: https://www.unaids.org/sites/default/files/media_asset/2021-global-aids-update_en.pdf.
2. National AIDS Control Organization (2021). National Guidelines for HIV Care and Treatment, 2021. New Delhi: NACO, Ministry of Health and Family Welfare, Government of India.
3. UNAIDS data. 2022. Available at https://www.unaids.org/en/regionscountries/countries/india.
4. Prenatal and perinatal human immunodeficiency virus testing. ACOG Committee Opinion No. 752. American College of Obstetricians and Gynecologists. *Obstet Gynecol*. 2018. 132:e138–42.
5. UNICEF data. Elimination of mother-to-child transmission. Available at https://data.unicef.org/topic/hivaids/emtct/.
6. HIV.gov. The Global HIV/AIDS Epidemic. Available at https://www.hiv.gov/federal-response/pepfar-global-aids/global-hiv-aids-overview/.
7. Government of India, MoHFW. Elimination of Vertical Transmission of HIV & Syphilis. Available at https://naco.gov.in/elimination-vertical-transmission-hiv-syphilis.
8. Landesman SH, Kalish LA, Burns DN, et al. Obstetrical factors and the transmission of human immunodeficiency virus type 1 from mother to child. The Women and Infants Transmission Study. *N Engl J Med*. 1996. 334:1617.
9. Cotter AM, Brookfield KF, Duthely LM, et al. Duration of membrane rupture and risk of perinatal transmission of HIV-1 in the era of combination antiretroviral therapy. *Am J Obstet Gynecol*. 2012. 207:482.e1.
10. Rousseau CM, Nduati RW, Richardson BA, et al. Association of levels of HIV-1-infected breast milk cells and risk of mother-to-child transmission. *J Infect Dis*. 2004. 190:1880.
11. Fowler MG, Qin M, Fiscus, et al. Benefits and risks of antiretroviral therapy for perinatal HIV prevention. *N Engl J Med*. 2016. 375:1726.
12. World Health Organization. WHO consolidated guidelines on the use of antiretroviral drugs for treating and preventing HIV infection: Recommendations for a public health approach. 2nd ed. 2016. WHO Press, Geneva.
13. Wade NA, Birkhead GS, Warren BL, et al. Abbreviated regimens of zidovudine prophylaxis and perinatal transmission of the human immunodeficiency virus. *N Engl J Med*. 1998. 339: 1409–1414.
14. British HIV Association guidelines for the management of HIV in pregnancy and postpartum, 2018. *HIV Med*. 2019.
15. Scott RK, Chakhtoura N, Burke MM, Cohen RA, Kreitchmann R. Delivery after 40 weeks of gestation in pregnant women with well-controlled human immunodeficiency virus. *Obstet Gynecol*. 2017. 130: 502–10.
16. Peters H, Byrne L, De Ruiter A, Francis K, Harding K, Taylor GP, Tookey PA, Townsend CL. Duration of ruptured membranes and mother-to-child HIV transmission: A prospective population-based surveillance study. *BJOG*. 2016. 123(6):975-81.
17. Cotter AM, Brookfield KF, Duthely LM, Gonzalez Quintero VH, Potter JE, O'Sullivan MJ. Duration of membrane rupture and risk of perinatal transmission of HIV-1 in the era of combination antiretroviral therapy. *Am J Obstet Gynecol*. 2012. 207: 482.e1–5.
18. Holmes WR, Hofmeyr GJ. Management of breech presentation in areas with high prevalence of HIV infection. *Int J Gynaecol Obstet*. 2004. 87: 272–276
19. Read JS, Tuomala R, Kpamegan E, et al. Mode of delivery and postpartum morbidity among HIV-infected women: The Women and Infants Transmission Study. *J Acquir Immune Defic Syndr*. 2001. 26:236–45. 89.
20. Marcollet A, Goffinet F, Firtion G, et al. Differences in postpartum morbidity in women who are infected with the human immunodeficiency virus after elective cesarean delivery, emergency cesarean delivery, or vaginal delivery. *Am J Obstet Gynecol*. 2002. 186:784–9.
21. Consolidated guidelines on HIV prevention, testing, treatment, service delivery and monitoring: Recommendations for a public health approach. 2021. WHO, Geneva.
22. National AIDS Control Organization & ICMR-National Institute of Medical Statistics. India HIV Estimates 2021: Fact Sheet. New Delhi: NACO, Ministry of Health and Family Welfare, Government of India. 2022.
23. World Health Organization. Antiretroviral drugs for treating pregnant women and preventing HIV infection in infants: Recommendations for a public health approach. 2010.
24. Bispo S, Chikhungu L, Rollins N, et al. Postnatal HIV transmission in breastfed infants of HIV-infected women on ART: A systematic review and meta-analysis. *J Int AIDS Soc*. 2017. 20: 1–8.
25. Taha T, Flynn P, Cababasay MP, et al. Maternal triple antiretrovirals (mART) and infant nevirapine (iNVP) prophylaxis for the prevention of mother-to-child transmission (MTCT) of HIV during breastfeeding (BF). International AIDS Conference. 2016. Durban, South Africa.

CHAPTER 43

Routine Care of the Newborn

SWATHI PADANKATTI

INTRODUCTION

Every day, approximately 67,385 babies are born in India. This accounts for about one-sixth of the total number of births in the world. Every minute, one of these babies dies. India's neonatal mortality rate of 22/1,000 live births is one of the highest in the world. 4 out of 5 newborn deaths result from preventable causes which include complications of childbirth such as perinatal asphyxia, infections, and complications of prematurity. Most neonatal deaths occur during delivery or on the day of birth [1,2,3].

Simple, cost-effective interventions employed soon after birth, including effective neonatal resuscitation, prevention of infection and hypothermia, early skin-to-skin contact, and successful breastfeeding, help to reduce neonatal mortality and therefore improve the chances of child survival and development in low- and medium-income countries (LMICs) including India. These interventions are the focus of **essential newborn care** as defined by the World Health Organization, and of various programmes undertaken by the Ministry of Health and Family Welfare, Government of India, such as the India Newborn Action Plan [4].

This chapter deals with newborn care at and immediately after birth in babies who cry at birth and do not need resuscitation. See **Chapter 44,** *Neonatal resuscitation*, for details of resuscitative procedures.

PRINCIPLES OF ROUTINE NEWBORN CARE

The transition from intrauterine to extrauterine life is a complex process, the failure of which can jeopardise the infant's life. In simple terms, the baby's first cry reassures the mother and the obstetrician that the baby has had a smooth, uncomplicated transition and has adapted to extrauterine life. Several steps need to be followed in the labour room to ensure the newborn's well-being.

Following birth, the routine care of the newborn usually includes the following:

- Noting the exact time of birth
- Preventing hypothermia
- Clearing the airway
- Documenting Apgar score
- Assessing the baby's breathing
- Skin-to-skin contact
- Cord clamping—delayed or immediate
- Prophylactic eye care
- Establishing patency of the esophagus and anal orifice
- Administering vitamin K
- Initiating breastfeeding

TIME OF BIRTH

The attending physician or nurse should record the time of birth as soon as the head is delivered. It is important to call out the time of birth aloud. This not only helps in the accurate recording of the time but also alerts other personnel about the delivery of the baby and the potential need for additional help [5].

The Golden Minute

The delivery of the entire body of the baby is considered the start of the golden minute, which is a critical window for establishing ventilation in a newborn. The first 30 seconds are used for the key interventions of drying, warming, stimulating, and auscultating the heart and assessing the respiratory rates. If the neonate still has not established spontaneous ventilation, there should be an escalation of ventilatory support (see **Chapter 44**, for further details).

> **Key Point**
>
> Though the golden minute is important, recent papers have questioned the ability to implement the recommended guidelines within this timeframe, even in high-resource countries, and especially in LMICs [6,7].

PREVENTING HYPOTHERMIA

Maintaining normal body temperature soon after birth is critical to reducing neonatal morbidity and mortality. Hypothermia can lead to hypoglycemia, bleeding diathesis, pulmonary hemorrhage, acidosis, apnea, respiratory failure, shock, and eventually, death [8].

Since 2015, the International Liaison Committee on Resuscitation (ILCOR) Neonatal Task Force [9] has recommended that the temperature of newly born non-asphyxiated babies be maintained between 36.5 and 37.5°C. However, several studies around the world have shown a high incidence of hypothermia in term and preterm babies soon after birth, in high- as well as low-resource settings.

The neonate loses heat from the surface of its body to the environment soon after birth by the following four mechanisms:

- **Evaporation** of amniotic fluid from the baby's wet skin, causing a drop in body temperature
- **Conductive heat loss** to any cold object that is in contact with the baby's body such as non-warmed towels or a cold resuscitative surface
- **Convective heat loss** due to air currents in which cold air from open windows or circulating air from the fan replaces warm air around the baby
- **Radiation**, by which, solid objects in the room like cold walls and metal cabinets bring down the ambient temperature.

Table 43.1 presents the interventions employed to prevent neonatal hypothermia in relation to the mechanism of heat loss [8]. A combination of these interventions will help prevent hypothermia, especially in preterm babies.

> **Key Point**
>
> Neonatal hypothermia is an important cause of neonatal morbidity and mortality. A combination of interventions aimed at reducing heat loss through evaporation, conduction, convection, and radiation have been shown to protect the newborn from hypothermia.

Concept of Warm Chain

The warm chain is a set of ten interlinked interventions carried out on the newborn baby at birth and afterwards, which reduce the likelihood of the development of hypothermia [10].

1. Warm delivery room
2. Warm resuscitation
3. Immediate drying
4. Skin-to-skin contact between baby and mother
5. Early breastfeeding
6. Postponement of bathing and weighing
7. Appropriate clothing and bedding
8. Keeping mother and baby together
9. Warm transportation
10. Raising awareness among healthcare providers

Drying the baby

Drying not only keeps the baby warm and prevents the ill effects of hypothermia, but also stimulates breathing. The newborn baby should be gently dried with a warm towel, wiping off only the amniotic fluid, blood, and meconium, and not the vernix caseosa. The vernix is an integral part of the newborn baby's transition from the intrauterine to extrauterine environment. It

Table 43.1 Mechanisms of heat loss in newborn babies and interventions to combat them

Mechanism of heat loss	Interventions
Evaporation	• Dry the baby immediately after birth • Wrap the baby in a plastic bag or cling film immediately after birth in preterm births ≤28 weeks' gestation
Conduction	• Use prewarmed linen for drying the baby • Remove wet linen immediately • Routine care to be provided on the mother's warm abdomen or chest • Use a warm resuscitation surface if resuscitation is required • Use a hat or cap to cover the baby's head • Use a thermal (exothermic) mattress, polyethylene plastic resealable bags, or cling film for preterm babies
Convection	• Close doors and windows to reduce draughts of cold air • Maintain delivery room temperature between 25 and 28°C • Use a plastic bag or cling film, hats, or caps • Use warm, humidified oxygen, if being administered
Radiation	• Switch off air conditioners and fans at least half an hour prior to delivery so that objects in the room slowly become warmer (in areas where the ambient temperature is <25°C) • Use a radiant warmer if the baby requires resuscitation

has been shown to protect the baby's skin from injury and helps to maintain its body temperature. The vernix can be left in place at birth as it gets absorbed on its own [5,11].

The baby's body, arms, legs, and head should be gently dried. The wet towel should be removed after drying and immediately be replaced with a clean, dry towel [10]. The baby's hands alone should not be dried as the newborn finds the mother's breasts through a sense of smell. The amniotic fluid on the baby's hands smells similar to secretions from the Montgomery glands in the mother's nipples. This facilitates the baby's 'breast crawl' when placed in skin-to-skin contact with the mother [12].

CLEARING THE AIRWAY

If there are any visible secretions from the baby's mouth or nose, they can be gently wiped using a clean cloth or gauze. There is no evidence for routine nasal and/or oral suctioning after birth, even for babies born through meconium-stained amniotic fluid. Some studies have also suggested possible adverse effects of routine nasal and/or oral suctioning including bradycardia, hypoxemia, impaired cerebral blood flow regulation, and infection.

If there are copious secretions (including blood or meconium), suctioning can be performed using a DeLee suction trap. The trap in this apparatus should be big enough (20 mL) to prevent aspirated fluid from going into the resuscitator's mouth. It is better not to use suction bulbs for suction because they are difficult to clean and might act as a source of cross-infection [5,10,13]. However, it may be the only suction device available in low-resource areas.

Key Point

There is no evidence to support routine nasal and/or oral suctioning after birth, even for babies born through meconium-stained amniotic fluid.

RECORDING OF APGAR SCORE

The Apgar score (Table 43.2) should be recorded at 1 and 5 minutes after birth. Although the Apgar score has limited value in guiding resuscitation and initial stabilisation, it provides an accepted and convenient method to report the newborn baby's status immediately after birth and is also helpful in documenting the response to resuscitation, if required. The score is affected by many factors including gestation, maternal medications, resuscitative efforts, and cardiopulmonary and neurologic conditions. The score does not predict neurological outcomes or neonatal mortality and cannot be used by itself to make a diagnosis of perinatal asphyxia. However, if the score is 7 or more at 5 minutes, it is unlikely that peripartum hypoxia–ischemia is the sole reason for neonatal encephalopathy [14].

> **Key Point**
>
> The Apgar score describes the condition of the newborn baby immediately after birth and can be used to document the response to resuscitation, if required. It cannot, however, be used as a predictor of neonatal mortality or neurologic outcome.

ASSESSMENT OF BREATHING

As the baby is being dried, his breathing should be assessed. A baby who is breathing well will cry lustily. A baby breathing regularly at a rate of 40–60 breaths per minute with good chest movements can be cared for on the mother's abdomen.

A baby who is not breathing, or is gasping (a series of deep, single, and irregular inspirations) will need resuscitation. Such a baby should have the umbilical cord clamped and cut immediately and must be taken to the newborn care corner to perform the initial steps of resuscitation [10] (see **Chapter 44** for further details).

IMMEDIATE SKIN-TO-SKIN CONTACT

Immediate **skin-to-skin contact (SSC)** is the practice of drying the baby and laying him directly on the mother's bare chest after birth, both of them covered in a warm sheet or blanket and left for at least an hour or until after the first feed [15], as shown in Fig. 43.1.

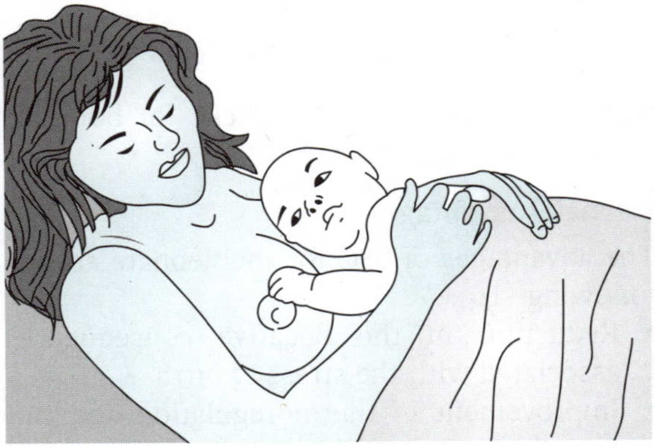

Fig. 43.1 Skin-to-skin contact between the mother and the baby immediately after birth

Table 43.2 Apgar scoring system

Sign	0	1	2
Colour	Blue or pale	Acrocyanotic	Completely pink
Heart rate	Absent	<100/minute	>100/minute
Reflex irritability	No response	Grimace	Cry or active withdrawal
Muscle tone	Limp	Some flexion	Active motion
Respiration	Absent	Weak cry, hypoventilation	Good cry

Being in continuous, uninterrupted SSC with the mother immediately after birth elicits the nine instinctive stages in the baby as described by Widström and colleagues [16]:

- Birth cry
- Relaxation
- Awakening
- Activity
- Rest
- Crawling
- Familiarisation
- Suckling and sleeping

The baby should be placed prone and lengthwise along the long axis of the mother's body, with the head turned to one side on the mother's chest, above her breasts. After a cesarean birth, the newborn infant might be positioned horizontally across the mother's breasts, above the drape, instead of vertically [16].

Advantages of SSC

Skin-to-skin contact is beneficial for both the newborn and the mother.

Neonatal advantages

The advantages of SSC for the neonate are the following [16]:

- Reduction in the negative consequences associated with the stress of birth
- Improvement in thermoregulation and cardiopulmonary stabilisation
- An increase in the chance of successful breastfeeding

Maternal advantages

The advantages for the mother are the following [16]:

- Earlier expulsion of the placenta
- Reduction in postpartum bleeding and pain
- Calming and relaxing effect on the mother

SSC has been incorporated in step 4 of the 2018 revision of the World Health Organization (WHO)/United Nations International Children's Emergency Fund (UNICEF) 'Ten Steps to Successful Breastfeeding' that form the basis of the Baby–Friendly Hospital Initiative [15].

Key Point

Immediate skin-to-skin contact refers to the practice of drying the baby and laying him directly on the mother's bare chest soon after delivery. The baby can be allowed to 'breast crawl' to initiate early breastfeeding while on SSC.

The Breast Crawl

Permitting the 'breast crawl' during SSC (Fig. 43.2a and b) as described by UNICEF and by the Breastfeeding Promotion Network of India (BPNI), promotes successful breastfeeding. The baby pushes up on his little elbows, sucks on his hand to get the taste of amniotic fluid which smells similar to the secretions of

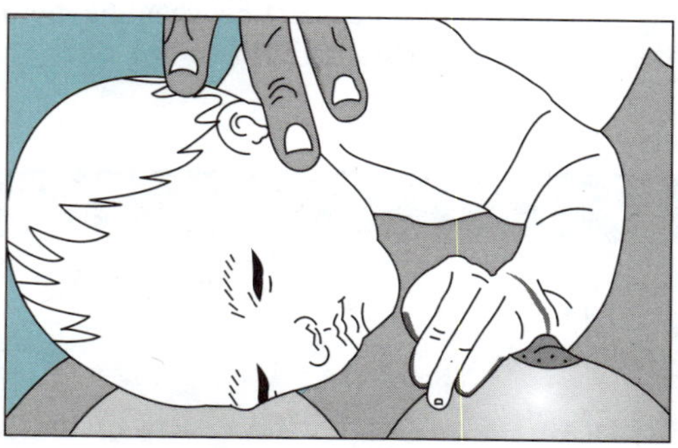

(a) Baby placed between mother's breasts

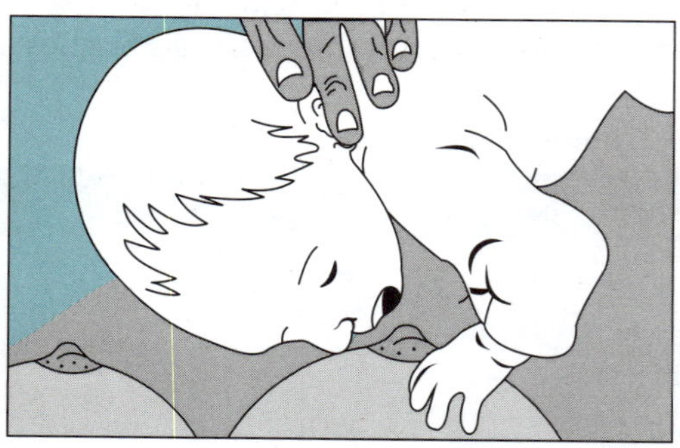

(b) Baby finds the mother's nipples

Fig. 43.2 The breast crawl is an element of skin-to-skin contact and involves the baby crawling in the direction of the breast, through leg and arm movements: (a) the baby is placed between the mother's breasts and (b) the baby finds the mother's nipple

the Montgomery glands on the mother's nipples, and uses the smell and taste as a guide to reach the nipple [12,16].

SSC should be continued for at least an hour in the delivery room. However, the mother–baby dyad should not be left alone during the period of SSC. The baby should be monitored for breathing, colour, and temperature every 15 minutes [5].

CLAMPING OF THE UMBILICAL CORD

Delayed Cord Clamping (DCC)

The ideal time for clamping the cord is the subject of ongoing research, but current evidence seems to suggest that in term and preterm newborns, delaying cord clamping for at least 1 minute after birth allows time for a passive physiological transfer of warm, oxygenated, fetal blood from the placenta to the baby at the time of birth (the process of 'placental transfusion').

The WHO recommends delaying cord clamping for 1–3 minutes in all stable term and preterm babies while initiating routine newborn care. Current research has also suggested that where adequate thermoregulation and initial resuscitation can be safely undertaken with an intact cord, it may even be possible to delay clamping whilst performing these interventions. The results of ongoing research are awaited [17].

Advantages of delayed clamping

The placental transfusion can provide the baby with 30% more blood volume and up to 60% more red blood cells. This increases the baby's hemoglobin and serum ferritin levels during the first 3–6 months of life, which may have a favourable effect on developmental outcomes. It also improves cardiopulmonary adaptation after birth and promotes breastfeeding.

A small increase in jaundice needing phototherapy has been found in term babies receiving DCC. This is not a contraindication for DCC. It is important, however, to ensure that these babies are monitored for neonatal hyperbilirubinemia and treated as needed [17,18]. The benefits of delayed cord clamping for infants and mothers are listed in Table 43.3.

Table 43.3 Benefits of delayed cord clamping for the infant and mother [17]

Infant				Mother
Immediate benefits		Long-term benefits		
Preterm/LBW babies	Full term babies	Preterm/LBW babies	Full term babies	
Decreases risk of: • Necrotising enterocolitis • Intraventricular hemorrhage • Late-onset sepsis	Provides adequate blood volume and birth iron stores	Increases hemoglobin at 10 weeks of age	Improves hemoglobin at 3–6 months of age	No effect on maternal bleeding or length of the third stage of labour
Decreases need for: • Surfactant • Mechanical ventilation • Blood transfusions	Increases: • Hemoglobin • Hematocrit	Improves neurodevelopmental outcomes in male babies	Improves iron status for up to 6 months of age	Less blood-filled placenta may shorten the third stage of labour and reduce the incidence of retained placenta

LBW, *low birth weight*

Milking of the Cord

Studies suggest that milking of the cord (physically squeezing out blood from the umbilical cord) may have similar benefits as DCC with regard to hemoglobin and iron stores, but the cardiovascular benefits are less certain. The need for inotropic support and transfusions is less with cord milking, but there is no overall reduction in morbidity and mortality of the preterm neonate. In neonates born before 28 weeks, cord milking is definitely **not** recommended because of the increased association with intraventricular hemorrhage [19].

The Resuscitation Council UK recommends umbilical cord clamping after at least 60 seconds, but if this is not possible, suggest that cord milking may be an option in babies born after 28 weeks' gestation [20].

As per the current standard of care, cord clamping should not be delayed in the following situations:

- Maternal hemorrhage or hemodynamic instability
- Placental circulation not intact (placental abruption, placenta previa, cord avulsion, fetal growth restriction with abnormal cord Doppler evaluation)
- Newborn requiring immediate resuscitation

Key Point

It is recommended that cord clamping be delayed for at least 1–3 minutes in all stable term and late preterm babies. This increases hemoglobin levels at birth, improves iron stores in the first few months of life and has a beneficial effect on cardiopulmonary adaptation after birth.

Procedure of Clamping the Cord

After a period of at least one minute, the umbilical cord should be clamped at a distance of 2–3 cm from the abdominal skin surface using a commercially available clamp, a sterile rubber band, or a string (Fig. 43.3). The clamp should be positioned away from the genitalia. Then, the cord should be cut using a sterile pair of scissors or a blade, with a sterile gauze held above to avoid splashing of blood. The stump should be left dry without applying any antiseptic. There is no evidence that applying an antiseptic to the cord stump prevents subsequent infections. The cord should be inspected every 15–30 minutes for the first few hours of life to detect any oozing [5,10].

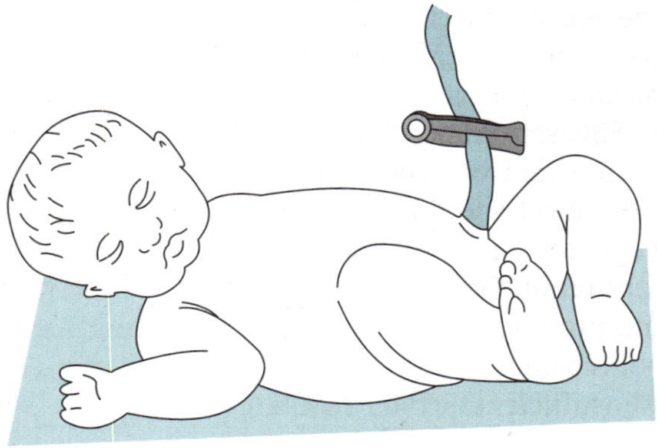

Fig. 43.3 Umbilical cord clamp

PROPHYLACTIC CARE OF THE EYES

Both the eyes of the baby should be gently cleaned using sterile cotton soaked in sterile water or normal saline, from the inner to the outer canthus as shown in Fig. 43.4. Prophylactic eye care is given shortly after birth as a

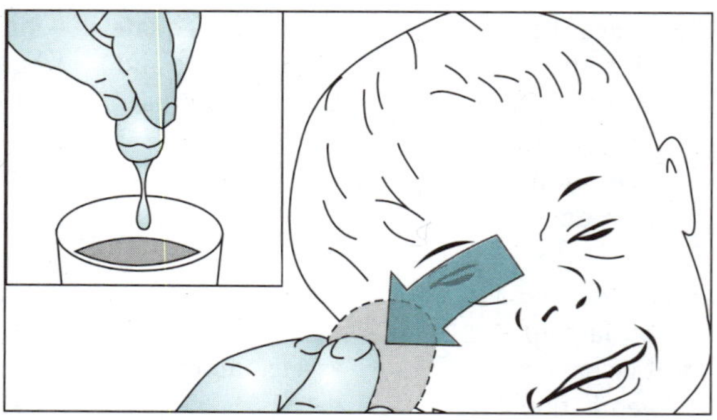

Fig. 43.4 Cleaning the eyes of a newborn baby using sterile cotton soaked in sterile water or normal saline, wiping from the inner to the outer canthus

preventive measure against developing gonococcal conjunctivitis. Any one of the following medications may be used:

- Silver nitrate solution
- Erythromycin ointment 0.5%
- Tetracycline ointment 1%
- Povidone–iodine solution 2.5%

Routine use of local antiseptic eye drops for the prophylaxis of ophthalmia neonatorum is not recommended in the Indian setting, as there is insufficient evidence to support this [5,10].

ESTABLISHING PATENCY OF THE ESOPHAGUS AND ANAL ORIFICE

Patency of the esophagus should be ascertained in all babies by passing an orogastric tube. This can be done during the initial examination of the baby. There is insufficient evidence to recommend routine stomach washing to prevent gastritis in the newborn baby, even if the baby is born through meconium-stained amniotic fluid [5,21].

Anal atresia can be ruled out by visual examination of the anal orifice.

PLACEMENT OF IDENTITY BAND

Utmost care should be taken to ensure the correct identity of the mother–baby dyad. An identity band must be placed on every baby (Fig. 43.5). This band should bear the name of the mother, the hospital registration number, the date of birth, and the gender and birth weight of the baby. This band can be placed on the baby's wrist or ankle [5]. This tagging should be done in the labour room, in front of the mother, after having her verify the data on the bands.

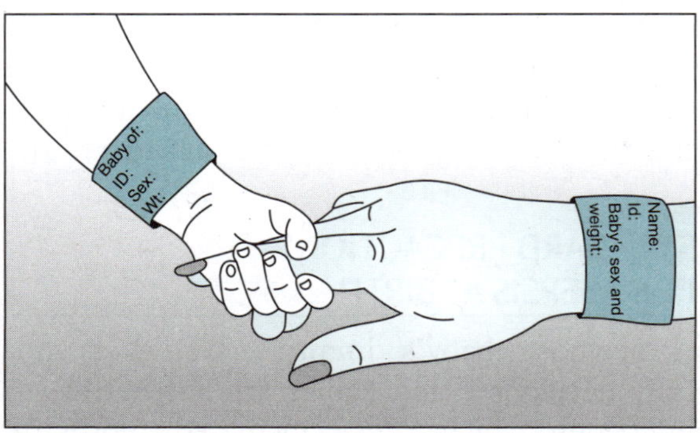

Fig. 43.5 Identity bands for the mother–baby dyad with the ID number and details of the mother and the baby

A matching adult-sized band with the same information is placed on the mother's wrist.

ADMINISTRATION OF VITAMIN K

All babies should be given vitamin K soon after birth by an intramuscular injection on the anterolateral aspect of the thigh, using a 1 mL syringe and 26G (1/2 inch) needle. This helps prevent hemorrhagic disease of the newborn and can be done with the baby in SSC. Babies with a birth weight <1000 g should receive 0.5 mg of vitamin K and those with a birth weight >1000 g should receive 1 mg. Vitamin K1 (phytomenadione) is preferred; however, K3 may be used if K1 is not available [5].

INITIATING BREASTFEEDING

After the umbilical cord has been cut after birth, the baby should be placed prone between the mother's breasts with SSC, and breastfeeding should be started as early as possible.

It has been well established that infants are born with an innate behaviour that enables them to find and self-attach to the breast. This is sometimes referred to as 'biological nursing or nurturing.' Milinko et al. [22] found that biologic nurturing lowered the incidence of sore nipples, cracked nipples, engorgement, and mastitis when compared to normal breastfeeding practices.

The baby may be allowed to initiate the 'breast crawl' and begin breastfeeding by himself (see section on *Skin-to-skin contact*). However, proactive support is required from the delivery room staff. They can support the baby when in SSC in the prone position so that the baby can suckle at the mother's breast. Mothers who deliver by cesarean delivery should also be supported for early breastfeeding.

The benefits of early breastfeeding include improved nutrition and immunity acquired by ingesting colostrum, the establishment of breastfeeding when the baby is still awake, and increased mother–baby bonding. Early breastfeeding also helps the mother with uterine involution (through the oxytocin hormone released in response to the suckling reflex) and reduces postpartum hemorrhage [5,10].

Key Point

Early breastfeeding established by allowing the infant to self-attach to the breast (biological nursing or nurturing) reduces breastfeeding problems for the mother.

DOCUMENTATION OF WEIGHT

The newborn baby should be weighed after stabilisation and after the temperature has been documented to be normal. It is best to use an electronic weighing scale for weighing the neonate. A single-use paper towel or sterile prewarmed cloth towel is placed on the weighing scale. The weighing scale is calibrated to zero reading and the baby is gently placed on the scale to check his weight. The weight must be recorded in the newborn records [5,10].

EXAMINATION OF THE NEWBORN BABY

First Examination

The first thorough physical examination of the baby should be conducted soon after birth, even as the baby is in SSC with the mother. This examination is necessary to identify babies at high risk of morbidity or mortality. Babies who may need to be cared for in the NICU or special care nursery include the following [5]:

- Babies with congenital malformations (cleft lip or palate, neck masses, omphalocele, hydrocephalus, diaphragmatic hernia, esophageal or anal atresia)
- Babies who are asphyxiated at birth and who need to be resuscitated
- Low-birth-weight (<2500 g) babies
- Preterm (<37 weeks) babies
- Babies with respiratory distress

Detailed Examination

Following the initial assessment in the delivery room, all newborn babies must have a detailed physical examination at 24 hours of age, and just prior to discharge.

Assessment Before Transfer Out of Delivery Room

All newborn babies should be assessed for stability before they are transferred out of the delivery room [5]. The baby should fulfil the following criteria to be shifted into the mother's room:

- Normal temperature (36.5–37.4°C)
- No respiratory distress
- No congenital malformations
- Pink colour
- Vigorous
- No oozing from the cord stump

IMMUNISATION

All newborn babies should receive the first dose of hepatitis B vaccine soon after birth, preferably within 24 hours. The zero-dose oral polio vaccine is recommended in all polio-endemic countries, and in countries where there is a potential for importation and spread of poliomyelitis. In LMICs such as India where tuberculosis is highly endemic, or in settings where there is a high risk of exposure to tuberculosis, the BCG vaccine should be given at birth [23].

STANDARD PRECAUTIONS FOR ASEPSIS AT BIRTH

A newborn baby's immune system is not fully developed, and babies are susceptible to infections which cause increased morbidity and mortality. Five simple, cost-effective interventions are mentioned below to prevent infection in the newborn.

Observing the following **five 'cleans'** will help prevent infection in the newborn baby [5]:

1. **Clean hands:** Perform appropriate hand hygiene and wear gloves before touching any of the sterile articles laid out for the routine care of the newborn or handling the baby.
2. **Clean surface**: Use a clean and sterile towel to dry and cover the baby and a clean resuscitation surface if the baby needs resuscitation.
3. **Clean clamp** or **tie**: The umbilical cord should be clamped with a clean and sterile clamp or tie.
4. **Clean cut**: The umbilical cord should be cut with a clean and sterile pair of scissors or a blade.
5. **Clean cord**: The stump of the umbilical cord should be kept clean and dry. Unless there is a high risk of contamination, no antiseptic solution needs to be applied to it.

PREPARATION FOR DELIVERY

Preparation for birth is the key to successful care of the newborn baby [5,10]. This includes the preparation of the delivery room, personnel, and the necessary equipment. It ensures that every eventuality is considered and planned for. Prevention of infection and hypothermia should be given utmost importance while preparing for delivery.

Preparation of the Delivery Room

Ambient temperature

Optimal delivery room temperature is of great importance in preventing hypothermia in the newborn baby and improving outcomes. The delivery room must be kept at an ambient temperature between 25 and 28°C. In cooler climates, air conditioning and fans should be switched off at least half an hour prior to delivery. This minimises the heat lost from the newborn's body due to convection and radiation. In cold areas, it is best to keep the doors and windows closed to prevent convective heat loss due to cold draughts of air.

Newborn care corner

Although the majority of newborn babies make the transition to extrauterine life without any difficulty and need not be separated from the mother at all, 10% may require some resuscitative assistance. The newborn care corner is a designated area in the delivery room to perform neonatal resuscitation. The radiant warmer in the newborn care corner (Fig. 43.6) should be switched on twenty minutes before delivery. Two sterile baby sheets or towels can be placed under the warmer so that the baby can be received in and dried with prewarmed sheets.

Preparation of Personnel

The personnel involved in the care of the newborn should be aware of the risks to be expected.

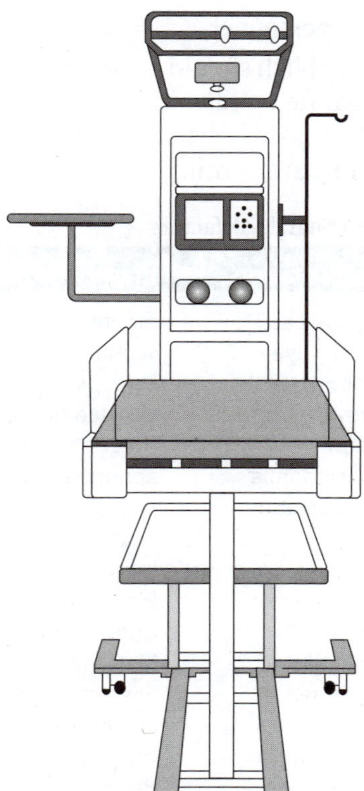

Fig. 43.6 Newborn care corner with radiant warmer

Antenatal assessment of risk

Every birth is a potential emergency; any newborn baby could require resuscitation. An accurate assessment of risk helps in anticipating the need for resuscitation, and in planning personnel and equipment accordingly.

- Preterm babies are more likely to need resuscitation at birth and may also need special follow-up care because of the higher risk of infection, hypothermia, and feeding problems.
- Although meconium-stained amniotic fluid does not mandate routine intubation or tracheal suctioning according to current neonatal resuscitation protocol, it is still a risk factor for abnormal transition, necessitating the presence of a person adept at neonatal resuscitation including endotracheal intubation.

Perinatal risk factors that can affect the outcome of the baby are listed in Table 43.4.

Presence of personnel

Ideally, every birth should be physically attended by one qualified individual who can perform the initial steps of resuscitation and establish positive pressure ventilation. If any of the risk factors mentioned in Table 43.4 are identified, more advanced neonatal resuscitation may be required. In these cases, at least two qualified personnel should be present solely for the care of the baby, at least one of whom has advanced resuscitation skills. A resuscitation team should be established with an identified role for each member of the team (see **Chapter 44**).

Team briefing

The team should get together before the delivery to discuss risk factors, potential problems, roles, and responsibilities.

Table 43.4 Perinatal risk factors

Antenatal risk factors	Intrapartum risk factors
• No prenatal care	• Emergency cesarean section
• Gestational age <37 weeks or >41 weeks	• Forceps or vacuum-assisted delivery
• Fetal growth restriction	• Breech or other abnormal presentation
• Fetal macrosomia	• Non-reassuring fetal heart rate pattern
• Multiple gestation	• Intrapartum bleeding
• Maternal hypertension, preeclampsia, or eclampsia	• Placental abruption
• Fetal anemia	• Chorioamnionitis
• Fetal hydrops	• Maternal general anesthesia or magnesium sulphate therapy
• Significant fetal malformations or anomalies	• Prolapsed umbilical cord
	• Shoulder dystocia

Preparation of Equipment and Supplies

Articles needed for routine newborn care (Fig. 43.7) include the following:

- Two prewarmed sheets or towels to receive and dry the baby
- Gauze to wipe the baby's mouth and nose
- DeLee suction trap (or suction bulb)
- Sterile scissors or blade to cut the umbilical cord
- Umbilical cord clamp or sterile cord tie
- Cotton swabs to clean the eyes

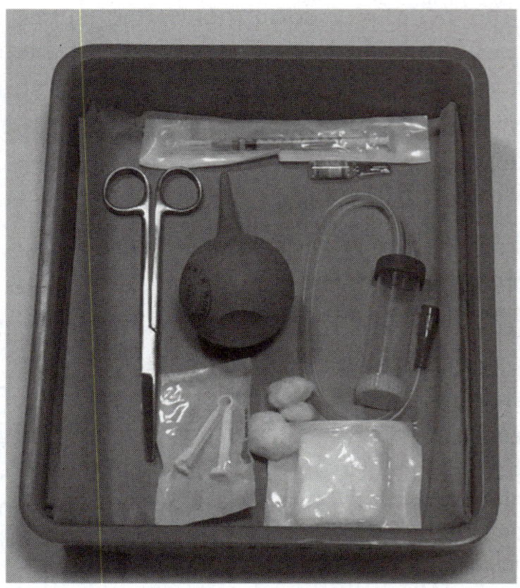

Fig. 43.7 Articles required for routine newborn care (*Image courtesy:* Dr Swathi Padankatti, Dr Rangarajan Memorial Hospital, Chennai)

- Vitamin K ampoule
- Syringe and needle

Neonatal resuscitation equipment will be covered in detail in **Chapter 44**.

CONCLUSION

Most neonatal deaths occur during delivery or in the first 24 hours after birth. Newborn deaths due to asphyxia, infection, and hypothermia can be prevented by providing essential routine newborn care to all babies.

REFERENCES

1. UNICEF. Key data [Internet]. www.unicef.org. Available from: https://www.unicef.org/india/key-data.
2. Paul VK, Kumar R, Zodpey S. Toward single digit neonatal mortality rate in India. *Journal of Perinatology.* 2016. 36(S3): S1–2.
3. WHO. Newborn Mortality [Internet]. www.who.int. 2022. Available from: https://www.who.int/news-room/fact-sheets/detail/levels-and-trends-in-child-mortality-report-2021.
4. India Newborn Action Plan (INAP): National Health Mission [Internet]. nhm.gov.in. Available from: https://nhm.gov.in/index4.php?lang=1&level=0&linkid=153&lid=174.
5. Ramesh A, Deorari A, Paul V, Sankar MJ, Sachdeva A. *AIIMS Protocols in Neonatology.* 2nd ed. Noble Vision. 2019.
6. McCarthy LK, Morley CJ, Davis PG, et al. Timing of interventions in the delivery room: Does reality compare with neonatal resuscitation guidelines? *J Pediatr.* 2013.163:1553–7.
7. Branche T, Perez M, Saugstad OD. The first golden minute - Is it relevant? *Resuscitation.* 2020. 156:284-285.
8. Trevisanuto D, Testoni D, de Almeida MFB. Maintaining normothermia: Why and how? *Seminars in Fetal and Neonatal Medicine.* 2018. 23(5): 333–9.
9. Aziz K, Lee HC, Escobedo MB, et al. American Heart Association Guidelines for Cardiopulmonary Resuscitation and Emergency Cardiovascular Care. *Pediatrics.* 2020. 21;e2020038505E.
10. NSSK Resource Manual: National Health Mission [Internet]. nhm.gov.in. [cited 2023 Apr 2]. Available from: https://nhm.gov.in/index1.php?lang=1&level=1&sublinkid=1427&lid=781.
11. Visscher MO, Narendran V, Pickens WL, LaRuffa AA, Meinzen-Derr J, Allen K, et al. Vernix Caseosa in Neonatal Adaptation. *Journal of Perinatology.* 2005. 14;25(7):440–6.
12. Varendi H, Porter RH, Winberg J. Does the newborn baby find the nipple by smell? *Lancet Lond Engl.* 1994. 344:989–90.
13. Fawke J, Wyllie J, Udaeta E, et al. International Liaison Committee on Resuscitation Neonatal Life Support Task Force. Suctioning of clear amniotic fluid at birth: A systematic review. *Resusc Plus.* 2022. 12:100298.
14. American Academy of Pediatrics Committee on Fetus and Newborn; American College of Obstetricians and Gynecologists Committee on Obstetric Practice. The Apgar Score. *Pediatrics.* 2015. 136(4):819-22.
15. UNICEF. Skin-to-skin contact - Baby Friendly Initiative [Internet]. Baby Friendly Initiative. UNICEF. 2023. Available from: https://www.unicef.org.uk/babyfriendly/baby-friendly-resources/implementing-standards-resources/skin-to-skin-contact/.
16. Widström AM, Brimdyr K, Svensson K, Cadwell K, Nissen E. Skin-to-skin contact the first hour after birth, underlying implications and clinical practice. *Acta Paediatr.* 2019. 108(7): 1192-1204.
17. Delayed umbilical cord clamping for improved maternal and infant health and nutrition outcomes. World Health Organization [Internet]. 2018. Available from: https://www.who.int/nutrition/publications/guidelines/cord_clamping/en/
18. American College of Obstetricians and Gynecologists' Committee on Obstetric Practice. Delayed Umbilical Cord Clamping After Birth: ACOG Committee Opinion, Number 814. *Obstet Gynecol.* 2020. 136(6): e100-e106.
19. Basile S, Pinelli S, Micelli E, Caretto M, Benedetti Panici P. Milking of the Umbilical Cord in Term and Late Preterm Infants. *Biomed Res Int.* 2019. 9185059.
20. Resuscitation Council UK. Newborn resuscitation and support of transition of infants at birth Guidelines [Internet]. Resuscitation Council UK. 2021. Available from: https://www.resus.org.uk/library/2021-resuscitation-guidelines/newborn-resuscitation-and-support-transition-infants-birth.
21. Deshmukh M, Balasubramanian H, Rao S, Patole S. Effect of gastric lavage on feeding in neonates born through meconium-stained liquor: A systematic review. *Arch Dis Child Fetal Neonatal Ed.* 2015. 100(5):F394-9.
22. Milinco M, Travan L, Cattaneo A, et al. Effectiveness of biological nurturing on early breastfeeding problems: a randomized controlled trial. *Int Breastfeed J.* 2020. 15:21.
23. WHO recommendations on newborn health: Guidelines approved by the WHO Guidelines Review Committee [Internet]. www.who.int. Available from: https://www.who.int/publications/i/item/WHO-MCA-17.07.

Neonatal Resuscitation

CHAPTER 44

V LAKSHMI

INTRODUCTION

Approximately 1 million newborns die within the first 24 hours of birth [1]. Birth asphyxia and birth trauma are the leading causes of neonatal death with Sub-Saharan Africa and Central and South Asia bearing the highest burden.

Most newborns make the transition to extra-uterine life without intervention. 85% of term newborns will initiate spontaneous breathing within 30 seconds of birth [2,3].

The need for resuscitation may be higher in babies born preterm and those with identified risk factors. However, the need for resuscitation cannot always be predicted. Hence, it is prudent to be prepared at every birth.

The Neonatal Resuscitation Program (NRP), established by the Indian Academy of Pediatrics in 1987, has helped healthcare providers acquire the skills and knowledge necessary to save the lives of asphyxiated newborns. In India, the NRP has become the training standard for pediatricians, neonatologists, and labour room care providers [4]. NRP teaches cognitive, technical, and teamwork skills to resuscitate and stabilise a newborn.

EFFECT OF ASPHYXIA ON THE FETUS OR NEONATE

Fetal Response to Asphyxia

Before birth, fetal respiratory function is performed by the placenta, which transfers oxygen from the mother to the fetus and CO_2 from the fetus to the mother. When placental circulation is interrupted, fetal oxygenation declines, CO_2 levels increase, and pH decreases, leading to asphyxia. This is reflected in the loss of fetal heart rate variability and/or the presence of decelerations, and the baby gasps in utero (**primary apnea**). If this asphyxia is not corrected, the fetus becomes apneic and bradycardic (**secondary apnea**).

Neonatal Response to Continuing Asphyxia

Primary apnea

Infants in a state of asphyxia will initially produce rapid respiratory efforts. These respiratory efforts slow down and eventually cease with continued asphyxia (**primary apnea**). Eventually, the heart rate and blood pressure drop, and the neuromuscular tone diminishes (Fig. 44.1). **During primary apnea, the infant will respond to tactile or noxious stimulation and re-initiate breathing.**

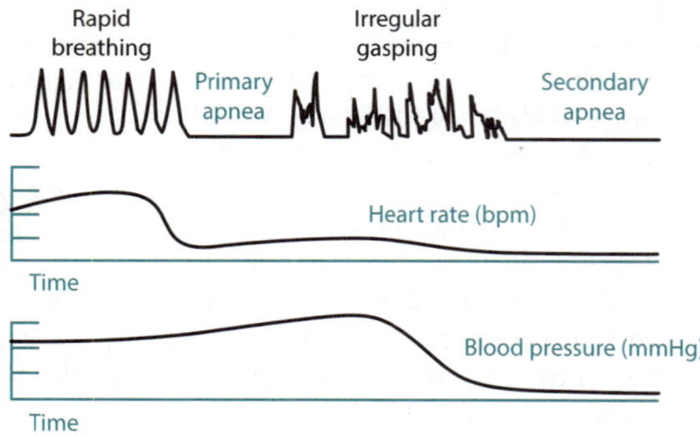

Fig. 44.1 Changes in breathing, heart rate, and blood pressure in the fetus or infant caused by fetal asphyxia

Secondary apnea

If primary asphyxia is not corrected, the infant starts taking deep, gasping breaths, which then slowly decrease in frequency and eventually cease (**secondary apnea**). The heart rate and blood pressure continue to drop, and the infant becomes flaccid. **Infants with secondary apnea do not respond to tactile or noxious stimulation and require positive-pressure ventilation (PPV) to restore breathing.**

> **Key Point**
>
> It is not clinically possible to differentiate between primary and secondary apnea. The diagnosis is based on whether the infant responds to stimulation (primary apnea) or requires positive-pressure ventilation (secondary apnea).

Irrespective of whether respiratory failure occurs before, at, or after birth, the primary problem is the lack of gas exchange. Therefore, the focus of neonatal resuscitation is on effective ventilation of the lungs.

CARDIORESPIRATORY TRANSITION FROM INTRA- TO EXTRAUTERINE LIFE

The transition from intrauterine to extrauterine life is a complex one. Any failure in this transition may endanger the infant's life. The following processes are involved in the transition:

- The fluid in the lung is replaced with air at birth as the baby takes its first breaths (cries).
- During fetal life, the pulmonary vessels are constricted and have high pressure. Most of the blood bypasses the lungs and is diverted through the patent foramen ovale and the ductus arteriosus as a right-to-left shunt to deliver the most oxygenated blood to the fetal head and heart. At birth, air in the lungs causes the pulmonary blood vessels to relax so that blood flows through the lung, and effective gas exchange takes place.
- Clamping of the cord results in the elimination of the low-pressure placental zone, and the systemic vascular resistance rises above the pulmonary circulation.
- Though these transitional changes occur in the first few minutes of life, it may take hours or days for the entire process to be completed.

The transition may not always be smooth, and the baby may demonstrate signs of respiratory distress. Neonatal resuscitation then becomes essential to help the infant breathe.

RESUSCITATION OF THE NEWBORN

It is important to remember that not all newborns will require help in transitioning to extrauterine life [3].

- 85% breathe spontaneously without intervention
- 10% respond after drying, stimulation and manoeuvres to open the airway
- Approximately 5% receive positive pressure ventilation
- Intubation rates vary between 0.4% and 2%
- Fewer than 0.3% of infants receive chest compressions
- Only 0.05% receive adrenaline

At birth, the baby is assessed and placed into one of three categories (Table 44.1). A baby who is not breathing or is gasping will require resuscitation. In such cases, the umbilical cord should be clamped and cut immediately, and the baby should be taken to the newborn care corner to initiate resuscitation.

Anticipation and Preparedness for Resuscitation

Ideally, every birth should be attended by at least one qualified individual who can initiate resuscitation [2]. In anticipated high-risk conditions, at least one or two qualified individuals should be present solely to manage the baby with a fully qualified team available on call. If advanced resuscitation is anticipated, a neonatal team should be present, which can perform endotracheal intubation and chest compression, provide vascular access, and administer drugs.

Equipment checklist

It is essential to maintain a checklist (Table 44.2) for the equipment required for resuscitation in order to ensure their availability beforehand.

Table 44.1 Assessment of the infant at birth and categorisation to decide on the need for resuscitation

Category	Neonatal findings	Action
I	• Healthy term baby • Cries within seconds • Good tone and activity • Heart rate of ≥100 bpm • Rapidly turns pink	• Dry the baby and wrap in a towel • Delay cord clamping • Skin-to-skin contact on mother's chest
II	• Irregular breathing • Heart rate ≥100 bpm • Central cyanosis	• Clamp cord • Dry, provide warmth, stimulate till normal respiratory effort initiated • Position and suction, if required
III	• Gasping or apneic • Heart rate <100 bpm • Pale • Poor tone/atony	• PPV indicated — Continue till HR >100 bpm — Chest moves with PPV • HR <60 bpm — Start chest compression

bpm, beats per minute; *HR*, heart rate; *PPV*, positive pressure ventilation

Identifying the high-risk pregnancy

The pregnancy at high risk of a newborn that requires resuscitation may be identified by the following questions [2,3]:

- What is the expected gestational age?
  - Premature and postdated pregnancies are high-risk
- Is the amniotic fluid clear?
  - The presence of significant meconium in the amniotic fluid is a risk factor (see **Chapter 16**, *Meconium-stained amniotic fluid: Assessment and management*)

Table 44.2 Checklist for the equipment required for the different aspects of infant resuscitation

Steps of resuscitation	Equipment required
Providing warmth	• Preheated warmer • Warm towels or blankets • Temperature sensor • Cap • Plastic wrap and thermal mattress at <32 weeks' gestation
Clearing airway	• Bulb syringe • 10–12 F suction catheter attached to wall suction set at 80–100 mmHg
Auscultation	• Pediatric stethoscope
Ventilation	• Equipment for free flow oxygen with flow meter set at 10 L/minute • Oxygen blender set at — 21% for term infant — 21–30% for preterm infant • Positive pressure ventilation device — Self-inflating bag — T-piece resuscitator, if available • Infant mask size 0 (preterm) and 1 (term) • Cardiac monitor and leads
Oxygenation	• Pulse oximeter • Target oxygen saturation table
Intubation	• Laryngoscope with straight blades — Size 0 for preterm infant — Size 1 for term infant — Size 00 for extremely preterm infant • Endotracheal tubes of different sizes • Measuring tape and endotracheal tube insertion depth table • Waterproof tape
Medication	• Adrenaline/epinephrine (0.1 mg/mL = 1 mg/10 mL) • Normal saline • Emergency tray for securing umbilical venous line

- Are there additional maternal or fetal risk factors?

  Risk factors that may lead to the baby requiring support for a smooth extrauterine transition are listed in Table 44.3.

Initial Steps of Resuscitation

Resuscitation in a baby that is not breathing begins with **rapid evaluation** and then proceeds to the assessment of the **airway, breathing, circulation,** and the **need for medications** [2,5].

Drying and providing warmth

- Cord clamping should not be delayed in a baby that is not breathing. The baby should immediately be moved to a preheated warmer after clamping and cutting the cord [4,6].
- The wet linen should be removed, and the baby should be wrapped in a dry towel. Preterm babies <32 weeks need not be dried before wrapping them in a polythene sheet.

Table 44.3 **Fetal and maternal factors that may necessitate resuscitation of the infant at birth**

Antepartum risk factors	Intrapartum risk factors
Maternal • Hypertensive disorders • Hyperglycemia in pregnancy • High BMI • Limited or no prenatal care ***Fetal*** • Gestational age <37 0/7 weeks • Gestational age ≥41 0/7 weeks • Multiple gestation • Fetal anemia • Polyhydramnios/ oligohydramnios • Fetal macrosomia/ FGR • Serious fetal anomaly • Fetal hydrops	• Forceps- or vacuum-assisted delivery • Emergency cesarean delivery • Breech or other abnormal presentation • Category II or III fetal heart rate pattern • General anesthesia • Magnesium therapy • Placental abruption • Intrapartum bleeding • Chorioamnionitis • Shoulder dystocia • Meconium-stained amniotic fluid • Cord prolapse • Opioid administered within 4 hours of delivery

BMI, body mass index; *FGR*, fetal growth restriction

> **Key Point**
>
> Temperature control is extremely important as hypothermia soon after birth is associated with higher mortality [7], especially in preterm infants [8].

Stimulation

- Breathing is stimulated by rubbing the baby's back or flicking its feet gently. Drying and suctioning the infant often provide enough stimulation.
- Efforts at stimulating the infant **should not last >30 seconds** before initiating the next resuscitative steps.

> **Key Point**
>
> Holding the baby upside down or slapping it is best avoided as these may harm the baby.

Positioning

- The head and neck should be positioned in a manner that opens up the airway and allows unrestricted air entry.
- The baby is positioned supine, keeping the head and neck slightly extended, with the face tilted to the ceiling in a 'sniffing position' (Fig. 44.2). A small, rolled towel may be placed under the baby's shoulders, especially if there is a rounded occiput.
- The neck should neither be hyperextended nor hyperflexed (neutral position).

Suctioning

- Secretions are suctioned from the mouth first, then the nose.

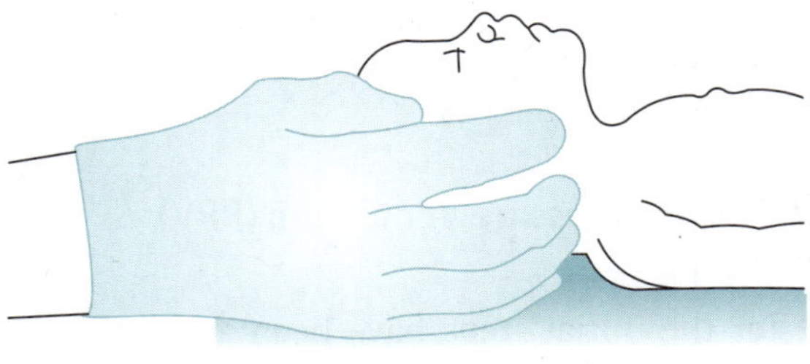

Fig. 44.2 The infant's head should be placed in a neutral position for successful airway management

- It is important to use the suction device gently to avoid injuring tissues and causing vagal stimulation, which may lead to apnea and bradycardia. If a wall-mounted suction device is used, negative pressure of <80–100 mmHg is recommended.

Administering oxygen

If the infant is breathing and has a heart rate (HR) of >100 bpm, but appears cyanosed, it should be checked for saturation. If the saturation is below target, free-flow oxygen should be administered.

Targets have been recommended for SpO_2 levels depending on the time after birth and help guide intervention with oxygen [2,9] (Table 44.4). The oximeter probe should be placed on the right upper extremity, ideally the wrist or medial surface of the palm [10].

Table 44.4 The target SpO_2 values for infants undergoing resuscitation in the delivery room

Time since birth of infant	SpO_2 to be achieved (%)
1 minute	60–65
2 minutes	65–70
3 minutes	70–75
4 minutes	75–80
5 minutes	80–85
10 minutes	85–95

Key Point

Immediately following birth, the neonate's oxygen saturation normally remains in the range of 70–80% for several minutes [2,3].

Positive Pressure Ventilation (PPV)

Indications

After the initial steps have been attempted for 30 seconds, PPV is initiated if:

- The baby is apneic or
- The heart rate is <100 bpm

Bag-and-mask ventilation

PPV may be initiated with a self-inflating bag [3,5]. A size 0 mask is chosen for a preterm infant and size 1 for a term infant (Table 44.2). In high-resource facilities, a T-piece resuscitator may be used. In LMICs like India, the self-inflating bag and mask are most commonly used.

- The mask is placed to cover the baby's face from the chin to the bridge of the nose, avoiding the eyes. Care should be taken to achieve an airtight seal (Fig. 44.3a).
- For infants >35 weeks of gestation, PPV is given for 30 seconds with room air.
- For infants <35 weeks of gestation, PPV is given for 30 seconds with 21–30% blended air.
- The bag is squeezed to raise the chest repeatedly (Fig. 44.3b).
- **The rate of PPV** should be 40–60 times per minute. A practical method of timing the PPV is to repeatedly say "breathe-2-3" and synchronising the squeezing with "breathe" and releasing while saying "2-3" [3].

Monitoring

In high-resource facilities, the infant is monitored continuously with pulse oximetry and continuous ECG. This provides a continuous assessment of the HR and oxygen saturation (SpO_2) during resuscitation [9].

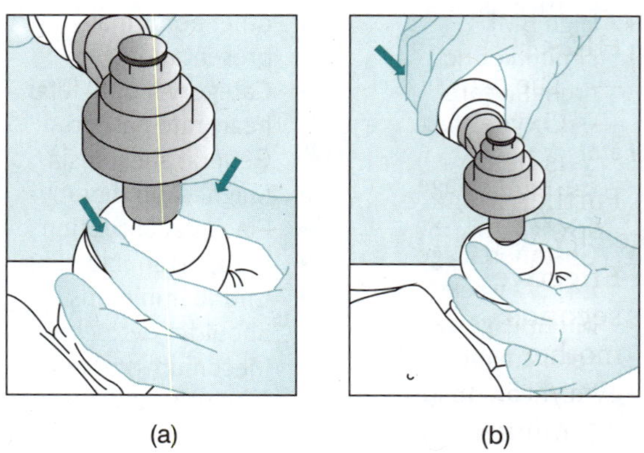

Fig. 44.3 (a) The mask is positioned so that it covers the face, while the fingers apply pressure (arrows) to create an airtight seal and (b) the bag is squeezed repeatedly (arrow) to move the chest

Effectiveness of PPV

If the PPV is effective, the following happen:
- The HR increases
- The chest moves with PPV, even if the HR is not increasing

Corrective action

If PPV does not achieve effective ventilation, corrective action should be taken. This includes the following measures (**MR SO P A**) [4]:
- **MR:** Readjust the **m**ask, **r**eposition the head and neck
- **SO:** **S**uction the mouth and nose and **o**pen the mouth to tilt the jaw forward
- **P:** Squeeze the bag harder and increase the delivered **p**ressure
- **A:** Use an **a**lternate method of keeping the airway open, such as intubation

Assessment of response and further management

- **Infant breathing well**
  - PPV is slowly weaned off
  - Oxygen is titrated till the target SpO_2 is reached
- **HR >100 bpm but infant not breathing well**
  - PPV is continued
  - Oxygen delivery is increased if saturation remains below target
  - Intubation is considered
- **HR <100 bpm**
  - The baby is intubated and PPV is continued
  - Oxygen delivery is increased if saturation is below the target

Further management depends on how long the PPV was required for the infant to recover.
- **Effective PPV provided only for 30 seconds:** The infant is observed at the mother's side with the monitoring of vitals every 15 minutes in the first hour and every 30 minutes in the second hour.
- **Effective PPV for >30 seconds:** After breathing has been established, the infant is observed in the nursery and provided post-resuscitation care (see section below on *Post-resuscitation care*).

Endotracheal Intubation

When direct access to the upper trachea is required for the delivery of invasive PPV, endotracheal intubation becomes necessary. Training should be provided for neonatal intubation. In high-risk pregnancies where neonatal support is anticipated, it would be prudent to have a neonatologist with intubation skills available.

Indications

Intubation is considered in the following situations:
- Prolonged PPV with bag and mask ventilation
- PPV with 100% oxygen for 60 seconds fails to obtain a good chest rise, even after corrective steps
- No increase in heart rate (<60 bpm) and saturation despite good chest movement with PPV
- Chest compression required
- Special circumstances
  - Congenital diaphragmatic hernia
  - Airway stabilisation of the extremely-low-birth-weight infant (<1000 g)
  - For administration of a surfactant

Equipment

- Laryngoscope with straight blades
  - For the term infant, blade size 1
  - For the preterm infant, blade size 0
  - For the extremely preterm infant, blade size 00
- Non-cuffed endotracheal (ET) tubes based on birth weight (Table 44.5)
- Tape to secure the endotracheal tube in position

Table 44.5 Choice of endotracheal tube based on the infant's weight and gestational age at birth

Weight	Gestational age	Endotracheal tube size
<1 Kg	<28 weeks	2.5 mm
1–2 Kg	28–32 weeks	3.0 mm
>2 Kg	>34 weeks	3.5 mm

Procedure

Endotracheal intubation must be performed by a clinician trained in the procedure. The laryngoscope blade is inserted into the mouth with the aim of visualising the vocal cords. An attempt to intubate should be limited to 30 seconds at a time, as prolonged and unsuccessful attempts may destabilise the baby. Effective PPV may be delivered by a bag and mask or LMA (laryngeal mask airway) between attempts to intubate.

The ET tube is inserted between the cords, and its endotracheal position is confirmed with the rise of the chest with PPV. Auscultation with a stethoscope will confirm equal air entry on both sides. The HR should also improve if it is in the right position. Once the correct position of the ET tube is confirmed, the tube is fixed in place with adhesive tape.

Depth of insertion: The ET tube is inserted to a depth equal to the nasal tragus length (NTL) + 1 cm. The NTL is the distance from the nasal septum to the tragus of the ear.

Assessment of response and further management

If clinical improvement is not seen despite the appropriate position of the ET tube, then the following causes **(DOPE)** should be ruled out:

- **D**isplaced tube
- **O**bstructed tube
- **P**neumothorax
- **E**quipment failure

After providing effective PPV with the ET tube for 30 seconds, the infant is assessed. Further management depends on the following:

- **HR >100 bpm and infant is breathing spontaneously:** Post-resuscitation care in the nursery
- **HR between 60–100 bpm:** PPV is continued
- **HR <60 bpm:** Chest compressions are intiated

Laryngeal Mask

If bag-and-mask ventilation is unsuccessful or if tracheal intubation is unsuccessful or not feasible, a laryngeal mask may be used as an alternative means of establishing an airway in infants of >34 weeks' gestation or weighing ≥2000 g [3].

Resuscitation in the Presence of Meconium-stained Amniotic Fluid (MSAF)

In the presence of significant MSAF and a non-vigorous infant, the infant is immediately transferred to the radiant warmer for initial steps. MSAF does not influence resuscitation. Routine intubation and tracheal suctioning of meconium do not have any benefit and are not recommended [2,3,4].

Chest Compressions (CC)

Indication

Chest compressions are indicated when the heart rate remains <60 bpm despite 30 seconds of PPV delivered through an ET tube, with good chest rise and ventilation.

Procedure

- The airway is secured with endotracheal intubation, if not already done, for better coordination of PPV and chest compression. The PPV is provided from the right side of the infant.
- 100% oxygen is started at 10 L/minute.
- Pressure is applied to the lower one-third of the sternum above the xiphisternum. Chest compressions are applied using the **two-thumb technique** (Fig. 44.4a). The **two-finger technique** is used if there is only one person available to resuscitate the infant (Fig. 44.4c). The two-thumb technique is preferred because it generates higher systolic and coronary perfusion pressure [10].
  - The torso is encircled with both hands and the back is supported with the fingers under the infant (Fig. 44.4b).
  - Downward pressure is used to depress the sternum by 1/3rd of the anteroposterior diameter. Care must be taken to see that pressure is applied to the centre and not laterally.

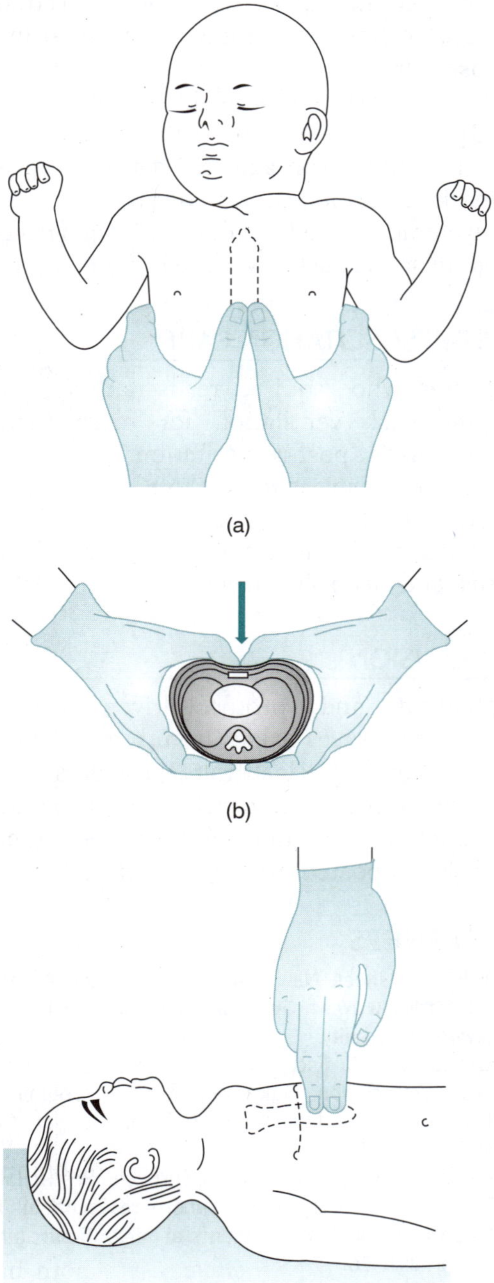

(a) (b) (c)

Fig. 44.4 Chest compression being provided with (a) two-thumb technique, where (b) pressure is provided at the centre (arrow) and not laterally; (c) the two-finger technique

— The compression rate should be 90/minute. The ratio of PPV:chest compression is 1 PPV:3 CC in 2 seconds or 30 PPV and 90 CC in 1 minute.

— A practical way of synchronising the two actions is to say, "1 and 2 and 3 and breathe", with the CCs being applied with the numbers and the PPV with the word "breathe" [4].

Assessment of response and further management

The heart rate is assessed after 60 seconds of starting chest compressions.

- **If HR is <60 bpm**
  - — Chest compressions and PPV through the ET tube are continued, as is oxygen. The baby is reassessed after 60 seconds.
  - — If the HR is still <60 bpm, medications are administered (see section below).
- **If HR is >60 bpm**
  - — Chest compressions are stopped and PPV is continued through the ET tube. Oxygen is also continued.
- **If HR is >100 bpm and SpO_2 has reached target range**
  - — The infant is shifted to the nursery for post-resuscitation care.

Medication

Infants with HR <60 bpm despite adequate ventilation and chest compressions should be given a dose of dilute adrenaline (epinephrine).

Obtaining IV access

Under aseptic precautions, the umbilical cord is tied and cut approximately 1 cm above the skin. The vein is identified, and an umbilical catheter (size 3.5–5 Fr) is inserted and secured at 2–4 cm after a backflow of blood is seen. Care should be taken to flush saline through the catheter before inserting it into the vein.

Dosage

Injection adrenaline is administered in 1:10,000 dilutions at the dose of 0.2 mL/Kg (0.1–0.3 mL/

Kg depending on weight and gestational age) followed by a saline flush of 3 mL. The dose may be repeated every three to five minutes if the HR remains <60 bpm.

ET tube access

Adrenaline may also be administered through the ET tube while waiting for vein access.

Dosage

ET adrenaline in 1:10,000 dilutions may be administered at a dose of 1.0 mL/Kg until umbilical venous access is established.

> **Key Point**
>
> 1 in 10,000 (0.1 mg/mL) adrenaline is reconstituted by adding 1 mL of adrenaline to 9 mL of normal saline. This is immediately labelled 1:10,000 and kept for further use.

Discontinuing Resuscitation

Resuscitative procedures may be discontinued after 10 minutes if the neonate has demonstrated no signs of life:

- No heartbeat
- No respiratory effort for >10 minutes

If they recover, the outcome in these infants is associated with early mortality and unacceptably severe motor and sensory disabilities.

Non-initiation of Resuscitation

In some situations, resuscitation may not be initiated because of the poor prognosis for the infant. This decision must be taken in consultation with the parents. These conditions include the following:

- Gestational age <24 weeks
- Birth weight <500 g
- Anencephaly or other lethal anomaly
- Chromosomal abnormalities incompatible with life such as trisomy 13 or 18

Special Situations

There are certain special situations where extra interventions may be required. These are as follows:

- Very preterm infant—surfactant administration
- Pneumothorax, pleural effusions—intercostal drain
- Airway obstruction as in choanal atresia, large goiter—oral airway/tracheostomy
- Congenital diaphragmatic hernia—bag and mask ventilation contraindicated
- Myelomeningocele/abdominal wall defects—warm saline packs over the lesion

POST-RESUSCITATION CARE

Neonates who required resuscitation beyond bag-and-mask ventilation for more than a minute need post-resuscitation care in the neonatal intensive care unit (NICU) along with frequent assessment of respiration, perfusion, blood glucose levels, urine output, neurological status, and electrolyte levels.

CONCLUSION

Methodical and protocol-driven neonatal resuscitation saves babies from birth asphyxia-related mortality. Healthcare providers in the delivery room should be trained in the neonatal resuscitation programme and also need to have their skills updated from time to time.

REFERENCES

1. WHO fact sheet. Newborn mortality. 2024. Accessed at https://www.who.int/news-room/fact-sheets/detail/newborn-mortality.
2. Aziz K, Lee HC, Escobedo MB, et al. 2020 American Heart Association Guidelines for Cardiopulmonary Resuscitation and Emergency Cardiovascular Care. *Pediatrics*. 2020.
3. Madar J, Roehr CC, Ainsworth S. European Resuscitation Council Guidelines 2021: Newborn resuscitation and support of transition of infants at birth. *Resuscitation*. 2021. 61:291-326.
4. Bharti LK, Prakash A, Jain, M. Neonatal Resuscitation Program. Standard treatment guidelines 2022. Accessed at https://iapindia.org/pdf/Ch-104-Neonatal-Resuscitation-Program.pdf
5. Yamada NK, Szyld E, Strand ML, et al. American Heart Association and American Academy of Pediatrics, 2023. Focused Update on Neonatal Resuscitation: An Update to the American Heart Association

Guidelines for Cardiopulmonary Resuscitation and Emergency Cardiovascular Care. *Pediatrics*. 2024. 153(2):e2023065030.

6. American Academy of Pediatrics. *Neonatal Resuscitation*. 8th ed, Weiner G, Zaichkin J (Eds). 2021. American Academy of Pediatrics, Itasca, IL.
7. Perlman JM, Wyllie J, Kattwinkel J, et al. Part 7: Neonatal Resuscitation: 2015 International Consensus on Cardiopulmonary Resuscitation and Emergency Cardiovascular Care Science With Treatment Recommendations. *Circulation*. 2015. 132(16 Suppl 1):S204-41.
8. Watkinson M. Temperature control of premature infants in the delivery room. *Clin Perinatol*. 2006. 33:43.
9. Noori S, Wlodaver A, Gottipati V, et al. Transitional changes in cardiac and cerebral hemodynamics in term neonates at birth. *J Pediatr*. 2012. 160:943.
10. Fernandes CJ. Neonatal resuscitation in the delivery room. Garcia-Prats JA (Ed). *UpToDate*. 2024. Waltham, MA.

CHAPTER 45

The Normal Puerperium

MATHANGI THIRUNAVAKARASU

INTRODUCTION

The puerperium or the postpartum period is defined as the time from the birth of the infant through the first six weeks after the delivery [1]. It is the period following childbirth during which most of the physiologic changes of pregnancy revert to the prepregnancy state; this usually takes 6 weeks but may extend to 8 weeks. Changes in the pelvic musculature and cardiovascular changes can take up to 12 weeks. The ACOG recommends that postpartum care should extend up to 12 weeks after delivery and has termed this the 'fourth trimester' [2].

The puerperium is arbitrarily divided into the following stages:

- **Immediate:** Within 24 hours
- **Early:** Up to 7 days
- **Remote:** Up to 6–8 weeks

This chapter will focus on physiological changes and maternal care in the normal puerperium.

POSTPARTUM PHYSIOLOGY AND CHANGES

Uterine Involution

Involution is the gradual reduction in the size of the pregnant uterus after delivery. First, hemostasis is established secondary to the contraction of the interlacing arterial smooth muscle bundles, causing the compression of the intramyometrial blood vessels. This is accompanied by thrombosis, hyalinisation, and endophlebitis of the vessels in the placental site during the first week of delivery.

The uterus weighs approximately 1000 g and has a volume of 5 L immediately after delivery, whereas the non-pregnant uterus weighs approximately 70 g with a volume of about 5–10 mL [3]. Soon after delivery, the height of the uterine fundus is halfway between the pubic symphysis and the umbilicus and feels firm, globular, and non-tender. The fundal height remains constant for the first 24 hours after delivery, following which there is a steady decline in height. This gradual decrease in the size of the uterus continues, and by the end of the second week of delivery, the uterus becomes a pelvic organ [4]. The rate of involution of the uterus hereafter slows down so that the uterus reaches the normal prepregnancy size in six weeks [5].

The endometrial surface rapidly decreases in size after delivery as the placenta gets separated from the decidual layer. The superficial layer is shed, and the deep layer regenerates to the prepregnancy state of the endometrium. By the seventh day, there is regeneration of the endometrial glands and stroma, and by the end of 16 days, the endometrium is almost completely restored [3].

Lochia

Lochia is the postpartum uterine discharge that commences as a bloody discharge and undergoes transformation to varying consistencies and colours through the weeks after delivery. The average duration of puerperal lochia is around one month and is unrelated to lactation [6].

- In the first 3–4 days after delivery, the discharge is called **lochia rubra** because it is

reddish-brown in colour. It contains erythrocytes, shredded decidua, epithelial cells, and bacteria.
- Over the next 2–3 weeks, the lochia becomes watery and loses colour to become pinkish-brown and is known as **lochia serosa**.
- Following this, the lochia is an admixture of leukocytes and reduced fluid content and assumes a white or yellow-white colour; this is known as **lochia alba**.

Key Point

Foul-smelling lochia is a sign of infection. It may be accompanied by fever. The mother should be informed at discharge to seek medical help if this occurs.

Changes in the Cervix, Lower Genital Tract, and Pelvic Muscles

The cervix

Within the first four days after delivery, the cervical epithelium starts to regress, and by six weeks, most pregnancy changes in the cervix resolve except for the external os, which never resumes its pregravid shape, and remains a large, transverse slit [3].

Lower genital tract

The vagina and the introitus gradually reduce in size after delivery but do not resume the prepregnancy size and shape. The hymen gets replaced by several small tags of tissue, which are known as **myrtiform caruncles** [1].

Pelvic muscles

After delivery, the pelvic floor is likely to have reduced tensile strength due to possible damage to the pelvic floor. It is important that perineal tears and sphincter injuries are identified at the time of delivery and repaired appropriately (see **Chapter 25**, *Prevention and management of perineal trauma occurring in childbirth*). The broad and round ligaments require significant time to recover from the stretching that occurs during pregnancy.

Ovarian Function

There is a period of amenorrhea and ovulation suppression in all women after delivery, though the time this takes can vary. In women who do not breastfeed, the mean time for ovulation to resume is 45–64 days [7]. The reason for ovulation suppression is a consistent elevation of serum prolactin in lactating women. Prolactin levels return to normal levels three weeks after delivery in non-lactating women but remain elevated longer in lactating women, which explains the late return of ovulation in the latter group. Menstruation resumes by 12 weeks in 70% of non-lactating women. In a woman who is exclusively breastfeeding, the likelihood of ovulation within the first six months postpartum is only about 1–5% [8].

Lactation

The breasts begin to secrete a thick, yellow liquid called **colostrum** during the first 2–3 days postpartum. This liquid is rich in immunological components, minerals, and amino acids with protein (mostly globulin), but contains less sugar and fat. It is important for babies to receive colostrum during the initial days of breastfeeding, and mothers must be educated about this. Colostrum secretion may continue for 5–7 days. It gradually gets converted to mature milk over the next 4–6 weeks [9].

Physiologic Weight Loss

A mean weight loss of 4–6 Kg immediately after delivery is expected because of the delivery of the infant, placenta, amniotic fluid, along with some blood loss [3]. Women lose half of their gestational weight gain by six weeks postpartum, and the remaining gradually over the next six months [1].

Hair and Skin

Women may have diffuse hair loss for 1–5 months postpartum. This is a transient phenomenon referred to as **telogen effluvium**. This phase is self-limiting, and normal hair growth pattern is eventually restored. Some of the skin changes such as striae are permanent but fade over time. Chloasma, on the other hand, disappears over a varying time period [10].

Cardiovascular System

There is a 60–70% increase in cardiac output and stroke volume due to the autotransfusion of uteroplacental blood to the intravascular space and the release of the mechanical compression of the vena cava by the gravid uterus. However, the plasma volume is reduced by 1 litre immediately after delivery, probably due to blood loss. Redistribution of extracellular fluid into the vascular space restores the plasma volume by three days postpartum. These changes are significant in women with pre-existing cardiac dysfunction.

There is also a manifestation of transient anemia as the blood volume tends to decrease by almost 15% of the predelivery levels. The hematocrit levels become normal by 8 weeks postpartum with the resumption of normalcy of the red cell mass. The rise in pulse rate, stroke volume, and cardiac output persist after delivery and may rise even higher during the first one hour of delivery. A transient rise of about 5% in both diastolic and systolic blood pressures may be observed in most women during the first 3–4 days postpartum [3].

Coagulation

The alterations in the coagulation system along with injury to the vessels combined with immobility may give rise to an increased risk of thromboembolism in the postpartum period, especially when the woman has had a cesarean delivery.

The maximum potential for coagulability is noted immediately after delivery and persists for the following 48 hours. Fibrinogen concentrations gradually fall over the first 2 weeks postpartum. Increased fibrinolytic activity is observed in the initial 4 days following delivery which returns to normal in a week as evidenced by plasminogen activation inhibitor levels. D-dimer levels are often higher than pregnancy levels, but this does not effectively reflect the chance of thrombus formation [11,3].

Urinary Tract

After delivery, the bladder is likely to have an increased capacity and a relative insensitivity to the increased intravesical pressure. This predisposes to **bladder dysfunction**, which may manifest as incomplete emptying, overdistension, and excessive residual urine in the postpartum period. The bladder mucosa may become edematous and show evidence of submucous extravasation of blood. Urinary stasis is seen in more than 50% of women, increasing the risk of postpartum urinary tract infection [3].

Gastrointestinal (GI) Tract

Delayed GI motility, mild ileus following delivery, along with perineal discomfort could cause **constipation** postpartum. Anal incontinence can develop in women who sustained anal sphincter injuries during labour [3].

POSTPARTUM MATERNAL CARE

The immediate postpartum period is one of significant physiological changes with the potential for complications. This is also a special time when mother–baby bonding and lactation are initiated. Therefore, it is very important that the mother is supported and monitored during the postpartum period.

Postpartum care focuses on the following:

- Restoring the health and well-being of the mother
- Promoting breastfeeding and care of the breasts
- Preventing infection/venous thrombosis
- Providing contraceptive advice

Immediate Puerperium

- **Postpartum hemorrhage:** Early identification of postpartum hemorrhage is important. Frequent fundal checks should be performed to confirm that the uterus is firm and well contracted below the level of the umbilicus; this rules out uterine atonicity. A perineal exam helps in assessing excess vaginal bleeding. These assessments should be performed hourly for the first 2 hours and then 4-hourly up to 24 hours after birth (see **Chapter 13**, *Abnormalities in the third stage of labour: Postpartum hemorrhage and retained placenta*).
- **Distended bladder:** An overdistended urinary bladder can be avoided by palpating the suprapubic area. If the uterus is felt above the level of the umbilicus, it may be an indication of retention or partial voiding of urine (see **Chapter 10**, *Immediate postpartum monitoring and care [including postpartum collapse]*). Documenting the first voided urine volume within six hours helps to ensure that there is no urinary retention [12].

Pain Management

Vaginal delivery

- **Perineal pain**: Perineal pain can be managed with paracetamol (650–1000 mg 3–4 times a day) and/or ibuprofen (400 mg every 6–8 hours). Warm compresses can help relieve pain. Some women may prefer ice packs. Local anesthetic ointments may help, particularly in the presence of an episiotomy or deep tear. If the episiotomy is very painful and the mother finds it difficult to sit, she may be advised to use a ring cushion, which is commonly used to manage hemorrhoids. However, if the woman complains of severe perineal, vaginal, or rectal pain, it is important to perform a careful inspection and palpation of the concerned area. In the immediate postpartum period, such pain could be due to a **hematoma**.
- **Perianal pain:** Congested or thrombosed hemorrhoids may become more prominent while pushing during delivery and this could cause perianal pain. Painful hemorrhoids may be treated with a high-fibre diet, stool softeners, and Sitz baths.

Cesarean section

See the section on *Pain relief* in **Chapter 10**, and **Chapter 22**, *Cesarean section: Procedure and technique*, for details.

After pains

As the uterus undergoes the process of involution, the woman may experience pronounced pain in the abdomen at varying intervals. The pain may be severe during nursing and is known as 'after pains'. The severity of pain varies with parity, with primigravidas experiencing more pain than multigravidas. It generally reduces by the third day postpartum. Paracetamol or ibuprofen may be administered if the pain is significant.

Perineal Care

Perineal hygiene is an important aspect of postpartum care. It is essential to advise the woman on good perineal and personal hygiene. An ice pack may be applied to the perineum immediately after delivery to relieve edema and pain during the first 24 hours, especially when there is a perineal laceration or an episiotomy.

Ambulation

Women should be encouraged to ambulate as soon as possible after delivery. This is also applicable to women who have had a cesarean birth. Early ambulation helps in the prevention of urinary retention, puerperal venous thrombosis, and pulmonary embolism. It is a crucial component of postpartum recovery.

Diet

The lactating mother requires a well-balanced diet. In the first six months postpartum, mothers require 330 Kcal/day more than non-lactating women and in the subsequent six months, they require 400 Kcal/day more than non-lactating women [14]. The recommended calorie intake in the postpartum period is presented in Table 45.1.

In a country like India where a large proportion of women is anemic, it is essential to include iron-rich foods in the diet. Iron supplementation in the postpartum period is important. There must be an emphasis on including fruits, vegetables, lentils, and protein sources daily. Traditional postpartum diets may be poor in protein and rich in calories. Appropriate counselling on dietary needs is an important aspect of postpartum care and should include the woman and her family.

Laboratory Testing

Evaluation of postpartum hemoglobin must be considered in symptomatic women with antepartum anemia and postpartum hemorrhage with estimated blood loss >500 mL [15]. The white blood cell count may not be a good predictor of infection. Hence, testing for WBC must be reserved for symptomatic women with suspicion of infection.

Table 45.1 Recommended calorie intake for postpartum women (adapted from the Institute of Medicine Panel on Dietary Antioxidants and Related Compounds and National Academy of Sciences)

Nutritional requirement	Age <19 years	Age >19 years
Total calories	2200 Kcal	2200–2400 Kcal
Protein	71 g (10–30% of Kcal)	71 g (10–30% of Kcal)
Carbohydrates	210 g (45–65% of Kcal)	210 g (45–65% of Kcal)
Fibre	14 g/100 Kcal	14 g/100 Kcal
Total lipids	25–35% of Kcal	25–35% of Kcal
Calcium	1300 mg	1000 mg
Iron	10 mg	9 mg
Vitamin D	600 IU	600 IU

Care of the Breasts

It is important to take care of the breasts during lactation. Women should be advised on lactation with a focus on latching and holding, hygiene, and the appropriate bra to use.

Mild breast engorgement, which can occur due to the stasis of milk, is common and usually resolves within a few days. Hot fomentation, expressing milk, cold compresses between feeds, and mild analgesics such as paracetamol help relieve the symptoms. A lactating woman must feed her baby at regular intervals to avoid engorgement of the breasts [8].

Mastitis or infection of the breast tissues caused by microorganisms like *Staphylococcus aureus*, Group A or B streptococci, β-*Haemophilus* species, and *Escherichia coli* may develop [1]. Sudden-onset fever, localised pain, and swelling in the breast are seen in cases of mastitis and breast abscess.

Prevention of Venous Thromboembolism (VTE)

VTE, which may occur in pregnancy, is more common in the postpartum period. There is a relative increase in the risk with cesarean birth when compared to vaginal delivery, especially in the first few weeks after birth. The risk reduces gradually until 12 weeks postpartum. Other added risk factors for VTE such as previous VTE, obesity, smoking, thrombophilias, postpartum hemorrhage, and sickle cell disease must be documented.

Pelvic Floor Muscle Exercises/Training (PFME/PFMT)

PFME to prevent urinary incontinence is recommended and should be initiated in pregnancy and continued postpartum. These exercises are performed multiple times a day. Studies have shown that initiating PFME in the antenatal period and continuing them postpartum has significant benefits in preventing urinary incontinence. PFME is contraindicated in the immediate postpartum period in women with levator ani muscle injury during delivery. Women with obstetric anal sphincter injuries (OASI) can ideally resume PFME two weeks after delivery; these exercises help to improve pelvic floor symptoms as well [2,3].

Mood Changes

It is quite common for postpartum women to exhibit some degree of depression a few days after delivery. This is termed 'postpartum blues'. Though often mild and self-limited to 2–3 days, it may sometimes last up to 10 days. Persistence or worsening of moods calls for an evaluation for symptoms of major depression [13]. It is important to be aware of the risk factors for postpartum depression and anxiety. Screening for these conditions is recommended, followed by appropriate referral and management [12].

Hospital Stay and Discharge

The WHO recommends observation of the mother and newborn in the facility for at least 24–48 hours after an uncomplicated birth [12]. The ACOG recommends a minimum hospital stay of 48 hours after vaginal delivery and 72 hours (excluding the day of delivery) after cesarean birth. If postpartum discharge is planned earlier, strict criteria must be adhered to before discharge. These include the following [15]:

- Normal vital signs in both mother and baby
- Contracted uterus with normal lochia
- Normal urination with adequate output
- Adequate pain relief and ambulation
- Normal diet
- Maternal comfort with the care of the newborn

At discharge, immunisation of the baby and where appropriate, anti-D immunoglobulin for the mother must be confirmed and documented.

The mother should be instructed on postpartum wound care, medications, diet, and exercise. She should also be asked to look out for various warning signs and triggers, which should prompt her to schedule a postnatal visit. These include the following:

- Excessive vaginal bleeding
- Worsening pelvic/perineal pain
- Dysuria
- Shortness of breath
- Leg pain/swelling
- Significant mood disturbances
- Breast pain or redness
- Signs of infection

Some neonates may require readmission for hyperbilirubinemia after being discharged early after delivery [1].

Key Point

Women who are discharged early should be educated about various warning signs—both for the mother and her baby—that should alert them to seek medical care. For their follow-up, they should be given clear instructions on the person they should contact for review.

Physical and Sexual Activity

Physical exercise

The most recent WHO recommendations for postpartum care [12] advise the following for maximum benefit for all postpartum women who have no contraindications:

- Regular physical activity throughout the postpartum period
- At least 150 minutes of physical activity throughout the week for substantial health benefits
- Physical and muscle-strengthening activities as well as gentle stretching

Though these activities need not be restricted in women who have had a cesarean delivery, some modifications are indicated for the first eight weeks, until fascial healing is complete [16]. On the other hand, abdominal exercises for rectus abdominis diastasis can be initiated any time after vaginal delivery.

Sexual intercourse

The couple may resume sexual activity 4–6 weeks after delivery or whenever the woman is comfortable. A decrease in libido is often noticed. This is due to hormonal changes, 'postpartum blues', and occasionally, postpartum depression. Dyspareunia due to episiotomy or perineal laceration, and vaginal dryness due to estrogen deficiency, are also common. The incidences of dyspareunia and sexual dysfunction are higher in women with operative vaginal delivery during the first six months postpartum compared to women who have had cesarean birth.

Some form of contraception should be used when resuming intercourse.

Contraception

Ideally, contraceptive advice should be discussed in the third trimester and reiterated before discharge and again during routine postnatal visits. Ovulation is unpredictable in women who are exclusively breastfeeding. After six months, the chances of pregnancy increase even when the woman is exclusively breastfeeding. For those who desire permanent contraception, tubal ligation can be performed in the puerperal period after 24 hours of birth or as an interval procedure. Vasectomy as an alternative permanent contraceptive method should also be discussed with the couple.

Key Point

Every postpartum woman should be counselled on different contraceptive options so that she can choose the one that works best for her. This conversation should be ideally initiated in the late third trimester and discussed before discharge and reiterated at the postnatal visit.

Follow-up visits

The WHO [12] recommends follow-up at 3 days, 1–2 weeks, and 6 weeks postpartum, especially in low-resource areas where perinatal complications are high. Clinical assessment of the mother and newborn baby must be performed during these visits. At these visits, the woman must be asked about adjustment to breastfeeding, and any concerns she might have should be addressed.

It is important to ask about the woman's mood at home and discuss contraceptive options, diet, and the resumption of physical and sexual activity. The physical exam should include checking the woman's breasts, perineum, and anal region for women who have had vaginal births and the abdominal wound for cesarean births.

Key Point

Routine follow-up visits are recommended at three points in the postnatal period. Women with complications need to be triaged and seen more often, if needed.

CONCLUSION

The puerperium is an important phase where the new mother goes through various physical and psychological changes. Appropriate support is required at this time to identify potential problems particularly for women with pregnancy complications.

REFERENCES

1. Berens F. Overview of the postpartum period: Normal physiology and routine maternal care. Prabhu M (Ed). *UpToDate*. 2024. Waltham, MA.
2. ACOG Committee Opinion No. 736: Optimizing postpartum care. *Obstet Gynecol.* 2018. 131:e140. Reaffirmed 2021.
3. Mark B Landon, Henry L Galan, Eric RM Jauniaux, et al. Postpartum care and long-term health considerations. *Gabbe's obstetrics: Normal and Problem Pregnancies.* 8th Edition. Philadelphia, PA, Elsevier, 459- 474.
4. Mulic-Lutvica A, Bekuretsion M, Bakos O, Axelsson O. Ultrasonic evaluation of the uterus and uterine cavity after normal, vaginal delivery. *Ultrasound Obstet Gynecol.* 2001.18(5):491-8. Erratum in: *Ultrasound Obstet Gynecol.* 2008. 29(8):1215. PMID: 11844171.
5. Willms AB, Brown ED, Kettritz UI, et al. Anatomic changes in the pelvis after uncomplicated vaginal

delivery: Evaluation with serial MR imaging. *Radiology.* 1995. 195:91.
6. Sherman D, Lurie S, Frenkel E, et al. Characteristics of normal lochia. *Am J Perinatol.* 1999. 16:399.
7. Jackson E, Glasier A. Return of ovulation and menses in postpartum non-lactating women: A systematic review. *Obstet Gynecol.* 2011. 117(3):657-662.
8. The World Health Organization Multinational Study of Breast-feeding and Lactational Amenorrhea. II. Factors associated with the length of amenorrhea. World Health Organization Task Force on Methods for the Natural Regulation of Fertility. *Fertil Steril.* 1998. 70:461.
9. Meek JY, Noble L, Section on breastfeeding. Policy Statement: Breastfeeding and the use of human milk. *Pediatrics.* 2022. 150 (1): e2022057988. 10.1542/peds.2022-057988.
10. Motosko CC, Bieber AK, Pomeranz MK, et al. Physiologic changes of pregnancy: A review of the literature. *Int J Womens Dermatol.* 2017. 3[4]:219-224.
11. Chandra S, Tripathi AK, Mishra S, et al. Physiological changes in hematological parameters during pregnancy. *Indian J Hematol Blood Transfus.* 2012. 28[3]:144-6.
12. World Health Organization. WHO recommendations on maternal and newborn care for a positive postnatal experience. 2022. Web annexes: WHO, Geneva. https://iris.who.int/handle/10665/352612. License: CC BY-NC-SA 3.0 IGO.
13. Butte NF, Stuebe A. Maternal Nutrition during lactation. Steven AB (Ed.). *UpToDate.* 2023. Waltham, MA. [Accessed January 2024].
14. Nicol B, Croughan-Minihane M, Kilpatrick SJ. Lack of value of routine postpartum hematocrit determination after vaginal delivery. *Obstet Gynecol.* 1997. 90:514.
15. Jones E, Stewart F, Taylor B, Davis PG, Brown SJ. Early postnatal discharge from hospital for healthy mothers and term infants. *Cochrane Database Syst Rev.* 2021. Issue 6. Art. No.:CD002958.
16. Minig L, Trimble EL, Sarsotti C, et al. Building the evidence base for postoperative and postpartum advice. *Obstet Gynecol.* 2009.114:892.

CHAPTER 46

Abnormalities in the Puerperium

MURALIDHAR V PAI

INTRODUCTION

The six weeks following childbirth—known as the puerperium—make up a critical phase in the lives of mothers and newborn babies. The majority of maternal and infant deaths occur during this time. However, this period is often overlooked, and women often do not receive quality care during this time, especially in low- and middle-income countries (LMICs).

The World Health Organization's (WHO) new postpartum care guidelines [1], focus on the importance of prompt identification and management of complications in the immediate postpartum period. They emphasise the need for continuous care and monitoring during the critical first 24 hours after childbirth to avoid maternal and neonatal morbidity and mortality. The guidelines also strongly recommend at least three postnatal care contacts during the first six weeks after delivery.

The puerperium can be complicated by various disorders either during the early or late postpartum period. In a recent study from a high-resource country, approximately 2.2% of women were reported to experience severe maternal morbidity (SMM) during hospitalisation for delivery and 15.7% developed SMM de novo within 6 weeks after hospital discharge [2]. Of these, the majority of complications occurred in the first two weeks after discharge.

Few studies have been carried out in resource-poor countries that have addressed early and late puerperal complications. A community-based study from India [3] found that life-threatening complications such as severe anemia, uterine infection, secondary postpartum hemorrhage (PPH), and severe hypertension or eclampsia occurred in 7.6% of women, of whom 5.7% had severe anemia, and 1.8% had one of the other conditions.

Reviews of hospital systems, both in high-resource and low-resource settings, have identified insufficient monitoring and delays in treatment initiation as important factors contributing to maternal mortality in the puerperium [4].

In the majority of LMICs, the morbidity and mortality resulting from these complications are due to the lack of consistent monitoring in the immediate postpartum period. In the Better Birth trial, which was a part of a WHO Safe Childbirth Checklist Programme in health facilities in Uttar Pradesh, India, only 7% of women across 15 control facilities had their blood pressure taken at any time between admission to the facility and 1 hour after delivery. Only 0.3% ever had their temperature taken [5].

COMPLICATIONS IN THE IMMEDIATE POSTPARTUM PERIOD

The following complications may present immediately or within 24 hours after delivery:

- Primary postpartum hemorrhage
- Genital tract injuries and hematomas
- Inversion of the uterus
- Sudden postpartum collapse
- Postpartum eclampsia
- Pubic symphysis diastasis

Primary Postpartum Hemorrhage

Primary postpartum hemorrhage (PPH) is one that occurs within 24 hours of the delivery. The incidence of PPH in India is 2–4% following vaginal delivery and 6% following cesarean section and is responsible for 25% of all maternal deaths in India [6].

For further details on primary postpartum hemorrhage, see **Chapter 13**, *Abnormalities in the third stage of labour: Postpartum hemorrhage and retained placenta.*

Genital Tract Injuries and Hematomas

Genital tract injuries

These may occur following uncontrolled vaginal delivery or instrumental delivery. Genital tract injuries should be suspected if there is persistent postpartum bleeding despite a well-contracted and retracted uterus. A prompt examination of the birth canal for injuries and their repair controls postpartum hemorrhage and prevents hematoma formation. Good lighting is essential for such examination and repair, which may occasionally require sedation or anesthesia.

- **Perineal tears and lacerations** are discussed in **Chapter 25,** *Prevention and management of perineal trauma occurring in childbirth.*
- **Periurethral and periclitoral lacerations** follow deliveries in which early extension of the fetal head occurs. They tend to bleed profusely and need immediate suturing with continuous locking sutures, followed by insertion of a Foley catheter to prevent retention of urine.
- **Vaginal lacerations** are commonly found in the posterolateral aspect. They are usually extensions from a perineal laceration or an episiotomy. Deep tears of the cervix may extend to the upper third of the vagina. Forceps delivery may cause isolated injuries of the middle third of the vagina. Prompt suturing of vaginal tears along with perineal and cervical tears should be performed. When deep lateral tears of the vagina are sutured, the sutures should include the deep tissues as there may be injury to the pelvic fascia and posterior fibres of the levator ani.
- **Cervical tears** that are actively bleeding or longer than 2 cm should be sutured.

Vulval and paravaginal hematoma

These occur following prolonged labour and operative vaginal delivery.

- **Vulval hematomas** present as extremely painful, tender, soft, fluctuating swellings in the region of the labium majus and appear deep purple in colour. They may attain considerable size and, at times, may produce symptoms and signs of internal hemorrhage such as restlessness, tachycardia, and pallor. They can also spread to the paravaginal tissues and the ischiorectal fossa.
- **Paravaginal hematomas** are not visible externally. Typically, the mother becomes restless and complains of pelvic pain, inability to pass urine, or rectal tenesmus a few hours after the delivery. She is often pale and has tachycardia and some degree of hypotension.

The management of hematomas includes incision under adequate sedation or anesthesia, evacuation of blood clots, identification and securing of bleeders, and obliteration of the cavity. A Foley catheter is inserted to drain the bladder, and the vagina is packed to exert pressure on the vaginal suture line. Both the catheter and the packing may be removed after 12–24 hours. Intravenous fluids and blood component therapy are considered, depending upon the condition of the mother. A single dose of a prophylactic antibiotic may be indicated.

Pelvic hematomas (broad ligament and retroperitoneal hematomas)

They are referred to as **supravaginal hematomas** and result from the rupture of vessels above the pelvic diaphragm following a cesarean delivery or rupture of the uterus.

Typical features are the following:

- Unexplained blood loss
- Unusual pelvic pain or pressure
- A palpable adnexal mass

A large, **broad-ligament hematoma** may be palpable as a swelling on one side of the uterus, pushing the uterus to the opposite side. Very large hematomas become palpable per abdomen above the pelvic brim. **Retroperitoneal hematomas** may grow rapidly and may rupture into the peritoneal cavity, causing hypovolemia and profound shock. Ultrasound or MRI will establish the diagnosis.

Supportive treatment including blood component therapy should be initiated without delay. Conservative management is enough if there is no progression of the hematoma on observation. However, if there is an increase in size or deterioration of the mother's condition, the following options need to be considered:

- Laparotomy to evacuate the hematoma, secure the bleeders, repair the rent in the uterus
- Internal iliac ligation, or in extreme cases, a hysterectomy
- Embolisation of the branches of the internal iliac vessels

Inversion of the Uterus

Uterine inversion is the collapse of the uterine fundus into the endometrial cavity, either completely or partially. Though rare, it can be a life-threatening obstetric complication. Obstetric healthcare providers should be aware of its causes, prevention, and management.

The incidence of uterine inversion ranges from 1 in 2000 to 1 in 23,000 deliveries. This wide variation may be due to the definition used, the population studied and the accuracy of reporting [7,8].

Based on the time of onset, it is categorised as follows:

- **Acute:** Within 24 hours of delivery (before cervical ring contraction)
- **Subacute:** >24 hours but <4 weeks of delivery (cervical ring has contracted)
- **Chronic:** ≥4 weeks postpartum

Depending on the extent of inversion, it can be categorised into one of the following groups:

- **First-degree (incomplete):** The fundus is within the uterine cavity, but not protruding through the cervix.
- **Second-degree (complete):** The fundus protrudes through the external os and into the vaginal canal.
- **Third-degree (prolapsed):** The fundus protrudes through the introitus and appears outside the vulva.
- **Fourth-degree:** Both the uterus and the vagina are inverted.

Precipitating factors

The process of uterine inversion always begins during the third stage of labour but is usually recognised late. The causes are as follows:

- **Spontaneous inversion** (40%), which may occur due to:
  - Precipitate labour
  - Atonic/overdistended uterus with raised intraabdominal pressure
  - Use of tocolytics/$MgSO_4$ just before labour
  - Pedunculated sub-mucous fibroid
- **Iatrogenic/induced inversion** (60%), which usually occurs due to mismanagement of the third stage of labour with the following:
  - Uncontrolled cord traction either at vaginal or cesarean delivery, especially in a relaxed uterus or undiagnosed adherent placenta
  - Excess traction on the baby with a short cord, especially in cases of fundal insertion of the placenta
  - Fundal pressure with or without cord traction when the placenta has not separated, and the uterus is relaxed
  - Following manual removal of the placenta (MRP), under general anesthesia, the manipulating hand is removed too soon, before the uterine tone has returned and the uterus has begun to contract

Clinical features

First-degree inversion may be asymptomatic, whereas in a second-/third-degree inversion, a purple-coloured mass is seen at the introitus along with the placenta. The woman has acute, excruciating abdominal pain and may collapse suddenly. She may complain of vaginal fullness with a bearing-down sensation after the delivery of the baby. PPH invariably ensues. Women with chronic inversion present with prolonged vaginal spotting, low backache, and offensive vaginal discharge.

Diagnosis

In addition to the obvious mass at the introitus, abdominal palpation reveals an absent uterine fundus in complete/prolapsed inversion. The diagnosis of incomplete inversion is usually made by ultrasound or an MRI, if ultrasound is inconclusive. In both, the transverse section shows a hyperechoic mass in the vagina with a central hypoechoic 'H'-shaped cavity, and the longitudinal section shows a 'U'-shaped depressed longitudinal groove extending from the uterine fundus to the centre of the inverted part.

Complications of inversion

The following complications are associated with uterine inversion:

- PPH
- Pulmonary embolism (due to air entering the circulation through exposed open sinuses)
- Cardiogenic shock
- Neurogenic shock (due to increased vagal tone from stretching of the pelvic parasympathetic nerves)
- Infection/sepsis (leading to endotoxic shock)
- Chronic inversion

Prognosis

If undiagnosed and not managed in time, death may occur from hemorrhage, embolism, or shock. Incomplete inversion may remain undiscovered without any symptoms and present later as chronic inversion with sepsis.

Prevention of inversion

- Controlled cord traction should be the method of placental delivery.
- Delivery of the unseparated placenta should not be attempted, especially when the uterus is relaxed.

Management

Supportive measures

These involve the management of shock using crystalloids and blood components.The bladder should be catheterised to monitor urine output. Prophylactic antibiotics should be started before any internal manipulation is attempted.

Definitive measures

These include the following:

- **Manipulative replacement of the uterus (Johnson's method)** is performed under deep general anesthesia to relax the constricted cervical ring through which the uterine fundus is prolapsed. Manual replacement should be attempted as soon as the diagnosis is made and before the formation of the constriction ring. The part that prolapsed last is reduced first and then the other parts are reduced successively (the cervical part, the lower segment, the lower body, and so on). Usually, the fundus goes back automatically once the majority of the uterus is reduced. The operator's fist is held in place until the uterus contracts over it; then, it is gently removed. With the other hand on the abdomen, the operator should apply counter-support to avoid overdoing the reduction. After the reduction, anesthesia is reversed, and an infusion of 20 units of oxytocin is started.

  If the placenta is unseparated, the uterus is reduced with the placenta in situ, and then the placenta is delivered by controlled cord traction or manually.
- **Hydrostatic replacement (O'Sullivan's method)** is performed with the woman in the lithotomy position. Under general anesthesia, warm sterile fluid is run into the posterior fornix from a height of approximately 3 feet, keeping the labia occluded to prevent leakage.

- **Laparotomy** may be required in women in whom the above measures have failed.
  - In **Huntington's method**, after laparotomy, the inverted cup of the uterus is gently pulled up using clamps, Allis forceps, or stay sutures on the fundus. An assistant may have to push the fundus up from the vagina [9].
  - The **Haultain's method** is used if there is a tough constriction ring. It involves making a vertical incision over the posterior cervical ring to relieve the constriction. Traction is then applied to the round ligaments, or an assistant may push the fundus up from below. The posterior incision is then repaired [9].
  - Antonelli and colleagues [10] reported using a **silastic vacuum cup** inserted into the inverted uterus at laparotomy, creating negative pressure, and then applying gentle traction upwards to reduce the inversion.
- **Laparoscopic-assisted reduction** of acute inversion has been reported [11].

Sudden Postpartum Collapse

Sudden postpartum collapse is an acute event that occurs due to several ill-described conditions. It involves the cardiorespiratory system and/or central nervous system, resulting in the woman experiencing reduced or absent consciousness. If maternal collapse not resulting from cardiac arrest is not treated effectively, maternal cardiac arrest may ensue. Though it is an uncommon event, the consequences are potentially catastrophic. It is essential that the clinical team is able to initiate effective resuscitation techniques immediately.

The risk of postpartum collapse can be minimised by closely monitoring all women throughout labour and after delivery.

See **Chapter 10**, *Immediate postpartum monitoring and care (including postpartum collapse)*, for further details.

Postpartum Eclampsia

Though the incidence of postpartum eclampsia is lower than that of antepartum eclampsia, it must be anticipated in all cases of preeclampsia, and one must be vigilant and prepared to initiate immediate treatment. The management of postpartum eclampsia is the same as that of antepartum eclampsia (see **Chapter 37**, *The hypertensive woman in labour*). A neurology consultation to rule out neurological conditions is also worth considering.

Headache

Postpartum headache is of concern if accompanied by the following symptoms:

- Altered mental status, seizures, papilledema, changes in vision, stiff neck, weakness, or focal neurological signs/symptoms
- Sudden onset of severe, unrelenting headache
- Change in headache characteristics (e.g., pain, pattern, severity) from usual headaches
- New-onset of migraine-type headache
- Headache that awakens the woman from sleep
- Headache unrelieved by pain medication

Postdural puncture headache

Women who have received spinal or epidural anesthesia are at risk for developing a severe headache due to a dural puncture. The headache is characterised by postural increase in pain when the woman attempts to sit up. It is treated by asking the woman to lie flat, ensuring hydration with intravenous fluids, and administering an autologous 'blood patch' (see **Chapter 9**, *Labour analgesia*).

Cerebral venous sinus thrombosis

Cerebral venous sinus thrombosis is a rare postpartum complication. In India, it has been reported to have an incidence of 450 per 100,000 deliveries [12].

The headache is intense and may be accompanied by vomiting. It is confirmed by imaging studies such as MRI. The severity of symptoms correlates with the degree of thrombosis and the vessel involved. It is treated with anticoagulation.

Pubic Symphysis Diastasis

During pregnancy, the pubic symphysis relaxes by about 3–7 mm, starting in the first trimester of pregnancy. This is the result of both mechanical pressure and the influence of the hormones progesterone and relaxin.

In some women, vaginal delivery results in separation of the right and left pubic rami to a width of **>10 mm**. This is known as diastasis, and the prevalence is reported as 1 in 300 pregnancies to 1 in 30,000 pregnancies [13].

Diastasis results in severe pain in the midline, directly over the pubic symphysis. If severe enough, the woman may find it very painful to walk. Though the symptoms and signs are enough to make the diagnosis, a plain X-ray can demonstrate the diastasis. An MRI is a definitive but expensive test.

Treatment

This condition is treated conservatively, using a brace or pelvic belt to stabilise the pelvis. Analgesics and anti-inflammatory medication are used to treat the pain as required.

COMPLICATIONS IN THE EARLY AND LATE POSTPARTUM PERIODS

The following complications may present in the first six weeks after delivery:

- Breakdown or disruption of the episiotomy/laceration following vaginal birth
- Secondary postpartum hemorrhage
- Puerperal infections
- Venous thromboembolism
- Mental health issues
- Other non-severe disorders and complications

Breakdown or Disruption of the Episiotomy/Laceration

An episiotomy or a second-degree laceration may break down occasionally. Though not common, it can be of great concern to the woman and her family. Repairs of third- and fourth-degree lacerations appear to be at an increased risk of infection and breakdown compared to repairs of first- and second-degree lacerations.

Management

Current clinical practice favours early re-repair [14]. This is usually done in the first two weeks postpartum. Delayed repair after 6–8 weeks does not seem to have any advantages and also causes the mother to suffer pain and discomfort for a longer period of time.

A single prophylactic dose of a second-generation cephalosporin (cefuroxime) is recommended at the beginning of the secondary repair of an episiotomy or second-degree laceration. For the repair following third- or fourth-degree laceration breakdown, antibiotic prophylaxis with aerobic and anaerobic coverage such as a second-generation cephalosporin plus metronidazole is recommended.

To reduce the risk of fecal contamination perioperatively, an enema the night before the surgery is considered good clinical practice.

Secondary Postpartum Hemorrhage

Secondary postpartum hemorrhage is defined as excessive bleeding that occurs more than 24 hours after delivery and up to 12 weeks postpartum [9]. However, it commonly occurs between days 5 and 10. The incidence is approximately 1% of deliveries. Some of the common causes include the following:

- Subinvolution of the placental site
- Retained placental bits, membranes, and blood clots
- Genital tract infection

- Trophoblastic disease
- Submucous myomas
- Chronic inversion of the uterus
- Inherited coagulation defects (e.g., factor deficiency such as von Willebrand)

Management

Apart from a thorough assessment of the vital parameters, uterine atony secondary to retained placental bits or membranes, and/or infection should be ruled out. Endometritis should be strongly suspected in the presence of uterine tenderness and a low-grade fever. One must assess the lochia, and if needed, it should be sent for culture. Inspection of the lower genital tract for signs of trauma and visualisation of the placental bits at the cervical os will help rule out other causes of secondary hemorrhage.

Investigations

A complete blood count, coagulation profile, and a cervical swab for culture and sensitivity should be performed. Pelvic ultrasound is performed to look for retained placental bits. Serial beta-hCG should be estimated to rule out persistent gestational trophoblastic disease.

Arrest of bleeding

To stop bleeding due to an atonic uterus, ergometrine 0.2 mg IM/IV and/or an oxytocin infusion (15–20 units in 500 mL of RL) is administered.

In suspected endometritis, pending the culture and sensitivity report, a parenteral broad-spectrum antibiotic is started. If retained placental bits are seen in the uterine cavity, suction evacuation may be required under antibiotic coverage. The tissues recovered should be sent for histopathological examination to rule out the rare possibility of a trophoblastic tumour. If there is evidence of gestational trophoblastic disease, either by histopathology examination or beta-HCG levels, single-dose or multiple-dose chemotherapy is considered as per the risk assessment.

Submucous pedunculated myomas may be excised after transfixing the pedicle.

Puerperal Infections

Puerperal infections occur in up to 8% of vaginal deliveries and are more common following a cesarean section.

Women may develop life-threatening complications such as pelvic cellulitis, pelvic abscess, peritonitis, pelvic thrombophlebitis, and septic shock syndrome.

> **Key Point**
>
> Puerperal sepsis is among the five leading causes of maternal deaths and remains the most important cause of morbidity following childbirth.

Puerperal pyrexia

It is a broad term used when the woman's temperature is higher than 38°C (100.4°F) on two separate occasions following the first 24 hours after delivery. Low-grade fever in the first 24 hours after delivery is of no significance and usually resolves spontaneously. After 24 hours, it may occur due to a variety of causes such as genital tract infection, breast engorgement, urinary tract infection, thrombophlebitis, wound infection, and even causes unrelated to pregnancy and childbirth such as typhoid, malaria, dengue, meningitis, or upper respiratory tract infection.

Puerperal sepsis

Maternal sepsis accounts for 11% of maternal deaths worldwide and is the third most common direct cause of maternal death. In South Asia (which includes India), puerperal sepsis accounts for 13.7% of maternal deaths [15].

It is a term specific to bacterial infection of the genital tract after delivery and includes endometritis, metritis with cellulitis, endomyometritis, and endoparametritis. Puerperal sepsis is one of the causes of puerperal pyrexia.

Etiology

Low socio-economic status, poor general health status of the mother, malnutrition, moderate to severe anemia, obesity, diabetes mellitus, multifetal deliveries, home deliveries, prolonged labour, frequent vaginal examinations in labour, premature rupture of membranes, intrauterine manipulations, instrumental vaginal delivery, and postpartum hemorrhage predispose to postpartum infection.

Causative microorganisms

Most puerperal infections are caused by commensals of the genital tract. Devitalised tissues due to genital tract trauma, suture materials and lochia provide an excellent culture medium for organisms ascending from the vagina. More than two-thirds of infections are mixed infections caused by both aerobic and anaerobic organisms.

Some common **aerobes** are gram-positive cocci such as group A, B, and D streptococci, *Enterococcus*, *Staphylococcus aureus*, and *Staphylococcus epidermidis*, gram-negative bacteria such as *Escherichia coli*, *Klebsiella*, and *Proteus* species and the gram-variable *Gardnerella vaginalis*. **Anaerobes** include *Peptostreptococcus*, *Peptococcus*, *Clostridium*, *Fusobacterium* species, and *Mobiluncus* species. Among others, *Mycoplasma* species, *Chlamydia* species, and *Neisseria gonorrhoea* are common. Of these, the lethal pathogens are group A-hemolytic *Streptococcus* (causing toxic shock syndrome) and community-acquired methicillin-resistant *S. aureus* (MRSA).

Morbidity

If not promptly and adequately treated, sepsis may progress directly or through the lymphatics to cause life-threatening pathology such as parametritis, salpingo-oophoritis, septic pelvic thrombophlebitis, pelvic abscess, generalised peritonitis, bacteremia, septicemia, endotoxic shock, and rarely, even death.

Clinical features

Symptoms and signs depend upon the severity and vary from mild temperature, lower abdominal discomfort, and mild uterine tenderness to spiking temperatures, chills, malaise, anorexia, abdominal pain, tender subinvoluted uterus, and foul-smelling lochia. As the infection progresses, there is an increased tenderness of the parametrium and later, signs of pelvic abscess. An ultrasound scan will help to localise the pathology.

Key Point

Blood cultures are the key investigation and should be obtained prior to antibiotic administration; however, empirical antibiotic treatment should be started without waiting for microbiology results.

Management

Antimicrobial treatment based on the culture and sensitivity is the mainstay of management and rapidly controls the infection. Intravenous broad-spectrum antibiotics should be started within one hour of suspicion of severe sepsis after obtaining blood for culture. The use of early, appropriate antibiotics is crucial in the management of maternal sepsis.

- **Puerperal pelvic abscess** may be drained with a needle under ultrasound guidance or by a posterior colpotomy, as it usually points towards the pouch of Douglas.
- **Septic pelvic thrombophlebitis** occurs due to an anaerobic infection and manifests with high, swinging temperature not responding to treatment. It is diagnosed by exclusion. Treatment includes both antimicrobial therapy and anticoagulation with heparin.
- **Episiotomy wound infection** is treated with antibiotics, Sitz baths, and warmth with a heat lamp. If there is evidence of pus or local fluctuation, the offending sutures need to be removed to permit drainage (see section above on *Breakdown or disruption of the episiotomy/laceration following vaginal birth*).
- **Cesarean wound infection** is managed by opening the wound and draining the purulent fluid. Appropriate antibiotics are administered. The wound is closed by secondary

intention after healthy granulation tissue has appeared.

Puerperal Mastitis and Breast Abscess

- **Mastitis** is a localised inflammation of the breast that is associated with fever, myalgia, breast pain, and redness. It is most common during the first six weeks postpartum and may follow a cracked or sore nipple. It is usually caused by *Staphylococcus aureus* from the infant's mouth. Both community and hospital-acquired methicillin-resistant *S. aureus* are now being commonly implicated in lactational mastitis.
- **Breast abscess** is a localised collection of pus in the breast tissue and may result when mastitis does not respond to antibiotic treatment. Clinically, there is redness, tenderness, and induration. High, spiking fever is characteristic. The causative organisms implicated are *Staphylococcus aureus, Streptococcus pyogenes, E. coli* and rarely, *Staphylococcus albus*.

It is important to perform an ultrasound examination to differentiate mastitis from a breast abscess. The following options are available for the treatment of a breast abscess:

- **Antibiotics** are initiated—the choice being one that will be effective against *S. aureus* or methicillin-resistant *S. aureus* based on culture and sensitivity.
- **Ultrasound-guided aspiration of the pus** is the current approach to the drainage of the abscess and ensures the complete removal of pus.
- **Surgical incision and drainage** are indicated for a very large abscess or one that has not responded to needle aspiration.

The mother should continue to breastfeed on the unaffected side and pump the affected side to relieve pressure and facilitate recovery.

Urinary Tract Infection

The mother presents with spiking temperature with chills, suprapubic discomfort, frequent and often painful micturition, and nausea and vomiting. The diagnosis is confirmed by a urine culture and sensitivity test. Treatment consists of high fluid intake and appropriate antimicrobial therapy.

Venous Thromboembolism (VTE)

Pregnancy is a state of hypercoagulability and predisposes to an increased incidence of VTE. The incidence of VTE is up to 10 times more common in pregnant than in non-pregnant women. About 30–50% of affected women have inherited thrombophilia. In most, there will be a past history of thromboembolism.

In the first month postpartum, the risk for phlebitis and thrombosis of the superficial veins of the lower extremity is increased. This may lead to deep vein thrombosis (DVT), which in turn, can result in pulmonary embolism (PE), with an increased risk of mortality.

In the postpartum period, the risk is increased with postpartum hemorrhage, anemia, stasis, local trauma to the vessel wall, and post-cesarean immobility. Other risk factors for developing thromboembolism during the postpartum period are advanced maternal age, obesity, multiparity, multiple gestation, preeclampsia, GDM, connective tissue disease, puerperal infection, and dehydration.

Deep vein thrombosis

Typical features are leg pain and discomfort (the left side is more commonly affected), swelling (increase in circumference >2 cm), calf muscle tenderness, edema, and increased local temperature. **Homan sign** (pain in the calf on dorsiflexion of the foot) is positive. The white cell count is raised. The D-dimer test is difficult to interpret during pregnancy and may not be useful.

Diagnosis

Proximal compression ultrasound with duplex scanning confirms the diagnosis.

Management

Rest and anticoagulant therapy with either unfractionated or low-molecular-weight heparin (LMWH) (Enoxaparin, 1 mg/Kg every 12 hours or dalteparin 200 units/Kg once daily) are the mainstay of treatment. Recovery is expected in a week. After the pain subsides, graded ambulation should be started, and elastic stockings should be fitted. The latter should be continued for at least two years to prevent post-thrombotic syndrome.

Pulmonary embolism (PE)

Though uncommon, the incidence of postpartum pulmonary embolism (not preceded by antenatal VTE) has been reported as 0.45 per 1000 deliveries [17]. It is more common up to 4 weeks postpartum and following a cesarean delivery.

Diagnosis

The typical presentation is the sudden onset of dyspnea, pleuritic chest pain, hemoptysis, and syncope. There can be severe hypotension, and the woman may collapse.

The clinical signs are tachypnea, tachycardia, and raised jugular venous pressure. Pulse oximetry may be useful. Normal SpO_2 parameters do not exclude the possibility of PE. However, abnormal oxygenation should raise further suspicion of PE.

The ECG shows S wave in lead I and Q wave along with T wave inversion in lead III in approximately 20% of cases. X-ray chest may reveal atelectasis, effusion, and loss of vascular markings in the lung region supplied by the obstructed artery. Arterial blood gases may show respiratory alkalosis and hypoxemia.

Management

Management includes immediate anticoagulation, and the drug of choice is low-molecular-weight heparin. After the acute phase, transition to warfarin is acceptable.

Mental Health Issues

Postpartum psychiatric disorders can be divided into three categories—postpartum blues, postnatal depression, and postpartum psychosis.

Postpartum blues

The prevalence of postpartum blues varies with reports. In a meta-analysis of 26 studies, the incidence ranged from 14 to 76% [18]. It is a common occurrence in the first few weeks after delivery.

Sleep deprivation and unfounded fears regarding their own health and that of the neonate are some of the factors implicated. The condition is self-limiting (usually resolves in 3–10 days) and is managed with reassurance and family support. If the depression persists, consultation with a psychiatrist may be sought.

Postnatal depression

Depressive episodes that first present in the first six weeks after birth are termed postpartum depression. Unplanned pregnancy, psychological disturbances during pregnancy, and problems in the marital relationship are some associations. Professional counselling and explanations help in most cases. An understanding partner and a supportive family go a long way in alleviating depression. Sedatives and tranquillisers help to break the fatigue cycle.

Postpartum psychosis

Though uncommon, there may be an exaggeration of psychosis during the postpartum period [19]. This is associated with depression, hallucinations, thought disturbances to a severe degree, infant abuse, infanticide, and suicide. Postpartum psychosis should be recognised and treated promptly with the help of psychiatrists to avoid calamities. These women need prompt admission and treatment with tricyclic antidepressants, phenothiazines, and lithium. Some may require anticonvulsive therapy.

Other Non-severe Disorders and Complications

Subinvolution of the uterus

Delayed involution of the uterus is called subinvolution. Retained bits of placenta or membranes, infection, thrombosed remodelled uteroplacental arteries, and anemia are some of the causes of this condition. The uterus is bigger and softer than expected. Complications include a prolonged period of lochial discharge and vaginal bleeding. An appropriate antibiotic should be started if there is evidence of infection. Anemia should be corrected.

Incomplete voiding and urinary retention

Some women may be unable to void spontaneously within six hours of vaginal delivery or removal of the Foley catheter after cesarean delivery. Voiding difficulty results from injury to the pudendal nerve during birth [20].

Voiding difficulty or urinary retention should be suspected when the mother presents with the following:

- An absence of voiding sensation
- Voiding small quantities of urine at a time
- Urinary frequency or urgency
- Bladder pain or discomfort
- Urinary incontinence

Clinically, bladder distension may be present, and may be recognised when the uterus is difficult to palpate abdominally, or if the uterus is felt above the umbilicus. An incompletely emptying bladder can be confirmed by a post-void ultrasound.

The following risk factors are associated with voiding difficulty [21]:

- Primiparity
- Instrument-assisted delivery
- Episiotomy
- Epidural analgesia

Management

Intermittent catheterisation every 4–6 hours may help resolve the issue. The mother can be taught self-catheterisation. Catheterisation can be stopped when the post-void residual urine is <150 mL.

If the mother is reluctant to perform self-catheterisation, she can be sent home with a Foley catheter and a urine bag. She should be instructed to clamp the catheter and release it to empty the bladder every 2–4 hours. At night, the Foley should not be clamped and should be left attached to the urine bag. Usually, the bladder function will return after 48–76 hours. The mother is usually readmitted to the hospital to remove the catheter and confirm that she is able to void spontaneously.

Hemorrhoids

Exacerbation of hemorrhoids may occur during the postpartum period, leading to pruritus, bleeding, pain, or prolapse. General management includes Sitz baths, a high-fibre diet, and plenty of fluids. Stool softeners/bulk-forming laxatives are prescribed. Topical astringent, anesthetic agents, corticosteroids, and vasoactive agents may relieve the symptoms.

Postpartum cardiomyopathy

This is unique to the latter half of pregnancy and the puerperium and occurs in 1:3500 and 1:5000 deliveries. The woman presents with congestive cardiac failure, cardiac arrhythmias, and cardiomegaly. The condition may have viral, toxic, immunologic, or genetic etiologies. Treatment is essentially medical and involves bed rest, digitalis, diuretics, salt restriction, and oxygen as required. In more than 60% of women, cardiac functions return to normal over a period of few weeks to 6 months.

CONCLUSION

The first 6 weeks following a delivery are an important period of significant physiological changes, during which mother-and-child bonding happens. Unfortunately, there can be complications during this period including bleeding, sepsis, wound breakdown, and mental health issues. Early identification and appropriate management are extremely important to reduce maternal morbidity.

REFERENCE

1. World Health Organization. WHO recommendations on maternal and newborn care for a positive postnatal experience. 2022. Available at:https://www.who.int/publications/i/item/9789240045989.
2. Chen J, Cox S, Kuklina EV, et al. Assessment of incidence and factors associated with severe maternal morbidity after delivery discharge among women in the US. *JAMA Netw Open*. 2021. 4:e2036148.
3. Iyengar K. Early postpartum maternal morbidity among rural women of Rajasthan, India: A community-based study. *J Health Popul Nutr*. 2012. 30(2):213-25.
4. Clarke-Deelder E, Opondo K, Oguttu M, Burke T, Cohen JL, McConnell M. Immediate postpartum care in low- and middle-income countries: A gap in healthcare quality research and practice. *Am J Obstet Gynecol MFM*. 2023. 5(2S):100764.
5. Semrau KEA, Hirschhorn LR, Marx Delaney M, **et al.** Outcomes of a coaching-based WHO safe childbirth checklist program in India. *N Engl J Med*. 2017. 377: 2313-2324.
6. Gora K, Depan A, Yadav K, Benwa D. Causes and management of post-partum hemorrhage at tertiary care center, Rajasthan, India. *International Journal of Reproduction, Contraception, Obstetrics and Gynecology*. 2019. 8(6):2425-2428.
7. Baskett TF. Acute uterine inversion: A review of 40 cases. *J Obstet Gynaecol Can*. 2002. 24:953.
8. Witteveen T, van Stralen G, Zwart J, van Roosmalen J. Puerperal uterine inversion in the Netherlands: A nationwide cohort study. *Acta Obstet Gynecol Scand*. 2013. 92:334.
9. Postpartum hemorrhage. Practice Bulletin No. 183. American College of Obstetricians and Gynecologists. *Obstet Gynecol*. 2017. 130:e168–86. Reaffirmed 2021.
10. Antonelli E, Irion O, Tolck P, Morales M. Subacute uterine inversion: Description of a novel replacement technique using the obstetric ventouse. *BJOG*. 2006. 113:846.
11. Vijayaraghavan R, Sujatha Y. Acute postpartum uterine inversion with hemorrhagic shock: Laparoscopic reduction: a new method of management? *BJOG*. 2006. 113:1100.
12. Srinivasan K: Cerebral venous and arterial thrombosis in pregnancy and puerperium: A study of 135 patients. *Angiology*. 1983. 34:731–46.
13. Parker JM, Bhattacharjee M. Images in clinical medicine. Peripartum diastasis of the symphysis pubis. *N Engl J Med*. 2009. 361(19):1886.
14. Dudley LM, Kettle C, Ismail KM. Secondary suturing compared to non-suturing for broken down perineal wounds following childbirth. *Cochrane Database Syst Rev*. 2013. Art. no.:CD008977.
15. Say L, Chou D, Gemmill A, et al. Global causes of maternal death: A WHO systematic analysis. *Lancet Glob Health*. 2014. 2(6):e323–e333. 10.1016/S2214-109X(14)70227-X.
16. McColl MD, Ramsay JE, Tait RC, et al. Risk factors for pregnancy associated venous thromboembolism. *Thromb Haemost*. 1997. 78:1183.
17. JM Morris, CS Algert, CL Roberts. Incidence and risk factors for pulmonary embolism in the postpartum period. *Journal of thrombosis and haemostasis*. Vol 8. Issue 5. 2010. 998-1003.
18. Rezaie-Keikhaie K, Arbabshastan ME, Rafiemanesh H, et al. Systematic review and meta-analysis of the prevalence of the maternity blues in the postpartum period. *J Obstet Gynecol Neonatal Nurs*. 2020.49:127.
19. VanderKruik R, Barreix M, Chou D, Allen T, Say L, Cohen LS. Maternal morbidity working group. The global prevalence of postpartum psychosis: A systematic review. *BMC Psychiatry*. 2017. 17(1):272.
20. Lee SJ, Park JW. Follow-up evaluation of the effect of vaginal delivery on the pelvic floor. *Dis Colon Rectum*. 2000. 43:1550.
21. Mulder FE, Hakvoort RA, Schoffelmeer MA, et al. Postpartum urinary retention: A systematic review of adverse effects and management. *Int Urogynecol J*.2014. 25:1605.

Index

17-Alpha-hydroxyprogesterone caproate (17-OHPC) 357

A

A, B, C of resuscitation 119
Abdominal examination 36
Absent cyclicity 90
Abuse 19
Acidosis 178
Acquired immunodeficiency syndrome (AIDS) 489
Active first stage 31,124
Active management of labour 58
Active management of the third stage of labour (AMTSL) 51
Active phase 16
- arrest of descent 129
- arrest of dilatation 129

Acute fatty liver of pregnancy (AFLP) 458
Acute hypoxia 179
- management of 181

Acyclovir 482
Afterpains 115
Amnioinfusion 198
Amniotic fluid 234
Amniotic fluid embolism (AFE) 119
Amniotomy 40,168
Analgesia 98
- fentanyl 102
- ketamine 102
- local infiltration 103
- non-opioid systemic analgesics 101
- non-pharmacological techniques 100
- paracervical block 103
- paracetamol 101
- pethidine 102
- pharmacological methods 101
- postdural puncture headache 109
- pudendal block 103
- regional neuraxial techniques 103
- remifentanil 102
- systemic opioids 102
- tramadol 102
- transcutaneous electrical nerve stimulation (TENS) 101

Angle of progression (AoP) 237
Antenatal education 23
Antenatal steroids 444
Antepartum fetal death 380
Antepartum hemorrhage 338
- causes of 338

Antibiotic prophylaxis 223
- characteristics of 223
- effect on neonatal oral and gut microbiome 227
- indications 223
- overuse and abuse 226
- principles of 223
- timing of 223,225

Antibiotics 35
- resistance 227

Antiepileptic drugs 461
Antiphospholipid syndrome (APS) 454
Apgar score 500,503
Artificial rupture of membranes (AROM) 40
Aseptic precautions 44
Asphyxia 83,512
- effect of 512

Asynclitism 14

B

Bacterial endocarditis 226
- prophylaxis 453

Balloon catheter devices 167
Bandl's ring 214
Birth companions 26
Bishop's score 165
Bladder emptying 35
Blood loss 111
B-Lynch compression 153
Braxton–Hicks contractions 2
Breast abscess 538
Breast crawl 504
Breech presentation 317
- complete breech 317
- complications of 318
- delivery 317
- diagnosis of 318
- etiology of 317
- footling 317
- frank breech 317
- management of 319
- mechanism of labour 318
- types of 317

Burns–Marshall technique: 323

C

Caput succedaneum 38
Cardiac disorders 449
- mechanical heart valves 453

Cardiorespiratory transition 513
Cardiotocography (CTG) 86
- admission CTG 94
- classification of 91
- misinterpretation of 186
- ominous CTG tracing 186
- suspicious or pathological CTG 93

Cerebral venous sinus thrombosis 534
Cerebroplacental ratio 395
Cervical cerclage 358
Cervical dilatation 34,58,236
Cervical effacement 15
Cervical length measurement 236
Cervical ripening 3,165
Cervix 9
- changes in 9

Cesarean section 256,260,274
- choice of suture 268
- classification of 257
- elective 258
- emergency 257
- factors contributing to 276
- intraoperative management 262
- maternal risks 275

- neonatal risks 275
- optimum rate 275
- overuse of 256
- postoperative care 270
- postoperative complications 271
- preoperative preparation 260
- rates in India 276
- Robson ten-group classification 277
- strategies to reduce 274,278
- surgical checklist 260
- technique 263
- types of 256
- unmet needs 256
- wound infection 537

Cervical softening 2
- initiation of 6
- lower uterine segment 3
- oxytocin 3
- phases of 1

Chickenpox 480
- medications 482

Cirrhosis 460
Classical cesarean section 256
Clearing the airway 502
Coagulation disorders 145
Combined spinal–epidural analgesia (CSEA) 105
Complicated twin pregnancy 210
Controlled cord traction (CCT) 53
Cord clamping 46
Coronavirus 465
Crede's manoeuvre 54
Crichton's manoeuvre 36

D

Damage control resuscitation (DCR) 160
Deeply impacted head 267
Deep vein thrombosis 538
Delayed cord clamping (DCC) 52,505
Delivery of the membranes 54
Descent 14
Descent and engagement 36
Diabetes 439
Dichorionic diamniotic (DCDA) pregnancy 210
Digital vaginal examination 231
- limitations of 231

Dilatation 16
Dinoprostone 169
Disrespect 19
Disseminated intravascular coagulopathy (DIC) 342
Doppler device 85

E

Early decelerations 88
Eclampsia 425
Elective repeat cesarean delivery (ERCD) 307
Electronic fetal monitoring (EFM) 86
Engagement 13
Entonox 102
Epidural 103
- patient-controlled epidural analgesia (PCEA) 105

Epilepsy 461
Episiotomy 74
- breakdown or disruption 535
- mediolateral 75
- midline 75
- perineal lacerations 74
- repair of 77
- suture material 79
- wound infection 537

Erb palsy 329
Estimation of fetal weight 33,327
Expulsive efforts 41
Extension 14
External cephalic version (ECV) 320,408
External rotation 14

F

Failed induction 173
False labour 125
Fentanyl 102
Fetal acidemia 447
Fetal acoustic stimulation test (FAST) 95
Fetal compromise 83
Fetal descent and station 38
Fetal distress 177
- clinical risk factors 178
- medicolegal issues 190

Fetal endocrine signals 6
Fetal growth charts 392
Fetal growth disorders 402
Fetal growth restriction 393,402
- classification of 393
- early-onset FGR 393
- late-onset FGR 394
- mode and timing of delivery 395

Fetal head position 235,237
Fetal heart rate (FHR) 85,87
- accelerations 87
- baseline FHR 87
- baseline variability 89
- cyclicity of the FHR 90
- decelerations 88
- monitoring 43
- sinusoidal pattern 88

Fetal lie 33,234
Fetal position 38
Fetal presentation 234
Fetal scalp blood sampling (FBS) 95
Fetal scalp stimulation test 95
Fetal surveillance 83
Fetus (passenger) 11
- attitude 11
- engaging diameter 12
- fetal lie 11
- fetal presentation 11

Fibroids 270,419
- management of labour 422
- postpartum complications 423
- potential effects 420
- red degeneration 420

First stage of labour 15,30,35
- supportive measures 35

Flexion 14,39
Flexion point 248
Forceps 241
- application and technique 249

Fourth stage of labour 111
Fractures 329
Friedman labour curve 30,58

G

Gaskin manoeuvre 334
Genital hematomas 117
Genital tract injuries 531
Growth-restricted fetus 392

H

Hair removal 262
Headache 534
Head–perineum distance (HPD) 237
HELLP syndrome 430
Hematoma 531
Hemorrhoids 540
Hemostatic resuscitation 159
Hepatic disorders 456
Hepatitis B (HBV) 459
Hepatitis C (HCV) 460
History 32
HIV 489
  mother-to-child transmission (MTCT) 491
Hygroscopic dilators 167
Hyperglycemia in pregnancy (HIP) 439
  intrapartum complications 439
  maternal surveillance 444
  route of birth 442
  timing of birth 440
Hyperstimulation 172
Hypertension 425
  management 430,433
  maternal early warning trigger tool (MEWT) 432
  modified early obstetric warning scores (MEOWS) 432
Hypothermia 501
Hypoxemia 83
Hypoxia 83,183
  gradually developing hypoxia 183
  subacute hypoxia 182
Hysterectomy 155
Hysterotomy 265,268

I

Iatrogenic childbirth-related postpartum fistula (ICRF) 297
Incomplete voiding 540
Induction 163
  augmentation 163
  cervical ripening 163
  checklist 164
  contraindications 164
  counselling 164
  indications 163
  prediction of successful induction 164
Infant feeding 496
Inflammatory mediators 6
Inhalational analgesia 102
Instrumental delivery 241
Intermittent auscultation (IA) 84
  intelligent structured intermittent auscultation (ISIA) 85
Internal iliac artery ligation 154
Internal podalic version 208,209
Internal rotation 14
International childbirth initiative 24
Intrahepatic cholestasis of pregnancy (ICP) 457
  bile acid 457
Intrapartum fetal death 380
Intrapartum fetal surveillance (IPFS) 84
Intrauterine fetal death (IUFD) 380
  diagnosis of 382
  follow-up visit 388
  management of labour and delivery 384
Inversion of the uterus 532

J

Jacquemier manoeuvre 332
Joel–Cohen technique 265

K

Kiwi handheld device 243

L

Labetalol 434
Labour 1
  analgesia 98,102
  breathing techniques 101
  continuous support 100
  diagnosis of 31
  epidural analgesia 103
  false labour 32
  history of 98
  in low- and middle-income countries 109
  mechanics of 8
  mechanism of 13
  water birth 101
  true labour 32
Labour Care Guide 62
Labour pain 98
  causes of 98
  effect of 99
  factors affecting 99
Lactation 523
LaQshya 19
Large-for-gestational age (LGA) 402
Late decelerations 88
Late fetal death (stillbirth) 381
Latent phase of labour 124
Late term 369
  management 374
  pregnancy dating 370
  prevention of 377
  recurrence risk 377
Lochia 522
Lower segment cesarean section (LSCS) 256
Low-lying placenta 233

M

Macrosomia 327,402
  effect on the progress of labour 407

mode of delivery 405
pathophysiology 403
prediction 404
risk factors 403
Magnesium sulphate 434
Malpositions 410
Malpresentations 413
Manual perineal protection 44
Manual rotation 42
Massive transfusion protocols 286
Mastitis 538
Maternal activity 36
Maternal forces 8
Maternal pelvis (passage) 9
classification of 11
diameters of 10
midpelvis 10
pelvic inlet 10
pelvic outlet 10
Mauriceau–Smellie–Veit technique 324
Maylard muscle-cutting technique 265
MCA–PI 395
McRoberts manoeuvre 331
Meconium 193
composition of 193
effect on the fetus 194
fetal maturation 194
grading system 194
hypoxia 195
maternal risk factors 195
Meconium-stained amniotic fluid 194
diagnosis of 196
fetal distress 196
management of 196
maternal complications 200
meconium aspiration syndrome (MAS) 200,201,203
neonatal outcomes 200
postnatal ward care 200
preterm meconium staining 196
Membranes 34,40
Membrane sweeping 166
Menticoglou manoeuvre 332
Midwifery care 23
Misoprostol 170
Modified Brandt–Andrews method 53
Modified Ritgen manoeuvre 44
Monochorionic diamniotic (MCDA) pregnancy 210
Monochorionic (MC) pregnancies 205
Moulding 38
Multiple pregnancy 205
adverse outcomes 206
mode of delivery 207
nomenclature 205
timing of delivery 209
Myocardial infarction 453
Myomas 419
Myomectomy 423

N

Neonatal complications 408
Neonatal hypoglycemia 447
Neonatal resuscitation 512
bag-and-mask ventilation 516
chest compressions 518
endotracheal intubation 517
equipment 514
medication 519
Nifedipine 434
Normal birth 30
Nuchal cord 45

O

Obstetric anal sphincter injuries 78
Obstetric fistula (OF) 297
Obstructed labour 213
diagnosis 215
etiology 214
management 216
risk factors 214
Occipitoposterior (OP) position 410
O'Leary suture 154
Operative vaginal delivery 241
classification of 244
contraindications to 245
indications for 244
prerequisites 246
prerequisites for 246
risks and complications 252
training in 254
Oral intake 35
Oropharyngeal suctioning 46
Ovarian mass 270
Oxytocin 131,132,170

P

Pain management in the postpartum period 115
Pain relief 36
Partogram 58
Partograph 58
action line 59
alert line 59
colour-coded partograph 59
composite partograph 59
modified partograph 59
WHO partographs 59
Pathological 92
Pelvic floor muscle exercises 526
Perimortem cesarean delivery (PMCD) 120
Perineal trauma 296
'buttonhole' tears 297
classification of 297
complications of 304
diagnosis of 297
dyspareunia 305
episiotomy 299
ethnicity 298
first-degree 296
fourth degree 296
management of 301
perineal massage 300
perineal support 300
prediction of 298
prevention 300

second-degree 296
second-degree tears 302
third- and fourth-degree tears 296,302
Peripartum hysterectomy 283
indications 285
risk factors 284
technique 285
uterine rupture 292
Personal protective equipment (PPE) 469
Pethidine 102
Pfannenstiel technique 265
Pinard manoeuvre 323
Piper's forceps 324
Placenta accreta spectrum (PAS) 234,283,285,347
diagnosis 348
management 348
risk factors 347
Placental abruption 338
clinical presentation 340
Couvelaire uterus 339
management 341
pathophysiology 339
recurrence of 342
risk factors 339
Placental cord drainage 56
Placental localisation 233
Placental separation 17,50
Placenta previa 233,343
classification 343
epidemiology 343
low-lying placenta 344
Portal hypertension 460
Position for delivery 44
Postdelivery evaluation of the fetus 386
Postdural puncture headache 534
Postnatal depression 539
Postpartum blues 539
Postpartum cardiomyopathy 540
Postpartum collapse 111,117
Postpartum eclampsia 534
Postpartum hemorrhage (PPH) 143,531
blood loss measurement 146
causes and risk factors 144
classification 144
management of 148
prevention 146
secondary 535
trauma 145
Postpartum monitoring 111
Postpartum psychosis 539
Postterm pregnancy 369
diagnosis of 370
etiology of 371
management 374
postmaturity syndrome 373
prevention of 377
recurrence risk 377
risk factors for 372
stillbirth 373
Post-vaginal delivery pain 115
Preeclampsia 425
Preterm birth 353
Preterm labour 352
definition of 352
diagnosis of 359
incidence of 353
management of 360
prediction of 354
prevention of 356
risk factors for 353
Preterm prelabour rupture of membranes (PPROM) 225,362
clinical features of 363
complications of 364
diagnosis of 363
incidence of 363
management of 364
pathophysiology of 363
risk factors for 363
Privacy 26
Progesterone 356
Prolonged deceleration 181
Prolonged latent phase 126
Prone positioning 476
Prophylactic antibiotics 262
Prophylactic anticoagulation 262
Prophylactic LMWH 455
Prostaglandin 3,5,169
intracervical PGE2 gel 169
Protracted active phase 129
Pubic symphysis diastasis 535
Puerperal pelvic abscess 537
Puerperal pyrexia 536
Puerperal sepsis 536
causative microorganisms 537
Puerperium 522,530
complications 530
Pulmonary embolism (PE) 539
Pushing 41

R

Radiant warmer 509
Record-keeping 94
Remifentanil 102
Respectful maternity care 30,124
Respectful obstetric care 19
Respectful vaginal examination 34
Restitution 14
Retained placenta 155
diagnosis of retained 156
epidemiology 156
management of 156
pathophysiology 156
Reverse Woods screw manoeuvre 333
Ritgen manoeuvre 45
Robson ten-group classification 277
Rotational instrumental delivery 251
Routine care of the newborn 500
Rubin II manoeuvre 333
Rubin I manoeuvre 331

S

SARS-CoV-2 465
care of the neonate 477
diagnosing 466
transmission 465
vaccination 468
Second stage of labour 15,31,40,134
active phase 134
duration of 135
latent 134
management of abnormalities 137
mechanism of 134

phases of 134
prolonged second stage 136
Separation of the membranes 50
Separation of the placenta 49
Septic pelvic thrombophlebitis 537
Septic shock 118
Sexual activity 527
Shaving of pubic hair 35
Shivering 112
Shock index 158
Shoulder dystocia 326,408
brachial plexus injury 328
complications of 328
diagnosis of 328
management of 330
mechanism of labour 326
prevention of 335
risk factors for 326
Shoulder presentation 415
Show 16
Skin-to-skin contact 503
Small for gestational age (SGA) 392,402
classification of 392
Standard universal precautions 498
Stillbirth 380
causes of 381
communicating the diagnosis 382
fetal postmortem 387
intrauterine fetal death 380
ST waveform analysis 95
Subacute hypoxia 182
Subinvolution of the uterus 540
Sudden postpartum collapse 534
Suture material 79

T

Tachysystole 172
Therapeutic low-molecular-weight heparin (LMWH) 455
Third stage of labour 15,31,49
Thrombocytopenia 108
Thromboembolism 118
Tocolysis 360,365
antenatal corticosteroids 366
nifedipine 365
Tokophobia 22
Torsion 420
Tramadol 102
Transducer 230
Transfusion therapy 158
Trial of labour after previous cesarean delivery (TOLAC) 307
delivery 313
failed 308
in special circumstances 314
intrapartum management 312
risks of 308
selecting women for 309
Triple P procedure 292

U

UA–PI 395
Ultrasound 229
transabdominal 232
transducer 232
transperineal 236
transvaginal 236
Umbilical cord milking 56
Universal precautions 44
Universal rights of women and newborns 20
Urinary retention 113,540
Urinary tract infection 538
Uterine artery embolisation 155
Uterine atony 144
Uterine compression sutures 153
Uterine contractions 2,8,36,91
Uterine dehiscence 218
Uterine involution 522
Uterine massage 51
Uterine rupture 213,217
diagnosis 219
in a scarred uterus 218
management 219
pregnancy after 220
unscarred uterus 218
Uterine segments 9
Uterine stretching 6
Uterotonics 51

V

Vaccine-induced thrombosis, thrombocytopenia (VITT) syndrome 468
Vacuum extractor 241
application and technique 247
Kiwi cup 243
rigid cups 242
soft cups 242
Vaginal birth after cesarean delivery (VBAC) 116,307,408
Valacyclovir 482
Variable decelerations 88
Varicella-zoster virus 480
varicella-zoster immunoglobulin (VZIG) 486
Vasa previa 234,346
diagnosed antenatally 347
diagnosis 346
management 347
presentation 346
Venous thromboembolism (VTE) 526,538
Vertical transmission 498
Vulval hematoma 114
VZV pneumonia 483

W

Warm chain 501
Window period 491
Woods screw manoeuvre 333
Work-up 383